T0257347

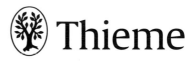

The Comprehensive Neurosurgery Board Preparation Book

Illustrated Questions and Answers

Paul V. Birinyi, MD, MS
Resident, Department of Neurosurgery
Saint Louis University
St. Louis, Missouri

Najib E. El Tecle, MD, MS
Resident, Department of Neurosurgery
Saint Louis University
St. Louis, Missouri

Eric Marvin, DO
Assistant Professor, Department of
    Neurosurgery
Virginia Tech Carilion School of Medicine
Assistant Professor, Department of
    Neurosurgery
Virginia College of Osteopathic Medicine
Roanoke, Virginia

Carlos Zamora, MD, PhD
Assistant Professor, Department of
    Radiology
University of North Carolina School of
    Medicine
Chapel Hill, North Carolina

Richard Prayson, MD, MEd
Section Head, Department of
    Neuropathology
Cleveland Clinic
Director of Student Affairs
Cleveland Clinic Lerner College of Medicine
Cleveland, Ohio

Samer K. Elbabaa, MD, FAANS, FACS
Reinert Endowed Chair in Pediatric
    Neurosurgery
Associate Professor, Department of
    Neurosurgery
Saint Louis University School of Medicine
St. Louis, Missouri

Matt Pierson, MD
Resident, Department of Neurosurgery
Saint Louis University
St. Louis, Missouri

Katie P. Huynh, DO
Attending Neurosurgeon
Kootenai Health
Coeur d'Alene, Idaho

Thieme

New York • Stuttgart • Delhi • Rio de Janeiro

Executive Editor: Timothy Hiscock
Managing Editor: Elizabeth Palumbo
Director, Editorial Services: Mary Jo Casey
Production Editor: Barbara Chernow
International Production Director: Andreas Schabert
Vice President, Editorial and E-Product Development:
    Vera Spillner
International Marketing Director: Fiona Henderson
International Sales Director: Louisa Turrell
Director of Sales, North America: Mike Roseman
Senior Vice President and Chief Operating Officer:
    Sarah Vanderbilt
President: Brian D. Scanlan
Compositor: Carol Pierson, Chernow Editorial Services, Inc.

Library of Congress Cataloging-in-Publication Data

Names: Birinyi, Paul V., author.
Title: The comprehensive neurosurgery board preparation
    book : illustrated questions and answers / Paul V.
    Birinyi [and 7 others].
Description: New York : Thieme Medical Publishers, [2017]
Identifiers: LCCN 2016017073 (print) | LCCN 2016018272
    (ebook) | ISBN 9781626232808 (alk. paper) | ISBN
    9781626232815 (ebook)
Subjects: | MESH: Neurosurgery | Neurosurgical Procedures
    | Examination Questions
Classification: LCC RD593 (print) | LCC RD593 (ebook) |
    NLM WL 18.2 | DDC 617.4/8—dc23
LC record available at https://lccn.loc.gov/2016017073

Important note: Medicine is an ever-changing science undergoing continual development. Research and clinical experience are continually expanding our knowledge, in particular our knowledge of proper treatment and drug therapy. Insofar as this book mentions any dosage or application, readers may rest assured that the authors, editors, and publishers have made every effort to ensure that such references are in accordance with **the state of knowledge at the time of production of the book.**

Nevertheless, this does not involve, imply, or express any guarantee or responsibility on the part of the publishers in respect to any dosage instructions and forms of applications stated in the book. **Every user is requested to examine carefully** the manufacturers' leaflets accompanying each drug and to check, if necessary in consultation with a physician or specialist, whether the dosage schedules mentioned therein or the contraindications stated by the manufacturers differ from the statements made in the present book. Such examination is particularly important with drugs that are either rarely used or have been newly released on the market. Every dosage schedule or every form of application used is entirely at the user's own risk and responsibility. The authors and publishers request every user to report to the publishers any discrepancies or inaccuracies noticed. If errors in this work are found after publication, errata will be posted at www.thieme.com on the product description page.

Some of the product names, patents, and registered designs referred to in this book are in fact registered trademarks or proprietary names even though specific reference to this fact is not always made in the text. Therefore, the appearance of a name without designation as proprietary is not to be construed as a representation by the publisher that it is in the public domain.

I dedicate this work to my wonderful wife and family, who have given everything to allow me to pursue my dreams and make my life and passion for neurosurgery possible.

—*Paul V. Birinyi*

To my wife to be, my parents, and my siblings, thank you for your unconditional support and for inspiring me everyday to be a better person. To my mentors for their unwavering encouragement and guidance. To those people who, in special circumstances in my life, made the impossible possible. To all neurosurgery residents—past, present, and future.

—*Najib E. El Tecle*

To Hajnalka, for her everlasting patience and unwavering support, and to Sophie and David, for the joy that they bring into our lives.

—*Carlos Zamora*

To my wife, Beth.

—*Richard Prayson*

To my beloved children, Kamal and Natalie. You touch my heart everyday, and you make it all worthwhile!

—*Samer K. Elbabaa*

Special thanks to my wife, Genie, my son, Tommy, and the baby girl on the way for their unending love and support, without which my endeavors would not be possible.

—*Matt Pierson*

This work is dedicated to my husband, Adam, and to my neurosurgery dad, Dan Miulli. They are my foundation and have been beside me throughout my journey to become a neurosurgeon.

—*Katie P. Huynh*

Contents

Section I.   Questions

Section II.   Answers

Section III.   Practice Exam

Foreword

The knowledge required to be a capable neurosurgeon is vast. A specialist who routinely operates on the body's most complex structures is expected to master the volumes written about the brain, spinal cord, and peripheral nerves and their disorders, in addition to having the dexterity and decision-making skills required during critical and delicate procedures. Thus, it is no accident that the training period in neurosurgery is the longest of any specialty, and even after spending seven years as a resident, many neurosurgeons are compelled to take a fellowship in a particular branch within the field to further prepare themselves for their career.

As part of this training, there must be an assessment of whether the knowledge delivered to the prospective neurosurgeon has been appropriately assimilated and can be recalled as needed. Questioning the trainee, a variant of the technique used by Socrates to explore ethical dilemmas, has been integral to medical education for centuries, as it represents the most direct method to confirm that knowledge has been transferred successfully. Even with tremendous advances in technology to simulate treatment situations and document the response of the trainee to medical scenarios, questioning the trainee about specific aspects of knowledge on a topic has no real alternative in the process of medical certification. As medical knowledge is constantly evolving and medical truths are changing as new information is obtained, the questions asked must also evolve and be updated as the need arises.

This new text from Dr. Paul Birinyi and colleagues is an excellent source for review to verify that one's neurosurgical knowledge is complete and up to date. Whether this volume is employed by residents in training taking their written boards for the first time to find out what they do not know, or by attendings who have been in practice for several years and are checking on new information prior to taking an exam to maintain their certification, the questions and answers found in this text address the needs of readers no matter where they stand in the educational spectrum.

To fully commit to neurosurgery is to commit to a life of education about the nervous system. This text provides the answers to the reader about the specific topics listed herein while addressing the larger question as to whether the reader has the information required to be a capable neurosurgeon. Should the questions indicate deficiencies in knowledge, this text can lead the way to addressing the deficiency and preparing one for perhaps the most rewarding career imaginable, that of being a neurological surgeon.

Richard D. Bucholz, MD, FACS, FAANS
KR Smith Professor of Neurological Surgery
Saint Louis University School of Medicine

Preface

The Comprehensive Neurosurgery Board Preparation Book: Illustrated Questions and Answers is intended to help the reader prepare for the neurosurgical primary board exam. It is one of the few contemporary review books to use the question-and-answer format, and it contains over 1,300 questions. Although some of the questions on the exam tend to be recycled each year, many new questions are added; therefore, we have incorporated the newer concepts that are addressed on the exam.

Many available review books are outdated and do not reflect the current trends in board question style and content; for instance, they do not provide examples of the color images that are now used on the exam. Furthermore, many question books and test banks do not follow the style of the board exam; for example, the exam does not use matching or negative questions (e.g., "All are true EXCEPT . . .").

This book differs from previous study books in that it provides a more accurate representation of the exam, its content, and its style. Brief explanations and pearls accompany each question to provide a good starting point for delving deeper into each topic. The questions are designed to be stud-ied either in a long study session or in briefer inter-mittent sessions as time permits during a busy day on the neurosurgical service. Finally, this book provides a full-length practice exam that can be taken with the same time constraints as the actual exam.

Due to copyright restrictions, and heeding the board exam's request that test takers not provide the questions to others following exam completion, the questions contained in this book are merely examples of the style and content of the questions appearing on past exams and are meant only as guides in studying for the exam. Any replication of an actual exam question or answer, or of its word-ing, is purely coincidental.

The authors want to acknowledge Dr. Miguel Guzman of Saint Louis University for providing invaluable assistance with the pathology/histology section.

This book is the comprehensive preparation tool that the authors wish had been available back when they prepared for the boards. This book is the single resource that you need to improve your confidence, knowledge, and, ultimately, your score. Happy studying!

About the Authors

Paul V. Birinyi, MD, MS

Dr. Birinyi is a resident of neurosurgery at Saint Louis University in St. Louis, Missouri. Originally hailing from the suburbs of Dallas, Texas, Dr. Birinyi completed his bachelor of arts and master of science degrees in cellular and molecular neuroscience at The Johns Hopkins University, where he pursued his interests in the genetics of alcohol and drug abuse at the National Institute on Drug Abuse and in restless leg syndrome at the Johns Hopkins Center for Restless Legs Syndrome. After returning home from Baltimore, Dr. Birinyi graduated from the University of Texas–Southwestern Medical School in Dallas, Texas, where he engaged extensively in anatomy education. In residency, Dr. Birinyi's interests include resident education and minimally invasive spinal surgery. Dr. Birinyi currently resides in the St. Louis, Missouri, area with his wife, Christina, and daughter, Aubrey. pbirinyi@gmail.com

Najib E. El Tecle, MD, MS

Dr. El Tecle is a resident of neurosurgery at Saint Louis University in St. Louis, Missouri. He completed his medical studies at the Lebanese University, Beirut, Lebanon, before joining Northwestern Memorial Hospital in Chicago, Illinois, for a post doctoral research fellowship in cerebrovascular surgery. Dr. El Tecle's neurosurgical interests include functional neurosurgery and spine surgery. Dr. El Tecle has a special interest in medical device development, and holds a master of science degree in biomedical engineering from Northwestern University. najibeltecle@gmail.com

Eric Marvin, DO

Dr. Marvin is an assistant professor of neurosurgery at Virginia Tech Carilion School of Medicine, and assistant professor of neurosurgery at Virginia College of Osteopathic Medicine in Roanoke, Virginia. He received his medical degree from Lake Erie College of Osteopathic Medicine, and completed his neurosurgery residency at Virginia Tech Carilion School of Medicine. His cerebrovascular and skull base fellowship was at Saint Louis University. Marvinea@slu.edu; Marvin.eric@gmail.com

Carlos Zamora, MD, PhD

Dr. Zamora is an assistant professor of radiology at the University of North Carolina School of Medicine in Chapel Hill, North Carolina. He received his medical degree from the Universidad de San Carlos in Guatemala, and subsequently obtained a Ph.D. in medical sciences at Kobe University in Japan. After a medical internship in New York, New York, he completed his residency in diagnostic radiology and a two-year fellowship in neuroradiology at Johns Hopkins Hospital in Baltimore, Maryland, where he also worked as a clinical instructor. Dr. Zamora is board certified in diagnostic radiology with an interest in all aspects of neuroradiology education including brain, head and neck, and spine, with a particular interest in skull base pathology. carlos_zamora@med.unc.edu

Richard Prayson, MD, MEd

Dr. Prayson is the section head of neuropathology at the Cleveland Clinic, and director of student affairs at the Cleveland Clinic Lerner College of Medicine in Cleveland, Ohio. praysor@ccf.org

Samer K. Elbabaa, MD, FAANS, FACS

Dr. Elbabaa is the Reinert Endowed Chair in Pediatric Neurosurgery, associate professor of neurosurgery, and director of pediatric neurosurgery at Saint Louis University School of Medicine in St. Louis, Missouri. He completed his internship and residency in neurological surgery at the University of North Carolina at Chapel Hill. He also completed a clinical fellowship in pediatric neurosurgery at the Cleveland Clinic. He is board certified by the American Board of Neurological Surgery. His clinical and research areas of interest include pediatric neurosurgery, brain and spinal cord tumors, skull base surgery, microneurosurgery, neuroendoscopy, fetal spina bifida surgery, craniocervical junctional anomalies, craniofacial surgery, and neurosurgical education. selbabaa@slu.edu

Matt Pierson, MD

Dr. Pierson is a resident of neurosurgery at Saint Louis University in St. Louis, Missouri. Mpierso8@slu.edu

Katie P. Huynh, DO

Dr. Huynh is a neurosurgeon in Coeur d'Alene, Idaho. Her fellowship is in cerebrovascular and skull base neurosurgery at Saint Louis University in St. Louis, Missouri. Dr. Huynh received her medical degree from the Western University of Health Sciences, and completed her neurological surgery residency at Arrowhead Regional Medical Center, both in Southern California. She loves spending time outdoors with her husband, Adam, and her three daughters, Kaitlin, Kara, and Isabella. huynhkp@slu.edu

Introduction to the Exam

Recently, the board exam was switched to a computer-based format, providing the test taker with the ability to window and zoom in on the color images. Thus, we recommend reviewing the electronic version of this book to prepare for the computer-based format.

The board exam is held on the second or third Friday in March for all neurosurgical residents in all programs.

The exam consists of five sections. The third section is followed by a 30-minute lunch break. The other sections are followed by a 10-minute break.

Each section contains approximately 75 questions, for a total of 375 questions on the exam. The sections contain a random assortment of questions covering all aspects of neurosurgery-related material. The test taker is allotted 60 minutes to complete each section. Previous sections cannot be returned to once they are completed.

The questions are multiple choice and typically have five, or sometimes four, answer choices. The four-choice questions more commonly address an image. The incorrect choices are designed to be distracters that are phrased with a similar level of complexity and generality.

On past exams, a few questions in each section were associated with an answer bank containing choices that can be used once, multiple times, or not at all. There have been fewer than ten of these questions on previous exams.

There are no "negative" questions (e.g., "All are true EXCEPT . . ."). Questions are in the "choose the best answer" style. There are no matching questions (e.g. when a series of questions uses a common bank of answer choices).

You are awarded points for correct answers; there is no penalty for guessing. Therefore, it is best to answer all questions and leave none blank.

The questions are designed to test important concepts in neurosurgery, and they require more than merely regurgitating memorized material.

I Questions

1 Physiology

1.

What allows for the voluntary retention of urine once a full bladder has induced an increase in bladder parasympathetic tone?

A. Inhibition of S2-S4 α-motor neurons causing relaxation of the external urethral sphincter striated muscle fibers

B. Inhibition of pelvic splanchnic nerves causing a compensatory increase in bladder sympathetic activity

C. Activation of S2-S4 α-motor neurons causing contraction of the external urethral sphincter striated muscle fibers

D. Activation of neurons in the inferior mesenteric ganglion and subsequent contraction of the internal urethral sphincter

E. Activation of neurons in the inferior mesenteric ganglion and subsequent contraction of the external urethral sphincter

2.

What neurotransmitter is used by preganglionic sympathetic fibers?

A. Norepinephrine
B. Epinephrine
C. Glutamate
D. Acetylcholine
E. GABA

Use the following answers for questions 3 and 4:

A. Botulism toxin
B. Tetanus toxin
C. Diphtheria toxin
D. Alpha bungarotoxin
E. Tetrodotoxin

3.

This toxin inhibits vesicle fusion in the presynaptic terminal at the neuromuscular junction.

4.

This toxin inhibits RNA translation.

5.

What decreases the rate of degradation of a passively conducted electrical signal in an axon?

A. Decreasing axonal diameter
B. Demyelinating an axon
C. Increasing axonal membrane resistance
D. Increasing extracellular resistance

6.

What substance releases factor VIII from von Willebrand factor?

A. Fibrinogen
B. Platelets
C. Factor IX
D. Antithrombin III
E. Thrombin

7.

In brain death, what happens to the intracranial pressure (ICP) as the mean arterial pressure (MAP) rises?

A. Cerebral autoregulation increases ICP.
B. Cerebral autoregulation decreases ICP.
C. The lack of cerebral autoregulation causes an increase in ICP.
D. The lack of cerebral autoregulation causes a decrease in ICP.
E. Cerebral autoregulation maintains a relatively constant ICP.

8.

The sensory nerves originating in the extremities with cell bodies in the dorsal root ganglia are examples of what classification of neuron?

A. Unipolar
B. Bipolar
C. Multipolar
D. Pyramidal
E. Multiaxonic

9.

To what type of motion/activity will the utricle respond?

A. Injecting cold water into the ear of a person sitting upright
B. Sleeping
C. Stopping at a stop sign in a motor vehicle
D. Beginning to spin in an office chair
E. Falling at terminal velocity while skydiving

10.

A patient has a hormone-producing pituitary microadenoma that puts him at risk (if left untreated) for peripheral neuropathies, cardiac arrhythmias, and sleep apnea. What hormone is the adenoma producing?

A. Adrenocorticotropic hormone (ACTH)
B. Growth hormone
C. Prolactin
D. Thyroid-stimulating hormone
E. Follicle-stimulating hormone

11.

What are the major proinflammatory cytokines?

A. TGF- α and VEGF
B. IL-1 and TNF-α
C. IL-6 and TGF-α
D. IL-6 and IL-13
E. IFN-γ and IL-10

12.

What is a miniature end-plate potential?

A. Inhibitory postsynaptic potential
B. Excitatory postsynaptic potential
C. Response of the postsynaptic terminal caused by the release of a single vesicle into the synaptic cleft
D. Response of the postsynaptic terminal caused by the release of a single molecule of neurotransmitter into the synaptic cleft
E. Response of the postsynaptic terminal caused by the release of the neurotransmitters from a single neuron only

13.

When do T-type calcium channels open during the action potential?

A. At the resting potential
B. Between the resting and threshold potentials
C. Between the threshold potential and maximal depolarization
D. Between maximal depolarization and the resting potential
E. Between the resting potential and "overshoot" phase (hyperpolarization)

14.

How do class 3 cardiac antiarrhythmics (potassium channel blockers) affect action potentials and conduction velocity?

A. Shorten action potential refractory period and increase conduction velocity
B. Shorten action potential duration and maintain normal conduction velocity
C. Prolong action potential refractory period and slow conduction velocity
D. Prolong action potential duration and maintain normal conduction velocity
E. Shorten action potential refractory period and slow conduction velocity

15.

What neurotransmitters never can be used to upregulate action downstream in a neural network?

A. GABA and glycine
B. Glutamate and acetylcholine
C. Norepinephrine and epinephrine
D. Dopamine and substance P
E. All neurotransmitters can be used to upregulate downstream neural network activation

16.

How does caffeine exert its effects?

A. GABA receptor antagonism
B. Phosphodiesterase inhibition
C. Adenosine receptor agonism
D. Acetylcholinesterase activation
E. Ryanodine receptor antagonist

17.

How does cocaine affect neurotransmission at the synaptic cleft?

A. Inhibition of the presynaptic uptake of monoamines
B. Induction of the release of monoamines
C. Prevention of the degradation of monoamines in the synaptic cleft
D. Blockade of the postsynaptic uptake of monoamines
E. Induction of the postsynaptic uptake of monoamines

18.

What are the degradation products of the reaction between acetylcholine and acetylcholinesterase on the postsynaptic membrane?

A. Phosphatidylcholine and choline
B. Phosphatidylcholine and acetate
C. Acetyl CoA and acetate
D. Choline and acetate
E. Choline and acetyl CoA

19.
What role do caspases play in necrosis?

A. Caspases signal and regulate the orderly fragmentation of DNA.
B. Caspases signal a cell to undergo necrosis.
C. Caspases typically are not part of necrosis.
D. Caspases inhibit necrosis and cell death.

20.
What molecules are needed to activate the ligand-gated component of NMDA receptors?

A. Glutamate and glycine
B. Magnesium and glycine
C. Magnesium and serine
D. Aspartate and zinc
E. Zinc and glycine

21.
What is the mechanism of action of bisphosphonates?

A. Increasing the body stores of calcium
B. Activation of osteocytes
C. Inhibition of osteocytes
D. Inhibition of osteoclasts
E. Recruitment of osteoblasts

22.
Where does GABA bind on the $GABA_A$ receptor?

A. On the α subunit
B. On the β subunit
C. Between the α and β subunits
D. On the γ subunit
E. Between the α and γ subunits

23.
A patient with a complete spinal cord injury has a patellar reflex in the acute period following his injury. What circuitry component must be intact?

A. Cell bodies in the midthoracic spinal cord
B. Dorsal columns between the brain and lumbar spinal cord
C. Cell bodies in the lumbar prominence of the spinal cord
D. Anterior horn cells between the brain and lumbar spinal cord

24.
What is the mechanism of action for temozolomide (Temodar)?

A. Microtubule inhibitor
B. DNA cross-linking
C. Anti-VEGF antibody
D. DNA alkylation
E. Topoisomerase inhibitor

25.
What are the first cleavage products of pro-opiomelanocortin?

A. β-lipotrophin, α-MSH, and γ-MSH
B. ACTH, α-MSH, and γ-MSH
C. α-MSH, β-MSH, β-endorphin
D. ACTH, β-lipotrophin, and γ-MSH
E. α-MSH, β-MSH, and γ-MSH

26.
What happens during testing of the H-reflex in electrophysiological studies when stimulation is increased to a supramaximal level?

A. The H-wave disappears.
B. The M-wave disappears.
C. The H-wave increases.
D. The M-wave decreases.
E. The F-wave remains constant.

27.
What is the substrate for nitric oxide synthetase?

A. Tyrosine
B. NADP
C. Citrulline
D. Arginine
E. Asparagine

28.
How does the isometric tension-length curve of smooth muscle compare to the curve of skeletal muscle?

A. Smooth muscle force is maximal in the tension trough.
B. The curve is wider with smooth muscle.
C. Maximal tension occurs at the point of maximal contraction in smooth muscle.
D. There is only a single peak of maximal tension with smooth muscle.

29.
What substance in excess in the extracellular space induces increased calcium ion flux through NMDA receptors on oligodendrocytes to cause excitotoxic damage?

A. Calcium
B. Glutamate
C. Acetylcholine
D. GABA
E. Epinephrine

30.
What component of the blood–brain barrier is most responsible for its integrity, creation, and maintenance?

A. Astrocytic foot processes
B. Arachnoid "cap" cells
C. Pericytes
D. Endothelial cells

31.
How do organophosphates cause accumulation of acetylcholine in the synaptic cleft?

A. Irreversible binding to and inhibition of acetylcholinesterase
B. Blockade of postsynaptic acetylcholine receptors
C. Blockade of presynaptic acetylcholine receptors
D. Stimulation of release of presynaptic acetylcholine
E. Temporary reduction in binding affinity for acetylcholine and acetylcholinesterase

32.
How does hemoglobin's affinity for oxygen change as blood passes through a capillary, and what shift occurs with the oxygen-hemoglobin dissociation curve?

A. The affinity of hemoglobin for oxygen decreases, and the oxygen-hemoglobin dissociation curve shifts to the left.
B. The affinity of hemoglobin for oxygen decreases, and the oxygen-hemoglobin dissociation curve shifts to the right.
C. The affinity of hemoglobin for oxygen increases, and the oxygen-hemoglobin dissociation curve shifts to the left.
D. The affinity of hemoglobin for oxygen increases, and the oxygen-hemoglobin dissociation curve shifts to the right.
E. The affinity of hemoglobin for oxygen remains the same, and the oxygen-hemoglobin dissociation curve does not shift.

33.
What is the approximate resting membrane potential of a neuron, and conductance of what ion is most responsible for determining this potential?

A. –65 mV; potassium
B. –60 mV; sodium
C. +60 mV; chloride
D. –90 mV; potassium
E. +20 mV; calcium

34.
Secretion of what proteins from the notochord establishes the ventral pole of the dorsal-ventral axis in the developing nervous system?

A. Bone morphogenic proteins
B. Wnt family proteins
C. Sonic hedgehog proteins
D. Patched proteins
E. Ras proteins

35.
How will a patient with severe myasthenia gravis affecting a particular neuromuscular junction react to organophosphate poisoning at that same junction?

A. No effect on postsynaptic activity
B. Increased postsynaptic activity
C. Decreased postsynaptic activity
D. Increased presynaptic activity
E. Decreased presynaptic activity

36.
If a resting neuron with only potassium permeability was taken from its normal extracellular space and placed in endolymph, what would happen to its resting state?

A. Its resting state would become more positive.
B. Its resting state would become more negative.
C. Its resting state would remain the same.
D. Its resting state would be too variable to predict.

37.
What is the mechanism of action of strychnine?

A. Blockade of GABA receptors
B. Activation of acetylcholine receptors on neurons in the spinal cord
C. Inhibition of neurons through activation of GABA receptors
D. Inhibition of glycine receptors
E. Potentiation of neurons through activation of glycine receptors

38.
What is the hourly rate of production of cerebrospinal fluid in the adult brain?

A. 10 mL/h
B. 14 mL/h
C. 18 mL/h
D. 22 mL/h
E. 26 mL/h

39.
What role do gamma motor neurons play in the muscle spindle?

A. Shorten the muscle spindles with skeletal muscle fiber contraction
B. Regulate beta motor neurons
C. Inhibit alpha motor neurons
D. Allow for the adaptation of type 2 afferents
E. Shorten the Golgi tendon organs with muscle contraction

40.
What enzyme promotes the conversion of 5-hydroxy-tryptophan to serotonin?

A. Tyramine β-hydroxylase
B. Aromatic amino acid decarboxylase
C. Tryptophan hydroxylase
D. Tyrosine hydroxylase
E. Catechol-O-methyl transferase

41.
How is presynaptic hyperpolarization of a neuron advantageous over postsynaptic hyperpolarization?

A. It allows for inhibition of the entire presynaptic and postsynaptic neuronal chain.
B. It allows for more precise temporal summation.
C. It reduces the amount of neurotransmitter degradation occurring in the synapse.
D. It allows for more precise spatial resolution.

42.
What role do L-type voltage-dependent calcium channels play in muscle contraction?

A. Release calcium from the sarcoplasmic reticulum
B. Allow for depolarization of the postsynaptic terminal
C. Reuptake calcium into the presynaptic terminal
D. Respond to depolarization and activate calcium channels on the sarcoplasmic reticulum
E. Binds to troponin to induce an allosteric change

43.
How does parathyroid hormone increase the serum calcium level?

A. Inhibits calcitonin production
B. Inhibits osteoblasts
C. Increases phosphate reabsorption in the kidneys
D. Blocks the formation of vitamin D
E. Inhibits osteoclasts

44.
A particular inhibitor is found to prevent the formation of L-dopa from tyrosine. Further studies show that the inhibitor only works once tyrosine hydroxylase has interacted with tyrosine. The inhibitor is a(n):

A. Competitive inhibitor
B. Noncompetitive inhibitor
C. Uncompetitive inhibitor
D. Mixed inhibitor

45.
What feature of excitatory synapses forces them to transmit in only one direction?

A. Absolute refractory period across the synaptic cleft
B. Postsynaptic clefts residing on multiple postsynaptic neurons
C. Presynaptic neurotransmitter reuptake receptors
D. Vesicles and corresponding receptors each on only one side of the synaptic cleft

46.
What is the brain's response to a rising PCO_2 with regard to cerebral blow flow (CBF) and intracranial pressure (ICP)?

A. Decrease CBF and increase ICP.
B. Increase CBF and decrease ICP.
C. Decrease CBF and decrease ICP.
D. Increase CBF and keep ICP constant.
E. Increase CBF and increase ICP.

47.
What makes an action potential propagate in only one direction once it has been initiated?

A. Absolute refractory period
B. Unidirectional protein transport
C. Saltatory conduction
D. Relative refractory period
E. Temporal summation

48.
How would hexamethonium administration affect postsynaptic parasympathetic neurons?

A. Reduction of the depolarization threshold
B. Favoring temporal instead of spatial summation
C. Selective inhibition of the parasympathetic nervous system
D. No postsynaptic blockade
E. Augmentation of the postsynaptic response

49.

How do steroid hormones pass through cell membranes?

A. Through membrane steroid channels
B. By simple diffusion
C. By facilitated diffusion
D. Through G proteins
E. By active transport

50.

What is the result of light falling upon the photo-receptor cells of the retina?

A. Phosphodiesterases inhibit the phototransduction cascade.
B. Retinal is converted from the trans to the cis isomer.
C. Molecules of cAMP are hydrolyzed.
D. Hyperpolarization of the retinal cells results in phototransduction.

51.

In which stage of the cell cycle does growth arrest by p53 occur?

A. G1 phase
B. S phase
C. G2 phase
D. M phase
E. G0 phase

52.

A motor unit is composed of:

A. A motor neuron and all of the muscle fibers innervated by that neuron
B. A muscle fiber and all of the motor neurons that innervate that fiber
C. All of the motor neurons within a peripheral nerve
D. A single motor neuron and a single muscle fiber innervated by that neuron
E. The motor and sensory neurons along with the muscle spindles associated with a single muscle fiber

53.

Where is norepinephrine synthesized?

A. Cytoplasm
B. Postsynaptic terminal
C. Neuronal membrane
D. Synaptic vesicle
E. Synaptic cleft

54.

How do cytotoxic and vasogenic edema differ?

A. Cytotoxic edema responds better to steroids than does vasogenic edema.
B. The blood–brain barrier is closed in cytotoxic edema and disrupted in vasogenic edema.
C. Cells shrink in vasogenic edema but expand in cytotoxic edema.
D. Cytotoxic but not vasogenic edema occurs after ischemic injury.
E. Proteins expand the extracellular space in cytotoxic edema.

55.

In rigor mortis, in what state are the myosin heads?

A. Myosin heads are unbound from actin with their heads uncocked.
B. Myosin heads are bound to actin following the power stroke.
C. Myosin heads are bound to actin before the power stroke.
D. Myosin heads are unbound from actin with their heads cocked.

56.

What enzyme is necessary for conversion of norepinephrine to epinephrine?

A. Monoamine oxidase
B. Tyrosine hydroxylase
C. Aromatic L-amino acid decarboxylase
D. Dopamine β-hydroxylase
E. Phenylethanolamine N-methyltransferase

57.

How would an isolated vitamin K deficiency affect the clotting cascade?

A. Upregulation of antithrombin activity
B. Reduced activity of factors XI and XII
C. Inhibition of synthesis of proteins C, S, and Z
D. Prolongation of bleeding time
E. Prolongation of the partial thromboplastin time without affecting the prothrombin time

58.

What typically prevents axonal regeneration in the central nervous system?

A. Reduced axonal growth factors following injury
B. Astrocytic scarring
C. Lack of progenitor cells
D. Lack of directional markers and/or architecture

59.
During the action potential, what does closing of the sodium channels cause?

A. Membrane depolarization
B. Opening of the potassium channels
C. The beginning of the relative refractory period
D. Membrane repolarization
E. Opening of the voltage-gated calcium channels

60.
What is the mechanism of action of hydrochlorothiazide?

A. Promotion of aquaporin channels in the distal convoluted tubules and collecting ducts
B. Inhibition of the sodium-potassium cotransporters in the distal tubules
C. Inhibition of the sodium-potassium-chloride symporters in the thick ascending limb of the loops of Henle
D. Reduction of sodium chloride and bicarbonate reabsorption in the proximal tubules
E. Inhibition of the sodium-chloride cotransporters in the distal tubules

61.
What are the two major characteristics of/associated with protein molecules that prevent them from being filtered into the Bowman capsule in the renal glomerulus?

A. Large size and negative charge
B. Low oncotic pressure and positive charge
C. Small size and negative charge
D. High hydrostatic pressure and positive charge
E. High hydrostatic pressure and negative charge

62.
Lateral geniculate cells have what type of receptive fields?

A. Concentric
B. Rectangular
C. Motion
D. Direction
E. No receptive fields

63.
What ion entering neurons during the secondary phase of traumatic brain injury accounts for the majority of the mitochondrial malfunctioning and damage?

A. Glutamate
B. Sodium
C. Potassium
D. Calcium

64.
What is the role of dynein in axoplasmic transport?

A. Slow anterograde transport
B. Both anterograde and retrograde transport
C. Fast anterograde transport
D. Inhibits transport
E. Retrograde transport

65.
What structure in the sarcomere is composed of myosin and actin filaments?

A. C-band
B. A-band
C. I-band
D. H-band
E. M-band

66.
What enzymes allow retroviruses to produce DNA from their RNA genomes?

A. RNA polymerases
B. DNA polymerases
C. Reverse transcriptases
D. Integrases
E. Helicases

67.
What is the rate-limiting step in dopamine synthesis?

A. Tyrosine availability
B. Tyrosine hydroxylase
C. Dopa decarboxylase
D. Dopamine β-hydroxylase
E. Tetrahydrobiopterin

68.
In addition to being synthesized in the neuron and being deactivated at the site of action, what other criterion is necessary to label a substance a neurotransmitter?

A. Released nonspecifically from the presynaptic terminal
B. Exogenous administration that mimics the endogenous activity
C. Presence throughout the nervous system
D. Ubiquitous effect throughout all neural networks
E. Exerting an effect at a distant site in the body

69.

What is the main role of orexin/hypocretin in the human body?

A. Promoting arousal
B. Promoting sleep
C. Inhibiting pain
D. Appetite suppression
E. Decreasing thermogenesis

70.

A patient receives an overdose of intravenous potassium. How would muscle action potentials be affected?

A. Resting membrane potential would increase, and the threshold to trigger an action potential would be reached with more miniature end-plate potentials (MEPPs)
B. Resting membrane potential would decrease, and the threshold to trigger an action potential would be reached with fewer MEPPs
C. Resting membrane potential would increase, and the threshold to trigger an action potential would be reached with fewer MEPPs
D. The threshold to trigger an action potential would become more negative
E. The threshold to trigger an action potential would become more positive

2 Anatomy

1.
A lesion in the pulvinar nucleus of the thalamus can result in:

A. Neglect syndromes
B. Anosmia
C. Contralateral sensory loss
D. Endocrine dysfunction and abnormalities
E. Memory difficulties

2.
A 67-year-old woman presents for follow-up 4 months after a stroke. She complains of her eyelids "twitching." She is found to have palatal myoclonus on physical exam. Her stroke likely involved what region of the brain?

A. Nucleus ambiguus
B. Tectospinal tract
C. Rubro-olivary tract/central tegmental tract (triangle of Mollaret)
D. Body of the caudate nucleus
E. Lateral lemniscus

3.
The ventral tegmental area sends projections through what neuroanatomic structure to the nucleus accumbens as part of the dopaminergic mesolimbic system (involved in reward circuitry)?

A. Medial forebrain bundle
B. Lateral hypothalamus
C. Ventral pallidum
D. Prefrontal cortex

Use the following answers for questions 4 and 5:

A. Area postrema
B. Nucleus tractus solitarius
C. Nucleus prepositus hypoglossi
D. Nucleus ambiguus
E. Inferior salivary nucleus

4.
What structure is the target for taste afferent fibers?

5.
What structure is the autonomic center for vomiting?

6.
What skin mechanoreceptors are best at sensing both rapid vibration and pressure?

A. Ruffini endings
B. Meissner corpuscles
C. Merkel disks
D. Pacinian corpuscles
E. Free nerve endings

7.
In what ventricular structure is cerebrospinal fluid not produced by the choroid plexus?

A. Roof of the fourth ventricle
B. Floor of the third ventricle
C. Lateral recess of the foramen of Luschka
D. Temporal horn of the lateral ventricle
E. Roof of the third ventricle

8.
The deep petrosal nerve is what type of nerve with what function?

A. Sensory nerve that unites with the greater superficial petrosal nerve to form the nerve of the pterygoid canal
B. Sympathetic nerve that unites with the lesser superficial petrosal nerve to form the vidian nerve
C. Sympathetic nerve that unites with the greater superficial petrosal nerve to form the vidian nerve
D. Sensory nerve that unites with the lesser superficial petrosal nerve to form the nerve of the pterygoid canal

9.
What nerve innervates the skin between the hallux and the second toe?

A. Superficial peroneal nerve
B. Medial dorsal cutaneous nerve
C. Intermediate dorsal cutaneous nerve
D. Deep peroneal nerve
E. Tibial nerve

10.
What is another name for the medial distal striate artery?

A. Tentorial artery (of Bernasconi and Cassinari)
B. McConnell capsular artery
C. Frontopolar artery
D. Recurrent artery of Heubner
E. Medial lenticulostriate artery

11.
What midbrain anatomic structure is responsible for pain modulation?

A. Superior colliculus
B. Substantia nigra
C. Crus cerebri
D. Red nucleus
E. Periaqueductal gray matter

12.
A patient has an intractable nosebleed following transsphenoidal pituitary surgery. What artery likely is injured?

A. Middle meningeal artery
B. Infraorbital artery
C. Internal maxillary artery
D. Superior hypophyseal artery
E. Anterior ethmoidal artery

13.
A patient presents with a winged scapula. What other nerve besides the long thoracic and dorsal scapular nerves may be injured?

A. Suprascapular nerve
B. Spinal accessory nerve
C. Thoracodorsal nerve
D. Lateral thoracic nerve

14.
What leptomeningeal structure is composed only of a single layer?

A. Intracranial dura
B. Spinal dura
C. Pia mater
D. Arachnoid

15.
In this spinal cord cross-sectional image, what letter corresponds to the location of the spinothalamic tract?

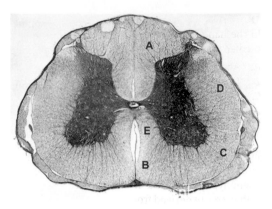

A. A
B. B
C. C
D. D
E. E

16.
The supplementary motor area is found at what location:

A. Along the midline surface of the cerebral hemisphere just anterior to the primary motor cortex leg area
B. In the parietal operculum just rostral to the lateral sulcus
C. Along the lateral surface of the cerebral hemisphere just anterior to the primary motor cortex arm area
D. Within the pars opercularis and pars triangularis of the inferior frontal gyrus
E. Along the medial surface of the cerebral hemisphere continuous with the postcentral gyrus of the parietal lobe

17.
Which structure runs through the petrotympanic fissure?

A. Pterygoid artery
B. Posterior deep temporal artery
C. Chorda tympani
D. Lingual nerve
E. Greater superficial petrosal nerve

18.
Which bone does not contribute to both the orbit and nasal septum?

A. Frontal bone
B. Ethmoid bone
C. Maxillary bone
D. Palatine bone

19.

In the hand, what muscles are innervated by the median nerve?

A. Abductor pollicis brevis
B. Lumbricals 3 and 4
C. Adductor pollicis
D. Opponens digiti minimi
E. Abductor pollicis longus

20.

Embryologically, the pituitary is composed of the adenohypophysis and neurohypophysis. Rathke cleft cysts are derived from the persistence of what primary germ layer?

A. Ectoderm
B. Neuroectoderm
C. Mesoderm
D. Endoderm

21.

The inferior aspect of the cuneus is bounded by what structure?

A. Tentorium
B. Parieto-occipital sulcus
C. Lingual gyrus
D. Collateral eminence
E. Calcarine sulcus

22.

From superior to inferior (rostral to caudal), what are the correct layers, in order, of the roof of the third ventricle?

A. Fornix, tela choroidea, velum interpositum, tela choroidea, and choroid plexus
B. Choroid plexus, velum interpositum, tela choroidea, and fornix
C. Fornix, velum interpositum, tela choroidea, choroid plexus, and tela choroidea
D. Tela choroidea, fornix, tela choroidea, velum interpositum, and choroid plexus
E. Fornix, velum interpositum, and choroid plexus

23.

What structure courses between the petrous temporal bone and basilar part of the occipital bone and drains blood from the cavernous sinus to the sigmoid sinus?

A. Superior petrosal sinus
B. Inferior petrosal sinus
C. Vein of Labbé
D. Basal vein of Rosenthal
E. Straight sinus

24.

Which structure primarily is responsible for carrying input to the cerebellum from the contralateral cerebral cortex?

A. Inferior cerebellar peduncle
B. Middle cerebellar peduncle
C. Superior cerebellar peduncle
D. Cerebral peduncle

25.

What structure in the medial limbic circuit is the major output of the thalamus?

A. Hippocampus
B. Amygdala
C. Fornix
D. Entorhinal cortex
E. Cingulate gyrus

26.

What is an accurate description of the location of the flocculonodular lobe of the cerebellum?

A. Rostral to the primary fissure
B. Caudal to the primary fissure
C. Anterior to and between the anterior and posterior cerebellar lobes
D. Midsagittal
E. Rostral to the anterior lobe and posterior to the sylvian aqueduct

27.

Afferents to the subthalamic nucleus originate in what structure?

A. Thalamus
B. Red nucleus
C. Globus pallidus
D. Cerebellum
E. Substantia innominata

28.

The lateral cord of the brachial plexus is formed from what structure(s)?

A. Anterior divisions of the upper and middle trunks
B. Nerve roots C5, C6, and C7
C. Posterior divisions of the superior, middle, and inferior trunks
D. Anterior division of the inferior trunk
E. Posterior division of the superior trunk

29.
The ventral posterior nucleus of the thalamus sends information to which Brodmann area(s)?

A. Areas 1, 2, and 3
B. Area 4
C. Area 17
D. Areas 39 and 40
E. Area 44

30.
The sural nerve provides sensation to the posterolateral surface of the leg, lateral foot, and the fifth toe. It is formed by contributions from which nerve(s)?

A. Tibial nerve
B. Common peroneal nerve
C. Tibial and common peroneal nerves
D. Superficial peroneal nerve
E. Tibial and superficial peroneal nerves

31.
If the facial nerve is sectioned just proximal to the nerve to the stapedius, what clinical finding would be expected other than paresis of the facial musculature?

A. Decreased lacrimation
B. Decreased taste in the anterior two thirds of the tongue
C. Increased salivation
D. Decreased sensation in the nasopharynx and palate mucous membranes

32.
What muscle is innervated by the anterior interosseous nerve?

A. Flexor pollicis brevis
B. Abductor pollicis brevis
C. Flexor carpi radialis
D. Pronator quadratus
E. Abductor pollicis longus

33.
Brodmann area 39 may be considered part of what cortical area?

A. Broca area
B. Visual cortex
C. Somatosensory association cortex
D. Wernicke area
E. Auditory cortex

34.
The inferior leaflet of the Liliequist membrane separates the interpeduncular from the prepontine cistern. The superior leaflet separates which two cisterns medially?

A. Chiasmatic and crural cisterns
B. Interpeduncular and crural cisterns
C. Interpeduncular and chiasmatic cisterns
D. Ambient and quadrigeminal cisterns
E. Interpeduncular and ambient cisterns

35.
Innervation of the facet joints in the lumbar spine is provided by what nerve?

A. Lateral branch of the dorsal ramus
B. Ventral ramus
C. Medial branch of the dorsal ramus
D. Ramus communicans
E. Dorsal root

36.
Which of the following is true regarding the cerebellothalamic tract (dentatothalamic tract)?

A. It is an uncrossed tract arising from the dentate nucleus that passes through the superior cerebellar peduncle and terminates in the ventral anterior nucleus of the thalamus.
B. It is an uncrossed tract arising from the dentate nucleus that passes through the middle cerebellar peduncle and terminates in the ventral anterior nucleus of the thalamus.
C. It is a crossed tract arising from the dentate nucleus that passes through the superior cerebellar peduncle and terminates in the ventral anterior nucleus of the thalamus.
D. It is a crossed tract arising from the dentate nucleus that passes through the middle cerebellar peduncle and terminates in the ventral anterior nucleus of the thalamus.
E. It is an uncrossed tract arising from the dentate nucleus that passes through the inferior cerebellar peduncle and terminates in the ventral anterior nucleus of the thalamus.

37.
Pain and temperature fibers from the face are relayed to what nucleus?

A. Mesencephalic nucleus of cranial nerve V
B. Ventral posterior lateral nucleus of the thalamus
C. Principal sensory nucleus of cranial nerve V
D. Solitary nucleus
E. Spinal nucleus of cranial nerve V

38.

What is the most proximal artery originating from the carotid artery distal to the ophthalmic artery?

A. Posterior communicating artery
B. Anterior choroidal artery
C. Superior hypophyseal artery
D. Inferior hypophyseal artery

39.

The vertebral artery often is divided into numbered segments. What segment exits the axis and curves posteromedially in a groove on the atlas and enters the foramen magnum?

A. V2
B. V3
C. V4
D. V5

40.

What type of nerve ending is slowly adapting?

A. Meissner corpuscle
B. Pacinian corpuscle
C. Merkel disk
D. Hair follicle receptor
E. A-delta free nerve ending

41.

What anatomic reference points form the stephanion?

A. Junction of the frontal, parietal, temporal, and sphenoid bones
B. Junction of the lambdoid, occipitomastoid, and parietomastoid sutures
C. Junction of the coronal and sagittal sutures
D. Junction of the coronal suture and superior temporal line

42.

The stria medullaris thalami connect what neural structures?

A. Globus pallidus and the field of Forel H
B. Septal nuclei and the habenular nuclei
C. Globus pallidus interna and the thalamic fasciculus
D. Amygdalae
E. Ventral tegmental area and the nucleus accumbens

43.

Corticospinal tracts terminate on which structures in the spinal cord?

A. Spinal gray interneurons in Rexed lamina IX
B. Alpha motor neurons in Rexed lamina VII

C. Gamma motor neurons in the anterior gray horn
D. Spinal gray interneurons in Rexed lamina VII
E. Gamma motor neurons in Rexed lamina IX

44.

Proprioception sense is carried in what decussating tract?

A. Spinothalamic tract
B. Posterior columns
C. Dorsal spinocerebellar tract
D. Ventral spinocerebellar tract
E. Corticobulbar tract

45.

The acoustic reflex to loud sound involves what circuitry?

A. Cranial nerve V to the tensor veli palatini muscle
B. Cranial nerve V to the stapedius muscle
C. Cranial nerve V to the levator palatini muscle and cranial nerve VII to the posterior belly of the digastrics muscle
D. Cranial nerve V to the tensor tympani muscle and cranial nerve VII to the stapedius muscle

46.

The transverse component of the transverse ligament of the atlas attaches to what structure?

A. Occipital condyle
B. Medial surface of the lateral mass of C1
C. Medial surface of the pars interarticularis of C2
D. Posterior aspect of the body of C2
E. Posterior arch of C1

47.

Damage to the anterior hypothalamus may cause what dysfunction?

A. Obesity
B. Cachexia
C. Hypothermia
D. Impaired memory
E. Hyperthermia

48.

The amygdala projects to which area of the insula?

A. Operculum
B. Anterior short gyri
C. Posterior long gyrus
D. Cingulate
E. Claustrum

49.
What deep cerebellar nucleus is located most laterally?

A. Dentate
B. Globose
C. Fastigial
D. Emboliform
E. Inferior olivary nucleus

50.
What percentage of people have a balanced configuration of the circle of Willis?

A. 5%
B. 20%
C. 40%
D. 60%
E. 80%

51.
The nucleus pulposus is the remnant of what embryonic structure?

A. Neural tube
B. Anterior neuropore
C. Posterior neuropore
D. Neural plate
E. Notochord

52.
What is the arterial supply for the optic tract?

A. Ophthalmic artery
B. Anterior communicating, posterior communicating, and posterior cerebral arteries
C. Posterior communicating, posterior cerebral, and anterior choroidal arteries
D. Lateral posterior choroidal artery

53.
What Brodmann area corresponds to primary visual cortex?

A. Area 41
B. Area 19
C. Area 17
D. Area 39

54.
How many primary ossification centers are present for the C1 (atlas) and C2 (axis) vertebrae, respectively?

A. One and three
B. Two and four
C. Three and five
D. Five and three
E. Three and one

55.
The afferent and efferent projections to and from the medial geniculate body, respectively, are from what structures?

A. Superior colliculus; visual cortex
B. Retina; visual cortex
C. Reticular formation; dorsal thalamic nuclei
D. Inferior colliculus; auditory cortex
E. Mammillary bodies; cingulum

56.
What blood vessel is at risk of injury during a Chiari decompression?

A. Lateral medullary segment of the posterior inferior cerebellar artery
B. Telovelotonsillar segment of the posterior inferior cerebellar artery
C. Tonsillomedullary segment of the posterior inferior cerebellar artery
D. Posterior spinal artery
E. V2 segment of the vertebral artery

57.
Number 2 in this image represents what structure?

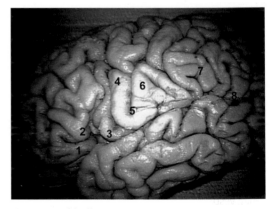

A. Pars orbitalis
B. Premotor gyrus
C. Pars triangularis
D. Angular gyrus
E. Supramarginal gyrus

58.
The largest intercostal artery is usually found at what location?

A. On the left side between the T9 and L2 levels
B. On the left side between the T1 and T4 levels
C. On the right side between the T9 and L2 levels
D. On the right side between the T1 and T4 levels
E. On the left side between the L2 and S1 levels

59.
The Kawase triangle also is known as a triangle by what other name?

A. Anteromedial middle cranial fossa triangle
B. Anterolateral middle cranial fossa triangle
C. Posteromedial middle cranial fossa triangle
D. Posterolateral middle cranial fossa triangle
E. Infratrochlear middle cranial fossa triangle

60.
What is the typical site and arterial segment involvement of traumatic internal carotid artery dissection?

A. At the carotid bifurcation with involvement of the carotid bulb
B. At the carotid bifurcation without involvement of the carotid bulb
C. Two centimeters above the carotid bifurcation with involvement of the carotid bulb
D. Two centimeters above the carotid bifurcation without involvement of the carotid bulb
E. In the supraclinoidal segment of the internal carotid artery

61.
The vertebral arch congenital defect with cystic distention of the meninges and structural/functional abnormalities of the spinal cord/cauda equina is also known by what term?

A. Spina bifida occulta
B. Myelomeningocele
C. Meningocele
D. Lipomyelomeningocele
E. Diastematomyelia

62.
Inputs from the dorsal spinocerebellar, cuneocerebellar, vestibulocerebellar, and pontocerebellar tracts are carried by what fibers?

A. Climbing
B. Mossy
C. Parallel
D. Purkinje
E. Association

63.
What nerve passes through the cavernous sinus and superior orbital fissure but does not go through the annulus of Zinn?

A. Superior division of the oculomotor nerve
B. Inferior division of the oculomotor nerve
C. Abducens nerve
D. Trochlear nerve
E. Optic nerve

64.
What muscle or muscle group allows for the abduction of the fingers?

A. Dorsal interossei
B. Lumbricals
C. Palmar interossei
D. Extensor digitorum
E. Flexor digitorum superficialis

65.
The anterior spinal artery arises from what artery or trunk?

A. Deep cervical artery
B. Costocervical trunk
C. Vertebral artery
D. Intercostal artery
E. Thyrocervical trunk

66.
The long thoracic nerve courses over the surface of what cervical muscle?

A. Anterior scalene
B. Middle scalene
C. Sternocleidomastoid
D. Omohyoid
E. Longus colli

67.
The motor nucleus for the trigeminal nerve is derived from what branchial arch?

A. First
B. Second
C. Third
D. Fourth
E. Sixth

68.
What structure extends from the supracondylar process of the humerus to the medial epicondyle?

A. Ligament of Struthers
B. Arcade of Struthers
C. Arcade of Frohse
D. Osborne ligament
E. Guyon canal

69.
The jugular foramen often is divided into two parts: the pars nervosa and the pars vascularis. What structures commonly are found in the anteromedial compartment?

A. Cranial nerves IX, X, and XI
B. Jugular bulb and inferior petrosal sinus
C. Cranial nerve IX, Jacobson's nerve, and inferior petrosal sinus
D. Cranial nerves X and XI, Arnold's nerve, and jugular bulb
E. Cranial nerves IX and X and Jacobson's nerve

70.
What is the only circumventricular organ that contains an intact blood–brain barrier?

A. Median eminence
B. Organ of the lamina terminalis
C. Subfornical organ
D. Area postrema
E. Subcommissural organ

71.
With respect to cytoarchitecture of the isocortex, what layer contains afferent fibers from the thalamus?

A. External granular
B. Internal granular
C. External pyramidal
D. Internal pyramidal
E. Multiform

72.
Corpus striatum refers to what structure(s)?

A. Caudate and putamen
B. Caudate, putamen, and globus pallidus
C. Putamen and globus pallidus
D. Caudate
E. Caudate and globus pallidus

73.
What cistern contains the anterior choroidal artery, posterior cerebral artery, medial posterior choroidal artery, and basal vein of Rosenthal?

A. Ambient
B. Quadrigeminal
C. Interpeduncular
D. Carotid
E. Crural

74.
The neurohypophysis contains axons that transport precursors of what hormones?

A. Adrenocorticotropic and thyroid-stimulating hormones
B. Luteinizing and follicle-stimulating hormones
C. Growth hormone and prolactin
D. Oxytocin and antidiuretic hormone
E. Oxytocin and growth hormone

75.
Which structure forms the roof of the temporal horn?

A. Amygdala
B. Hippocampus
C. Tapetum
D. Choroidal fissure
E. Collateral eminence

76.
The spinocerebellar tract (SCT) conveys proprioceptive information from the body to the cerebellum. Which pathway is correct?

A. Fibers from the ventral SCT often cross contralaterally in the spinal cord and cross again contralaterally in the superior cerebellar peduncle to reach the cerebellum.
B. Fibers entering the dorsal SCT synapse in the Clarke column and then ascend to travel to the cerebellum through the contralateral inferior cerebellar peduncle.
C. Fibers entering the ventral SCT often cross contralaterally in the spinal cord and cross again contralaterally in the inferior cerebellar peduncle to reach the cerebellum.
D. Fibers entering the dorsal SCT cross contralaterally in the spinal cord and then ascend to travel to the cerebellum through the contralateral superior cerebellar peduncle.
E. Fibers entering the ventral SCT synapse in the Clarke column and then ascend to travel to the cerebellum through the ipsilateral inferior cerebellar peduncle.

77.
Where do climbing fibers originate?

A. Vestibular nucleus
B. Dentate nucleus
C. Cerebellar glomeruli
D. Inferior and superior colliculi
E. Inferior olivary nucleus

78.

What extraocular muscle is innervated by a contralateral nucleus?

A. Inferior oblique
B. Inferior rectus
C. Superior rectus
D. Medial rectus
E. Lateral rectus

79.

What brain structure is rich in acetylcholine?

A. Locus coeruleus
B. Raphe nucleus
C. Basal nucleus of Meynert
D. Substantia nigra
E. Suprachiasmatic nucleus

80.

What Rexed lamina contains motor neurons?

A. II
B. IV
C. VII
D. IX
E. X

81.

What are Renshaw cells?

A. Inhibitory interneurons found in the spinal cord that release GABA
B. Inhibitory interneurons found in the spinal cord that release glycine
C. Excitatory interneurons found in the spinal cord that release glutamate
D. Excitatory interneurons found in the spinal cord that release acetylcholine
E. Inhibitory interneurons found in the brainstem that releases GABA

82.

Schaffer collateral branches consist of what fibers?

A. Fibers projecting from CA3 to CA1
B. Fibers projecting from CA3 to the fornix
C. Fibers projecting from the dentate gyrus to CA3
D. Fibers projecting from the cingulum to the parahippocampal gyrus
E. Fibers projecting from the lateral olfactory stria to the pyriform cortex

83.

What two veins provide immediate contributions to the vein of Galen?

A. Anterior septal and thalamostriate veins
B. Inferior sagittal sinus and internal cerebral vein
C. Superior sagittal and straight sinuses
D. Basal vein of Rosenthal and internal cerebral vein
E. Basal vein of Rosenthal and straight sinus

84.

A patient with a stroke of the occipital lobe sparing the most caudal area of the visual cortex would have what visual findings?

A. Congruent homonymous hemianopsia without sparing of central vision
B. Congruent homonymous hemianopsia with sparing of central vision
C. Incongruent homonymous hemianopsia
D. Bitemporal hemianopsia
E. Junctional scotoma

85.

The vertical crest (Bill's bar) separates what two structures?

A. Facial nerve and cochlear nerve
B. Superior vestibular nerve and inferior vestibular nerve
C. Cochlea and anteromedial turn of the carotid
D. Facial nerve and superior vestibular nerve
E. Pars nervosa and pars vascularis of the jugular foramen

86.

The nasociliary nerve innervates what areas/structures?

A. Lacrimal gland
B. Ethmoid sinuses
C. Forehead and frontal sinuses
D. Iris dilator muscle
E. Cornea

87.

What connective tissue structure prevents separation of the sciatic nerve into fascicles?

A. Perineurium
B. Endoneurium
C. Epineurium
D. Deep fascia
E. Superficial fascia

3 Adult Neurosurgery

1.
Which tumor is associated with hydrocephalus and sudden death?

A. Colloid cyst
B. Glioblastoma multiforme
C. Lymphoma
D. Pilocytic astrocytoma

2.
Complex regional pain syndrome type 2 (formerly known as causalgia) is defined by what symptoms?

A. Burning pain, autonomic dysfunction, and trophic changes following obvious nerve damage
B. Increased perspiration in excess of what is required for regulation of body temperature
C. Burning pain, autonomic dysfunction, and trophic changes without obvious nerve damage
D. An initial lack of sensation and tingling on one side of the body followed later by severe, chronic dysesthesias or allodynia
E. Recurrent hospitalizations with dramatic, untrue, and extremely improbable tales of past experiences

3.
What factors contribute to the intracranial hemorrhage (ICH) score for a patient with a hemorrhagic stroke?

A. Patient age, Glasgow Coma Scale (GCS) score, acuity of ICH
B. ICH volume, GCS score, acuity of ICH
C. Intraventricular hemorrhage (IVH), position of ICH, patient age
D. Position of ICH, patient age, baseline Karnofsky Scale score
E. Patient age, IVH, hemiplegia

4.
A patient with a history of intravenous drug use is seen in clinic with new-onset severe back pain. An MRI is obtained that demonstrates bony erosion and collapse of the L2/L3 disk. What is the next step in the management of this patient?

A. Perform a lumbar puncture, and send spinal fluid cultures.
B. Obtain a CT scan of the spine.
C. Obtain blood cultures.
D. Obtain a bone scan.
E. Schedule follow-up with a repeat MRI in 4 to 6 weeks.

5.
How is mechanical back pain associated with activity?

A. Improves with activity
B. Worsens with activity
C. Relieved by standing
D. Worsens with axial unloading

6.
Where should the dissection take place during a transpsoas approach to the lumbar spine in order to minimize the risk of nerve injury?

A. Anterior to the psoas major
B. Posterior to the psoas major
C. Through the bulk of the psoas major
D. Along the medial aspect of the psoas major
E. Along the lateral aspect of the psoas major

7.
A 17-year-old girl presents to the neuro-ophthalmology clinic with complaints of episodic diplopia that has been present for the past week. The episodes occur about every hour and last around 1 minute each time. The patient has a history of a transsphenoidal resection of a craniopharyngioma 3 years ago followed by radiation. Postoperative ophthalmologic exams including visual fields have been unremarkable. An MRI from 1 month ago demonstrated no evidence of recurrent disease. The patient is examined during one of these episodes and is found to have an exotropia of her right eye that resolves spontaneously. She is prescribed carbamazepine, and her symptoms improve. What is her most likely diagnosis?

A. Craniopharyngioma recurrence
B. Myasthenia gravis
C. Ocular neuromyotonia
D. Seizures

8.
A man presents to clinic with results from an electromyographic (EMG) study showing fibrillations and reduced motor unit potentials in his gluteus medius and extensor digitorum longus. He has no abnormal EMG findings in his biceps femoris (short head). Weakness of foot eversion and numbness on the dorsum of the foot are noted on his exam. What nerve(s) is/are being affected?

A. L4 nerve root only
B. L5 nerve root only
C. S1 nerve root only
D. Common peroneal nerve proximal to the fibular head only
E. L5 nerve root and common peroneal nerve at the fibular head

9.
A malignant peripheral nerve sheath tumor is discovered in a patient's left upper extremity. Where should screening first be focused to detect distant metastases?

A. Brain
B. Other extremities
C. Axial skeleton
D. Lungs
E. Lymph nodes

10.
What type of spinal arteriovenous malformation typically is associated with low blood flow?

A. Dural
B. Juvenile
C. Extramedullary/intradural
D. Glomus

11.
Multiple sclerosis is a contraindication to what procedural treatment for trigeminal neuralgia?

A. Microvascular decompression
B. Percutaneous radiofrequency rhizotomy
C. Percutaneous glycerol injection into the Meckel cave
D. Percutaneous balloon microcompression
E. Stereotactic radiosurgery

12.
What is the major complication of a stereotactic mesencephalotomy for medically intractable right upper extremity pain?

A. Ipsilateral weakness
B. Anesthesia dolorosa
C. Memory deficits

D. Diplopia
E. Hypothalamic dysfunction

13.
A patient undergoing a craniotomy for resection of a vestibular schwannoma has a reasonable chance of losing serviceable hearing following surgery if the preoperative speech discrimination is below what percentage?

A. 50%
B. 65%
C. 75%
D. 85%
E. 95%

14.
A woman with a known pituitary macroadenoma presents to the emergency room with a sudden, intense headache and a new-onset ophthalmoplegia with her chronic visual field cuts. She endorses photophobia. After imaging confirms the most likely diagnosis, what is the next step in her management?

A. Sumatriptan administration
B. Follow-up with repeat imaging in 6 weeks
C. Repeat pituitary lab work as an outpatient
D. Observation
E. Preparation for transsphenoidal decompression immediately

15.
A woman is referred to you for treatment of a cerebellopontine angle tumor. She has obvious weakness of the right side of her face. She does have some motion but has no motor contraction over her forehead, she cannot close her eye completely, and she has noticeable asymmetry of her mouth when attempting to smile. What is her House-Brackmann classification grade?

A. 2
B. 3
C. 4
D. 5
E. 6

16.
What form of nicotine potentially will not decrease spinal fusion rates?

A. Cigarette smoking
B. Chewing tobacco
C. Nicotine gum
D. Nicotine patches
E. No form of nicotine avoids the risk of decreased spinal fusion rates.

17.

What is the recommended torque used on a halo pin on an adult skull?

A. 4 in-lbs
B. 8 in-lbs
C. 12 in-lbs
D. 20 in-lbs
E. 30 in-lbs

18.

Injury to the subthalamic nucleus during a functional lesioning procedure classically produces what type of movement disorder?

A. Myoclonus
B. Hemiballism
C. Pill-rolling tremor
D. Fixed posture of limbs
E. Chorea

19.

Deep brain stimulation in the setting of Parkinson disease is expected to result in brief minimal improvement to what characteristic of the disease?

A. Dyskinesia
B. Balance
C. Tremors
D. Rigidity
E. Cognitive impairment

20.

What electromyography/nerve conduction study finding supports a diagnosis of lumbar radiculopathy from a herniated disk?

A. Paraspinal muscle fibrillations
B. Abnormal sensory nerve action potentials (SNAPs)
C. Increased motor fiber recruitment with volitional activity
D. Absence of spontaneous sensory nerve activity

21.

A patient presents with a blunt cerebrovascular injury after a motor vehicle collision. The patient has no intracranial hemorrhage. CT angiogram reveals an internal carotid artery luminal irregularity with < 25% stenosis. What is the next step in the management of this patient?

A. No acute intervention; repeat imaging in 4 to 6 weeks.
B. Initiate a heparin drip if there are no contraindications.
C. Perform endovascular stenting.
D. Perform a ligation/occlusion of carotid artery.
E. Initiate antiplatelet therapy if there are no contraindications.

22.

Halo bracing is least effective for what type of cervical fractures?

A. Odontoid fractures
B. Levine type 2 pars fractures
C. Midcervical spine fractures
D. C1 fractures with a type 3 odontoid fracture
E. Teardrop fractures

23.

What artery often is associated with hemifacial spasm?

A. Posterior inferior cerebellar artery
B. Anterior inferior cerebellar artery
C. Superior cerebellar artery
D. Posterior cerebellar artery
E. Vertebral artery

24.

For nonemergent neurosurgical procedures, it is recommended that a patient's INR be less than or equal to what value?

A. 1.0
B. 1.2
C. 1.4
D. 1.6

25.

With pituitary tumors, what optic chiasm position is most associated with optic nerve compression?

A. Prefixed chiasm
B. Postfixed chiasm
C. Chiasm superior to the sella turcica
D. Neutral position chiasm

26.

Over 95% of vestibular schwannomas present with progressive unilateral or asymmetric sensorineural, high-frequency hearing loss. In general, what is considered the definition of serviceable hearing?

A. Pure tone audiogram of 40 dB or less; speech discrimination score of at least 40%
B. Pure tone audiogram of 60 dB or less; speech discrimination score of at least 60%
C. Pure tone audiogram of 60 dB or less; speech discrimination score of at least 40%
D. Pure tone audiogram of 40 dB or less; speech discrimination score of at least 60%
E. American Academy of Otolaryngology–Head and Neck Surgery (AAO-HNS) class C or D

27.

A 50-year-old woman presents with an acute onset of severe headache, bitemporal hemianopsia, and cranial nerve III palsy. She is alert and conversant. What is the most appropriate next step in this patient's management?

A. Rapid administration of corticosteroids

B. Cerebral angiography

C. Administration of nimodipine

D. Obtaining an erythrocyte sedimentation rate, C-reactive protein concentration, and blood cultures

E. Intracranial pressure monitoring

28.

A 19-year-old man presents following a motor vehicle collision complaining of lower extremity weakness. He is found to have a thoracic spine Chance fracture. He has full strength in his upper extremities. He has sensation in his lower extremities and perineum, and his motor strength in his lower extremities ranges from 4–/5 to 4/5. What is his American Spinal Injury Association (ASIA) impairment scale score?

A. A

B. B

C. C

D. D

E. E

29.

What incomplete spinal cord injury syndrome is associated with a poor prognosis for recovery and dissociated sensory loss?

A. Central cord syndrome

B. Anterior cord syndrome

C. Brown-Séquard syndrome

D. Posterior cord syndrome

E. Cauda equina syndrome

30.

When placing a C2 pedicle screw, what is the trajectory of the screw?

A. Superior and medial

B. Superior and lateral

C. Inferior and medial

D. Inferior and lateral

E. Parallel to the spinous process

31.

What is a relative contraindication for the placement of an anterior odontoid screw that may make surgery technically very difficult?

A. Type 2 odontoid fracture

B. Combined 5-mm overhang of the lateral masses of C1 on C2

C. Acute fracture

D. Reducible fracture

E. Barrel chest

32.

A patient presents in the emergency room with a cervical spine fracture and the following radiographic findings: a triangular bone fragment fractured off the anterior inferior vertebral body, retrolisthesis of the caudal vertebrae, and disruption of the facet joints and the disk space. What type of fracture is suspected?

A. Avulsion fracture

B. Clay-shoveler fracture

C. Jefferson fracture

D. Teardrop fracture

E. Locked facets

33.

A patient presents after a significant fall from a ladder with an L2 burst fracture that has a 70% loss of height, 50% canal stenosis due to retropulsion, and 15 degrees of angulation. How would you reduce this fracture with ligamentotaxis?

A. Removing ligaments such as the ligamentum flavum that would allow for easier manipulation of the fracture

B. Distracting pedicle screws to reduce indirectly the retropulsed segment by putting tension on the posterior longitudinal ligament

C. Compressing pedicle screws to reduce the retropulsed fragment by releasing tension on the posterior longitudinal ligament

D. Placing a strut or cage to reduce the loss of height of the vertebral body

E. Positioning the patient to utilize the anterior longitudinal ligament to reduce the kyphotic angulation associated with the fracture

34.

In what zone is a sacral fracture that occurs in the region of the sacral foramina?

A. Zone 1

B. Zone 2

C. Zone 3 (vertical)

D. Zone 4 (transverse)

E. Zone 5

35.

Fisher grade 3 is differentiated from Fisher grade 2 for aneurysmal subarachnoid hemorrhage by what characteristic?

A. Greater than 1 mm of blood
B. Presence of hydrocephalus
C. Intracerebral or intraventricular clot
D. Presence of vasospasm
E. Greater than 1 cm of blood

36.

A 37-year-old man presents with a sudden onset of the "worst headache of my life." The CT shows intraventricular hemorrhage that you suspect resulted from hemorrhage entering through the lamina terminalis. You are suspicious of an aneurysm at what location?

A. Middle cerebral artery bifurcation
B. Posterior communicating artery
C. Internal carotid artery terminus
D. Anterior communicating artery
E. Basilar artery tip

37.

A patient presents with subacute bacterial endocarditis. Evaluation and workup includes a CT angiogram followed by a cerebral angiogram that demonstrates two small aneurysms on distal left middle cerebral artery branches. What treatment modality is indicated?

A. Endovascular coiling
B. Surgical clipping
C. Antibiotics and serial imaging
D. Observation

38.

Following the standard of care, what role does brachytherapy play as an adjunctive treatment for high-grade gliomas?

A. Brachytherapy is a viable alternative to whole brain radiation.
B. Brachytherapy is superior to stereotactic radiosurgery.
C. Brachytherapy has no role as an adjuvant to whole brain radiation.
D. Brachytherapy can be useful in addition to whole brain radiation.
E. Brachytherapy can substitute for whole brain radiation.

39.

Following resection of a low-grade oligodendroglioma, what is the next step in adjuvant therapy?

A. Intravenous chemotherapy
B. Focused radiation
C. Whole brain radiation
D. Intrathecal chemotherapy

40.

What is the complication rate for shunting a patient with normal pressure hydrocephalus?

A. 5 to 10%
B. 10 to 25%
C. 25 to 40%
D. 40 to 55%

41.

A woman is referred to your office for symptoms consistent with carpal tunnel syndrome. She has had a nerve conduction study showing that the proximal median nerve latency is shorter than the distal median nerve latency. What is the explanation for this finding?

A. Poor quality/erroneous nerve conduction study
B. Lesion of the proximal median nerve
C. Presence of a Martin-Gruber anastomosis
D. Marinacci syndrome
E. Diabetic neuropathy

42.

A 17-year-old boy is brought to the emergency room following a motor vehicle collision with multiple fatalities. He is alert, awake, and oriented. He denies neck pain, has no midline tenderness, and does not have any other injuries. The neurologic exam is unremarkable. He has not used alcohol or drugs. What is the minimum radiographic study needed to clear the cervical spine?

A. Radiographs are not indicated
B. Upright lateral and AP X-rays
C. Flexion-extension X-rays
D. Lateral and AP X-rays with CT imaging of areas that are suspicious or not easily seen on plain films
E. Thin-cut axial CT scan from the occiput to T1 with sagittal and coronal reconstructions

43.

A 63-year-old diabetic man with a remote history of vertebral osteomyelitis presents to the hospital with low back pain and pain down the anterior part of the thigh for the past 3 weeks. Neurologic exam is unremarkable. MRI suggests a psoas and epidural abscess without severe compression. What is the next appropriate step in this patient's management?

A. Discharge home on oral antibiotics with follow-up with an infectious disease specialist.

B. Admit to the floor, place on antibiotics, and consult interventional radiology for culture and biopsy of the epidural abscess.

C. Consult interventional radiology for culture and biopsy of the epidural space prior to starting antibiotics.

D. Admit to the floor, obtain blood cultures, and consult interventional radiology for biopsy of the psoas abscess prior to administering antibiotics (if the biopsy can be done in a timely manner).

E. Perform a decompressive laminectomy with evacuation of the abscess.

44.

An 82-year-old woman presents to the neurosurgery clinic with typical trigeminal neuralgia. She has substantial medical comorbidities and would like to avoid surgery. The patient opts for stereotactic radiosurgery. What factor would predict a favorable outcome?

A. Absence of atypical pain

B. Using a radiation dose less than 60 Gy

C. Prior successful surgical microvascular decompression

D. Decreased sensation in the affected nerve prior to treatment

E. Trigeminal neuralgia related to multiple sclerosis

45.

What is the most effective surgical option for the treatment of glossopharyngeal neuralgia in the absence of vascular compression?

A. Cranial nerve IX rhizotomy alone

B. Cranial nerve X rhizotomy alone

C. Cranial nerve IX rhizotomy with sectioning the upper one third of cranial nerve X

D. Extracranial nerve ablation of cranial nerve IX

E. Cranial nerve XI rhizotomy alone

46.

A teenager suffering from a defect in his L5 pars interarticularis as a result of an insufficiency fracture of the pars can be characterized as having what type of spondylolisthesis?

A. Dysplastic

B. Isthmic

C. Degenerative

D. Traumatic

E. Pathological

47.

You perform a stereotactic-guided biopsy of a thalamic lesion. You notice bleeding from the cannula. What is the next step?

A. Perform an emergent craniotomy and exploration.

B. Immediately abort the procedure, and obtain a CT.

C. Abort the procedure, wake the patient, and obtain a neurologic exam.

D. Elevate the head of the bed, decrease the blood pressure, and irrigate the cannula.

E. Insert a Fogarty catheter into the cannula, inflate the balloon, and obtain a CT.

48.

What is the most common location of mycotic aneurysms?

A. Distal middle cerebral artery branches

B. Proximal anterior cerebral artery

C. Distal anterior cerebral artery

D. Basilar tip

E. Posterior inferior cerebellar artery

49.

A 35-year-old woman presents with spontaneous neck pain. A noncontrast head CT demonstrates subarachnoid hemorrhage, and an angiogram reveals a lesion suspicious for an intradural vertebral artery dissection. What is the appropriate treatment for this finding?

A. Observation if asymptomatic

B. Immediate heparinization followed by oral anticoagulation

C. Immediate surgery or endovascular treatment

D. Delayed surgery to allow for swelling resolution

E. Nonoperative treatment followed by a delayed angiogram in 5 to 7 days to assess healing

50.
A 32-year-old man presents with slurred speech and a hypoglossal palsy. He reported that he was involved in a motor vehicle collision 3 weeks prior for which he did not pursue medical evaluation. He reports that he has had neck pain since the accident. What is the suspected diagnosis?

A. Atlanto-occipital dislocation
B. Vertebral artery dissection with stroke
C. Odontoid fracture
D. Clival fracture
E. Condyle fracture

51.
A 43-year-old woman presents to the neurosurgery clinic complaining of hand clumsiness. A neurologic exam reveals wasting and weakness of the abductor pollicis brevis and hand intrinsics. There is sensory loss over the medial forearm, but sensation in the hand is normal. According to the above findings, what is the next appropriate test for diagnosis?

A. MRI of the brain
B. Cerebrospinal fluid studies
C. Chest radiograph
D. MRI of the cervical spine
E. Cervical spine radiographs with oblique and apical lordotic views

52.
What tumor often arises from the "roof" of the fourth ventricle?

A. Ependymoma
B. Juvenile pilocytic astrocytoma
C. Brainstem glioma
D. Choroid plexus papilloma
E. Medulloblastoma

53.
A 38-year-old man presents with seizures, and workup reveals an arteriovenous malformation that is 6.4 cm in size, involves the posterior fronto-parietal and occipital lobes, and drains into the galenic system. What is the preferred treatment option for this lesion?

A. Embolization alone
B. Stereotactic radiosurgery alone
C. Surgical resection
D. Observation
E. Embolization and stereotactic radiosurgery

54.
After elective clipping of an unruptured anterior communicating artery aneurysm, the patient wakes up with dysarthria and contralateral paresis of his face and arm. What vessel likely is incorporated into the aneurysm clip?

A. Anterior choroidal artery
B. Recurrent artery of Heubner
C. Middle cerebral artery
D. Distal anterior cerebral artery

55.
The most common primary, intra-axial posterior fossa tumor in adults is associated with what condition?

A. Smoking
B. Tumor suppressor gene inactivation on chromosome 9q34
C. Tumor suppressor gene inactivation on chromosome 7q21
D. Tumor suppressor gene inactivation on chromosome 3p25

56.
A 21-year-old man presents with a brachial plexus avulsion type injury. What is the recommended treatment option?

A. Periodic electromyography/nerve conduction studies starting 3 to 12 weeks following the injury with consideration of surgical neurotization at 3 to 6 months if there is no improvement
B. Periodic electromyography/nerve conduction studies starting 3 to 12 weeks following the injury with consideration of surgical neurolysis at 3 to 6 months if there is no improvement
C. Periodic electromyography/nerve conduction studies starting 3 to 12 weeks following the injury with consideration of a spinal cord stimulator if pain remains after 3 to 6 months
D. Exploration and surgical repair within 3 days
E. Exploration at 2 to 3 weeks

57.
What type of basal skull fracture is associated with an increased risk of mortality?

A. Longitudinal temporal bone fracture
B. Transverse temporal bone fracture
C. Fracture through the planum sphenoidale
D. Clival fracture

58.
During decompression of an ulnar nerve, the surgeon wishes to ensure that the nerve is decompressed distally. The ulnar nerve can be found entering the forearm in relation to what structure?

A. Deep to the pronator teres
B. Deep to the flexor carpi radialis
C. Deep to the flexor digitorum profundus
D. Lateral to the ulnar artery
E. Between the two heads of the flexor carpi ulnaris

59.
During a carotid endarterectomy, what is the correct order of vessel occlusion?

A. External, common, and then internal carotid artery
B. Internal, common, and then external carotid artery
C. Common, internal, and then external carotid artery
D. Internal, external, and then common carotid artery
E. External, internal, and then common carotid artery

60.
A 63-year-old woman presents with ruptured anterior communicating artery aneurysm and an intracranial hemorrhage in the gyrus rectus. What is her Fisher grade?

A. 0
B. 1
C. 2
D. 3
E. 4

61.
What approach characterizes a far lateral craniotomy?

A. Suboccipital craniotomy including opening of the foramen magnum and drilling of the occipital condyle
B. Suboccipital craniotomy with exposure of the transverse and sigmoid sinus
C. Suboccipital craniotomy with pre- and post-sigmoid exposure
D. Subtemporal craniotomy with removal of the petrous apex
E. Retrosigmoid craniotomy with removal of the lamina of C1 and C2

62.
What characteristics (location and size) of a cerebral abscess are a surgical indication?

A. Subcortical location; 2.5 cm in diameter
B. Brainstem location; 1.0 cm in diameter
C. Small lesion in the early cerebritis stage; 0.5 cm in diameter
D. Periventricular location; 2.0 cm in diameter

63.
A patient presents with subarachnoid hemorrhage due to a ruptured aneurysm. What is the approximate risk of re-rupture over the next 14 days if the aneurysm is not treated?

A. 1 to 2%
B. 5 to 10%
C. 15 to 20%
D. 50%
E. 75%

64.
What is the most definitive treatment for atonic seizures?

A. Ethosuximide
B. Adrenocorticotropic hormone
C. Multiple subpial transections
D. Hemispherectomy
E. Corpus callosotomy

65.
What is the most effective thalamic target during deep brain stimulation to control tremor associated with Parkinson disease?

A. Medial nucleus
B. Ventralis intermedius nucleus
C. Nucleus accumbens
D. Anterior nucleus
E. Pedunculopontine nucleus

66.

How is the C7 plumb line measured?

A. Originates at the posterior vertebral body of C7 and is measured from the anterior vertebral body of S1

B. Originates at the mid-vertebral body of C7 and is measured from the mid-vertebral body of S1

C. Originates at the mid-vertebral body of C7 and is measured from the posterior superior corner of S1

D. Originates at the anterior vertebral body of C7 and is measured from the mid-vertebral body of S1

E. Originates at the anterior vertebral body of C7 and is measured from the anterior vertebral body of S1

67.

A patient with L4/L5 degenerative spondylolisthesis presents with radiculopathy. The L4 vertebral body is approximately 60% anterolisthesed. What grade is this spondylolisthesis according to the Meyerding grading scale?

A. Grade 1

B. Grade 2

C. Grade 3

D. Grade 4

E. Grade 5

68.

A middle-aged woman presents to the emergency room with complaints of a sudden onset of the "worst headache of my life." She complains of photophobia and nuchal rigidity. The head CT was negative for subarachnoid hemorrhage, and the CT angiogram did not reveal an aneurysm. What would be the most reasonable next step in this patient's management?

A. Discharge the patient home with pain medications.

B. Admit the patient with aneurysm precautions, and repeat the CT angiogram in 5 to 7 days.

C. Obtain a lumbar puncture.

D. Repeat the head CT in 4 to 6 hours.

E. Obtain a brain MRI.

69.

This diagram attempts to define which parameter?

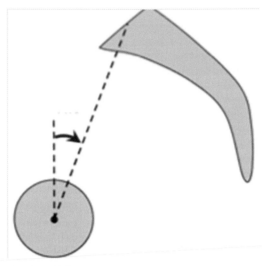

A. Sacral slope

B. Pelvic tilt

C. Pelvic incidence

D. Sagittal vertical axis

E. T1 tilt

70.

In the repair of peripheral nerve lesions with large gaps, the standard graft material is:

A. Autologous anterior interosseus nerve

B. Autologous sural nerve

C. Silicone

D. Cadaveric nerve

E. Autologous vein

71.

During a percutaneous trigeminal radiofrequency rhizotomy for a patient with trigeminal neuralgia, after inserting the electrode into the oral mucosa, the initial trajectory is:

A. Toward a point on a line intersecting the external auditory meatus and medial aspect of the pupil

B. Toward a point on a line intersecting 3 cm anterior to the external auditory meatus and medial aspect of the pupil

C. Toward a point on a line intersecting the external auditory meatus and contralateral medial aspect of the pupil

D. Toward a point on a line intersecting the clivus and posterior clinoid

E. Toward a point > 8 mm beyond the clival line

72.

With regard to vertebral artery injury and C2 neuralgia, what is the difference (if any) between utilizing a C1 lateral mass–C2 pedicle/pars screw construct for C1 to C2 fixation versus placement of transarticular screws?

A. Less chance of vertebral artery injury and C2 neuralgia with transarticular screw fixation compared with the C1 lateral mass–C2 pedicle/pars screw approach

B. Less chance of vertebral artery injury and more C2 neuralgia with transarticular screw fixation compared with the C1 lateral mass–C2 pedicle/pars screw approach

C. More chance of vertebral artery injury and C2 neuralgia with transarticular screw fixation compared with the C1 lateral mass–C2 pedicle/pars screw approach

D. More chance of vertebral artery injury and less C2 neuralgia with transarticular screw fixation compared with the C1 lateral mass–C2 pedicle/pars screw approach

E. Same chance of vertebral artery injury with both approaches with more C2 neuralgia with the C1 lateral mass–C2 pedicle/pars approach

73.

A 29-year-old woman underwent a cervical lymph node biopsy for persistent lymphadenopathy. Postoperatively, she complained of an inability to abduct her arm. What condition is suspected?

A. Hysteria

B. Carotid injury and stroke

C. Injury to the C5 nerve root

D. Injury to the spinal accessory nerve

E. Injury to the long thoracic nerve

74.

A 61-year-old woman presents with an acute, severe headache with nausea and vomiting. CT of the brain revealed cisternal subarachnoid hemorrhage. Cerebral angiography revealed an aneurysm not amenable to coiling. The patient was taken for an open craniotomy and clipping of the aneurysm. After surgery, the patient was noted to have an oculomotor nerve palsy. Where was the patient's aneurysm most likely located?

A. At the internal carotid artery bifurcation

B. At the origin of the posterior inferior cerebellar artery

C. At the middle cerebral artery most proximal bifurcation

D. At the junction of the anterior cerebral artery A1 segment and anterior communicating artery

E. At the junction of the basilar and superior cerebellar arteries

75.

The most common deficit associated with a corpus callosotomy is:

A. Intracerebral hemorrhage

B. Hyperthermia

C. Memory problems

D. Speech irregularities

E. Visual problems

76.

A 52-year-old man presents to the emergency room after a fall from his porch. The neurologic exam shows weakness more pronounced in the upper extremities compared with the lower extremities, with distal weakness greater than proximal weakness. Imaging suggests severe cervical stenosis with an associated cord signal change. After 24 hours, the patient's neurologic exam is worse. What is the appropriate next step in the treatment of this patient?

A. High-dose steroid administration

B. Bracing and physical therapy

C. Surgical decompression with or without fixation

D. Dynamic radiographs to rule out instability

E. Neurology service consultation

77.

A man incurs an injury to the musculocutaneous nerve during a car accident. Three months following the accident, the electrophysiological studies of the patient's biceps show fibrillations and motor unit potentials. What is this patient's Sunderland peripheral nerve injury classification?

A. First degree

B. Second or third degree

C. Fourth degree

D. Fifth degree

78.
A punctate midline myelotomy can be valuable for patients with intractable pain associated with malignancy in the abdominal or pelvic regions. A myelotomy for these purposes commonly is performed at what spinal level?

A. L2
B. T2
C. T8
D. T10
E. T12

79.
Anterior choroidal artery aneurysms usually have what orientation compared to the parent vessel?

A. Oriented superiorly/superolaterally
B. Oriented medially
C. Oriented inferiorly/inferomedially
D. Oriented anteriorly
E. Oriented posteriorly

80.
How much of the superior sagittal sinus can be sacrificed without a high risk of inducing venous infarctions?

A. Anterior two thirds
B. No more than one third of any portion
C. Anterior one third
D. Entire sinus as long as the cortical bridging veins are left intact
E. None of the sinus but all of the cortical bridging veins can be sacrificed without risk of venous infarctions.

81.
A man presents with an infarct of the artery of Percheron. What are his expected deficits?

A. Obtundation, coma, variable degrees of hemiplegia or hemisensory loss, a vertical gaze palsy, and memory impairment
B. Hemiparesis, hemisensory loss, and a homonymous hemianopsia
C. Hemiparesis of the upper extremity and face, dysarthria, and hemichorea
D. A cranial nerve III palsy, Parinaud syndrome, abulia, and somnolence
E. Ipsilateral sensory loss in the face and contralateral sensory loss in the body without pyramidal findings or a change in sensorium

Use the following answers for questions 82, 83, and 84:

A. Dorsal root entry zone lesioning
B. C1-C2 cordotomy
C. Spinal cord stimulation
D. Selective dorsal rhizotomy
E. Midline myelotomy

82.
What pain procedure is best for pelvic visceral cancer pain?

83.
What pain procedure is best for intractable severe upper extremity cancer pain?

84.
What pain procedure is best for diplegic spasticity?

85.
When accessing the third ventricle through a transcallosal, transchoroidal surgical approach, what layers, in order, are passed through as the roof of the third ventricle is traversed?

A. Fornix, vascular layer, superior layer of the tela choroidea, inferior layer of the tela choroidea, choroid of the third ventricle
B. Superior layer of the tela choroidea, fornix, vascular layer, choroid plexus of the third ventricle, inferior layer of the tela choroidea
C. Superior layer of the tela choroidea, fornix, vascular layer, inferior layer of the tela choroidea, choroid plexus of the third ventricle
D. Choroid plexus of the third ventricle, superior layer of the tela choroidea, vascular layer, fornix, inferior layer of the tela choroidea
E. Fornix, superior layer of the tela choroidea, vascular layer, inferior layer of the tela choroidea, choroid plexus of the third ventricle

86.

A 40-year-old man presented to the emergency room with complaints of left-hand numbness. Further workup revealed the lesion on MRI that is shown in this image. He was taken to surgery for resection. Postoperatively, the patient awoke with a dense left hemiparesis. Supplementary motor area (SMA) syndrome was suspected. What is the expected prognosis of SMA syndrome?

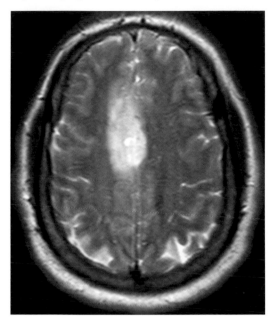

A. Permanent left hemiparesis/hemiplegia
B. Temporary decreased spontaneous and voluntary movements of the left upper and lower extremities with spontaneous recovery
C. Permanent decreased spontaneous and voluntary movements of the left upper and lower extremities with aphasia without spontaneous recovery
D. Temporary left lower extremity paresis with loss of muscle tone with spontaneous recovery
E. Temporary left upper and lower extremity paresis and hemisensory loss with spontaneous recovery

87.

A 63-year-old man wakes from anesthesia following an anterior cervical diskectomy and fusion (ACDF). Postoperatively, he complains of unilateral blurry vision, and ptosis is noted on the same side. What is the most common cause of Horner syndrome following an ACDF?

A. Retractor placement
B. Carotid dissection
C. Recurrent laryngeal nerve injury
D. Vertebral artery injury

88.

In the event of trauma, what finding on a skull radiograph best indicates the possible need for emergent surgical intervention?

A. Fluid level in the sphenoid sinus
B. Pneumocele
C. Double density sign
D. Fluid level in the frontal sinus
E. Linear temporal fracture

89.

According to the Asymptomatic Carotid Artery Stenosis (ACAS) trial, what are the recommendations regarding performing a carotid endarterectomy (CEA)?

A. There is a moderate benefit to performing an immediate CEA compared with medical management in patients under 75 years of age with asymptomatic carotid stenosis > 60%.
B. Patients with symptomatic moderate (50 to 69%) and severe (≥ 70%) carotid stenosis should be considered for a CEA.
C. Carotid stenting and CEA are associated with similar rates of death and disabling strokes, with an increased stroke incidence associated with stenting and an increased myocardial infarction incidence associated with CEA.
D. Patients with carotid stenosis > 80% or symptomatic lesions > 50% and who are at high risk for surgery have equal outcomes when treated by stenting compared with a CEA.
E. In patients with good health and asymptomatic carotid stenosis > 60%, a CEA is beneficial if the surgeon maintains perioperative morbidity/mortality rates less than 3%.

90.

During a subtemporal approach, the greater superficial petrosal nerve often is divided. What deficit is expected upon sectioning this nerve?

A. Decreased salivation
B. Miosis
C. Decreased tearing
D. Mydriasis
E. Hyperacusis

91.

What is/are the contraindication(s) for traction with a cervical spine injury?

A. Atlanto-occipital dislocation and a type 2A hangman fracture
B. C4/C5 locked facets and a type 2A hangman fracture
C. Atlantoaxial rotatory subluxation and a type 2A hangman fracture
D. Atlanto-occipital dislocation and atlantoaxial rotatory subluxation
E. C4/C5 locked facets and atlantoaxial rotatory subluxation

92.

After what age does the chance of a spontaneous subarachnoid hemorrhage become more likely to be due to an aneurysm than due to an arteriovenous malformation?

A. 18 years old
B. 30 years old
C. 45 years old
D. 55 years old
E. 68 years old

93.

A 67-year-old woman presents to the emergency room following a motor vehicle collision with a large right-sided subdural hematoma and uncal herniation seen on CT. The Glasgow Coma Scale score is 5. She has a dilated and nonreactive right pupil. She has flexor posturing on the left side and is hemiplegic on the right side. What is the most likely explanation for her right-sided hemiplegia?

A. Uncal compression of the right midbrain
B. Compression of the left midbrain
C. Diffuse axonal injury involving the right internal capsule
D. Spinal cord injury
E. Left-side Duret hemorrhages in the pons

94.

What is the most effective means of sterilization for operating room procedures involving Creutzfeldt-Jakob disease?

A. Boiling
B. Immersion in 1 N NaOH for 15 minutes
C. Ultraviolet radiation
D. Immersion in sodium hypochlorite
E. Steam autoclaving for 1 hour at 132°C

95.

What is the most common location for dural arteriovenous fistulae to drain?

A. Superior sagittal sinus
B. Junction of the transverse and sigmoid sinus
C. Cavernous sinus
D. Inferior petrosal sinus
E. Junction of the sigmoid sinus and jugular vein

96.

With subthalamic nucleus deep brain stimulation, the adverse effect of flushing and sweating following surgery indicates current spread to what direction relative to the intended target?

A. Anterior
B. Posterior
C. Lateral
D. Medial
E. Anterolateral

97.

What is a contraindication to performing an anterior lumbar interbody fusion?

A. Unilateral pars defect
B. Bilateral pars defect
C. Grade 3 or 4 spondylolisthesis
D. Severe loss of disk space height
E. Grade 1 isthmic spondylolisthesis

98.

A 65-year-old woman presents with headache. She describes scalp tenderness in the temporal region, with her jaw being stiff when she chews. She also describes chronic fatigue, muscle aches, and weight loss. Headache treatment is started, and she is scheduled for surgery. With what complication can a delay in the treatment of her suspected diagnosis be associated?

A. Blindness
B. Re-rupture
C. Contiguous intracranial spread
D. Herniation
E. Corneal abrasions

99.

A 22-year-old man presents after a motorcycle accident complaining of neck pain and lower extremity paraplegia. He has a cervical burst fracture. His exam demonstrates 0/5 strength in the lower extremities. He has 4/5 strength in the biceps and wrist extensors bilaterally. He has 0/5 strength in the triceps, grip, and hand intrinsics. What is the American Spinal Injury Association (ASIA) motor score?

A. 8
B. 16
C. 42
D. 58
E. 92

100.

What is the benign lesion seen in this intraoperative image with a gross pearly white appearance?

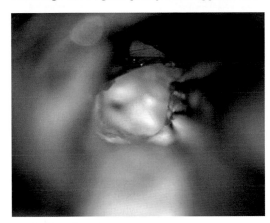

A. Epidermoid cyst
B. Dermoid cyst
C. Lipoma
D. Adamantinomatous craniopharyngioma

101.

A patient presents with complaints of a herniated disk that correlates with imaging. MRI demonstrates a far lateral disk herniation at L4/L5. What nerve root should be affected?

A. L4 traversing nerve root
B. L4 exiting nerve root
C. L5 traversing nerve root
D. L5 exiting nerve root

102.

Isthmic spondylolisthesis is found in what group of patients?

A. HLA-B27 histocompatability complex positive individuals
B. Truck drivers
C. Rheumatoid arthritis patients
D. Gymnasts, football linemen, and weight lifters
E. Black people, diabetics, and women over 40 years old

103.

This image shows what type of intracranial lesion?

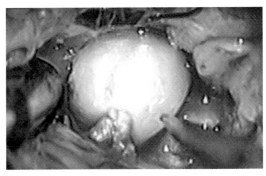

A. Arachnoid cyst
B. Epidermoid cyst
C. Dermoid cyst
D. Neurenteric cyst

104.

A 70-year-old woman presents with large, enhancing frontoparietal mass suspicious for a glioblastoma. She is unable to work but is able to live at home and care for some of her personal needs. She requires considerable assistance and frequent medical care. What is the estimated Karnofsky Scale score?

A. 10
B. 30
C. 50
D. 70
E. 90

105.

Ankylosing spondylitis is associated with what human leukocyte antigen?

A. HLA-DQA1
B. HLA-DRB1
C. HLA-B27
D. HLA-DR2
E. HLA-B47

106.
Current spread in what direction during subthalamic nucleus deep brain stimulation will cause
double vision and pupillary constriction?

A. Anterior
B. Posterior
C. Lateral
D. Medial
E. Inferomedial

107.
During a carotid endarterectomy, the internal
carotid artery (ICA) is identified coursing posterior
to the external carotid artery (ECA). What land-
mark is used to differentiate the external from the
internal carotid artery during surgery?

A. Lingual artery arising from the ECA
B. Superior thyroid artery arising from the ECA
C. Ascending pharyngeal artery arising from the
   ECA
D. Facial vein coursing over the ECA
E. Ascending pharyngeal artery arising from the
   ICA

108.
Prior to cross-sectional imaging, a named point was
used to identify the fourth ventricle and determine if any midline shift was present. Where is
this point located?

A. Where the septal and thalamostriate veins
   converge
B. At the arterial branch from the inferior extent
   (caudal loop) of the tonsillomedullary segment
   of the posterior inferior cerebellar artery
C. Where the posterior choroidal artery enters
   the velum interpositum
D. At the arterial branch from the superior extent
   (cranial loop) of the telovelotonsillar segment
   of the posterior inferior cerebellar artery
E. Where the anterior choroidal artery enters the
   choroidal fissure of the lateral ventricle

109.
What recess is indicated by the *arrow* in this image?

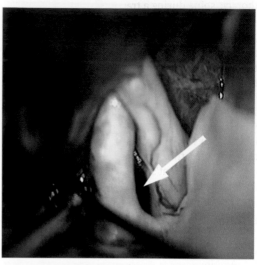

A. Opticocarotid cistern
B. Carotico-oculomotor cistern
C. Interpeduncular cistern
D. Lamina terminalis
E. Cerebellopontine angle

110.
In the adult patient, subdural effusions are associated with what entity?

A. Chronic subdural hematomas
B. Tuberculosis
C. Syphilis
D. *Haemophilus influenzae* meningitis
E. Skull fractures

111.
A patient is referred to the neurosurgical clinic for
a dural arteriovenous fistula (dAVF). An angiogram
shows anterograde drainage into a venous sinus
with retrograde flow into subarachnoid veins. What
is the Borden classification for this dAVF?

A. 1
B. 2
C. 3
D. 4
E. 5

112.

What structure impedes the caudal exposure of the thoracic spine during a transthoracic approach?

A. Vena cava
B. Aorta
C. Diaphragm
D. Liver
E. Twelfth rib

113.

After a proximal shunt revision surgery, a patient is unable to void and requires straight catheterization. What is the most appropriate next step in treating this patient's condition?

A. Obtain a urology consultation for possible bladder injury.
B. Administer bethanechol.
C. Administer diazepam
D. Administer oxybutynin.
E. Administer morphine.

114.

Occlusion of a dAVF is most effective with what minimally invasive method?

A. Transvenous coil embolization
B. Transarterial embolization with Onyx glue
C. Minimally invasive keyhole endoscopic microsurgical clip ligation of feeding arteries
D. Stereotactic radiosurgery

115.

During an endonasal transsphenoidal approach, what structure limits the working space and maneuverability of the instruments?

A. Inferior turbinate
B. Middle turbinate
C. Superior turbinate
D. Anterior nasal septum

116.

Patients flying soon after major intracranial surgery may be theoretically at risk for what complication?

A. Blindness
B. Wound infection
C. Pneumonia
D. Tension pneumocephalus
E. Spontaneous hemorrhage

117.

What is the most common site of ulnar nerve compression around the elbow?

A. Arcade of Struthers
B. Cubital tunnel
C. Medial epicondyle
D. Medial intramuscular septum
E. Deep flexor aponeurosis

118.

Although not always conclusive, what imaging sequence is most helpful in differentiating a cerebral abscess from a tumor?

A. CT with contrast
B. MR T1 with contrast
C. MR FLAIR
D. Diffusion-weighted imaging
E. MR angiography

119.

What components constitute the system for indocyanine green video angiography?

A. Incandescent tungsten-halogen light source projecting light through the collector lens and into the substage condenser
B. Mercury vapor arc lamp with a monochromatic light source expanded in the near-ultraviolet
C. Argon ion emission at 488 to 514 nm used in confocal source emission
D. Near-infrared light source with an optical filter to block ambient and excitation light
E. Electronic flash 5500 K illumination to capture specimens with high-speed daylight transparency film

120.

A bilateral thalamotomy is contraindicated due to the possibility of what side effects?

A. Hemiparesis and homonymous hemianopsia
B. Dysarthria and cognitive impairment
C. Myosis and anhydrosis
D. Quadriparesis and respiratory depression
E. Hemiparesis and bladder dysfunction

121.

What are the Surgical Care Improvement Project (SCIP) prophylactic antibiotic guidelines?

A. All surgical patients must receive cefazolin prior to the skin incision.
B. Prophylactic antibiotics must be received within 1 hour prior to the surgical incision.
C. Prophylactic antibiotics should be continued for 24 hours after the surgery end time.
D. Prophylactic antibiotics should be continued for at least 48 hours after the surgery end time.

122.

What procedure is best at relieving the symptoms associated with a traumatic brachial plexus nerve root avulsion?

A. Cordotomy
B. Midline myelotomy
C. Dorsal root entry zone lesioning
D. Cingulotomy
E. Rhizotomy

123.

Superior hypophyseal artery aneurysms usually have what orientation compared to the parent vessel?

A. Oriented superolaterally
B. Oriented posterolaterally
C. Oriented inferolaterally
D. Oriented inferomedially
E. Oriented posteromedially

124.

How does melanoma in the central nervous system respond to radiation?

A. Melanoma is entirely radiation insensitive and should not be treated by radiation.
B. Melanoma is mostly radiation insensitive, but radiation may be somewhat effective.
C. Melanoma is mostly radiation sensitive, and radiation typically may be effective.
D. Melanoma is entirely radiation sensitive and should be treated primarily by radiation.

125.

A 58-year-old woman underwent an uneventful single-level anterior cervical diskectomy and fusion (ACDF). Six months later, she presented with a low-grade fever, dysphagia, anorexia, and neck pain. The symptoms had been ongoing for a month. MRI showed osteomyelitis at the surgical site. What is the most appropriate diagnostic test to find the source of infection?

A. Panorex imaging to look for dental abscesses
B. Echocardiogram
C. Blood cultures
D. Upper gastrointestinal imaging
E. Nuclear bone scan

126.

What bone product is primarily an osteoinductive agent?

A. Demineralized bone matrix
B. Bone morphogenic protein
C. Cadaveric fibular strut
D. Tricalcium phosphate
E. Hydroxyapatite

127.

What size must an aneurysm be to be considered giant?

A. 0.7 cm
B. 1.0 cm
C. 1.5 cm
D. 2.5 cm
E. 4.0 cm

128.

Ophthalmic artery aneurysms usually have what orientation and origin compared with the parent vessel?

A. Oriented medially and arising from the posterior wall
B. Oriented superiorly and arising from the anterior wall
C. Oriented anteriorly and arising from the posterior wall
D. Oriented superiorly and arising from the superior wall
E. Oriented anteriorly and arising from the anterior wall

129.

Anterior communicating artery (ACOM) aneurysms usually have what orientation and origin compared with the parent vessel?

A. Directed laterally and arising from the branch point of the dominant A1 segment and the ACOM
B. Directed laterally and arising from the nondominant A2 segment
C. Directed laterally and arising from the dominant A2 segment
D. Directed contralaterally and arising from the branch point of the nondominant A1 segment and the ACOM
E. Directed contralaterally and arising from the branch point of the dominant A1 segment and the ACOM

130.
What is the most common location for the "pearly" tumor shown in this image?

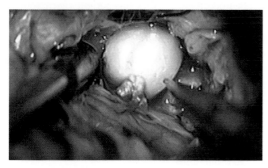

A. As part of the dural along the cerebral convexities
B. Cerebellopontine angle
C. Thalamus
D. Extra-calvarial
E. Pineal gland

131.
A man underwent a long-segment spine surgery while positioned supine with the lower extremity externally rotated at the hip with the knee flexed. Iatrogenic injury to what nerve is most likely to result from this operative position?

A. Common peroneal nerve
B. Deep peroneal nerve
C. Superficial peroneal nerve
D. Obturator nerve
E. Lateral femoral cutaneous nerve

132.
A 50-year-old woman presents to the hospital after a new onset of seizures. She describes headache and poor vision. Her family notes that her memory has been worsening, and she is becoming more confused. Neurologic exam reveals a loss of smell on the left side. Ophthalmologic exam reveals a pale left optic disk. The right optic disk is congested and edematous. What is her most likely diagnosis?

A. Pituitary adenoma
B. Posterior reversible encephalopathy syndrome
C. Olfactory groove meningioma
D. Brainstem cavernoma
E. Central pontine myelinolysis

133.
The roof of the third ventricle is composed of how many layers?

A. Two
B. Three
C. Four
D. Five
E. Six

134.
When harvesting the sural nerve, what structure accompanies the nerve as it courses lateral to the Achilles tendon?

A. Superficial peroneal nerve
B. Great saphenous vein
C. Small saphenous vein
D. Posterior tibial artery
E. Posterior tibial vein

135.
What is the primary disadvantage of approaching a pineal region tumor using an infratentorial supracerebellar approach?

A. Difficulty may be encountered navigating around the deep venous system.
B. Morbidity may be associated with positioning.
C. Visual deficits are likely.
D. Seizures may be induced.
E. Disconnection syndrome may occur.

136.
What are the current recommendations (level 2 evidence) for use of prophylactic anticonvulsants in the setting of a traumatic brain injury?

A. The use of prophylactic anticonvulsants is recommended for 30 days following injury to decrease the risk of posttraumatic seizures.
B. Prophylactic anticonvulsants have not been shown to decrease the risk of posttraumatic seizures.
C. Prophylactic anticonvulsant use for 6 months following injury has been shown to decrease the incidence of late posttraumatic seizures.
D. Prophylactic anticonvulsants are indicated to decrease the incidence of early posttraumatic seizures.
E. Prophylactic anticonvulsants are indicated to decrease the incidence of late posttraumatic seizures occurring more than 6 months following injury.

137.

A 36-year-old woman is diagnosed with a rup-tured, wide neck posterior communicating aneu-rysm with a fetal posterior cerebral artery. After an uneventful clipping of the aneurysm, she wakes up with contralateral weakness and numbness and a homonymous hemianopsia. What event likely caused the postoperative symptoms?

A. Incorporation of the posterior communicating artery into the aneurysm clip
B. Prolonged placement of temporary clips
C. Thromboembolic event
D. Vasospasm
E. Incorporation of the anterior choroidal artery into the aneurysm clip

138.

What are the resection limits of the dominant and nondominant temporal lobes, respectively, as mea-sured along the middle temporal gyrus from the temporal pole in an anterior-posterior direction?

A. 2 to 3 cm; 6 to 7 cm
B. 4 to 5 cm; 4 to 5 cm
C. 6 to 7 cm; 8 to 9 cm
D. 4 to 5 cm; 6 to 7 cm
E. 3 to 4 cm; 8 to 9 cm

139.

A patient with a baclofen pump presents with a high-grade fever, hyperreflexia, and seizures. What is the underlying cause of this patient's symptoms?

A. Infected hardware
B. Baclofen toxicity
C. Meningitis
D. Baclofen withdrawal

140.

Scheuermann disease is defined as:

A. Nontraumatic anterior wedging of at least 5 degrees in at least three adjacent thoracic ver-tebral bodies
B. Hypermobility of the craniovertebral junction
C. Congenital fusion of two or more cervical vertebrae
D. Nontraumatic subluxation of the atlantoaxial joint caused by inflammation or infection
E. Compression of the esophagus and dysphagia resulting from a cervical osteophyte

4 Pediatric Neurosurgery

1.

What structure is indicated by the *arrow* in this image from an endoscopic third ventriculostomy?

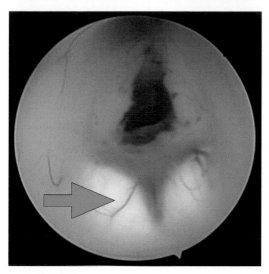

A. Optic chiasm
B. Pituitary stalk
C. Tip of basilar artery
D. Fornix
E. Mammillary bodies

2.

During an infratentorial supracerebellar approach to a pineal tumor, what vein in the galenic draining group may be sacrificed safely without negative sequelae?

A. Basal vein of Rosenthal
B. Posterior mesencephalic vein
C. Straight sinus
D. Precentral cerebellar vein
E. Internal cerebral vein

3.

A premature neonate's head ultrasound demonstrates intraventricular hemorrhage. The ventricles are dilated mildly. What is the infant's subependymal hemorrhage grade?

A. Grade 1
B. Grade 2
C. Grade 3
D. Grade 4

4.

A 3-year-old boy presents with a history of spinal cord de-tethering and excision of a thoracic dermal sinus tract during infancy. What is the most likely spinal cord lesion seen on the current T2 MRI shown in this image?

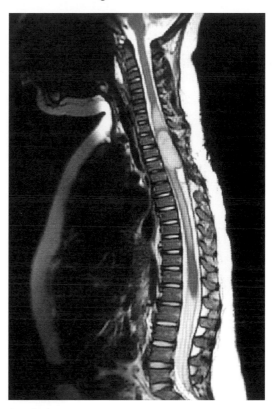

A. Syrinx
B. Ependymoma
C. Astrocytoma
D. Dermoid tumor
E. Epidermoid tumor

5.

What component is necessary to classify a Chiari malformation as type 3?

A. Cervical cord syrinx
B. Occipital encephalocele
C. Lumbar myelomeningocele
D. Cerebellar vermian agenesis
E. Platybasia

6.

A 2-year-old boy presents with gait imbalance and progressive headaches. MRI suggests a posterior fossa tumor. Gross total resection and pathological analysis reveal an average risk medulloblastoma. The next adjuvant therapy step is:

A.   Chemotherapy alone
B.   Radiation therapy alone
C.   Concomitant chemotherapy and radiation
D.   No need for further adjuvant therapy

7.

An 8-year-old child with a history of myelomeningocele repair after birth presents with progressive leg weakness and a neurogenic bladder. An MRI of lumbar spine, shown in this image, suggests:

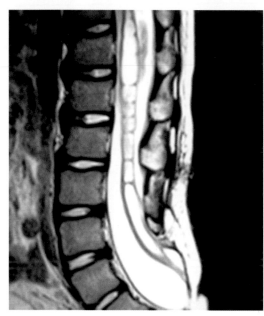

A.   Syringomyelia secondary to a tethered spinal cord
B.   Idiopathic syringomyelia
C.   Spinal lipoma
D.   Dermoid tumor
E.   Thickened filum terminale

8.

A 2-month-old baby has a slowly growing midline mass over the anterior fontanelle, as shown in the MRI in this image. The most likely diagnosis is:

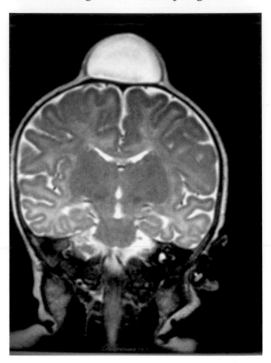

A.   Dermoid cyst
B.   Eosinophilic granuloma
C.   Epidermoid cyst
D.   Fibrous dysplasia
E.   Hemangioma

9.

A 3-month-old baby has an abnormal head shape. Based on the 3D reconstruction imaging of the skull, shown in this image, what syndrome is suspected?

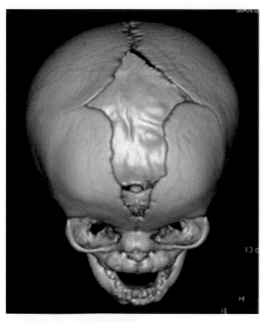

A. Pierre Robin syndrome
B. Treacher Collins syndrome
C. Pfeiffer syndrome
D. Goldenhar syndrome
E. Moebius syndrome

10.

The normal level of conus medullaris in infants and children is at the level of:

A. L1-L2
B. L3-L4
C. L4-L5
D. L5-S1
E. T12-L1

11.

The most common postoperative complication encountered after selective dorsal rhizotomy for spasticity is:

A. Cerebrospinal fluid leak
B. Paraplegia
C. Bladder incontinence
D. Bowel incontinence
E. Lower extremity hyperesthesia

12.

The most life-threatening complication during endoscopic third ventriculostomy for obstructive hydrocephalus is secondary to:

A. Forniceal injury
B. Thalamic injury
C. Injury to the basilar artery bifurcation
D. Meningitis
E. Oculomotor nerve injury

13.

The most common location of atypical teratoid/rhabdoid tumors during infancy and childhood is in the:

A. Suprasellar region
B. Spinal cord
C. Posterior fossa
D. Frontal lobe
E. Temporal lobe

14.

What surgical procedure should be considered as a treatment option in pediatric patients with disabling drop attacks and generalized seizures?

A. Anatomic hemispherectomy
B. Functional hemispherectomy
C. Mesial temporal lobectomy
D. Amygdalohippocampectomy
E. Corpus callosotomy

15.

The most common symptomatic intracranial vascular anomaly in children is a(n):

A. Arteriovenous malformation (AVM)
B. Cavernoma
C. Venous angioma
D. Berry aneurysm
E. Mycotic aneurysm

16.

What particular spinal feature is associated with achondroplasia?

A. Scalloping of the vertebrae
B. Hemivertebrae
C. Foramen magnum stenosis
D. Os odontoideum
E. Dermal sinus tract

17.

An 11-month-old boy presents with macrocrania and failure to thrive. An MRI of the brain, shown in this image, confirms what likely type of hydrocephalus?

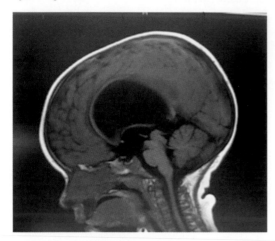

A. Communicating hydrocephalus
B. Obstructive hydrocephalus secondary to a Dandy-Walker malformation
C. Obstructive hydrocephalus secondary to aqueductal stenosis
D. Obstructive hydrocephalus secondary to a posterior fossa tumor
E. Obstructive hydrocephalus secondary to a vein of Galen aneurysm

18.

A 10-year-old boy presents with progressive weakness of his bilateral wrist and finger extensors (wrist drop). He also has abdominal pain. What is the most likely source of his chemical poisoning?

A. Lead
B. Arsenic
C. Mercury
D. Copper
E. Iron

19.

What molecular subgroup of medulloblastoma is associated with the best 5-year overall survival rate?

A. Wnt subgroup
B. SHH subgroup
C. Group 3
D. Group 4

20.

Trilateral retinoblastoma describes bilateral ocular retinoblastomas and a(n):

A. Astrocytoma
B. Medulloblastoma
C. Neurofibroma
D. Optic nerve sheath tumor
E. Pineoblastoma

21.

A pregnant woman presents after a pelvic MRI, shown in this image, evaluated a fetal spina bifida lesion detected by ultrasound. She is being considered for a fetal in-utero repair. What are the gestational age limits (minimum and maximum) for consideration of fetal repair per the MOMs trial criteria?

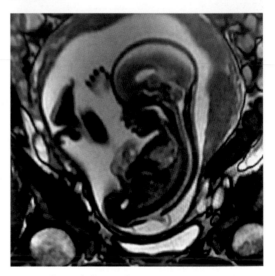

A. 15 through 20 weeks
B. 19 through 26 weeks
C. 20 through 25 weeks
D. 25 through 28 weeks
E. 30 through 35 weeks

22.

A 10-year-old boy presents with chronic neck pain. The CT shown in this image suggests atlantoaxial instability due to:

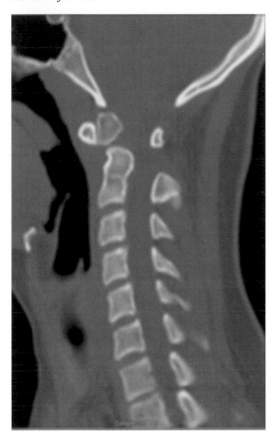

A. Acute odontoid fracture
B. Os odontoideum
C. Clival chordoma
D. Condylar fracture
E. Ligamentous injury

23.

What is the most common pathogen implicated in neonatal meningitis?

A. *Haemophilus influenzae*
B. *Listeria* species
C. *Neisseria meningitidis*
D. *Staphylococci*
E. *Streptococci*

24.

What is the most common asymptomatic side effect of ventriculopleural shunts?

A. Pleural effusion
B. Shunt disconnection
C. Subdural hematoma
D. Shunt infection
E. Tension pneumothorax

25.

The MRI shown in this image suggests that the cause of the cervicothoracic syringomyelia in this child is due to:

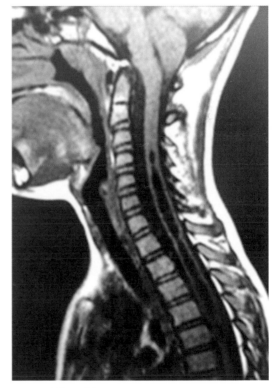

A. An idiopathic cause
B. Trauma
C. A Chiari malformation
D. Tethered cord due to a cervical dermal sinus tract
E. A craniocervical ependymoma

26.

What intracranial tumor is associated with polycythemia?

A. Ependymoma
B. Pilocytic astrocytoma
C. Medulloblastoma
D. Hemangioblastoma
E. Choriocarcinoma

27.
What percentage of children with agenesis of the corpus callosum have developmental delays?

A. 10%
B. 30%
C. 50%
D. 70%
E. 90%

28.
A child presents with a second episode of middle cerebral artery stroke. The cerebral angiogram, shown in this image, suggests:

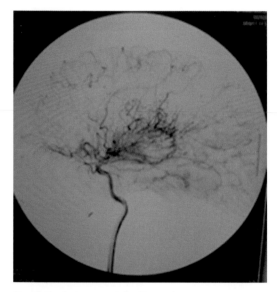

A. Anterior communicating artery aneurysm
B. Arteriovenous malformation
C. Cavernous malformations
D. Moyamoya disease
E. Vein of Galen malformation

29.
What skull suture is involved in the post-shunting craniosynostosis shown in this image of an 18-month-old toddler?

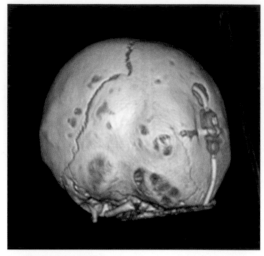

A. Left coronal suture
B. Sagittal suture
C. Right lambdoid suture
D. Metopic suture
E. Left lambdoid suture

30.
A 9-year-old boy presents with headache, upgaze paresis, and a pineal region tumor. A cerebrospinal fluid analysis is performed showing elevated levels of β-HCG. What tumor type is suspected?

A. Choriocarcinoma
B. Embryonal carcinoma
C. Germinoma
D. Teratoma
E. Yolk sac tumor

31.
What is the approximate incidence of Chiari 2 malformations when a myelomeningocele is present at birth?

A. 100%
B. 75%
C. 50%
D. 25%
E. < 5%

32.
What is the average head circumference for a newborn and an adult?

A. 29 and 49 cm
B. 31 and 51 cm
C. 33 and 53 cm
D. 35 and 55 cm

33.
A newborn girl presents with congestive heart failure. She is noted to have an increased head circumference and dilated scalp veins. Imaging demonstrates a large mass with obstructive hydrocephalus in the area of the posterior third ventricle/pineal region. Your next step in the management of this patient is to:

A. Perform a lumbar puncture
B. Perform an endoscopic third ventriculostomy with biopsy
C. Plan for surgical resection of the lesion
D. Perform an angiogram
E. Plan for radiation

34.
Selective dorsal rhizotomy (SDR) classically is considered a surgical treatment for children with spasticity. What type of spasticity is best managed by SDR?

A. Spastic diplegia
B. Spastic quadriplegia
C. Mixed spasticity and dystonia
D. Hereditary spastic paraparesis
E. Severe head injury

35.
What genetic condition carries the highest risk of developing intracranial meningiomas in the pediatric population?

A. Tuberous sclerosis
B. Sturge-Weber disease
C. Neurofibromatosis type 1
D. Neurofibromatosis type 2
E. von Hippel–Lindau disease

36.
Trigonocephaly is caused by premature closure of what skull suture during infancy?

A. Coronal suture
B. Sagittal suture
C. Lambdoid suture
D. Metopic suture
E. Frontosphenoidal suture

37.
Hypsarrhythmia is an electroencephalographic chaotic appearance classically seen in children with what condition?

A. Lennox-Gastaut syndrome
B. Infantile spasms
C. Absence seizures
D. Juvenile myoclonic epilepsy
E. Mesial temporal lobe epilepsy

38.
What fetal spinal anomaly commonly is associated with maternal hyperglycemia?

A. Dandy-Walker malformation
B. Holoprosencephaly
C. Sacral agenesis
D. Encephalocele
E. Chiari malformation

39.
What supplement during the first trimester of pregnancy is considered preventive for myelomeningocele?

A. Vitamin A
B. Vitamin B12
C. Vitamin D
D. Zinc
E. Folic acid

40.
An endoscope-assisted strip craniectomy procedure for an infant with sagittal craniosynostosis, shown in this image, followed by helmet therapy will have the best cosmetic outcome if it is performed at what age?

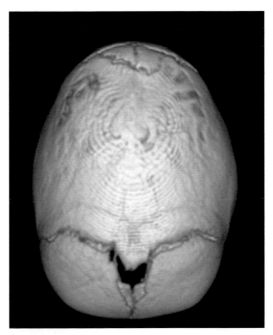

A. 18 months
B. 12 months
C. 9 months
D. 6 months
E. 3 months

41.
What cranial nerves most commonly are affected in a symptomatic Chiari type 2 malformation?

A.   VII and VIII
B.   V
C.   VI
D.   XII
E.   IX and X

42.
According to the Food and Drug Administration (FDA), vagal nerve stimulation is indicated for use in partial-onset seizures refractory to medical therapy in patients of what age?

A.   Any age
B.   Older than 6 years
C.   Older than 8 years
D.   Older than 12 years
E.   Older than 18 years

43.
What dose of intrathecal baclofen is used during the screening trial prior to pump insertion for children with spastic quadriplegia?

A.   50 µg
B.   100 µg
C.   200 µg
D.   500 µg
E.   750 µg

44.
A 7-year-old boy presents with a skull mass. A skeletal survey, shown in this image, reveals multiple other bony osteolytic lesions. The most likely diagnosis of his skull mass is:

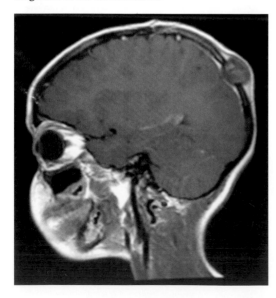

A.   Dermoid cyst
B.   Epidermoid tumor
C.   Eosinophilic granuloma
D.   Osteoma
E.   Ewing sarcoma

45.
An absolute contraindication to performing an endoscopic third ventriculostomy is:

A.   Fourth ventricle outlet obstruction
B.   Aqueductal stenosis
C.   Presence of intraventricular hemorrhage
D.   Patient age younger than 1 year
E.   Suspected infection of the cerebrospinal fluid

46.
The most common intramedullary spinal cord tumor in children is:

A.   Ependymoma
B.   Hemangioblastoma
C.   Astrocytoma
D.   Cavernoma
E.   Ganglioglioma

47.
At what age does the metopic suture typically close?

A.   1 to 2 months
B.   3 to 9 months
C.   9 to 18 months
D.   24 months
E.   36 months

48.
Endoscopic third ventriculostomy has the highest success rate in children over the age of 12 months with what pathology?

A.   Shunt infection
B.   Posterior fossa tumor
C.   Myelomeningocele
D.   Idiopathic aqueductal stenosis
E.   Communicating hydrocephalus

49.
What is the most common pineal region tumor in children?

A.   Ependymoma
B.   Astrocytoma
C.   Germinoma
D.   Mature teratoma
E.   Meningioma

50.

A 6-month-old girl has recurrent urinary tract infections. Urodynamic studies suggest that she has a neurogenic bladder. MRI of lumbar spine likely will demonstrate what associated pathology?

A. Low-lying conus and fatty filum terminale
B. Arachnoiditis
C. Anterior sacral meningocele
D. Lumbar hemivertebrae
E. Klippel-Feil syndrome

51.

The majority of spinal neurenteric cysts are found in what location?

A. Anterior to the spinal cord and extradural
B. Posterior to the spinal cord and extradural
C. Intradural and extramedullary
D. Intradural and intramedullary
E. Craniocervical junction

52.

Patients with split cord malformation type 1 have what anatomy?

A. Two hemicords in one dural sac
B. Two hemicords in two separate dural sacs
C. Open myelomeningocele
D. Anterior sacral meningocele
E. Thoracic dermal sinus tract

53.

A 6-year-old boy presents to the emergency department after a motor vehicle collision. He denies pain and weakness and has an unremarkable neurologic exam. Lateral X-rays identify 3 mm of C2 on C3 anterolisthesis with angulation. What is the next step in the management of this patient?

A. Flexion-extension X-rays of the cervical spine if there are no other cervical spine injuries or fractures
B. Hard orthosis for suspected Effendi type 1 hangman fracture
C. MRI to evaluate for ligamentous injury
D. Surgical reduction and stabilization for suspected Effendi type 2 hangman fracture
E. Closed reduction with craniocervical traction

54.

What initial weakness develops during the infectious neuropathy associated with diphtheria?

A. Visual accommodation paralysis
B. Facial paralysis
C. Oropharyngeal paralysis
D. Distal sensorimotor polyneuropathy
E. Ascending paralysis

55.

A 6-year-old boy presents with new-onset seizures. MRI of the brain, shown in this image, demonstrates an enhancing temporal mass. What is the most likely diagnosis?

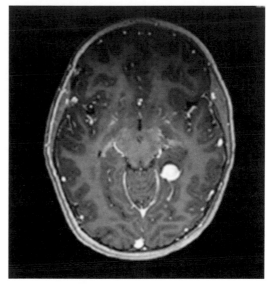

A. Anaplastic astrocytoma
B. Ependymoma
C. Ganglioglioma
D. Meningioma
E. Primitive neuroectodermal tumor

56.

What is the most common complication during resection of a lipomyelomeningocele during infancy?

A. Neural injury
B. Aseptic meningitis
C. Cerebrospinal fluid leak and infection
D. Neurogenic bladder
E. Hydrocephalus

57.

Pediatric patients with ventricular shunt catheters are at risk for developing ventriculitis. What bacteria most commonly are associated with shunt infections?

A. *Staphylococcus epidermidis*
B. *Staphylococcus aureus*
C. *Streptococcus pneumoniae*
D. *Streptococcus milleri*
E. *Escherichia coli*

5 Neurology

1.

A boy is found to have patches of retinal pigmentation after he is brought to clinical attention because of several episodes of seizures. He subsequently is diagnosed with Aicardi syndrome following an MRI of the brain and cervical spine. What abnormality was seen on imaging to prompt the diagnosis of Aicardi syndrome?

A. Absence of the septum pellucidum
B. Dandy-Walker malformation
C. Fusion of the cervical vertebrae
D. Agenesis of the corpus callosum
E. Chiari type 3 malformation

2.

A positive Romberg sign indicates a disturbance of what structure(s)?

A. Posterior columns
B. Cerebellar vermis
C. Lateral geniculate body
D. Cerebellar hemisphere
E. Corticospinal tract

3.

A 7-year-old boy presents to the emergency department after suffering a first-time seizure at home. His mother says that he had been febrile recently and seemingly slightly confused. On exam, the child is lethargic without focal deficits. Mild papilledema is seen on funduscopic examination. Routine laboratory studies are unremarkable, but a lumbar puncture reveals cerebrospinal fluid with leukocytosis and an elevated protein content. Multiple cultures are sent to the lab. An MRI with FLAIR sequence reveals an abnormality within the left temporal lobe. Electroencephalography demonstrates periodic lateralizing epileptiform discharges from the left temporal lobe. What are the most likely diagnosis and next step in the patient's management?

A. Varicella zoster encephalitis; begin intravenous acyclovir
B. Varicella zoster encephalitis; await culture results before initiating treatment
C. Herpes simplex encephalitis; begin intravenous acyclovir
D. Herpes simplex encephalitis; await culture results before initiating treatment

4.

Apert syndrome is distinguished from Crouzon syndrome as individuals with Apert, and not Crouzon, syndrome tend to have:

A. Absence of a cleft palate
B. Normal intelligence
C. Mental retardation
D. Complex syndactyly
E. Craniosynostosis

5.

Damage to what neural structure(s) is most associated with prosopagnosia?

A. Mid-fusiform gyrus and inferior occipital gyrus
B. Bilateral amygdalae
C. Mesial temporal lobe
D. Calcarine sulcus and dominant angular gyrus
E. Superior parietal lobule and supramarginal gyrus

6.

A 62-year-old man presents with masked facies without tremor. His family members report that over the past year, the patient had multiple falls, dysarthria, and dysphagia. They report he has had some personality changes. On exam, he has a hyperactive jaw jerk, axial dystonia, and downgaze paresis. You suspect the patient has what condition?

A. Parkinson disease
B. Olivopontocerebellar degeneration
C. Progressive supranuclear palsy
D. Multiple system atrophy

7.

Bilateral periodic lateralizing epileptiform discharges (PLEDs) that are not reactive to painful stimulation are suggestive of what condition?

A. Subacute sclerosing panencephalitis
B. Creutzfeldt-Jakob disease
C. Herpes simplex encephalitis
D. Hepatic encephalopathy

8.

Transcranial Doppler can detect changes in flow velocities in the cerebral arteries. Vasospasm is differentiated from a hyperemic state by:

A. A mean flow velocity greater than 120 cm/s, indicating vasospasm
B. Measuring the middle cerebral to internal carotid artery velocity ratio
C. Checking for flow symmetry on the contralateral side
D. Measuring the velocity/vessel diameter ratio
E. Determining the direction of flow

9.

What involuntary movement disorder typically persists during sleep?

A. Hemifacial spasm
B. Blepharospasm
C. Athetosis
D. Facial myokymia

10.

The Cantu system for concussion grading uses what three variables to determine severity?

A. Loss of consciousness, transient confusion, and symptom duration
B. Loss of consciousness, posttraumatic amnesia, and neurologic deficits
C. Eye opening, motor response, and verbal response
D. Loss of consciousness, posttraumatic amnesia, and symptom duration

11.

A 49-year-old man presents with left elbow pain. His symptoms have not improved with rest, ice, splinting, and analgesics. He has noticed progressive weakness in extension of his thumb and fingers without weakness of his wrist or arm. There is no sensory loss. What is the suspected diagnosis?

A. Radial nerve neuropathy in the upper arm
B. Tennis elbow
C. Posterior interosseous neuropathy
D. C8 radiculopathy
E. Radial tunnel syndrome

12.

A 28-year-old woman presents to the emergency room with a severe orbital headache. What findings would support a diagnosis of spontaneous internal carotid artery dissection?

A. Complete Horner syndrome with hemisensory loss, dysphagia, ataxia, and vertigo
B. Complete Horner syndrome with shoulder and arm pain
C. Complete Horner syndrome with neck pain and delayed contralateral weakness and sensory loss
D. Incomplete Horner syndrome with neck pain and delayed contralateral weakness and sensory loss
E. Mydriasis with contralateral weakness and sensory loss

13.

A 15-year-old boy presents with significant discharge from the left ear with severe headache, facial pain, and diplopia. On exam, he is noted to have a left-sided lateral gaze palsy. What is the patient's suspected diagnosis?

A. Venous sinus thrombosis
B. Tolosa-Hunt syndrome
C. Raeder paratrigeminal neuralgia
D. Gradenigo syndrome
E. Ramsay-Hunt syndrome

14.

A patient has a cerebellar lesion causing symptoms including a wide and staggering gait with little impairment of arm or hand movement. What is the likely location of such a lesion?

A. Vestibulocerebellum
B. Cerebellar tonsils
C. Cerebrocerebellum
D. Spinocerebellum
E. Dentate nucleus

15.

What is the Wartenberg sign?

A. Wasting of the interossei muscles in the hand
B. Grasping a sheet of paper resulting in extension of the proximal phalanx and flexion of the distal phalanx
C. Hyperextension at the metacarpophalangeal joints and flexion at the interphalangeal joints in digits four, five, and partially three
D. Abduction of fifth digit due to weakness of the third palmar interosseous muscle
E. Sensory loss over the hypothenar eminence, fifth finger, and ulnar half of the fourth finger on the palmar aspect only

16.

A 53-year-old man with a heavy smoking history comes to the office complaining of right upper extremity pain and weakness. Physical examination reveals a small right pupil and right eye ptosis. What disease process likely explains this finding?

A. Perineural spread of metastatic disease
B. Tumor compression of the stellate ganglion
C. Cerebral metastatic tumor compressing the hypothalamus
D. Spinal metastatic disease

17.

An 8-year-old girl is brought to the emergency room by her grandmother after 1 week of fever and lethargy and a 2-day history of progressive right-sided weakness. A head CT is normal, and an MRI with FLAIR sequence of the brain and spine demonstrates a subtle abnormality within the subcortical white matter. Cerebrospinal fluid studies show an elevated white blood cell and protein count. Further studies are pending. What is the most likely diagnosis?

A. Juvenile-onset multiple sclerosis
B. Progressive multifocal leukoencephalopathy
C. Adrenoleukodystrophy
D. Acute disseminated encephalomyelitis

18.

Fill in the blanks.
Korsakoff psychosis results from deficiency of _____ (nutrient), is _____ (reversible/irreversible), and affects the _____ (anatomic structure).

A. Folate; irreversible; medial dorsal thalamic nuclei
B. Folate; reversible; mammillary bodies
C. Thiamine; irreversible; medial dorsal thalamic nuclei
D. Thiamine; reversible; mammillary bodies
E. Thiamine; irreversible; cerebellum

19.

The nurse calls you to evaluate a recently admitted patient with Guillain-Barré syndrome. The patient initially had only lower extremity weakness but now has a weak quality of voice and is taking shallow, rapid breaths. What is the next most appropriate step in this patient's management?

A. Initiate plasmapheresis.
B. Give intravenous dexamethasone.
C. Intubate the patient.
D. Give intravenous immunoglobulin.

20.

A 72-year-old woman was admitted to the hospital for severe vertigo of 1 day's duration. She subsequently developed nausea, vomiting, dysphagia, hoarseness, and loss of left facial pain sensation. The patient is alert and oriented to time, space, and person. She has no motor deficits but does have ptosis on the left and clumsiness of the left arm. The patient also has decreased proprioception in the left foot and loss of pain and temperature sensation on the right side. The patient's MRI demonstrates an ischemic stroke. What is the most likely localization of the stroke?

A. Right lateral medulla
B. Left lateral medulla
C. Right medial medulla
D. Left medial medulla
E. Right and left lateral medulla

21.

An 81-year-old man with a history of hip replacement 3 weeks ago complicated by a mild myocardial infarction is brought to the hospital with an acute-onset middle cerebral artery stroke. The patient has been maintained on warfarin, and the INR is 2.3. The platelet count is 120,000. In this patient, what is an absolute contraindication to thrombolysis?

A. Age over 80 years
B. Hip replacement within 3 weeks of presentation
C. Recent history of myocardial infarction
D. INR of 2.3
E. Platelets count of 120,000

22.

A 3-year-old boy who was previously healthy develops a red, scaly rash over his face, neck, hand, and legs. He then starts having emotional liability and episodic cerebellar ataxia, and eventually experiences developmental delay. After being worked up, he is treated with high doses of nicotinamide. What is the patient's diagnosis?

A. Hartnup disease
B. Phenylketonuria
C. Homocystinuria
D. G6PD deficiency
E. Tetrahydrobiopterin deficiency

23.

A 48-year-old woman presents with a sudden onset of blurred vision and pain on movement of her right eye. She reports that 2 years ago, she had loss of sensation in the hands that progressed over a couple of weeks to motor involvement limiting her ability to write with the left hand. At the time, she was afraid to seek medical attention. What is the most likely diagnosis?

A. Multiple sclerosis
B. Guillain-Barré syndrome
C. Transient ischemic attack
D. Myasthenia gravis
E. Amyotrophic lateral sclerosis

24.

A 30-year-old man with a history of homocystinuria develops a headache followed by hemiparesis and focal epilepsy. He is brought to the emergency room for evaluation. What is the most sensitive imaging modality to detect this patient disease?

A. Noncontrast CT scan
B. T2-weighted MRI
C. Angiogram
D. Whole body PET CT
E. Perfusion-weighted imaging

25.

When examining a man, you notice that he has difficulty maintaining balance when his feet are together and his eyes are closed. He also struggles to rub accurately the heel of one foot along the shin of the opposite leg. What system is most likely malfunctioning?

A. Vision
B. Proprioception
C. Vestibular system
D. Cerebellum

26.

A retired boxer with a history of more than 20 bouts comes to your office for evaluation of "abnormal behavior" reported by the family. On exam, the patient has a resting tremor, decreased coordination, poor attention span, no focal weakness, and subtle paranoia upon questioning. You suspect chronic traumatic encephalopathy. What would you expect to find on pathological examination of his cerebral tissue?

A. Normal cerebral architecture
B. Loss of pigmentation in the substantia nigra
C. Caudate atrophy
D. Deposition of β-amyloid plaques

27.

What is the most effective mean of aborting a cluster headache?

A. Inhaled 100% O_2
B. Sublingual nitroglycerin
C. Ergotamine
D. Methysergide
E. Intravenous nonsteroidal anti-inflammatory agents

28.

A 4-month-old boy with psychomotor retardation develops repetitive, generalized limb extension and neck flexion spasms that occur more than 10 times daily. These episodes are associated with altered consciousness. Electroencephalographic evaluation demonstrates high-voltage polyspike and slow wave discharges between spasms and suppression of these bursts during the spasms. What is the patient's most likely diagnosis?

A. Absence seizures
B. West syndrome
C. Epilepsia partialis continua
D. Complex partial seizures
E. Juvenile myoclonic seizures

29.

A 27-year-old man is involved in a motor vehicle collision. The patient is brought to the emergency room and stabilized, and imaging demonstrates a lower cervical spinal cord injury. On exam, the patient is hypotensive and lethargic with minimal movements of the upper extremities. You suspect spinal shock and initiate pressor support. Spinal shock occurs when there are injuries to the spinal cord above what level, and the hypotension observed is due to interruption of what element of the nervous system?

A. T6; sympathetics
B. T1; sympathetics
C. T6; parasympathetics
D. T1; parasympathetics

30.

When looking at an electromyogram, you notice that the motor unit potentials are demonstrating decreased amplitudes and durations. What process(es) exhibit these changes?

A. Denervation
B. Reinnervation
C. Myopathy and neuromuscular junction disease
D. Myopathy but not neuromuscular junction disease

31.

The pathology of acute disseminated encephalomyelitis in humans is similar to an animal model of experimental allergic encephalomyelitis. How is this model typically developed?

A. Injection of central nervous system proteins into animal brain parenchyma
B. Injection of whole blood into the subarachnoid space of an animal
C. Injection of penicillin into animal brain parenchyma
D. Injection of white blood cell extracts into the subarachnoid space of an animal
E. Injection of prions into animal brain parenchyma

32.

What is classically described as the cause of an immediate coma in a patient after a head injury without evidence of an intracranial mass or ischemia?

A. Severe concussion
B. Diffuse axonal injury
C. Dural sinus thrombosis
D. Atlantoaxial dislocation

33.

A 13-year-old boy presents to his physician because his parents are concerned about an enlarging abdomen and increasing fatigue over the course of 2 months. The patient's father is noted to have slurred speech and difficulty with balance as he enters the exam room. On physical exam, spider nevi are noted on the boy's chest, and there are some corneal abnormalities in the eyes. What is the best treatment for the patient's condition?

A. Dimercaprol
B. Penicillamine
C. L-dopa
D. Interferon
E. Splenectomy

34.

A patient is referred for nervus intermedius neuralgia. Based on this diagnosis, what clinical findings are expected?

A. Paroxysmal, lancinating pain in the lower one third of the face
B. Loss of taste to the anterior two thirds of the ipsilateral tongue
C. Periorbital vesicular rash, conjunctivitis, keratitis, and uveitis with involvement of the tip of the nose

D. Paroxysmal, lancinating pain in the upper one third of the face
E. Paroxysmal, lancinating pain in the depth of the ear with loss of taste in the anterior two thirds of the tongue with possible increased salivation

35.

What is the most common side effect of vagal nerve stimulation, and when does this effect typically occur during device discharge?

A. Bradycardia; during device discharge
B. Neck pain; following device discharge
C. Gastrointestinal irritation; regardless of device discharge
D. Voice change; during device discharge

36.

What finding suggests a clinical diagnosis of Creutzfeldt-Jakob disease?

A. Rapid mental deterioration, myoclonus, and 1- to 2-Hz periodic electroencephalography complexes
B. Cerebrospinal fluid positive for 14-2-2 protein
C. Increased signal on T1 MRI sequences in the basal ganglia and striatum
D. Periodic lateralized epileptiform discharges on electroencephalography not responsive to noxious stimuli
E. Serum assay positive for S-100

37.

When utilizing brainstem auditory evoked potentials, what finding can a vestibular schwannoma demonstrate?

A. Loss of amplitude of waves IV and V
B. Flattened waves I and II
C. Increased interpeak latency in waves I through V
D. Increased interpeak latency between waves VI and VI

38.

What are the neurologic manifestations of Lyme disease?

A. Cranial neuritis, meningitis, radiculopathy
B. Dorsal column dysfunction, pupil dysfunction, general paresis
C. Encephalopathy, dementia, myelopathy
D. Dementia, ataxia, and myoclonus

39.
What is the most likely diagnosis in an HIV-positive patient with subependymal enhancement?

A. Glioblastoma
B. Ventriculitis
C. Lymphoma
D. Toxoplasmosis

40.
A 7-year-old boy is referred to your office by his endocrinologist after an MRI was obtained during a workup for precocious puberty. The MRI reveals a nonenhancing T1 isointense and T2 isointense lesion within the hypothalamus. Other than precocious puberty, there are no focal findings on exam. While you are interviewing his parents, you notice that the patient occasionally has brief episodes of laughter. What is the most likely diagnosis, and what is the natural history of the described seizures?

A. Low-grade astrocytoma; good seizure control with dietary modifications
B. Germ cell tumor; excellent control of seizures with ethosuximide
C. Hypothalamic hamartoma; poor seizure response to medications
D. Lipoma; good control of seizures with topiramate

Use the following answers for questions 41 and 42:

A. Weakness of dorsiflexion and ankle inversion
B. Weakness of plantarflexion and ankle eversion
C. Weakness of dorsiflexion and ankle eversion
D. Weakness of plantarflexion and ankle inversion

41.
What deficit is expected with a common peroneal nerve injury?

42.
What deficit is expected with an L5 nerve injury?

43.
Subacute necrotizing leukoencephalitis is a side effect most commonly associated with what chemotherapeutic agent?

A. Cisplatin
B. Bevacizumab
C. Temozolomide
D. Methotrexate
E. Vincristine

44.
A corn farmer presents with a rash and complains of reduced sensation in his fingertips and lower extremity weakness bilaterally. His wife is concerned that he has been confused lately. What is his likely vitamin deficiency?

A. Thiamine
B. Niacin
C. B6
D. B12
E. Vitamin A

45.
Following trauma to his arm, a patient is unable to abduct and oppose his thumb. He has weakness in forearm pronation and wrist and finger flexion. What other physical exam findings is this patient expected to have?

A. Benediction sign and claw hand deformities
B. Ape hand and benediction sign deformities
C. Claw hand and wrist drop deformities
D. Wrist drop and benediction sign deformities

46.
What are the symptoms seen in dorsal midbrain syndrome?

A. Upward gaze paralysis, eyelid retraction, and "setting sun" sign
B. Upward gaze paralysis, Argyll-Robertson pupils, and nystagmus
C. Lateral gaze paralysis, eyelid retraction, and "setting sun" sign
D. Lateral gaze paralysis, Argyll-Robertson pupils, and nystagmus
E. Upward gaze paralysis, Argyll-Robertson pupils, and visual field cuts

47.
What metabolic disorder causes vertical supranuclear ophthalmoplegia mimicking Parinaud syndrome?

A. Niemann-Pick disease
B. Gaucher disease
C. Von Gierke disease
D. Cori disease
E. Pompe disease

48.

A 48-year-old woman has a history of twisting movements of the head. These twistings are painful and have resulted in hypertrophy of the sternocleidomastoid and trapezius muscles. What is the most likely diagnosis?

A. Meigs syndrome
B. Tardive dyskinesia
C. Spasmodic torticollis
D. Hemifacial spasm
E. Malingering

49.

A 69-year-old man incidentally was found to have 85% stenosis of his right internal carotid artery. According to the North American Symptomatic Carotid Endarterectomy Trial (NASCET), what management option is the most likely to prevent a future stroke in the patient?

A. Warfarin therapy
B. Carotid angioplasty
C. Statin therapy
D. Carotid endarterectomy
E. Aspirin therapy

50.

A 44-year-old woman is diagnosed with trigeminal neuralgia. What is the current first-line treatment option for her pain?

A. Microvascular decompression
B. Oxcarbamazepine
C. Mechanical balloon compression
D. Lamotrigine
E. Pimozide

51.

For what should a screening test be designed to detect before starting an Asian patient with trigeminal neuralgia on oxcarbamazepine?

A. HLA-A*30 allele
B. HLA-B*1502 allele
C. Chromosome 14 deletions
D. Chromosome 21 trisomy
E. Chromosome 6 monosomy

52.

Injury to the recurrent artery of Heubner may result in what deficits?

A. Hemianesthesia, hemiparesis, and homonymous hemianopsia
B. Altered mental status, vertical gaze palsy, and memory impairment

C. Ipsilateral lower extremity weakness and sensory loss
D. Monocular blindness
E. Hemiparesis of the contralateral upper extremity and face with dysarthria

53.

Follow transection of her spinal cord, a patient is found to have flaccid quadriplegia and areflexia. How long does it usually take following this type of injury for areflexia and flaccidity to change into hyperreflexia and spasticity?

A. 24 hours
B. 1 to 2 days
C. 3 to 21 days
D. 2 to 6 months
E. 1 year

54.

Spasticity following a spinal cord injury usually can be alleviated by baclofen. What is the mechanism of action of baclofen?

A. GABA agonism
B. Anticholinergic effects
C. Antimuscarinic effects
D. α-Adrenergic agonism
E. Unknown mechanism of action

55.

A man is found to have profound weight loss, hyperactivity, hypoglycemia, and a euphoric affect. He is diagnosed with an infiltrating glioma likely centered in what location?

A. Anterior thalamus
B. Anterior hypothalamus
C. Posterior thalamus
D. Midbrain
E. Pituitary gland

56.

A patient presents with bilateral trigeminal neuralgia that developed a week ago during a tropical vacation. What other neurologic disease should be a part of the differential diagnosis?

A. Epilepsy
B. Multiple sclerosis
C. Herpes zoster
D. Glossopharyngeal neuralgia
E. Bell palsy

57.
A 30-year-old man is stabbed in the lateral chest beneath his left arm. On presentation, he had a pneumothorax for which he received a chest tube. On follow-up, the patient is found to have a scapula that projects posteriorly and is closer to the midline on the injured side. The patient also complains that he cannot reach forward as much as he could prior to the injury. What nerve is injured in the patient?

A. Axillary
B. Long thoracic
C. Musculocutaneous
D. Radial
E. Lower subscapular

58.
A 58-year-old man has left-sided hemiplegia, right-sided deviation of the tongue on attempted protrusion, and loss of discriminative touch and vibration sensation on the left side. Occlusion of what artery is responsible for this patient's symptoms?

A. Basilar
B. Left anterior spinal
C. Right anterior spinal
D. Left posterior inferior cerebellar
E. Right posterior inferior cerebellar

59.
A patient presents with a severe headache and is found to have superior sagittal sinus thrombosis after long-term oral contraceptive use. After discontinuing the patient's medications, what is the best treatment option?

A. Anticoagulation
B. Antiplatelet therapy
C. Intra-sinus thrombolytic therapy
D. Mechanical aspiration of the thrombus
E. Steroids

60.
A 19-year-old woman with a history of epilepsy is brought to the emergency room for continuous generalized tonic-clonic seizures for the past 15 minutes. Intravenous access is achieved quickly, and the patient is given 2 mg of intravenous lorazepam but fails to stop seizing. What is the next best step in the patient's management?

A. Continuous intravenous fosphenytoin
B. Continuous intravenous propofol
C. Continuous intravenous midazolam
D. Bolus of intravenous phenobarbital
E. Obtain an electroencephalogram

61.
A 21-year-old woman presents with right-sided facial weakness of 1 day's duration. A brain MRI is unremarkable, as is an infectious workup. A chest radiograph is normal, as is the angiotensin-converting enzyme level. What is the patient's most likely diagnosis?

A. Bell palsy
B. Stroke
C. Transient ischemic attack
D. Sarcoidosis
E. Lyme disease

62.
A 55-year-old black woman presents with bilateral cranial nerve VII and VII palsies. A brain MRI is negative for mass lesions. A chest radiograph is abnormal. What is the next most appropriate test in the workup of this patient?

A. ELISA for IgM or IgG antibodies to *B. burgdorferi*
B. Cerebrospinal fluid analysis for oligoclonal bands
C. Serum angiotensin-converting enzyme level
D. Whole body PET scan

63.
Gaze disorders often follow a vascular episode. What finding would localize a lesion to the pons?

A. Deviation of both eyes toward a jerking limb
B. Deviation of both eyes away from a hemiparetic limb
C. Each eye abducted (wall eyes)
D. Deviation of both eyes toward a hemiparetic limb
E. Cranial nerve III palsy with a contralateral hemiparetic limb

64.
What is the definition of dysdiadochokinesia?

A. Lack of voluntary coordination of muscle movements
B. Breakdown of movements with "overshooting" when performing specific motor tasks such as the finger-to-nose test
C. Inability to perform rapid, alternating movements
D. Dilation and elongation of an artery often resulting in tortuosity
E. Slowness in the execution of movements

65.

Classically, what does a positive Romberg sign indicate?

A. Cerebellar dysfunction
B. Corticospinal tract dysfunction
C. Extrapyramidal dysfunction
D. Frontal lobe dysfunction (Bruns ataxia)
E. Posterior column dysfunction

66.

A patient presents with a stroke and gaze preference toward the right. The patient has a dense right-sided hemiparesis. Where is the patient's lesion?

A. Right frontal lobe
B. Left frontal lobe
C. Left paramedian pontine reticular formation
D. Right paramedian pontine reticular formation
E. Right thalamus

67.

A patient presents with speech difficulties and is found to have poor fluency but good comprehension with intact repetition. How would this patient's aphasia be classified?

A. Broca aphasia (expressive)
B. Wernicke aphasia (receptive)
C. Conduction aphasia
D. Transcortical motor aphasia
E. Transcortical sensory aphasia

68.

A woman presents with a complaint of weakness. During an electromyographic study, the compound muscle action potential amplitude significantly increased with sustained contraction. What is the suspected diagnosis?

A. Myasthenia gravis
B. Botulism
C. Polymyalgia rheumatica
D. Lambert-Eaton syndrome
E. Neuralgic amyotrophy

69.

A characteristic 3-Hz spike and wave pattern lasting more than 2 seconds is suggestive of what underlying diagnosis?

A. Creutzfeldt-Jakob disease
B. Absence seizures
C. Lennox-Gastaut syndrome
D. Subacute sclerosing panencephalitis
E. Herpes encephalitis

70.

A lesion of the nucleus ambiguus would result in what clinical findings?

A. Vertigo, nystagmus, ipsilateral ataxia, contralateral loss of pain and temperature from the body, and ipsilateral loss of pain and temperature from the face
B. Nystagmus to the contralateral side and ipsilateral ataxia
C. Increased heart rate
D. Loss of taste from the ipsilateral anterior two thirds of the tongue
E. Nasal speech, dysphagia, dysphonia, diminished gag reflex, and deviation of the uvula toward the contralateral side

71.

A 78-year-old woman presents to the emergency room after experiencing dizziness and syncope. A neurologic exam revealed decrease pain/temperature sensation on the right side of the body, a left facial palsy, decreased pain/temperature sensation on the left side of the face, left-sided hearing loss, ptosis, nausea, vomiting, and vertigo. An infarction in what vessel is suspected?

A. Vertebral/posterior inferior cerebellar artery
B. Anterior inferior cerebellar artery
C. Superior cerebellar artery
D. Short circumferential pontine basilar perforators
E. Artery of Percheron

72.

What type of gait abnormality may be associated with extrapyramidal disorders?

A. Scissor gait
B. Magnetic gait
C. Antalgic gait
D. Steppage gait
E. Festinating gait

73.

A lesion in the medial longitudinal fasciculus rostral to the abducens nuclei will cause an internuclear ophthalmoplegia. If the lesion affects the left medial longitudinal fasciculus, what will be the neurologic findings?

A. Looking left, the left eye will fail to abduct, and the right eye will have nystagmus.
B. Looking right, the left eye will fail to adduct, and the right eye will have nystagmus.
C. Looking left, the left eye will have nystagmus, and the right eye will fail to adduct.
D. Looking right, the left eye will have nystagmus, and the right eye will fail to abduct.
E. Looking left, the left eye will fail to abduct, and the right eye will fail to adduct.

74.

What is the site of injury in patients with Anton-Babinski syndrome?

A. Bilateral visual cortices and corpus callosum
B. Bilateral retinae with preservation of the visual cortex
C. Unilateral visual cortex and splenium of the corpus callosum
D. Unilateral visual cortex and Broca area
E. Bilateral visual cortices

75.

In patients with alexia without agraphia, what is the most common site of injury?

A. Broca area and left visual cortex
B. Left visual cortex only
C. Splenium of the corpus callosum and right visual cortex
D. Splenium of the corpus callosum and left visual cortex
E. Broca area and splenium of the corpus callosum

76.

For individuals working in loud and noisy environments, what injury can be avoided with hearing protection?

A. Hearing loss and tinnitus
B. Hearing loss and vertigo
C. Ataxia and tinnitus
D. Vertigo and tinnitus
E. Hearing loss and ataxia

77.

A 15-year-old patient has middle ear disease and is complaining of decreased hearing. Relative to a patient without middle ear disease, how are sounds transmitted by air and bone affected in this patient?

A. Normal conduction in air with diminished bone conduction
B. Normal conduction in air and bone
C. Diminished conduction in air with normal bone conduction
D. Diminished conduction in air and bone
E. Increased conduction in air with normal bone conduction

78.

A woman with multiple sclerosis notices that the symptoms worsen when she exercises. What is the reason of this worsening?

A. Increased body temperature
B. Activation of the sympathetic nervous system
C. Deactivation of the parasympathetic nervous system
D. Movement during exercise
E. Decreased oxygen availability

79.

A 45-year-old woman is referred for follow-up. She has been told that she sustained a brachial plexus injury. On exam, she has good bilateral inspiratory function and the scapulae are symmetric, but abduction of the arm cannot be initiated unless the arm is helped through the first 45 degrees of abduction. What is the patient's likely site of injury?

A. Axillary nerve
B. Posterior cord
C. Cervical nerve roots
D. Upper trunk
E. Suprascapular nerve

80.

A 48-year-old homeless man with a history of alcoholism, heroin abuse, smoking, hypertension, and diabetes was brought to the emergency room for evaluation of 3 days of recurrent nausea and vomiting. The patient states that he was not able to keep any food down since his symptoms started. After the patient was started on maintenance intravenous fluids, he started to complain of progressively worsening blurry vision and became increasingly disoriented, ataxic, and dysarthria. What in this patient's history predisposes him to developing this symptomatology?

A. Alcoholism
B. Smoking
C. Substance abuse
D. Hypertension
E. Diabetes

81.

A patient with lateral medullary syndrome has dysphagia secondary to involvement of what structure?

A. Nucleus solitarius
B. Nucleus ambiguus
C. Descending tract of cranial nerve V
D. Inferior cerebellar peduncle
E. Middle cerebellar peduncle

82.

A woman with multiple sclerosis was treated with steroids then maintained on interferon β-1A. After 2 years, she developed another flare of symptoms. What is the most appropriate treatment at this time?

A. Interferon β-1B
B. Corticosteroids
C. Intravenous immunoglobulin
D. Glatiramer
E. Pramipexole

83.

What artery is most likely to be occluded in a patient with lateral medullary syndrome?

A. Basilar
B. Vertebral
C. Superior cerebellar
D. Anterior inferior cerebellar
E. Anterior spinal

84.

A 65-year-old man was found to have a small stroke in the left medial lemniscus. What finding is expected on physical exam?

A. Loss of sensation in the left face and trunk and right upper and lower extremities
B. Loss of sensation in the right face, trunk, and upper and lower extremities
C. Loss of proprioception of the left trunk and upper and lower extremities
D. Loss of proprioception of the right trunk and upper and lower extremities
E. Loss of pain and temperature sensation in the left trunk and upper and lower extremities

85.

What evoked response pattern most often is abnormal in patients with multiple sclerosis?

A. Visual evoked potentials
B. Far field somatosensory evoked responses
C. Brain auditory evoked responses
D. Jolly test
E. Sensory nerve conduction test

86.

A 34-year-old man with HIV on HAART presents with the "worst headache of my life" after sexual intercourse. The patient is found to have a large parietal lobe hematoma. What is the most likely diagnosis?

A. Mycotic aneurysm rupture
B. Hypertensive hemorrhage
C. Traumatic hemorrhage
D. Amyloid angiopathy
E. Berry aneurysm rupture

87.

A 58-year-old man presents for neurologic evaluation. He has a history of chronic renal failure and has been on dialysis for 10 years. What is the most common neurologic complication expected in this patient?

A. Peripheral neuropathy
B. Seizures
C. Stroke
D. Dementia
E. Delirium

6 Radiology

1.

A 56-year-old man presents to the emergency room with 1 week of altered mental status. His medical history is significant for a glioblastoma treated with resection followed by temozolomide therapy and whole brain radiation 1 year ago. An MRI is performed, and contrast-enhanced, diffusion-weighted, and apparent diffusion coefficient sequences are shown in these images. Perfusion maps (not shown) demonstrate decreased relative cerebral blood volume. What is the likely cause of his new symptoms?

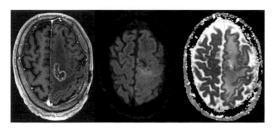

A. Radiation necrosis
B. Recurrent glioblastoma
C. Secondary tumor caused by chemotherapy regimen
D. Encephalomalacia from tumor resection

2.

The lesion shown in these images depicts a(n):

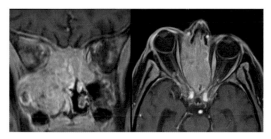

A. Optic nerve glioma
B. Meningioma
C. Chordoma
D. Esthesioneuroblastoma

3.

What likely is associated with the imaging findings on the MR susceptibility-weighted imaging (SWI) sequence shown in these images?

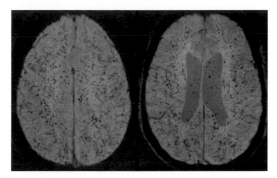

A. Shearing injury from rotational acceleration
B. β-amyloid peptide deposits
C. Mutations in the *CCM1* gene
D. Long bone fractures

4.

A 22-year-old man without a significant medical history presents with progressive midthoracic pain. An MRI examination of the spine is shown in these images. What is the most likely diagnosis?

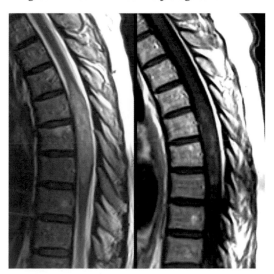

A. Astrocytoma
B. Ependymoma
C. Metastasis
D. Tumefactive demyelination

5.

A neonate underwent an MRI of his brain, shown in this image. What may be an associated finding?

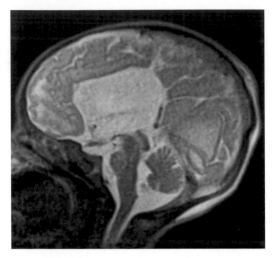

A. Interhemispheric cysts
B. Collapse of ventricular atria and occipital horns
C. Low-riding third ventricle
D. Curvilinear pericallosal lipomas

6.

What is a characteristic of the lesion depicted in the MRI study shown in these images?

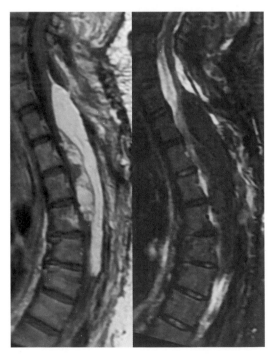

A. Results from premature disjunction of the cutaneous ectoderm from the neuroectoderm during neurulation
B. Infiltrative hypercellular lesion with variable degrees of mitosis/atypia
C. Results from clonal transformation of cells of B-cell origin
D. May be associated with endolymphatic sac tumors, renal cell carcinomas, and retinal angiomas

7.

A 30-year-old woman with a history of recurrent genital and oral aphthae and erythema nodosum underwent an MRI of the brain. What is a likely imaging finding in this patient?

A. Enhancing lesion involving the brainstem
B. Fluid-attentuated inversion recovery (FLAIR) hyperintense lesion sparing red nuclei and substantia nigra
C. Lesions with a leading edge of restricted diffusion
D. Lesions involving the pulvinar and dorsomedial thalamic nuclei
E. Lesions with an incomplete rim of enhancement

8.

A 54-year-old man underwent an MRI of the spine. Sagittal and axial postcontrast T1-weighted images are shown in these images. What is the patient's likely diagnosis?

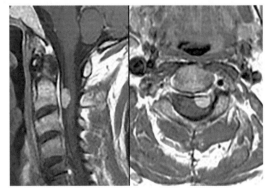

A. Leptomeningeal metastasis
B. Neurofibroma
C. Schwannoma
D. Meningioma

9.

The lesion shown in this image *(arrow)* can result from injury to what structure?

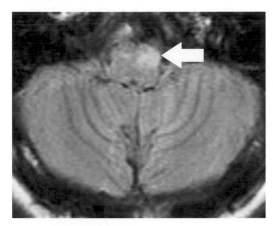

A. Central tegmental tract
B. Lateral lemniscus
C. Spinothalamic tract
D. Reticulospinal tract

10.

Axial T2 and postcontrast T1-weighted imaging of the lumbar spine are shown in these images. To what does the abnormality indicated by the arrow correspond?

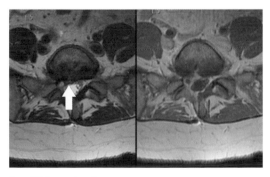

A. Disk protrusion
B. Epidural scar
C. Disk extrusion
D. Epidural abscess
E. Sequestered disk

11.

A 12-year-old girl is brought to the emergency department in an obtunded state following an episode of seizures. Based on these images, what is the diagnosis?

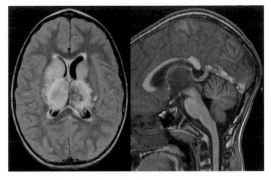

A. Cortical venous thrombosis
B. Deep venous thrombosis
C. Mitochondrial encephalopathy
D. Hypoxic ischemic encephalopathy
E. Arterial infarction

12.

A woman underwent a head CT, shown in these images. What is the likely diagnosis?

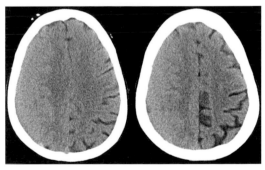

A. Infiltrative tumor
B. Acute infarct
C. Intracranial hemorrhage
D. Meningitis

13.

A boy with truncal ataxia and abnormal eye movements undergoes an MRI of the brain, which shows continuation of the cerebellar hemispheres and dentate nuclei and absence of the vermis. What is the most likely diagnosis?

A. Pontine tegmental cap dysplasia
B. Rhombencephalosynapsis
C. Joubert syndrome
D. Dandy-Walker malformation

14.

A 38-year-old man who sustained a gunshot wound to the head underwent an emergent CT scan, shown in this image. What finding portends the worst prognosis?

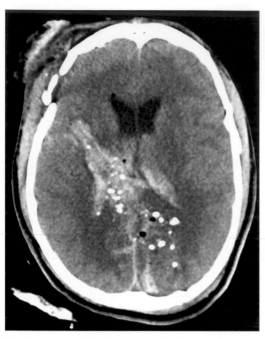

A. Presence of both entry and exit wounds
B. Involvement of the inner and outer tables of the calvaria
C. Bullet tract crossing the deep midline structures
D. Presence of metallic fragments along the bullet trajectory
E. Presence of an open comminuted fracture

15.

The axial CT scan in this image shows the level of termination of bilateral cerebral deep brain stimulation leads. What is the anatomic location of these leads?

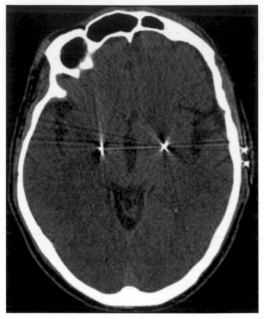

A. Globus pallidus interna
B. Subthalamic nuclei
C. Ventral intermediate nuclei
D. Red nuclei

16.

A man is reported to have a "string of pearls" appearance on his angiogram. What is the likely diagnosis?

A. Severe carotid artery stenosis
B. Dural arteriovenous fistula
C. Fibromuscular dysplasia
D. Arteriovenous malformation
E. Carotid artery dissection

17.

A sagittal T2-weighted image of a patient with a tethered cord is shown in this image. What is a characteristic of the pathology represented here?

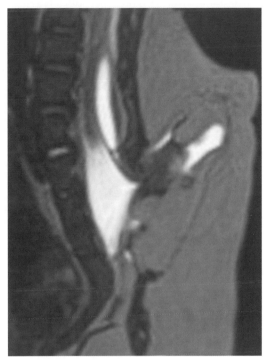

A. Reduced risk following folic acid supplementation

B. Associated with Chiari 2 malformations

C. Secondary to premature disjunction of the neural ectoderm

D. Most cases are familial

18.

What is the origin of the lesion on the contrast-enhanced T1 image shown here?

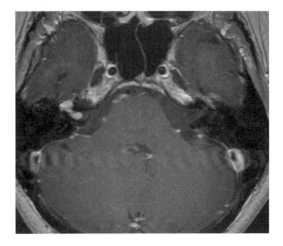

A. Facial nerve

B. Vestibular nerve

C. Aberrant carotid artery

D. Inferior petrosal sinus

19.

A falcotentorial arteriovenous malformation is noted to have its primary vascular supply from an enlarged tentorial artery. What is the usual origin of this vessel?

A. Meningohypophyseal trunk

B. Inferolateral trunk

C. Neuromeningeal trunk

D. Posterior cerebral artery

20.

Sagittal CT and MRI STIR sequences of the cervical spine are shown in these images. What is the injury type demonstrated?

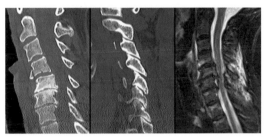

A. Hangman fracture

B. Clay-shoveler fracture

C. Jefferson fracture

D. Flexion-distraction injury

E. Locked facets

21.

What MRI features would favor a metastatic (pathological) compression fracture over a benign osteoporotic fracture?

A. Horizontal low signal intensity bands

B. Convex posterior vertebral margins

C. Areas of spared vertebral marrow

D. Retropulsion of a bone fragment

E. Enhancement of the involved vertebra

22.

A man with a history of depression presents with rapid and involuntary movements involving his face and limbs. The clinical exam is notable for hypotonia, hyperreflexia, and mild bradykinesia. A noncontrast CT of the head is shown in this image. What mutation is the likely cause of the patient's presentation?

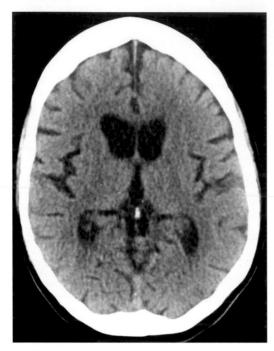

A. Trinucleotide repeat expansion
B. Point mutation
C. Frameshift mutation
D. Deletion

23.

Gradient echo MRI sequences are particularly useful for the detection or evaluation of what process or pathology?

A. Myelin injury
B. Purulence
C. Acute ischemia
D. Glucose metabolism
E. Blood products

24.

A man without a history of trauma is brought to the emergency department with nausea, vomiting, and ataxia. Axial T2-weighted images of the neck and posterior fossa are shown here. What is a characteristic of the lesion in the neck?

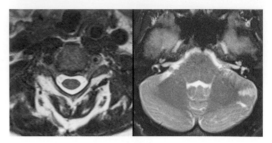

A. It may be related to connective tissue disorders.
B. The majority occur in patients older than 60 years of age.
C. Intradural lesions are more common.
D. Rupture is more common in extradural than intradural lesions.

25.

A 56-year-old patient involved in a motor vehicle collision underwent a cervical spine CT scan, shown in these images. What is true of the osseous abnormality demonstrated?

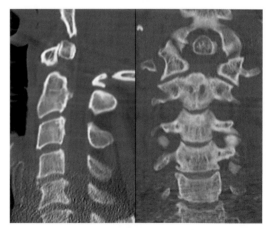

A. It is consistent with an acute type 2 odontoid fracture.
B. It results from failure of fusion of the ossiculum terminale.
C. It is associated with Morquio syndrome and multiple epiphyseal dysplasia.
D. Orthotopic lesions are more likely to be unstable than dystopic lesions.

26.
A 52-year-old obese woman with a history of head-aches presents to clinic. An MRI of the brain was obtained, and is shown in these images. What additional radiographic finding may be seen?

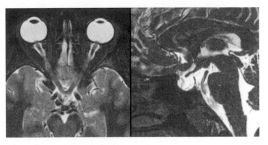

A. Dural venous sinus stenosis
B. Venous sinus engorgement
C. Brainstem sagging
D. Decreased mammillopontine distance

27.
A woman who was involved in a motor vehicle collision underwent a CT of the cervical spine, which shows a fracture involving an occipital condyle. What structure is likely to be affected?

A. Cranial nerve IX
B. Cranial nerve X
C. Cranial nerve XI
D. Cranial nerve XII

28.
The lesion shown in this image is associated with a chromosome 13q deletion. What is a characteristic of this lesion?

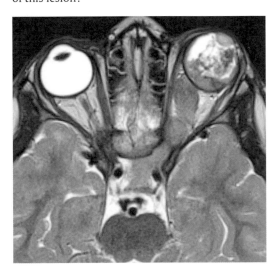

A. Has a tendency for leptomeningeal spread
B. Anterior eye segment enhancement indicates disease infiltration
C. Likely has high apparent diffusion coefficient values
D. Likely has high signal intensity on susceptibility-weighted imaging

29.
What is true regarding the lesion shown in this CT image?

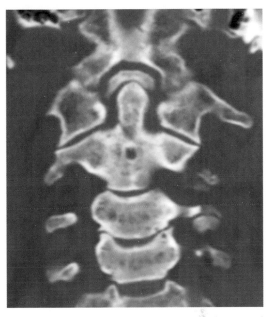

A. Usually heals well with traction and immobilization
B. Usually considered stable
C. Constitutes the most common type of fracture at this site
D. Fracture occurs above the transverse band of the cruciform ligament
E. Most likely fracture type to progress to nonunion

30.

A patient with left-sided cranial neuropathies underwent a brain MRI study, shown in these images. What is a likely complication of this lesion?

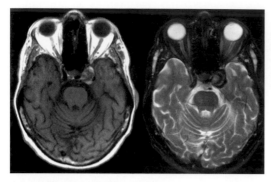

A. Malignant transformation
B. Carotid-cavernous fistula
C. Subarachnoid hemorrhage
D. Posterior circulation infarcts

31.

What is a characteristic of the entity depicted on the digital subtraction angiographic images shown here?

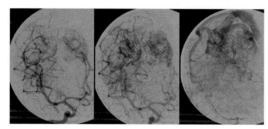

A. Cortical venous reflux denotes increased bleeding risk.
B. Multiple lesions may be seen in Klippel-Trenaunay-Weber syndrome.
C. Deep venous drainage connotes increased surgical risk.
D. Most have a primarily dural vascular supply.

32.

What is a characteristic of the injury shown on this CT scan?

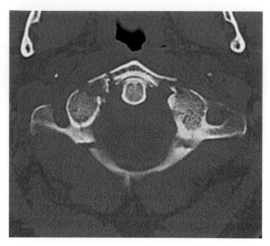

A. Combined offset of the lateral C1 masses relative to C2 greater than 6 mm, which suggests disruption of the alar ligaments
B. Frequently associated with diving head first into shallow water
C. High frequency of neurologic injury
D. Most commonly occurs in infants and young children
E. Usually warrants emergent surgical fixation

33.

The abnormality in the left frontal lobe on the CT of the head shown in this image is consistent with what process?

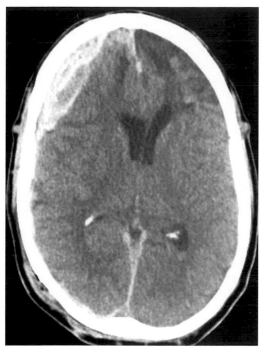

A. Acute infarction
B. Cortical contusion
C. Remote injury
D. Neoplasm
E. Abscess

34.

What entity is compatible with the abnormality indicated by the arrow on the MRI shown in this image?

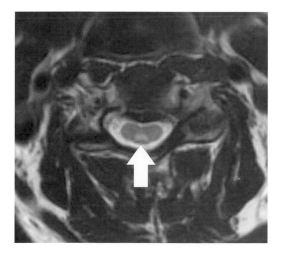

A. Ependymoma
B. Neuromyelitis optica
C. Subacute combined degeneration
D. Infectious myelitis

35.

A patient with extensive T2 hyperintensity and enhancement of the skull base shows a "black turbinate" sign on postcontrast T1 MRI sequences. What is the likely etiology of these findings?

A. Bacterial infection
B. Invasive fungal infection
C. Nasopharyngeal carcinoma
D. Osseous infarction

36.

What explains the development of the abnormality demonstrated on the brain MRI shown in these images?

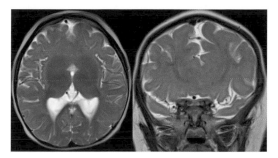

A. Failure of closure of the rostral neuropore
B. Failure of diverticulation
C. Nondisjunction of the neural ectoderm
D. Premature disjunction of the neural ectoderm

37.

What tumor type would be expected to show the lowest apparent diffusion coefficient (ADC) values on an MRI of the brain?

A. Atypical teratoid rhabdoid tumor
B. Juvenile pilocytic astrocytoma
C. Ependymoma
D. Dysembryoplastic neuroepithelial tumor
E. Diffuse astrocytoma

38.

What is a characteristic of acute demyelinating encephalomyelitis?

A. Most cases occur following vaccination.
B. Deep gray nuclei usually are spared.
C. Most lesions show contrast enhancement.
D. It is typically a monophasic process.

39.

A 5-year-old boy with visual and hearing deficits and loss of developmental milestones presents for evaluation. MRI of the brain shows occipitoparietal periventricular demyelination with a leading edge of enhancement. What is the patient's likely diagnosis?

A. Adrenoleukodystrophy
B. Canavan disease
C. Alexander disease
D. Krabbe disease
E. Pelizaeus-Merzbacher disease

40.

The spinal cord lesion in the T2-weighted MRI shown in this image is consistent with what disease process?

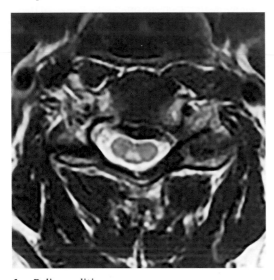

A. Poliomyelitis
B. Amyotrophic lateral sclerosis
C. Guillain-Barré syndrome
D. Subacute combined degeneration

41.

A brain MRI shows a small lesion in the pons that is slightly hyperintense on T2-weighted imaging and shows "brush-like" enhancement and signal dropout on gradient echo sequences. There is no surrounding edema. This lesion is consistent with what disease process?

A. Demyelinating plaque
B. Metastasis
C. Cavernous malformation
D. Capillary telangiectasia

42.

Where is a type C carotid-cavernous fistula located according to the Barrow classification?

A. Between meningeal branches of the external carotid artery and cavernous sinus
B. Between meningeal branches of the internal carotid artery and cavernous sinus
C. Directly between the cavernous internal carotid artery and cavernous sinus
D. Between meningeal branches of both the external and internal carotid arteries and cavernous sinus

43.

What is a characteristic of the lesion depicted in the MRI shown in these images?

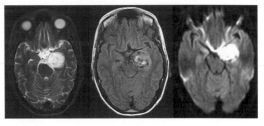

A. Lined by arachnoid cells resulting in accumulation of cerebrospinal fluid
B. Most are intraventricular
C. Show complete signal suppression on MR FLAIR sequences
D. Usually show areas of patchy enhancement
E. Associated with a risk of malignant transformation

44.

A 12-year-old boy presented to the emergency department with progressive headaches, nausea, and vomiting. Axial T2 and contrast-enhanced T1-weighted imaging and apparent diffusion coefficient maps are shown in these images. What is the patient's likely diagnosis?

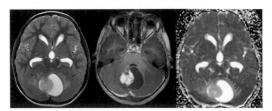

A. Medulloblastoma
B. Ependymoma
C. Pilocytic astrocytoma
D. Hemangioblastoma
E. Metastasis

45.

A 74-year-old woman presents to the emergency room complaining of vertigo and nausea increasing in severity over the past several hours. CT and MRI studies were performed, and representative images are shown here. This lesion likely represents a(n):

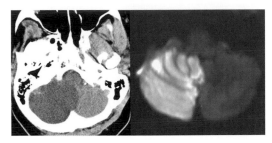

A. Primary neoplasm
B. Acute infarction
C. Metastatic disease
D. Arachnoid cyst
E. Epidermoid cyst

46.

A man who was found lying on the ground underwent an emergent CT of the head, shown in these images. What is the likely diagnosis?

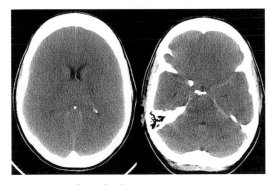

A. Ruptured cerebral aneurysm
B. Acute arterial infarction
C. Global anoxic injury
D. Venous thrombosis

47.

A young woman underwent an MRI study, shown in these images. What tumor is she at risk of developing?

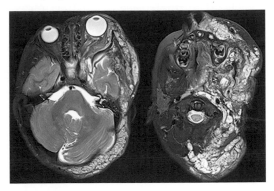

A. Glioma
B. Meningioma
C. Ependymoma
D. Endolymphatic sac tumor
E. Subependymal giant cell tumor

48.

What factor favors an epidural versus a subdural empyema?

A. Restricted diffusion
B. Crescentic shape
C. Crosses sutures
D. Less common cerebral edema
E. Peripheral enhancement

49.
A mass, shown in this image, was discovered in a 29-year-old woman presenting with progressive bitemporal hemianopsia and hyperprolactinemia. Immunohistochemistry and electron microscopy following resection demonstrated chromophobic tumor cells and "misplaced exocytosis" with extrusion of secretory granules. What neuroimaging feature is highly suggestive of cavernous sinus invasion?

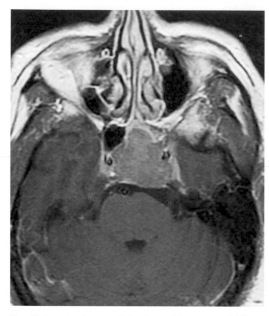

A. Extension beyond the lateral intercarotid line
B. Carotid encasement greater than 180 degrees
C. Obliteration of the superior venous compartment
D. Obliteration of the inferolateral venous compartment

50.
What is a characteristic of the lesion depicted in this angiogram?

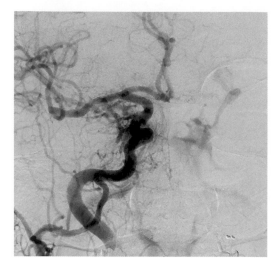

A. Fibromuscular dysplasia predisposes to an increased risk of direct-type lesions.
B. Spontaneous intracranial hemorrhage is the most common presentation.
C. Dural-type lesions commonly present with a subjective bruit.
D. A majority of direct-type lesions result from venous thrombosis.
E. Dural-type lesions most commonly present in young males.

51.
The tumor depicted in the MRI shown in these images demonstrated microcysts and mild pleomorphism on histological examination and stained positive for glial fibrillary acidic protein, neuron-specific enolase, and neuronal cell adhesion molecule. What is true about this lesion?

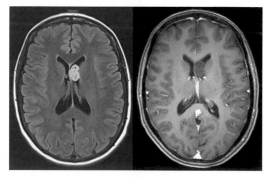

A. Associated with a high recurrence rate
B. Presents most commonly in young adults
C. Frequently complicated by hemorrhage
D. Associated with *TSC-1* and *TSC-2* gene mutations
E. Usually shows minimal to no contrast enhancement

52.

What is a feature of the focal areas of signal intensity (FASI) or unidentified bright objects (UBOs) in neurofibromatosis type 1?

A.   They are most common in basal ganglia and dentate nuclei.

B.   They are premalignant lesions.

C.   A small proportion show contrast enhancement.

D.   The presence of mass effect is characteristic.

53.

What MRI sequence specifically should be included to evaluate a patient with suspected cerebral abscess?

A.   Susceptibility weighted

B.   Diffusion weighted

C.   Time of flight

D.   Constructive interference in steady state (CISS)

E.   FLAIR

54.

A 74-year-old man underwent a CT study of the chest, which demonstrated the lesion shown in these images. This lesion is compatible with what diagnosis?

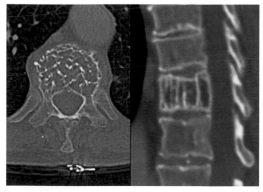

A.   Metastasis

B.   Paget disease

C.   Hemangioma

D.   Plasmacytoma

55.

A 67-year-old man with left L5 radiculopathy underwent MRI of the lumbar spine, shown in this image. This lesion likely represents a(n):

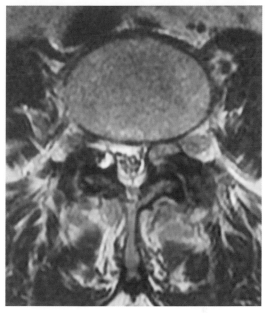

A.   Extruded disk

B.   Synovial cyst

C.   Ligamentum flavum hypertrophy

D.   Uncovertebral joint hypertrophy

56.

What is true regarding the lesion indicated by the arrow in the contrast-enhanced T1-weighted MRI shown in this image?

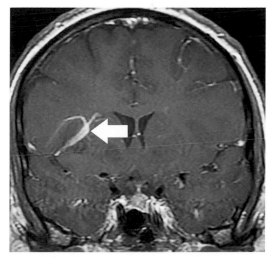

A.   It is usually angiographically occult.

B.   It is composed of radially arranged medullary veins emptying into a dilated draining vein.

C.   High flow from shunting may result in flow-related aneurysms.

D.   A larger nidus is associated with an increased surgical risk.

57.
A patient presents to clinic for follow-up after suffering from a nontraumatic retinal detachment. The lesion shown in these images is found on a subsequent MRI. The patient should be screened for:

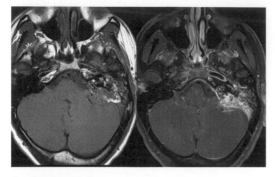

A. Lisch nodules
B. Bilateral vestibular schwannomas
C. Subependymal giant cell astrocytoma
D. Renal cell carcinoma
E. Low levels of serum ceruloplasmin

58.
What is a characteristic of the condition depicted in the T2-weighted MRI shown in this image?

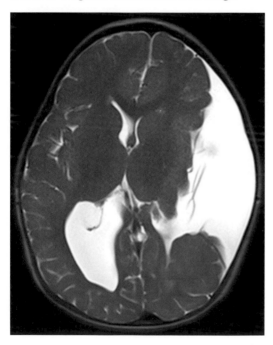

A. Lined by dysplastic white matter
B. Frequently accompanied by microcephaly and other cerebral anomalies
C. Lined by endodermal endothelium
D. May show variable signal intensities depending on its contents
E. Results from a bilateral vascular insult to the anterior cerebral circulation in utero

59.
A 12-year-old boy with progressive headaches and lower cranial nerve palsies underwent an MRI scan, shown in these images. Which is the likely diagnosis?

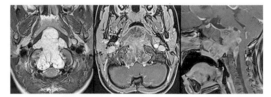

A. Chondrosarcoma
B. Chordoma
C. Nasopharyngeal carcinoma
D. Meningioma
E. Lymphoma

60.
A man presented with dysfunction of the left cranial nerves V and VI. T1- and T2-weighted MRI and the corresponding apparent diffusion coefficient (ADC) map are shown in these images. What is the patient's likely diagnosis?

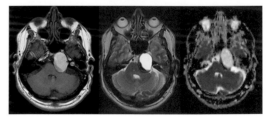

A. Cholesterol granuloma
B. Cholesteatoma
C. Trapped secretions within pneumatized petrous cells
D. Trigeminal schwannoma

61.

What is the likely mechanism that caused the injury shown in this image?

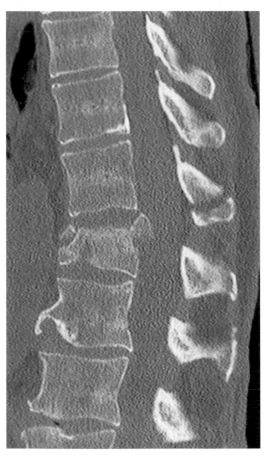

A. Lateral bending and compression
B. Axial rotation
C. Abrupt extension
D. Axial loading
E. Flexion and distraction

62.

A 37-year-old man who is an intravenous drug user presented with headaches. An MRI of the brain was performed, shown in these images. What is an additional expected imaging finding?

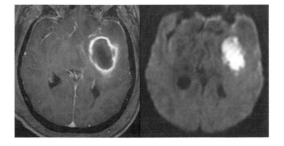

A. Presence of lactate and amino acids on MR spectroscopy
B. Hyperintense capsule on T2 sequence
C. Increased apparent diffusion coefficient values in the center of the lesion
D. High relative cerebral blood volume ratio in the capsule relative to white matter

63.

A 75-year-old man underwent a CT scan of the head. Representative images are shown here. What is the patient's likely diagnosis?

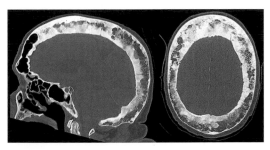

A. Multiple myeloma
B. β-thalassemia
C. Prostate cancer metastases
D. Paget disease

64.

The digital subtraction angiogram shown here depicts a(n):

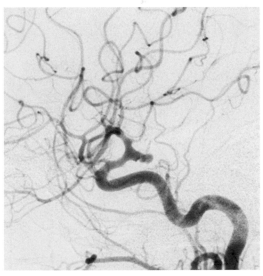

A. Middle cerebral artery/anterior cerebral artery bifurcation aneurysm
B. Posterior communicating artery aneurysm
C. Basilar tip aneurysm
D. Ophthalmic artery aneurysm

65.

A 53-year-old man is status post–glioblastoma resection and radiation therapy with concomitant temozolomide. A brain MRI shows an increasing enhancing lesion. What neuroimaging finding would favor the presence of recurrent tumor over radiation necrosis/pseudoprogression?

A. Increased apparent diffusion coefficient (ADC) values
B. Increased relative cerebral blood volumes
C. "Cut green pepper" appearance
D. Decreased FDG uptake on PET

66.

A 48-year-old woman with a history of HIV underwent a brain MRI, shown in this image. The MRI findings are consistent with:

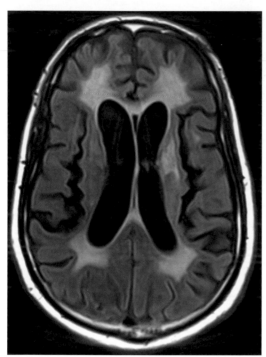

A. Lymphoma
B. Progressive multifocal leukoencephalopathy
C. HIV encephalopathy
D. Cerebritis

67.

What MRI sequences are necessary for the evaluation of Hirayama disease?

A. Gradient echo sequences
B. Delayed contrast sequences
C. Diffusion-weighted sequences
D. Flexion/extension sequences

68.

A 45-year-old immigrant presents with a several month history of back pain and malaise. There is no history of fever. An MRI was performed, shown in this image. What is the likely diagnosis?

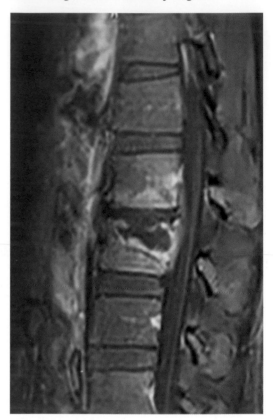

A. Pyogenic diskitis/osteomyelitis
B. Tuberculous spondylitis
C. Degenerative disk disease
D. Osseous metastases

69.

The presence of a "swirl" sign is described on a CT of the head. This finding indicates:

A. Thrombosis
B. Malignant transformation
C. Acute extravasation
D. Abscess formation

70.

A coronal noncontrast CT reformat of a 35-year-old woman is shown in this image. What process is likely to be directly related to the represented disease?

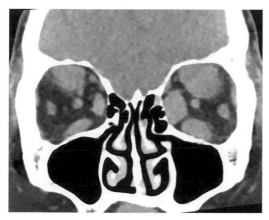

A. Cytokine release and production of muco-polysaccharides
B. Hematogenous spread of poorly differentiated adenocarcinoma
C. IgG4-positive lymphoplasmacytic infiltration
D. Monoclonal B-cell population

71.

What is an expected radiographic finding in tension pneumothorax?

A. Ipsilateral diaphragmatic elevation
B. Contralateral increased intercostal spaces
C. "Deep sulcus" sign
D. Mediastinal deviation to the contralateral side
E. Tracheal deviation to the ipsilateral side

72.

A CT of the lumbar spine shows a squared vertebra with a "picture frame" appearance. This finding is consistent with what disease process?

A. Paget disease
B. Vertebral hemangioma
C. Lytic metastasis
D. Blastic metastasis

73.

What structure is supplied by the arteries shown in this image *(arrows)*?

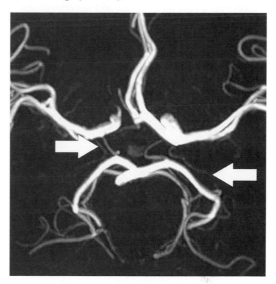

A. Posterior limb of the internal capsule
B. Anterior limb of the internal capsule
C. Anteromedial caudate nucleus
D. External capsule
E. Thalamus

74.
A 23-year-old man is brought to the emergency department following a high-velocity motor vehicle collision. An emergent CT of the cervical spine is shown in this image. What is a characteristic of this lesion?

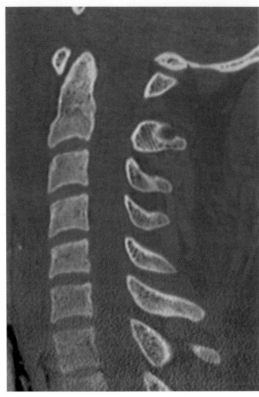

A. Uncommon in children
B. High incidence of neurovascular injury
C. Occurs secondary to axial loading
D. May be identified by a basion-dental interval greater than 7 mm

75.
A 45-year-old woman with history of breast cancer underwent an MRI study of the brain. What is a common clinical manifestation of the process presented in these images?

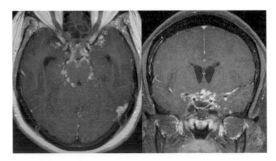

A. Meningismus
B. Headache
C. Ischemia
D. Diabetes insipidus
E. Dysarthria

76.
Axial noncontrast CT and T2-weighted MRI are shown in these images. What is the likely diagnosis?

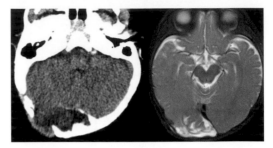

A. Langerhans cell histiocytosis
B. Epidermoid
C. Abscess
D. Leptomeningeal cyst

77.
A 48-year-old man underwent CT and MR studies after presenting with left-sided ophthalmoplegia. The lesion enhanced following the administration of intravenous contrast material and did not show restricted diffusion. Representative images are shown here. What is correct regarding this entity?

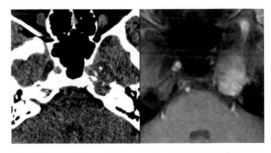

A. Commonly produces a chondroid matrix
B. Consists of granulation tissue and cholesterol crystals
C. Represents trapped secretions within the petrous apex
D. Arises from aberrant ectoderm within petrous apex cells
E. Commonly demonstrates low apparent diffusion coefficient values

78.

A 42-year-old man with back pain underwent an MRI examination of the lumbar spine, shown in this image. What is an expected imaging finding in this patient?

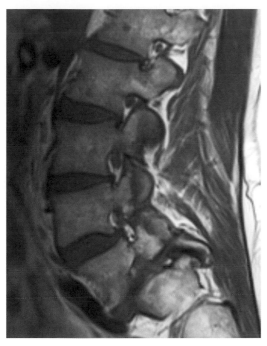

A. Expansion of the L5 vertebra
B. Sclerosis of the contralateral pars inter-articularis
C. Widening of the spinal canal on a midsagittal image
D. Widening of the neural foramina

79.

A 40-year-old woman with a history of an intra-cranial aneurysm was brought to the emergency department after being found lying on the ground. An emergent CT scan showed diffuse sulcal and cisternal hyperdensity. Images from a CT angio-gram and cerebral blood volume (CBV) perfusion map performed 5 days later are shown here. What complication is seen?

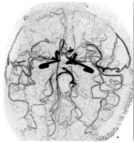 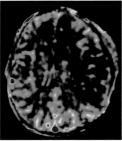

A. Embolic infarcts following angiography
B. Cerebritis
C. Venous thrombosis
D. Vasospasm

80.

A 14-year-old boy with a history of stroke presented for evaluation. 3D time-of-flight and T2-weighted sequences at the level of the circle of Willis are shown in these images. What is a characteristic of this disease?

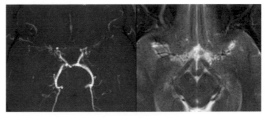

A. It most commonly presents in the elderly population.
B. It may show abnormal MRI signal in engorged pial vessels.
C. Dystonia and choreoathetosis are the most common clinical manifestations.
D. The posterior circulation is most commonly affected.

81.

A 32-year-old woman with a long-standing his-tory of intractable epilepsy underwent a contrast-enhanced MRI of the brain, shown in these images. What is a characteristic of this lesion?

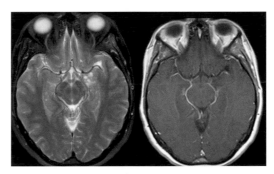

A. Classified as a WHO grade II tumor
B. Commonly associated with focal cortical dysplasia
C. Shows low signal on apparent diffusion coeffi-cient maps
D. Most demonstrate contrast enhancement
E. Has a propensity for leptomeningeal spread

82.

What is routinely a non-enhancing neural structure on contrast-enhanced MRI?

A. Area postrema
B. Organum vasculosum
C. Fornix
D. Anterior pituitary
E. Pineal gland

83.

A patient status post–resection of a right vestibular schwannoma underwent a noncontrast MRI study, shown in these images. What vessel has been injured?

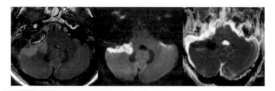

A. Superior cerebellar artery
B. Posterior inferior cerebellar artery
C. Anterior inferior cerebellar artery
D. Superior cerebellar vein
E. Inferior cerebellar vein

84.

A brain MRI shows a small lesion in the pons that is slightly hyperintense on T2-weighted images and shows "brush-like" enhancement and signal dropout on gradient echo sequences. There is no surrounding edema. This is consistent with what pathology?

A. Demyelinating plaque
B. Metastasis
C. Cavernous malformation
D. Capillary telangiectasia

85.

An axial FLAIR image is shown here. What diagnosis is represented?

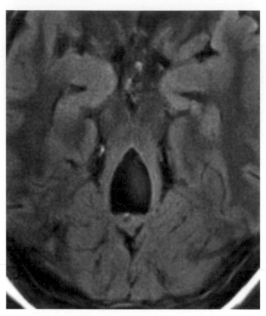

A. Rhombencephalosynapsis
B. Dandy-Walker malformation
C. Blake pouch cyst
D. Mega cisterna magna
E. Joubert syndrome

86.

A 9-year-old girl with a long-standing history of seizures and mental retardation presented to the emergency room with nausea, vomiting, and papilledema. Physical examination demonstrated a rash in the malar region and thick, nodular plaques with a leathery texture on the lower back. T2-weighted and contrast-enhanced T1-weighted MRI of the brain are shown in these images. What is a characteristic of the lesion depicted on the MRI scan?

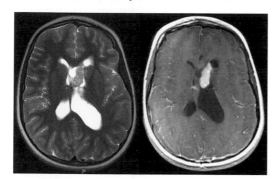

A. Histologically consists of balloon cells with prominent nucleoli
B. Categorized as a WHO grade II tumor
C. Usually develops after the fourth decade of life
D. Fifty percent are associated with malignant transformation
E. Typical bubbly appearance and attachment to the septum pellucidum

87.

An axial noncontrast CT and a sagittal contrast-enhanced T1-weighted MRI of the head are shown in these images. The lesion depicted likely represents a(n):

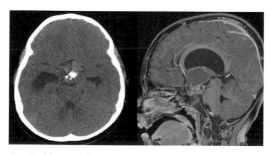

A. Epidermoid
B. Craniopharyngioma
C. Germinoma
D. Thrombosed aneurysm
E. Pituitary adenoma

88.

What is a radiological finding in syntelencephaly?

A. Absent body of the corpus callosum
B. Non-separation of the frontal and occipital poles
C. Absent sylvian fissure
D. Absent interhemispheric fissure

89.

Contrast-enhanced T1 and diffusion-weighted (b = 1,000) imaging with a corresponding apparent diffusion coefficient map are shown in these images. What is a characteristic of the lesion shown?

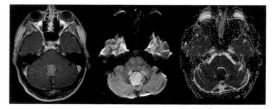

A. Ependymal rosettes may be seen.
B. It is a low-grade, capillary-rich neoplasm.
C. It is formed by sheets of small round blue cells.
D. Rosenthal fibers may be present.

90.

What is a characteristic of neurocysticercosis?

A. Lesions commonly occur at gray matter–white matter junctions.
B. It is acquired by ingesting undercooked pork.
C. Contrast enhancement is the hallmark of the vesicular stage.
D. It has an increased incidence in AIDS patients.
E. Spinal cord involvement is seen in 20% of cases.

91.

A 23-year-old otherwise healthy man presents with first-onset seizures. What is a characteristic of the lesion depicted in the MRI study shown here?

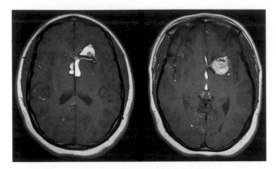

A.   Can result in vasospasm after rupture
B.   Does not contain dermal appendages
C.   Demonstrates increased alanine on MR spectroscopy at short TE
D.   Chemical meningitis is a frequent complication.
E.   May degenerate into a high-grade glial tumor

92.

The lesion depicted in the MRI shown in these images was found incidentally and has been stable over many years. What is a characteristic of this lesion?

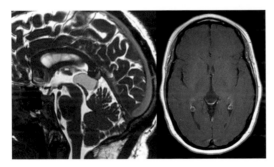

A.   More common in women
B.   Should suppress on FLAIR sequences
C.   Generally demonstrate restricted diffusion
D.   Two thirds eventually are complicated by hydrocephalus
E.   Lined by ependymal cells

93.

What is a characteristic imaging finding in spinal paragangliomas?

A.   "Target" sign
B.   Intrinsic T1 hyperintensity
C.   Flow voids
D.   Intramedullary expansion

94.

A 9-month-old girl with a prior finding of ventriculomegaly on a prenatal ultrasound study underwent half Fourier acquisition single shot turbo spin echo (HASTE) T2-weighted sequences of the brain. What is a characteristic of the entity shown in this image?

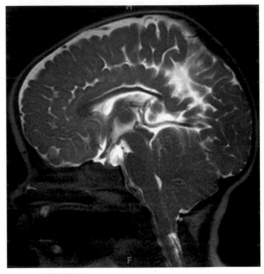

A.   The presence of a skin-covered myelomeningocele is a requisite for its development.
B.   It is not clinically significant unless peg-like tonsils descend greater than 5 mm below the foramen magnum.
C.   Gray matter heterotopia is present in 10 to 30% of cases.
D.   It may be associated with a monoventricle.

95.
Axial T2 images of the cervical spine are shown here. What is the likely diagnosis for this pathology?

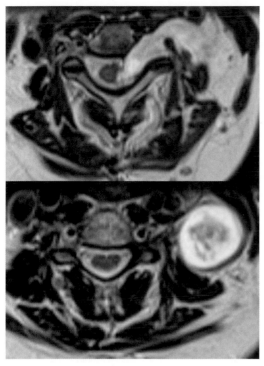

A. Paraganglioma
B. Ependymoma
C. Meningioma
D. Peripheral nerve sheath tumor

96.
A patient with an intracerebral hemorrhage is noted to have a positive "spot sign" on a CT angiogram. This indicates a(n):

A. Underlying neoplasm
B. Underlying arteriovenous malformation
C. Increased risk of hemorrhage expansion
D. Hypertensive hemorrhage
E. Underlying arteriovenous fistula

97.
A man status post–resection of a meningioma complains of shortness of breath. The chest radiograph shows bilateral "bat-wing" pulmonary opacities, Kerley lines, peribronchial cuffing, and blunting of the costophrenic angles. What is the likely cause of his symptoms?

A. Pneumonitis
B. Pulmonary edema
C. Aspiration
D. Infection

98.
A patient with a history of seizures is found to have left-sided cerebral hemiatrophy and ipsilateral cortical/subcortical calcifications, some of which show a "tram track" configuration. What are the expected additional features of this disease entity?

A. Leptomeningeal angiomatosis
B. Atrophy of the ipsilateral choroid plexus
C. Facial capillary malformation sparing the ophthalmic and maxillary division territories of the trigeminal nerve
D. Aplasia of the ipsilateral frontal sinuses
E. Thinning of the ipsilateral calvaria

99.
What finding is suggestive of cryptococcal infection?

A. Concentric T2 FLAIR "target" sign
B. Eccentric "target" sign
C. Pseudocysts
D. Enhancing nodules with low T2 signal intensity

100.

A 52-year-old man with long-standing symptoms underwent a CT of the cervical spine, shown in this image. What is the most common clinical manifestation of the condition shown?

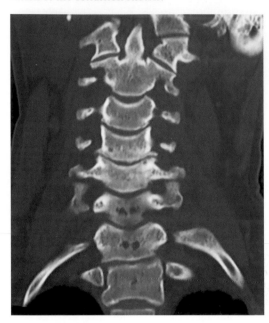

A. Hand ischemia
B. Hand and arm dysesthesia
C. Muscle atrophy
D. Upper extremity swelling
E. Collateral vein formation

101.

A man with a history of seizures undergoes an MRI of the brain, which shows numerous non-enhancing and mildly expansile cortical/subcortical lesions and subependymal nodules. There also are T2 hyperintense radial white matter lines and small parenchymal cysts. What gene is involved in this patient's process?

A. *NF1*
B. *TSC1/TSC2*
C. *NF2*
D. *VHL*
E. *SMARCB1*

102.

A woman is noted to have an "empty delta" sign on a contrast-enhanced CT of the head. This finding likely is secondary to:

A. Cortical vein thrombosis
B. Dural venous thrombosis
C. Subdural blood along the posterior falx
D. Deep venous thrombosis
E. Subarachnoid hemorrhage

103.

The "scalpel" sign in the spine is used to describe what pathological condition?

A. Epidural hematoma
B. Spinal cord herniation
C. Arachnoid cyst
D. Dorsal arachnoid web

104.

The lesion shown on this diffusion-weighted image no longer was present on a follow-up MRI performed 1 month later. What may be associated with such an abnormality?

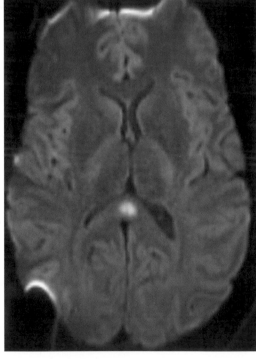

A. Demyelinating plaque
B. Embolic infarct
C. Antiepileptic drug usage
D. Acute disseminated encephalomyelitis

105.
A child presents for evaluation and undergoes a CT scan of the head. A surface-rendered 3D reconstruction is shown in this image. What gene may be altered in the patient's disorder?

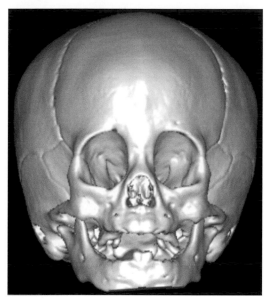

A. *TSC1*
B. *NOTCH3*
C. *FGFR*
D. *SMARCB1*

106.
A woman undergoes a myelogram of the lumbar spine, which shows an "empty sac" sign. This appearance is described in what entity?

A. Arachnoid cyst
B. Arachnoiditis
C. Intradural tumor
D. Epidural collection
E. Subdural collection

107.
An MRI on a patient with a left preauricular squamous cell carcinoma invading the parotid gland shows new tumor infiltration of the mandibular branch of the left trigeminal nerve and the Meckel cave. Along what nerve is the likely route of the tumoral spread?

A. Maxillary nerve
B. Greater superficial petrosal nerve
C. Vidian nerve
D. Auriculotemporal nerve

108.
A 65-year-old man presenting with a relatively rapid progression of left limb ataxia and intention tremors underwent an MRI examination. Axial postcontrast T1 and diffusion-weighted (b = 1,000) images and corresponding apparent diffusion coefficient map are shown here. What is the likely diagnosis?

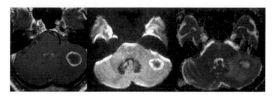

A. Metastasis
B. Glioblastoma
C. Tumefactive demyelination
D. Abscess
E. Toxoplasmosis

109.
The lesion found on the contrast-enhanced MRI shown here demonstrates a *1p36* deletion on fluorescence in situ hybridization. What is a characteristic of this lesion?

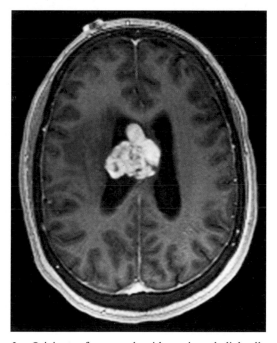

A. Originates from arachnoid meningothelial cells
B. Most common in the pediatric population
C. Associated with mutations in or inactivation of hamartin
D. Arises from the ependymal lining of the ventricular system
E. Usually stains positive for glial fibrillary acidic protein

110.

A frontal view digital subtraction angiogram following a right carotid artery injection is shown in this image. What is the likely etiology of the lesion demonstrated?

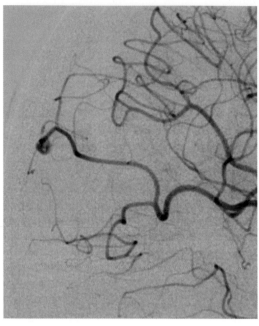

A. Atherosclerosis
B. Immune vasculitis
C. Congenital
D. Endocarditis

111.

A man with altered mental status has necrosis of the retinae and optic disks. An MRI of the brain shows necrosis of the lateral putamina and white matter edema bilaterally. What is the patient's most likely diagnosis?

A. Creutzfeldt-Jakob disease
B. Methanol intoxication
C. Carbon monoxide intoxication
D. Wernicke encephalopathy

112.

A 43-year-old man involved in a motor vehicle collision underwent an emergent CT scan of the head, shown in this image. What is a characteristic of this lesion?

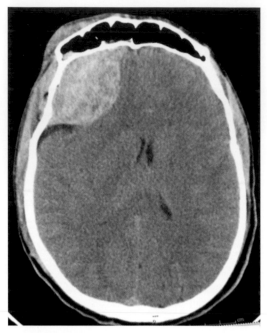

A. Often respects cranial sutures
B. Does not cross the midline
C. Mixed density contents predict stability
D. Most commonly occurs secondary to venous injury
E. Develops between the inner and outer layers of the dura

113.

What is a characteristic of the midbrain lesion shown in these images?

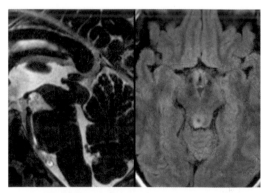

A. Focal radiotherapy is the initial treatment of choice.
B. The majority are low-grade lesions.
C. It is the most common cause of congenital hydrocephalus.
D. It may be related to mutations in the *L1CAM* gene.

114.

Axial FLAIR images of the brain of a 43-year-old woman are shown here. What ancillary laboratory finding may be present?

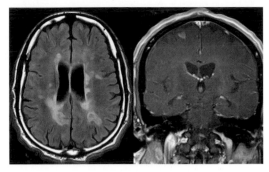

A. Serum aquaporin-4 antibodies
B. Serum cryptococcal antigen
C. Cerebrospinal fluid anti–*Borrelia burgdorferi* antibodies
D. Cerebrospinal fluid IgG and IgM oligoclonal bands

115.

A 17-year-old boy with progressive facial swelling underwent a noncontrast CT scan, shown in this image. This imaging finding is consistent with:

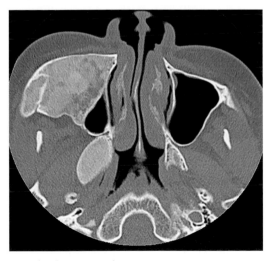

A. Blastic metastasis
B. Paget disease
C. Fibrous dysplasia
D. Plasmacytoma

116.

A 60-year-old man with gait ataxia and nystagmus underwent an MRI of the brain that showed a "hot cross bun" sign. What is an additional finding in this disease entity?

A. Molar tooth configuration
B. Thin middle cerebellar peduncles
C. "Hummingbird" sign
D. Nonvisualization of nigrosome-1

117.

An MRI of the brain is performed, and the report describes the presence of a lesion in the cerebellar hemisphere with a "corduroy" appearance. This lesion likely represents:

A. Cerebellitis
B. A medulloblastoma
C. A subacute posterior inferior cerebellar artery infarct
D. A dysplastic cerebellar gangliocytoma

118.

What imaging characteristic would favor lymphoma over toxoplasmosis in a patient with AIDS?

A. Concentric T2 FLAIR "target" sign
B. Eccentric "target" sign
C. Increased perfusion on an MR relative cerebral blood flow map
D. Decreased uptake on thallium-201 SPECT
E. Lipid peak on MR spectroscopy

119.

A 33-year-old woman presents to the emergency department with an abrupt-onset, recurrent "thunderclap" headache. The initial CT scan of the head shows a small-volume, convex subarachnoid hemorrhage. Lateral view digital subtraction angiography is shown in this image. What is the patient's diagnosis?

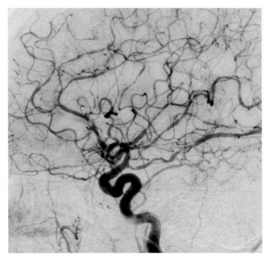

A. Venous infarction
B. Reversible cerebral vasoconstriction syndrome
C. Aneurysmal rupture
D. Acute vascular occlusion

120.

A 1-year-old boy undergoes an MRI of the chest and thoracic spine, which shows a paravertebral mass resulting in scalloping of the adjacent vertebrae and ribs. The mass demonstrated avid uptake on ^{123}I-metaiodobenzylguanidine (^{123}I-MIBG) scintigraphy. What is the patient's likely diagnosis?

A. Giant cell tumor
B. Eosinophilic granuloma
C. Neuroblastoma
D. Aneurysmal bone cyst

121.

A 42-year-old patient presents to the emergency department with focal back pain not relieved by rest. He underwent an MRI examination, shown in these images. What is/are likely to be found in the patient's history?

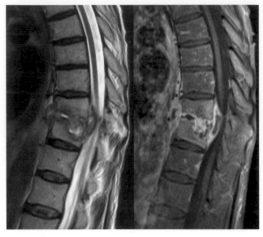

A. Lung cancer
B. Intravenous drug use
C. Fall from a height
D. Anemia, hypercalcemia, and renal failure
E. Seronegative spondyloarthropathy

122.

A 61-year-old man presents to the emergency department with 1 day of fever, seizures, and a decreased level of consciousness. FLAIR and diffusion-weighted images from an emergent MRI scan are shown here. What is a characteristic of this entity?

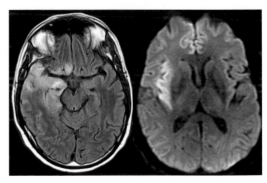

A. Most commonly caused by herpes simplex virus type 2
B. Typically involves the basal ganglia
C. Associated with hemorrhagic necrosis
D. Mediated by paraneoplastic antineuronal (anti-Hu) nuclear antibodies
E. Characterized by diffuse neoplastic glial cell infiltration

123.

A non-enhancing, cystic-appearing extra-axial lesion is seen on an MRI of the brain. What is the most important sequence that likely will aid in the characterization of this lesion?

A. FLAIR
B. Susceptibility weighted
C. Gradient recalled echo
D. T2 weighted
E. Dynamic susceptibility contrast perfusion

124.

Occlusion of the vessel shown in this image *(arrow)* may result in infarction of what territories?

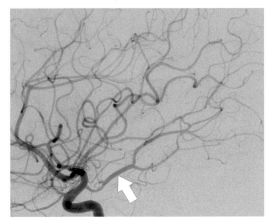

A. Superior cerebellum, superior vermis, dentate nuclei, and part of the midbrain
B. Posteroinferior cerebellum, inferior cerebellar vermis, and lateral medulla
C. Occipital lobe, thalamus, and part of the midbrain
D. Anterior aspect of the right cerebellar hemisphere and middle cerebellar peduncle

125.

A 65-year-old man patient underwent an MRI of the brain, shown in these images. What is the patient's likely diagnosis?

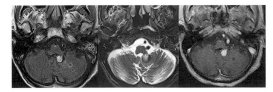

A. Aneurysm
B. Meningioma
C. Choroid plexus tumor
D. Subependymoma

126.

A woman underwent an MRI of the brain, shown in these images) for evaluation of headaches. What is the likely diagnosis?

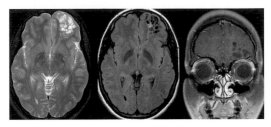

A. Giant perivascular space
B. Dysembryoplastic neuroepithelial tumor
C. Metastasis
D. Cystic glioma

127.

A 9-year-old girl with a history of uncontrollable laughing spells underwent an MRI scan and was found to have the lesion depicted in this image that was isointense to the cerebral cortex on T1-weighted images (not shown). What is an additional expected diagnostic feature of this entity?

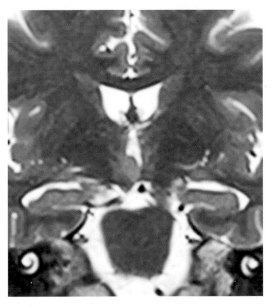

A. Precocious puberty
B. Moderate contrast enhancement
C. Progressive growth
D. Coarse calcifications

128.

A brain MRI of a 32-year-old man shows numerous parenchymal lesions of various sizes that have a "popcorn" or "berry" appearance and show signal loss on susceptibility-weighted sequences. There is no history of prior radiation. What is a possible germline gene mutation in this patient?

A. *ENG*
B. *CCM1*
C. *ACVRL1*
D. *RASA1*

129.

A sagittal MRI of the brain is shown in this image. What is the likely diagnosis?

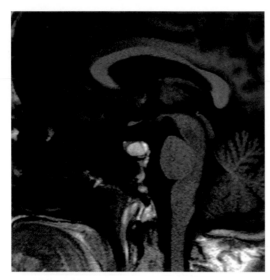

A. Craniopharyngioma
B. Rathke cleft cyst
C. Lymphocytic hypophysitis
D. Granular cell tumor
E. Neurosarcoidosis

130.

What characteristic is more common in adult craniopharyngiomas compared with those that occur in children?

A. Cystic changes
B. Solid appearance
C. Calcifications
D. Heterogeneous contrast enhancement
E. Lower apparent diffusion coefficient values

131.

A high-resolution axial CT of the left temporal bone is shown in this image. To what structure does the arrow point?

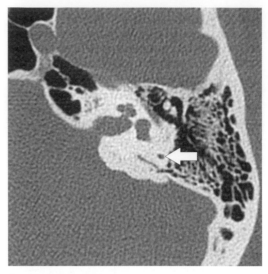

A. Singular canal
B. Facial nerve canal
C. Vestibular aqueduct
D. Semicircular canal

132.

What is an imaging characteristic of progressive multifocal leukoencephalopathy?

A. Symmetric signal abnormalities
B. Prominent edema
C. Leading edge of high diffusion-weighted imaging signal
D. Heterogeneous enhancement
E. Sparing of subcortical U fibers

133.

The lesion shown in these images demonstrates sheets of densely packed cells, hyperchromatic nuclei, and Homer-Wright rosettes. What is a common neuroimaging feature of this lesion?

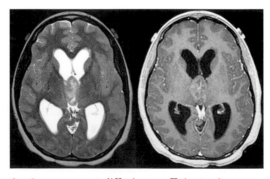

A. Low apparent diffusion coefficient values
B. "Engulfed" calcifications
C. Low density on CT
D. Dural tail

134.

A 28-year-old woman presents with acute-onset severe headache and diplopia. Representative MR images are shown here. What is the patient's likely diagnosis?

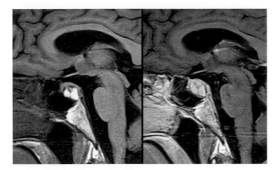

A. Pituitary apoplexy
B. Craniopharyngioma
C. Epidermoid
D. Aneurysmal rupture

135.

The lesion shown here, found in a 25-year-old woman, was hyperdense to gray matter on non-contrast CT and showed restricted diffusivity on apparent diffusion coefficient maps. A normal pituitary gland was identified on sagittal MRI (not shown). Pathology demonstrated sheets of large, polygonal primitive cells with clear, glycogen-rich cytoplasm and abundance of lymphocytes. How does this lesion respond to radiation?

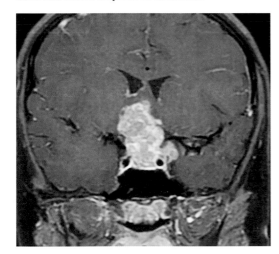

A. The pathology is entirely radiation insensitive and should not be treated by radiation.
B. The lesion is mostly radiation insensitive, but radiation may be somewhat effective.
C. The lesion is mostly radiation sensitive, and radiation typically may be effective.
D. The lesion is entirely radiation sensitive and should be treated primarily by radiation.

136.

What presentation is consistent with the MRI shown in this image?

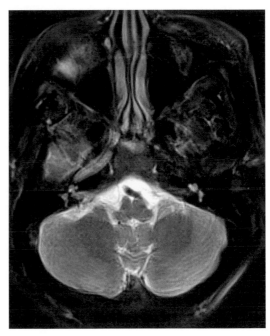

A. Vision loss
B. Hemiparesis
C. Gait ataxia
D. Wallenberg syndrome
E. Locked-in syndrome

137.

An otherwise healthy child underwent an MRI examination under general anesthesia for evaluation of sensorineural hearing loss. The study showed mild, diffuse sulcal FLAIR nonsuppression. The patient is otherwise asymptomatic and fully alert after recovery from the anesthesia. What is the likely cause of this imaging finding?

A. Leptomeningeal tumor spread
B. Meningitis
C. Subarachnoid blood
D. High FiO_2 concentration

138.

What is a neuroimaging feature of uncomplicated cystic hydatid disease of the brain?

A. Perilesional edema
B. Well-circumscribed margins
C. Restricted diffusion
D. Enhancement
E. Calcification

139.

A 5-year-old otherwise healthy girl presents with a several-week history of neck pain. An MRI of the cervical spine was performed, and a sagittal T2 image is shown here. What is the patient's likely diagnosis?

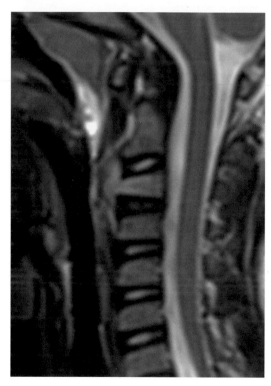

A. Metastasis
B. Eosinophilic granuloma
C. Telangiectatic osteosarcoma
D. Diskitis-osteomyelitis
E. Fracture

140.

What is the structure indicated by the arrow on this lateral view digital subtraction angiogram?

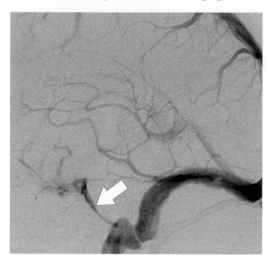

A. Sphenoparietal sinus
B. Superior petrosal sinus
C. Inferior petrosal sinus
D. Inferior anastomotic vein
E. Marginal sinus

141.

What is a characteristic of intracranial lipomas?

A. The curvilinear type is associated with callosal dysgenesis.
B. They arise from anomalous differentiation of the meninx primitiva.
C. They show increased signal on STIR sequences.
D. They almost never calcify.
E. Approximately 20% arise at the midline.

142.
What grade is the intraventricular hemorrhage demonstrated on the cranial ultrasound image shown here?

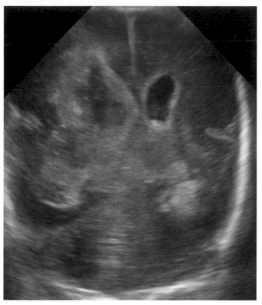

A. Grade 1
B. Grade 2
C. Grade 3
D. Grade 4
E. Grade 5

143.
Representative MR images of the brain are shown here. What is the likely diagnosis?

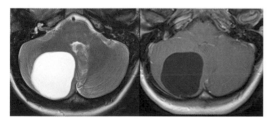

A. Arachnoid cyst
B. Giant perivascular space
C. Neuroglial cyst
D. Cysticercal cyst

144.
A coronal T2-weighted image of the brain of a pediatric patient is shown here. What may be seen in the depicted disease entity?

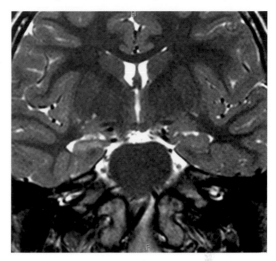

A. Increased N-acetylaspartate on MR spectroscopy
B. Increased FDG uptake interictally
C. Hypertrophy of the ipsilateral fornix
D. Atrophy of the ipsilateral mammillary body

145.
What is a characteristic of the lesion depicted on the CT and MR images shown here?

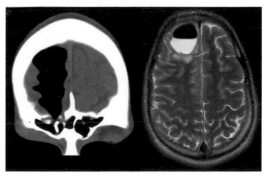

A. Requires a pial-arachnoid defect
B. Majority are iatrogenic
C. Lined by true epithelium
D. Lined by an arachnoid membrane

146.

T2-weighted MR images of the cervical spine in a patient with history of trauma are shown here. What is an additional imaging finding that may be seen?

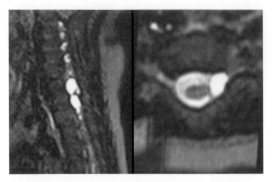

A.   Contrast enhancement of the ovoid lesions
B.   Signal suppression of the ovoid lesions on STIR images
C.   Enhancement of the paraspinal musculature
D.   Restricted diffusion in the ovoid lesions

147.

What anatomic structure is indicated by the arrow in this image?

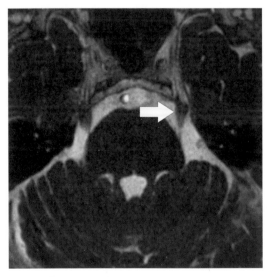

A.   Oculomotor nerve
B.   Trochlear nerve
C.   Trigeminal nerve
D.   Abducens nerve
E.   Glossopharyngeal nerve

148.

A 23-year-old man sustained trauma to the right side of his neck during a motor vehicle collision. The CT angiogram is shown here. What is the patient's diagnosis?

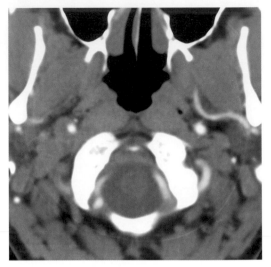

A.   Vertebral artery dissection
B.   Carotid artery pseudoaneurysm
C.   Carotid artery dissection
D.   Vertebral artery pseudoaneurysm
E.   Node of Rouvière

149.

The lesion in the right sacrum on the noncontrast CT study shown in this image likely represents:

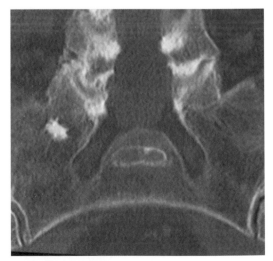

A.   Blastic metastasis
B.   Osteoid osteoma
C.   Enostosis
D.   Osteoblastoma

150.

What skull lesion characteristically is lytic without sclerotic margins?

A. Chondroblastoma
B. Epidermoid
C. Eosinophilic granuloma
D. Osteoid osteoma

151.

A 56-year-old woman with left hemiballismus undergoes an MRI of the brain. Noncontrast T1 images show hyperintensity in the right lentiform nucleus and caudate nucleus head. What is the patient's likely diagnosis?

A. Carbon monoxide intoxication
B. Hyperglycemia
C. Methanol intoxication
D. Liver disease

152.

The "white cerebellum" sign indicates what process?

A. Anoxic-ischemic brain injury
B. Cerebellitis
C. Cerebellar neoplasm
D. Rhombencephalosynapsis

153.

What anatomic variant is shown on the time-of-flight MR angiography in this image?

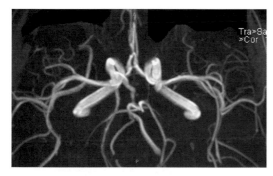

A. Persistent hypoglossal artery
B. Persistent trigeminal artery
C. Persistent otic artery
D. Persistent stapedial artery
E. Persistent pro-atlantal artery

154.

A 50-year-old woman is brought to the hospital with altered mental status and a vertical gaze palsy. Diffusion-weighted MRI sequences (b = 1,000) are shown in these images. What is the patient's likely diagnosis?

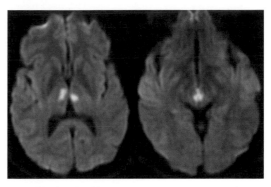

A. Bithalamic glioma
B. Percheron artery infarct
C. Deep venous thrombosis
D. Top of the basilar syndrome

155.

A 35-year-old woman with acute myelopathy has evidence of longitudinally extensive signal abnormality involving most of the cervical cord, with patchy areas of enhancement on a spine MRI. An MRI of the brain shows white matter lesions with "cloud-like" enhancement, "pencil-thin" ependymal enhancement, and abnormal T2/FLAIR signal in the optic chiasm and prechiasmatic optic nerves. What is an additional expected finding in this disease process?

A. Dawson fingers
B. Hilar adenopathy
C. Enhancement of ventral cauda equina roots
D. Aquaporin-4 IgG seropositivity
E. Decreased levels of B12

156.

A patient is reported to have a "string of pearls" appearance on his angiogram. What is the likely diagnosis?

A. Severe carotid artery stenosis
B. Dural arteriovenous fistula
C. Fibromuscular dysplasia
D. Arteriovenous malformation
E. Carotid artery dissection

157.

What is correct regarding the imaging features of hangman fractures according to the Effendi classification (as modified by Levine and Edwards)?

A. Type 4 fractures present with severe angulation and displacement and facet dislocation.
B. Type 2a fractures present with minimal displacement and severe angulation.
C. Type 1 fractures present with severe displacement and no angulation.
D. Type 3 fractures present with severe displacement and severe angulation without facet dislocation.

158.

An arteriogram is performed, and the report mentions that an infundibulum is present. What is a lesion consistent with this finding?

A. 3-mm funnel-shaped segment at the posterior communicating artery origin
B. Triangular-shaped segment more than 3 mm from the origin of the anterior communicating artery
C. Spherical dilation of the basilar artery tip
D. 3- to 4-mm focal dilation located adjacent to the anterior choroidal artery
E. Narrow-necked 7-mm middle cerebral artery aneurysmal dilation

159.

What is a characteristic of the lesion shown on these pre- and postcontrast CT images?

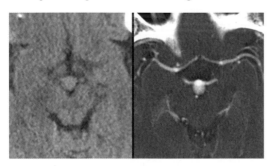

A. It is treated primarily with open microsurgery.
B. It has a lower rate of hemorrhage compared with anterior circulation lesions.
C. It hemorrhages primarily into the interhemispheric fissure.
D. The apex is the most common location.

160.

The lesion illustrated on this MR image *(arrow)* showed syncytial and epithelial cells with indistinct cytoplasmic borders and whorl-like structures on histopathological analysis. What is the diagnosis represented?

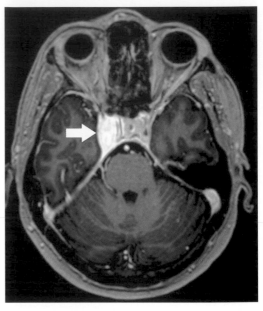

A. Hemangiopericytoma
B. Lymphoma
C. Schwannoma
D. Meningioma

161.

What is the origin of the lesion depicted on these MR images?

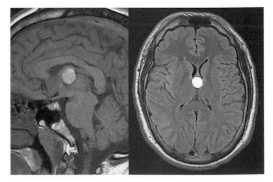

A. Embryonic endoderm
B. Embryonic ectoderm
C. Notochord
D. Mesoderm
E. Arachnoid cap cells

162.

What is a characteristic of the pericallosal lesion on these MR images of the brain?

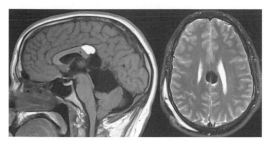

A. Arises from arachnoid cap cells
B. Calcification is common
C. Contains dermal appendages
D. Demonstrates an alanine peak on MR spectroscopy

163.

The head CT shown in this image is compatible with what pathology:

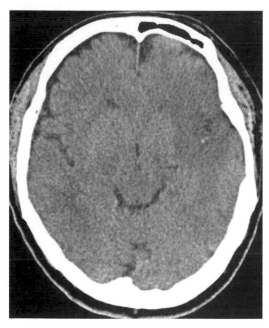

A. Abscess
B. Neoplasm
C. Acute infarct
D. Contusion
E. Old infarct

164.

A man with lethargy, confusion, and one episode of seizures underwent an MRI of the brain, shown in these images. What is the likely diagnosis?

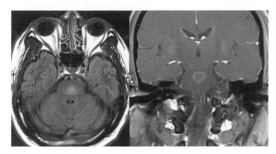

A. Infiltrative glioma
B. Acute infarct
C. Osmotic demyelination
D. Brainstem encephalitis

165.

A woman complaining of neck pain undergoes a cervical spine CT. The exam shows a 1.5-cm lucent vertebral lesion with a calcified core and surrounding sclerosis. What is a characteristic of this lesion?

A. Increased incidence in the elderly
B. More commonly develops along the end plates
C. Shows increased uptake on bone scintigraphy
D. Pain increases with activity

166.

An infant involved in a motor vehicle collision is brought to the emergency department where he underwent a CT examination of the head, shown in this image. There is no evidence of intracranial hemorrhage, and the patient is neurologically intact. What is a characteristic of this patient's lesion?

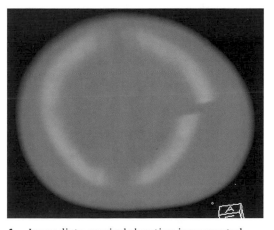

A. Immediate surgical elevation is warranted.
B. There is an increased risk of dural tears.
C. Elevation decreases the incidence of posttraumatic seizures.
D. There is a low risk of cortical laceration.
E. It represents the most common type of pediatric skull fracture.

167.

An MRI of the orbits shows a "tram track" sign. What is a characteristic of this lesion?

A. It is a small round blue cell tumor.
B. It is associated with neurofibromatosis type 1.
C. It derives from arachnoid cap cells.
D. It is related to deposition of mucopoly-saccharides.

168.

A contrast-enhanced T1-weighted MR image of the thoracic spine is shown here. What is the likely diagnosis?

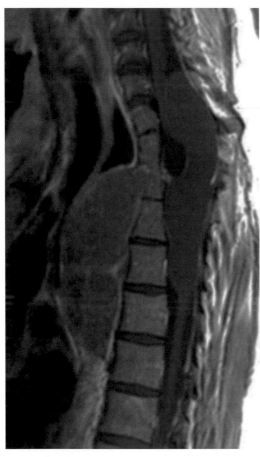

A. Epidermoid
B. Traumatic pseudomeningocele
C. Arachnoid cyst
D. Neurenteric cyst

169.

What normal intracranial component demonstrates high signal intensity on a T1-weighted sequence of the brain?

A. Unmyelinated white matter
B. Melanin
C. High vascular flow
D. Deoxyhemoglobin

170.

In the setting of a large extra-axial hematoma or other significant supratentorial space-occupying lesion, the Kernohan notch phenomenon refers to:

A. Contralateral hydrocephalus secondary to obstruction of the foramen of Monro
B. Compression of the ipsilateral cerebral peduncle against the cerebellar tentorium
C. Compression of the anterior cerebral artery against the falx cerebri
D. Compression of the contralateral cerebral peduncle against the cerebellar tentorium

171.

The lesions demonstrated on these MR images likely represent:

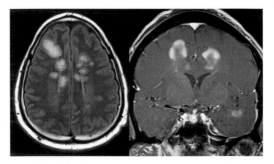

A. Acute demyelination
B. Metastases
C. Multifocal glioblastoma
D. Multifocal abscesses
E. Vasculitis

Use the following answers for questions 172 and 173:

A. McRae line
B. Chamberlain line
C. Wackenheim line
D. McGregor line

172.

What is the line that is drawn along the clivus and extrapolated posteroinferiorly to the upper cervical spinal canal?

173.

What is the line that connects the basion to the opisthion?

174.

A 55-year-old man became confused and hypotensive following a diagnostic angiographic procedure with difficult groin access. Emergent CT of the head was noncontributory. A noncontrast CT of the abdomen is shown here. What is the patient's most likely diagnosis?

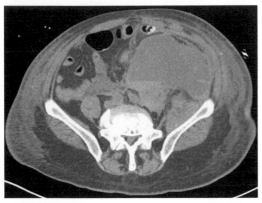

A. Urinoma
B. Bowel infarction
C. Ascites
D. Hematoma

175.

What is a characteristic of the lesion depicted in this CT image?

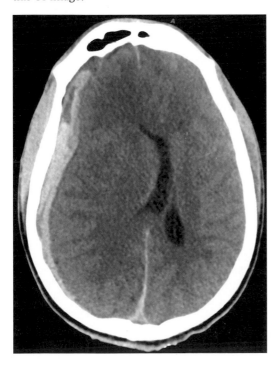

A. Limited by sutures
B. Usually crosses the midline
C. Most commonly due to an arterial injury
D. Occurs between the inner and outer layers of the dura
E. Limited by dural reflections

176.

What is a characteristic of oligodendrogliomas?

A. It is more common in the occipital lobes.
B. Calcification is present in 10% of cases.
C. High cerebral blood flow on perfusion MRI correlates with high histological grade.
D. Preferential involvement of the cortex is a distinctive feature.
E. Tumors with *1p/19q* deletions respond poorly to treatment.

177.

A man with sickle cell disease and secondary moyamoya-type vascularity underwent an MRI study of the brain, which demonstrates an "ivy" sign. This sign is related to:

A. Pial collateral circulation
B. Leptomeningeal carcinomatosis
C. Meningitis
D. Cerebral microhemorrhages
E. Areas of acute ischemia

178.

What imaging feature favors a pilocytic astrocytoma over a hemangioblastoma?

A. High relative cerebral blood volumes
B. Presence of small vascular flow voids
C. Enhancing nodule abutting the pia
D. Enhancement of the cyst wall

179.

What characteristic neuroimaging feature has been described in angiocentric gliomas?

A. Enhancing nodule abutting the meningeal surface
B. Bubbly appearance on T2 images
C. Intrinsic T1 hyperintensity
D. Triangular morphology

180.

A 17-year-old boy is brought to the emergency department with dysarthria and ataxia. An MRI of the brain shows increased T2/FLAIR signal and restricted diffusion involving the lateral putamina and tectum. On clinical exam, he has peripheral brownish rings in his corneas, and the liver function tests are elevated. Mutations in what gene likely is involved in this patient's disease process?

A. *ATP7B*
B. *NOTCH3*
C. *SMARCB1*
D. *FGFR*
E. *PTEN*

181.

The "eye of the tiger" sign is described on an MRI of the brain. This is seen in what entity?

A. Pantothenate kinase–associated neuro-degeneration
B. Huntington disease
C. Wilson disease
D. Carbon monoxide intoxication

182.

A woman with multiple cranial neuropathies undergoes an MRI of the brain, which shows a well-circumscribed mass in the cavernous sinus. The lesion has areas of profound T2 hypointensity and prominent band-like artifact propagating along the phase encoding direction. What is the patient's likely diagnosis?

A. Aneurysm
B. Meningioma
C. Chordoma
D. Chondrosarcoma

183.

A patient is noted to have "harlequin-eye" deformities on a craniofacial CT. What cranial suture is fused?

A. Sagittal
B. Coronal
C. Lambdoid
D. Metopic

184.

A 52-year-old woman with a history of decompressive left hemicraniectomy for a large middle cerebral artery territory infarction presents with new-onset headache, vomiting, and lethargy. Her CT scan is shown in this image. What is the next appropriate step for her management?

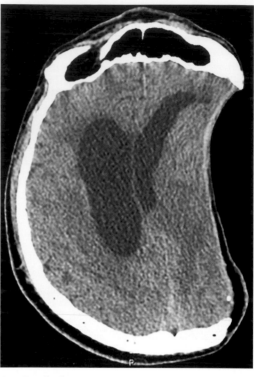

A. Cranioplasty
B. Surgical evacuation
C. Contralateral craniectomy
D. Lumbar spinal fluid drain

185.

What feature favors a spinal cord ependymoma over an astrocytoma?

A. Association with neurofibromatosis type 1
B. Ill-defined margins
C. Heterogeneous enhancement
D. Central location

186.

A man was brought to the emergency room following a high-speed motor vehicle collision. CT of the cervical spine showed a fracture of the pars inter-articularis of C2 bilaterally. What finding would indicate an unstable fracture?

A. More than 2 mm between fragments
B. Greater than 10 degrees of angulation
C. Subluxation of C2 on C3
D. Lateral offset more than 6 mm

187.

A lumbar spine radiograph from a patient with a history of posterior spinal fusion surgery and progressive back pain is shown in this image. What surgical procedure is indicated?

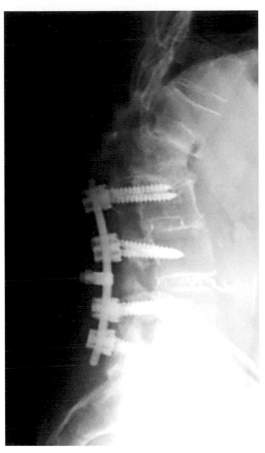

A. Hardware removal due to diskitis/osteomyelitis
B. Pedicle subtraction osteotomy
C. Hardware revision due to loosening
D. Anterior interbody fusion

188.

What is a characteristic of Sturge-Weber syndrome?

A. Multifocal arteriovenous malformations
B. Port-wine stain along the cranial nerve VII distribution
C. Glioneuronal hamartomas
D. Progressive hemifacial atrophy
E. Sporadic presentation

189.

A 56-year-old woman with a history of progressive headaches presented after a seizure episode. An MRI examination of the brain was performed, shown in this image. What is an expected imaging feature of the lesion?

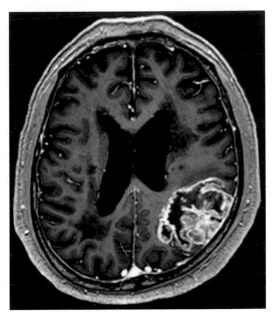

A. Increased relative cerebral blood volume
B. Elevated apparent diffusion coefficient values
C. Elevated N-acetylaspartate levels
D. Decreased choline levels
E. Elevated alanine levels

190.

A previously healthy 35-year-old man presented to clinic complaining of new headaches for several months. An MRI examination of the brain revealed a large, extra-axial, heterogeneous, and avidly enhancing supratentorial mass with prominent internal flow voids, corkscrew vessels, parenchymal edema, and erosion of the adjacent bone without hyperostosis. There was no alanine peak on spectroscopy. The tumor was resected and stained positive for vimentin and CD34, with histological analysis demonstrating uniform spindle cells and stag horn vessels. This lesion is consistent with what tumor diagnosis?

A. Hemangioblastoma
B. Meningioma
C. Lymphoma
D. Hemangiopericytoma

191.

What is a characteristic of optic pathway gliomas?

A. Sporadic gliomas are more frequently chiasmatic or postchiasmatic.
B. They are associated with neurofibromatosis type 2.
C. Calcification is common.
D. Hemorrhage is common.
E. Contrast enhancement correlates with tumor grade.

192.

What is the Evans ratio?

A. Ratio of the largest width of the frontal horns divided by the internal diameter of the skull at the same level
B. Ratio of the largest width of the temporal horns divided by the largest width of the frontal horns
C. Ratio of the largest width of the frontal horns divided by the maximum internal diameter of the skull
D. Occipital-frontal circumference divided by age (in months) of the child

193.

What skull lesion shows a lytic lesion without sclerotic margins?

A. Hemangioma
B. Epidermoid
C. Eosinophilic granuloma
D. Osteoid osteoma

194.

What is Pott's puffy tumor?

A. Osteomyelitis of the skull with subperiosteal abscess
B. Tuberculosis of the spine
C. Suprasellar tumor associated with moyamoya syndrome
D. Dermoid cyst of the skull

195.

What is the typical distribution of T2/FLAIR signal abnormalities in patients with Wilson disease?

A. Medial thalami, periaqueductal gray, tectum, and mammillary bodies
B. Red nuclei and substantia nigra
C. External capsules and temporal poles
D. Lateral putamina and tectum
E. Globi pallidi, subcortical white matter, hippocampi, and cerebral cortex

196.

A man with a dermal sinus tract in the lower back undergoes an MRI of the spine and is found to have a mass in the region of the conus medullaris and cauda equina. What imaging finding would support the diagnosis of superimposed infection of the mass?

A. Thickening and enhancement of the cauda equina
B. Markedly increased diffusion-weighted imaging signal within the mass
C. Increased signal within the mass on the post-contrast T1 sequences
D. Signal dropout on gradient echo sequences

197.

An MRI of the lumbar spine shows diffuse and homogeneous thickening and enhancement preferentially involving the ventral nerve roots. What is the likely diagnosis, given these findings?

A. Leptomeningeal carcinomatosis
B. West Nile virus infection
C. Dural arteriovenous fistula
D. Sarcoidosis

7 Pathology/Histology

1.

In cerebral amyloid angiopathy, what typically occurs with respect to the basal membrane and the internal elastic lamina of the affected vessels?

A. The basal membrane thins, and the internal elastic lamina thickens.
B. The basal membrane thickens, and the internal elastic lamina fragments.
C. The basal membrane fragments, and the internal elastic lamina thickens.
D. The basal membrane is unaffected, and the internal elastic lamina fragments.
E. The basal membrane thickens, and the internal elastic lamina is unaffected.

2.

This image shows a specimen from cerebral white matter. What is the underlying pathology?

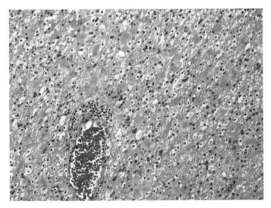

A. Creutzfeldt-Jakob disease
B. Multiple sclerosis
C. Subacute infarction
D. Sarcoidosis

3.

Malignant peripheral nerve sheath tumors commonly have what set of immunohistochemical features?

A. Alterations in chromosome 17, S-100, and nestin
B. Alteration in chromosome 22, GFAP, and CD10
C. Alterations in chromosome 6, vimentin, MIB-1
D. Alterations in chromosome 4, AFP, and CD20
E. Alterations in chromosome 18, HCG, and desmin

4.

A pathologist reports that a resected mass displays basophilic psammoma bodies with mesenchymal and epithelial cells that stain for vimentin and epithelial membrane antigen. Dural feeders in a sunburst pattern were noted in the lesion on preoperative angiogram. What is the likely pathology?

A. Dural arteriovenous fistula
B. Arteriovenous malformation
C. Meningioma
D. High-grade glioma
E. Hemangioblastoma

5.

What type of craniopharyngioma occurs in children, and with what type of keratin is it typically associated?

A. Adamantinomatous; dry
B. Adamantinomatous; wet
C. Papillary; dry
D. Papillary; wet
E. Both adamantinomatous and papillary; dry

6.

The most common neurologic manifestation of HIV infestation is:

A. Toxoplasmosis
B. Primary central nervous system lymphoma
C. AIDS dementia complex
D. Encephalitis
E. Vacuolar myelopathy

7.

What neurotoxic agent is responsible for causing primarily a myelinopathy?

A. Amiodarone
B. Bismuth
C. Lead
D. Mercury
E. Methanol

8.

What type of hematoma occurs in the loose connective tissues of the scalp that may cross sutures, may require blood transfusions, and does not calcify?

A. Subgaleal hematoma
B. Subperiosteal hematoma
C. Subdural hematoma
D. Temporalis contusion

9.
A 43-year-old patient presents with a large, enhancing mass with a necrotic center with mass effect and significant vasogenic edema. Following resection, histology demonstrated neovascularization with endothelial proliferation and pseudopalisading around areas of necrosis. Histopathology was significant for a *TP53* mutation. What is the most likely diagnosis?

A. Primary glioblastoma
B. Secondary glioblastoma
C. Rhabdoid meningioma
D. Medulloblastoma
E. Chordoma

10.
What syndrome is associated with tumors in the optic/visual pathways with histology demonstrating Rosenthal fibers?

A. Von Hippel–Lindau
B. Neurofibromatosis type 1
C. Neurofibromatosis type 2
D. Tuberous sclerosis
E. Sturge-Weber

11.
The sellar mass shown in this image, if hormonally active, most likely secretes:

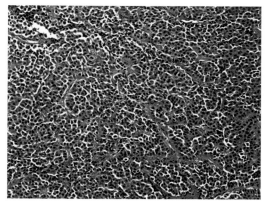

A. Adrenocorticotrophic hormone
B. Follicle-stimulating hormone
C. Growth hormone
D. Prolactin
E. Vasopressin

12.
The eosinophilic cytoplasmic inclusion shown in this image of a patient with Alzheimer disease represents what histological entity?

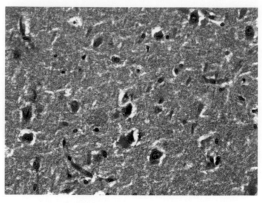

A. Amyloid body
B. Granulovacuolar degeneration
C. Hirano body
D. Lewy body
E. Neurofibrillary tangle

13.
A 65-year-old man has diffuse muscle wasting with spasticity, slowed movements, and muscle cramping. The section shown in this image was taken from the anterior horn cell region of the lumbar spinal cord. The most likely diagnosis is:

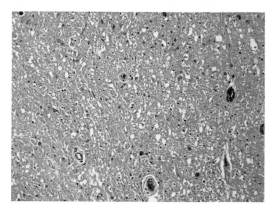

A. Amyotrophic lateral sclerosis
B. Multiple system atrophy
C. Spinal muscular atrophy type 1
D. Spinal muscular atrophy type 2
E. Syphilis

14.
A germinal matrix hemorrhage with intraventricular hemorrhage and ventricular enlargement represents what grade of lesion?

A. Grade 1
B. Grade 2
C. Grade 3
D. Grade 4
E. Grade 5

15.

Small, round, eosinophilic neuronal cell inclusions known as Bunina bodies are associated with what disease?

A. Alzheimer disease
B. Amyotrophic lateral sclerosis
C. Huntington chorea
D. Machado-Joseph disease
E. Olivopontocerebellar atrophy of Menzel

16.

A bruise of the skin and underlying tissue on the scalp with hemorrhage defines a(n):

A. Abrasion
B. Avulsion
C. Contusion
D. Laceration
E. Scrape

17.

What immunohistochemical profile is most consistent with metastatic melanoma, shown in this image?

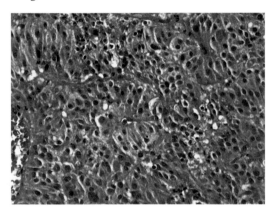

A. Epithelial membrane antigen and cytokeratin AE1/3 positivity
B. Glial fibrillary acidic protein and S-100 protein positivity
C. Melan-A and HMB-45 positivity
D. S-100 protein and progesterone receptor positivity
E. TTF-1 and synaptophysin positivity

18.

The neoplasm shown in this image arises from what cellular origin?

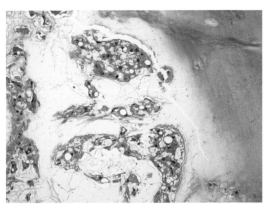

A. Chondrocytes
B. Ependymal cells
C. Epithelial cells
D. Nevoid cells
E. Notochord remnants

19.

A biopsy is taken targeting a midline mass. The frozen section appearance of the biopsy is shown in this image. The best diagnosis for the frozen section is:

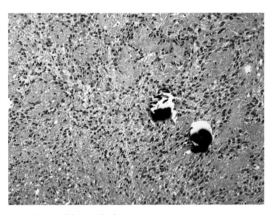

A. Normal hypothalamus
B. Normal neurohypophysis
C. Normal pineal gland
D. Optic chiasm
E. Pilocytic astrocytoma

20.

This fontal convexity mass shown in this image is thought to represent an eosinophilic granuloma. The best stain to prove that the macrophage cells are Langerhans histiocytes is one staining:

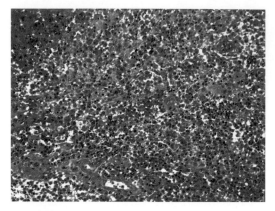

A. CD1a
B. CD15
C. CD45RB
D. CD68
E. HAM56

21.

The paraspinal soft tissue mass shown in this image was diagnosed as a granular cell tumor. The granular quality of the cytoplasm is due to an increased number or amount of:

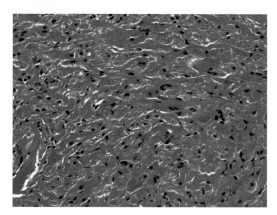

A. Endoplasmic reticulum
B. Lysosomes
C. Mitochondria
D. Neurofilaments
E. Ribosomes

22.

The cerebellopontine angle mass shown in this image is associated with alterations in what gene?

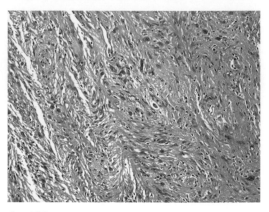

A. *NF2*
B. *TP53*
C. *PTEN*
D. *SOD1*
E. *TSC2*

23.

What type of metastatic brain tumor generally is considered radiosensitive to whole brain radiation therapy?

A. Thyroid
B. Renal
C. Melanoma
D. Breast
E. Sarcoma

24.

A 32-year-old man with mental retardation and a history of seizures presents for resection of a tumor associated with hydrocephalus. Histology shows fibrillary areas alternating with large cells containing generous amounts of eosinophilic cytoplasm. On what chromosome(s) can abnormalities associated with this disease be found?

A. Chromosome 17p
B. Chromosomes 9q and 16p
C. Chromosomes 1p and 19q
D. Chromosomes 3q, 7q, and 7p
E. Chromosome 15

25.

The lesion shown in this image is best classified as a(n):

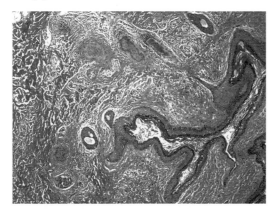

A. Craniopharyngioma
B. Colloid cyst
C. Dermoid cyst
D. Endodermal cyst
E. Epidermoid cyst

26.

The tumor shown in this image represents what pathology?

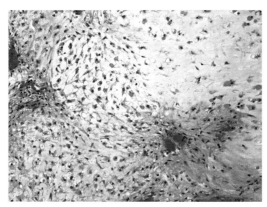

A. Chondroma
B. Chondrosarcoma
C. Chordoid meningioma
D. Chordoma
E. Teratoma

27.

A 7-year-old previously healthy girl presented with progressive ataxia and palsy of cranial nerves VI and VII. Representative scans from an MRI study are shown in these images. What is a characteristic of this entity?

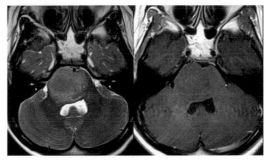

A. There is a high incidence of distal metastases.
B. Hydrocephalus is an early complication.
C. Most pontine tumors have high-grade histology.
D. Calcifications frequently are identified.

28.

The dural-based, glial fibrillary acidic protein (GFAP) negative mass shown in this image represents a(n):

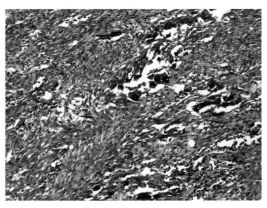

A. Chondrosarcoma
B. Gliosarcoma
C. Hemangiopericytoma
D. Metaplastic meningioma
E. Osteosarcoma

29.

On the histological level, the morphological changes of hypoxic ischemia typically are first observed how soon after the precipitating event?

A. 3 hours
B. 6 hours
C. 12 hours
D. 36 hours
E. 48 hours

30.

The chromogranin positive staining mass shown in this image is most likely to arise in what location?

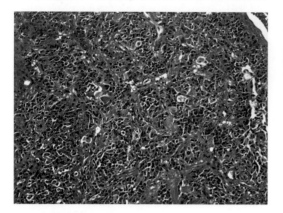

A. Cerebellum
B. Filum terminale
C. Frontal lobe
D. Lateral ventricle
E. Pons

31.

The lytic skull lesion shown in this image was biopsied in a 72-year-old man who also has a history of recently developing renal failure. The lesion most likely will stain with what antibody?

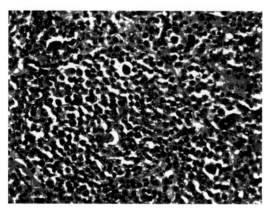

A. CD3
B. CD5
C. CD45
D. CD79
E. CD138

32.

What is the most common site of origin of the cystic mass shown in this image?

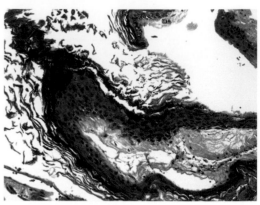

A. Cerebellopontine angle
B. Foramen of Monro
C. Lumbar cord
D. Temporal lobe
E. Sella

33.

A tear in the middle meningeal artery is most likely responsible for a hemorrhage in what space or location?

A. Epidural space
B. Intraventricular space
C. Subarachnoid space
D. Subdural space
E. Thalamus

34.

How long after a diffuse axonal injury can dystrophic axons be visualized with β-amyloid precursor protein staining?

A. 2 hours
B. 4 hours
C. 8 hours
D. 12 hours
E. 24 hours

35.
The pathological findings seen in the vastus lateralis muscle shown in this image from a 32-year-old woman are consistent with what pathology?

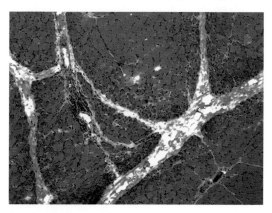

A. Dermatomyositis
B. Inclusion body myositis
C. Polyarteritis nodosum
D. Polymyositis
E. Sarcoidosis

36.
The muscle shown in this image is from a 4-year-old boy who has proximal muscle weakness, a positive Gower sign, and calf muscle hypertrophy. Abnormal staining with what antibody is anticipated?

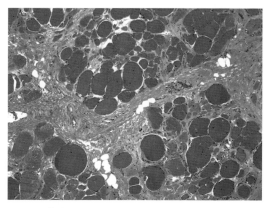

A. Dysferlin
B. Dystrophin
C. Merosin
D. Sarcoglycan alpha
E. Spectrin

37.
This right temporal lobe cyst shown in this image is classified best as a(n):

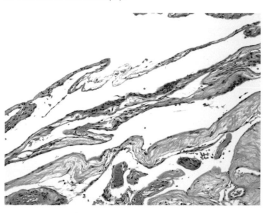

A. Arachnoid cyst
B. Choroid plexus cyst
C. Cystic meningioma
D. Ependymal cyst
E. Epidermoid cyst

38.
A 72-year-old man presents with muscle weakness, atrophy, and a biopsy shown in this image. The pathological process is likely to respond to what therapy?

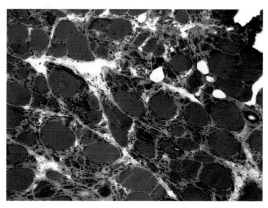

A. Statins
B. Intravenous IgG
C. Methotrexate
D. Steroids
E. No available therapies

39.

The findings in the NADH-stained section of skeletal muscle shown in this image are associated with what underlying pathological process?

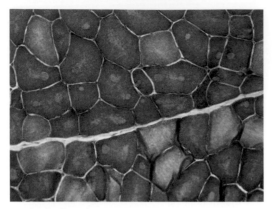

A. CCTG repeats
B. Loss of myosin filaments
C. Mitochondrial myopathy
D. Nemaline rod myopathy
E. Ryanodine receptor gene mutation

40.

A 2-year-old boy presents with vacuolar changes on muscle biopsy. The vacuoles are filled with glycogen and stain with acid phosphatase, as shown in this image. The patient's most likely diagnosis is:

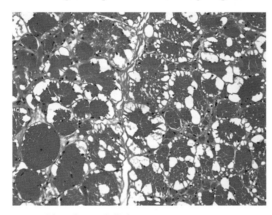

A. Acid maltase deficiency
B. Debrancher enzyme deficiency
C. Hypokalemic periodic paralysis
D. Myophosphorylase deficiency
E. Phosphofructokinase deficiency

41.

What protein is unlikely to form cerebral amyloid?

A. Cystatin C
B. Gelsolin
C. Kappa light chain protein
D. Prion protein

42.

A CAG trinucleotide repeat in what gene is associated with Huntington disease?

A. *Ataxin-2* gene
B. *CACNAIA* gene
C. *Chorein* gene
D. *HTT* gene
E. *Myotonin* gene

43.

The pathology illustrated with the Bielschowsky stain shown in this image is encountered most commonly in what disease process?

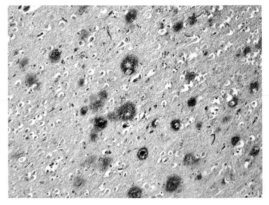

A. Alzheimer disease
B. Diffuse Lewy body disease
C. Ganglioglioma
D. Mitochondrial encephalopathy
E. Pick disease

44.

An antibody for what protein best highlights the structures shown in this Bielschowsky stain image?

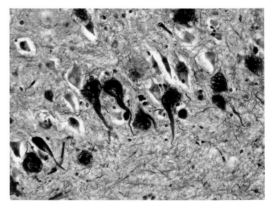

A. α-synuclein
B. Congo red
C. Glial fibrillary acidic protein
D. Tau
E. Thioflavin S

45.

What tumor pathology consists of tumor cells forming cuffs around blood vessels?

A. Germinoma
B. Ependymoma
C. Chordoma
D. Lymphoma
E. Hemangioblastoma

46.

The presence of xanthochromia, high protein, and clotting of the cerebrospinal fluid is referred to as:

A. Queckenstedt syndrome
B. Coup de poignard of Michon
C. Froment sign
D. Froin syndrome
E. Foix-Alajouanine

47.

The cyst shown in this image is situated near the foramen of Monro. What is an unlikely presenting symptom for the most likely lesion?

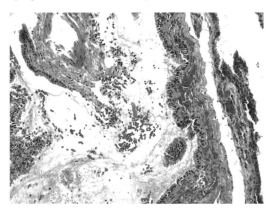

A. Headache
B. Incontinence
C. Personality change
D. Seizure
E. Sudden death

48.

The eosinophilic deposits shown in this image represent amyloid accumulation in a patient with suspected Alzheimer disease. What is the single best stain to prove the diagnosis?

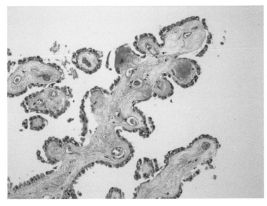

A. β-amyloid
B. Luxol fast blue
C. Mucicarmine
D. Prussian blue
E. Trichrome

49.

A lesion with a vascular nature is resected, and the pathology lab reports that the lesion is consistent with a vascular hamartoma with irregular thick- and thin-walled sinusoidal vascular channels without intervening brain tissue. What is the diagnosis for this lesion?

A. Capillary telangiectasia
B. Cavernous malformation
C. Venous angioma
D. Arteriovenous malformation
E. Dural arteriovenous fistula

50.

Sturge-Weber disease is inherited in what fashion?

A. Autosomal dominantly
B. Autosomal recessively
C. X-linked recessively
D. Sporadically with no obvious genetic transmission

51.
The cytoplasmic inclusion shown in this image is most likely associated with a mutation in what gene?

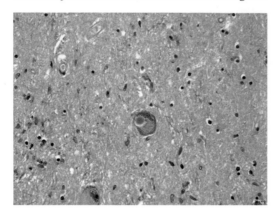

A. *SNCA*
B. *PARK1*
C. *PARK2*
D. *PARK5*
E. *PARK8*

52.
A man presents for genetic counseling with deafness, skeletal abnormalities, mental retardation, and coarse facial features. He is found to have an autosomal recessive mucopolysaccharidosis. What is the patient's enzyme deficiency?

A. L-iduronidase
B. Iduronate sulfatase
C. Galactose 6-sulfatase and β-galactosidase
D. Sulfatase B
E. β-glucuronidase

53.
Klippel-Feil syndrome is associated with what common findings?

A. Low posterior hairline, brevicollis, and decreased neck motion
B. Sebaceous adenomas, mental retardation, and seizures
C. Anorectal malformation, anterior sacral defects, and presacral masses
D. Dementia, urinary incontinence, and gait instability

54.
Axonal spheroids are seen with what neurologic pathology?

A. Friedreich ataxia
B. Huntington disease
C. Cerebral infarction
D. Amyotrophic lateral sclerosis

55.
The best diagnosis for the mucin and glial fibrillary acidic protein (GFAP)-positive spinal cord mass shown in this image, presenting in a 33-year-old man with a 4-year history of lower back pain, is:

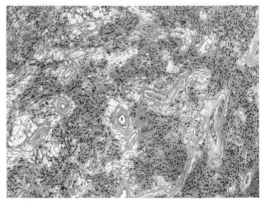

A. Meningioma
B. Metastatic adenocarcinoma
C. Myxopapillary ependymoma
D. Paraganglioma
E. Schwannoma

56.
The Prussian blue stain shown in this image highlights increased iron accumulation in a patient with a *PANK2* gene mutation. The iron accumulation most commonly is seen in what location in the central nervous system?

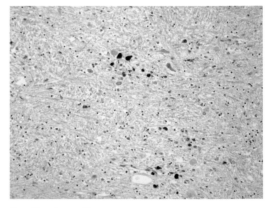

A. Basal ganglia
B. Cerebellum
C. Cervical and lumbar spinal cord
D. Hippocampus
E. Pons

57.

A 22-year-old woman with seizures for 12 years has hippocampal sclerosis pathology, as shown in this image. What two regions of the hippocampus usually are affected most severely?

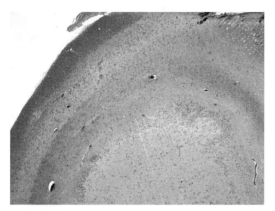

A. CA1 and CA2
B. CA1 and CA3
C. CA1 and CA4
D. CA2 and CA4
E. CA3 and CA4

58.

Multisystem atrophy (cerebellar predominant type) is characterized by what pathological or clinical finding?

A. Atrophy of the putamen
B. Dysautonomia
C. Neuronal loss in the striatonigral system
D. Rigidity and dystonia
E. Ubiquitin positive tangles

59.

A mutation in what gene is associated with 20% of familial cases of amyotrophic lateral sclerosis?

A. *PTEN*
B. *SMN1*
C. *SMN2*
D. *SOD1*
E. *TARDBP*

60.

The optic nerve shown in this image was sampled at autopsy. The most likely pathology observed is:

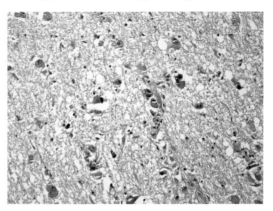

A. Cytomegalovirus infection
B. Diffuse astrocytoma
C. Fungal infection
D. Pilocytic astrocytoma
E. Sarcoidosis

61.

The vascular changes seen in the recurrent glioblastoma shown in this image are most likely due to what process?

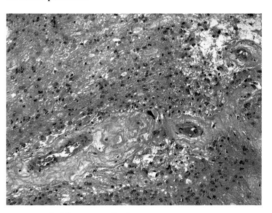

A. Amyloid accumulation
B. Chemotherapy effects
C. Radiation effects
D. Tumor involution
E. Tumor progression

62.

This lesion shown in this image most commonly arises in what central nervous system location?

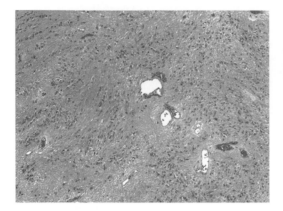

A. Cervical spinal cord
B. Fourth ventricle
C. Frontal lobe
D. Lumbosacral spinal cord
E. Temporal lobe

63.

The lateral ventricular mass shown in this image, presenting in a 26-year-old woman, is associated with what mutation or disease?

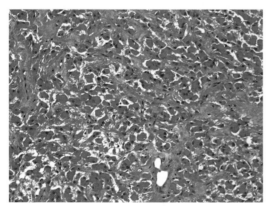

A. *Notch3* mutation
B. *PTEN* mutation
C. Tuberous sclerosis
D. Turcot syndrome
E. Von Hippel–Lindau disease

64.

The IDH-1–positive staining tumor shown in this image also is likely to show what characteristic?

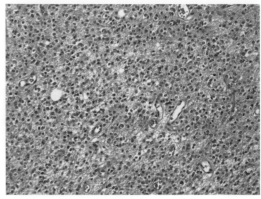

A. ATRX protein staining
B. Chromosome 10p deletion
C. EGFR protein staining
D. P53 protein staining
E. PTEN protein mutation

65.

What is the best predictor of prognosis for the focally enhancing, frontal lobe tumor shown in this image, arising in a 45-year-old man?

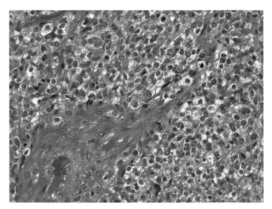

A. Mitotic count
B. EGFRvIII mutation
C. Ki-67 labeling index
D. Deletion on chromosome 1p
E. Necrosis

66.

What antibody is most useful in differentiating between a low-grade fibrillary astrocytoma and gliosis?

A. GFAP
B. IDH-1
C. Ki-67
D. p53
E. S-100

67.

Degeneration of the posterior columns of the spinal cord shown in this image most likely is associated with a deficiency of what vitamin?

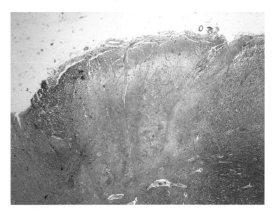

A. B1
B. B2
C. B6
D. B12
E. C

68.

What gene alterations are most likely encountered in the tumor shown in this image, presenting in the brainstem of a 16-year-old girl?

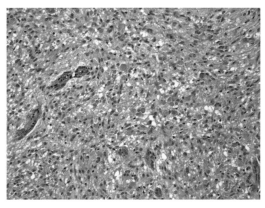

A. *BRAF*
B. *EGFR*
C. *IDH-1*
D. *TP53*

69.

What is true regarding the multinodular, cortical-based tumor shown in this image?

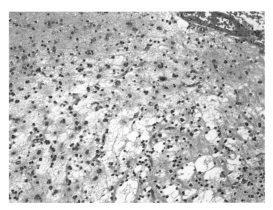

A. Associated with focal cortical dysplasia
B. Has a cyst with an enhancing mural nodule appearance on imaging
C. Most commonly arises in the cerebellum
D. Often has a Ki-67 labeling index of 5 to 10%
E. Is a WHO grade II neoplasm

70.

The structures shown in this image are characteristic of what spinal cord mass?

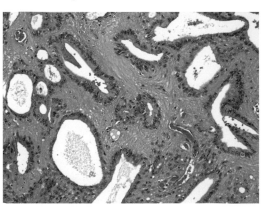

A. Ependymoma
B. Lymphoma
C. Myxopapillary ependymoma
D. Retinoblastoma
E. Subependymoma

71.

What is the most common pathogen found in brain abscesses across all demographics?

A. *Streptococcus* species
B. *Staphylococcus* species
C. *Bacteroides* species
D. *Proteus* species
E. Enteric bacilli

72.

What is the most common source of the pathogen found in brain abscesses across all demographics?

A. Heart valve vegetations
B. Open cranial wounds and injuries
C. Iatrogenic from surgery or catheter placement
D. Adjacent sinus or ear infections
E. Bacteremia due to remote infections

73.

An astrocytoma is resected, and pathological analysis reveals pseudopalisading necrosis without frank necrosis, in addition to mild vascular proliferation and moderate pleomorphism. What is the likely WHO grade of this astrocytoma?

A. Grade I
B. Grade II
C. Grade III
D. Grade IV

74.

A patient has a known familial syndrome associated with brain tumors and is found to have a supratentorial primitive neuroectodermal tumor (S-PNET). The patient also has breast cancer and a soft tissue sarcoma. What is the likely familial syndrome/genetic/protein mutation in the patient?

A. Turcot syndrome
B. Merlin protein mutation
C. Neurofibromin 1 protein mutation
D. P53 protein mutation
E. Von Hippel–Lindau tumor suppressor gene mutation

75.

Antibodies to what marker would be most useful in confirming a diagnosis of a central neurocytoma for the tumor shown in this image?

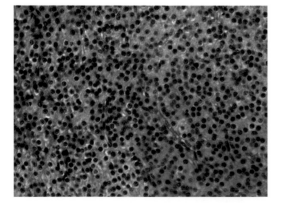

A. CD34
B. Epithelial membrane antigen
C. Glial fibrillary acidic protein
D. S-100 protein
E. Synaptophysin

76.

The Ki-67 labeling index shown in this image is most likely associated with what central nervous system tumor?

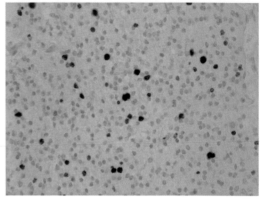

A. WHO grade I meningioma
B. WHO grade I pilocytic astrocytoma
C. WHO grade II gemistocytic astrocytoma
D. WHO grade II pleomorphic xanthoastrocytoma
E. WHO grade III anaplastic astrocytoma

77.

What is the WHO grade designation for the reticulin rich, temporal lobe mass shown in this image, presenting in a 17-year-old boy with a history of seizures?

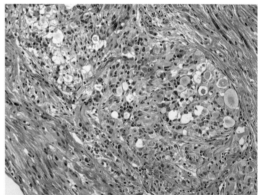

A. WHO grade I
B. WHO grade II
C. WHO grade III
D. WHO grade IV

78.
A 12-year-old girl with seizures undergoes resection of the epileptogenic region, shown in this image. What is her most likely diagnosis?

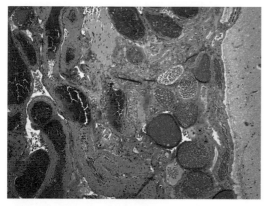

A. Angiomatous meningioma
B. Arteriovenous malformation
C. Cortical tuber
D. Normal brain parenchyma
E. Sturge-Weber syndrome

79.
The nasal mass shown in this image presented in a 17-year-old boy. Imaging showed no connection of this lesion to the brain. The best diagnosis for this lesion is:

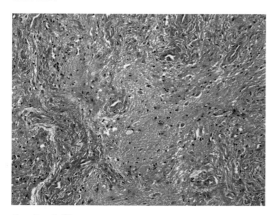

A. Angiofibroma
B. Encephalocele
C. Meningioma
D. Nasal glioma
E. Pituitary adenoma

80.
INI1 and chromosome 22 abnormalities in young children suggest what brain tumor type?

A. Medulloblastoma
B. Ependymoma
C. Astrocytoma
D. Atypical teratoid/rhabdoid tumor
E. Schwannoma

81.
A 46-year-old man presents with hypodense lesions in the mammillary bodies. At autopsy, he has shrunken and dusky discolored mammillary bodies. The underlying cause of these changes is:

A. Carbon monoxide poisoning
B. Dilantin toxicity
C. Methanol ingestion
D. Reye syndrome
E. Thiamine deficiency

82.
A glial-lined cavity within the parenchyma of the medulla is referred to as:

A. Diplomyelia
B. Hydromyelia
C. Iniencephaly
D. Syringobulbia
E. Syringomyelia

83.
The organism highlighted on the GMS-stained section shown in this image most commonly presents in the brain with what pattern of injury?

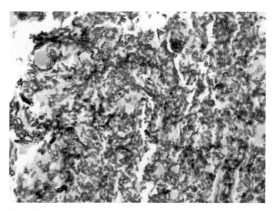

A. Abscess
B. Hemorrhagic infarct
C. Empyema
D. Encephalitis
E. Meningitis

84.

Elevated amniotic fluid levels of α-fetoprotein and acetylcholinesterase are associated with what developmental abnormality?

A. Dandy-Walker malformation
B. Focal cortical dysplasia
C. Macrocephaly
D. Open neural tube defect
E. Polymicrogyria

85.

A 7-year-old boy presents with acute hydrocephalus and precocious puberty. The histological findings of a biopsy of a pineal mass are shown in this image. The most likely diagnosis is:

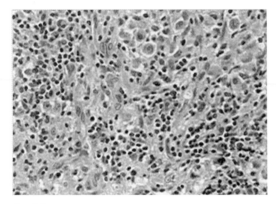

A. Mature teratoma
B. Pineoblastoma
C. Germinoma
D. Sarcoidosis
E. Pineal cyst

86.

The histological findings of a biopsy of a cerebellar mass in a 27-year-old woman are shown in this image. The imaging findings describe a cystic mass with a homogeneously enhancing nodule. The most likely diagnosis is:

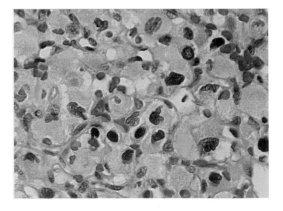

A. Pilocytic astrocytoma
B. Hemangioblastoma
C. Medulloblastoma
D. Ependymoma
E. Oligodendroglioma

87.

The pathology shown in this image is associated with:

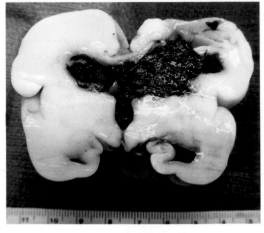

A. Intrauterine cytomegalovirus infection
B. Congenital toxoplasmosis
C. Prematurity
D. Gestational diabetes
E. ABO histoincompatibility

88.

The most accurate diagnosis of the tumor shown in this image is:

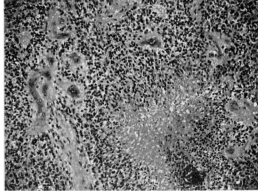

A. Anaplastic astrocytoma, WHO grade III
B. Diffuse astrocytoma, WHO grade II
C. Gemistocytic astrocytoma, WHO grade II
D. Glioblastoma, WHO grade IV
E. Oligodendroglioma, WHO grade II

89.

A 50-year-old woman presents to clinic with complaints of pain in her left calf. The pain is associated with a palpable mass. The surgical pathological report states that the mass "reveals spindled proliferation with both cellular and loose stroma with some areas of spindle cells arranged in a palisading fashion without necrosis." No axons are seen coursing through the lesion. Radiological images of the lesion are shown here. What is the patient's most likely diagnosis?

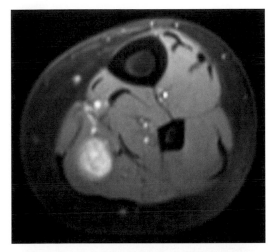

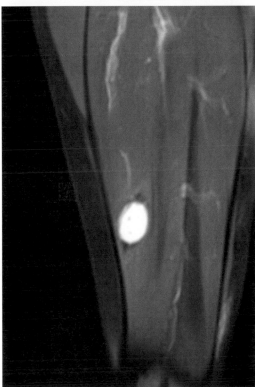

A. Neurofibroma

B. Schwannoma

C. Malignant peripheral nerve sheath tumor (MPNST)

D. Metastatic tumor

E. Lipoma

90.

What cerebral disorder presents with extracellular deposits of β-amyloid?

A. Alzheimer disease

B. Pick disease

C. Creutzfeldt-Jakob disease

D. Dementia with Lewy bodies

E. Huntington disease

91.

What is the most common location for hypertensive hemorrhage?

A. Putamen

B. Cerebral hemispheres

C. Thalamus

D. Pons

E. Cerebellum

92.

The most common chromosomal abnormality associated with the tumor shown in this image is:

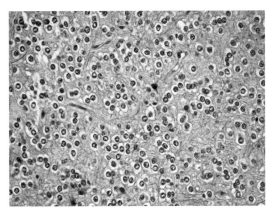

A. Chromosome 10p deletion

B. Chromosomes 1p and 19q co-deletion

C. Gain of chromosome 7q34

D. Monosomy of chromosome 6

E. Monosomy of chromosome 22

93.
The temporal lobe mass shown in this image presented in a 20-year-old man with seizures. The lesion represents a(n):

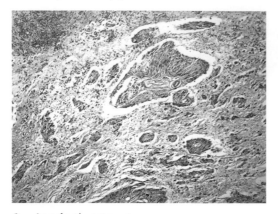

A. Anaplastic astrocytoma
B. Angiocentric glioma
C. Ependymoma
D. Ganglioglioma
E. Gliomatosis cerebri

94.
In what type of tumor are Homer-Wright rosettes found?

A. Ependymoma
B. Craniopharyngioma
C. Pineocytoma
D. Neuroblastoma
E. Subependymoma

95.
What meningioma subtypes are classified as WHO grade III?

A. Angiomatous and secretory
B. Clear cell and chordoid
C. Meningothelial and transitional
D. Psammomatous and fibrous
E. Papillary and rhabdoid

96.
The most common histological type of optic pathway/hypothalamic glioma in children is:

A. Anaplastic astrocytoma
B. Glioblastoma
C. Pilocytic astrocytoma
D. Xanthoastrocytoma
E. Ganglioglioma

97.
The microscopic finding shown in this image is seen in the setting of:

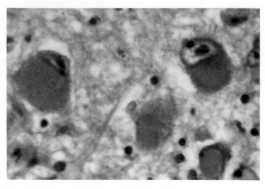

A. Amyotrophic lateral sclerosis
B. Frontotemporal dementia
C. Cytomegalovirus infection
D. Parkinson disease
E. Rabies

98.
What tumor often is described by its "chicken wire" vasculature and "fried egg" histological appearance?

A. Germinoma
B. Cellular ependymoma
C. Pleomorphic xanthoastrocytoma
D. Subependymal giant cell astrocytoma
E. Oligodendroglioma

99.
What is the most common organism found in cerebral abscesses?

A. *Streptococcus* species
B. *Escherichia coli*
C. *Bacteroides*
D. *Actinomyces*
E. *Staphylococcus epidermidis*

100.

A 9-year-old boy presents with a posterior fossa mass. This image is a representative section of the tumor. The most likely diagnosis is:

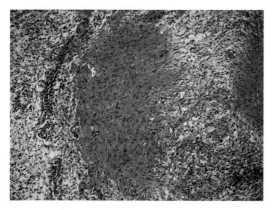

A. Ependymoma
B. Hemangioblastoma
C. Medulloblastoma
D. Oligodendroglioma
E. Pilocytic astrocytoma

101.

The most common primary tumor of the central nervous system is:

A. Glioblastoma
B. Lymphoma
C. Meningioma
D. Metastatic carcinoma
E. Schwannoma

102.

The tumor shown in this image presented as a frontal lobe mass in a 74-year-old man. The tumor had positive immunostaining with TTF-1 antibody. The most likely diagnosis is:

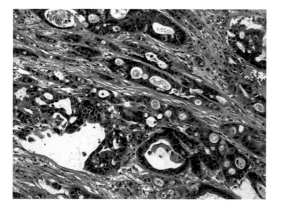

A. Glioblastoma
B. Lymphoma
C. Medulloblastoma
D. Metastatic carcinoma
E. Meningioma

103.

What histologic features would be most important in determining that the tumor shown in this image is an anaplastic astrocytoma (WHO grade III)?

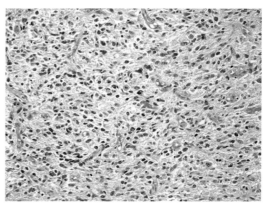

A. Calcifications
B. Infiltrative border
C. Mitotic activity
D. Necrosis
E. Vascular proliferation

104.

The best diagnosis for the p53 mutated tumor shown in this image is:

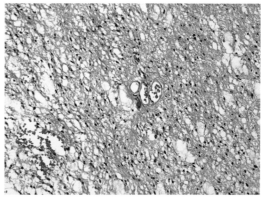

A. Anaplastic astrocytoma
B. Low-grade diffuse astrocytoma
C. Low-grade oligodendroglioma
D. Pilocytic astrocytoma
E. Pleomorphic xanthoastrocytoma

105.

Epidermal growth factor receptor (EGFR) amplification or overexpression, shown in this image, is most likely encountered in what variant of glioblastoma, as shown in this image.

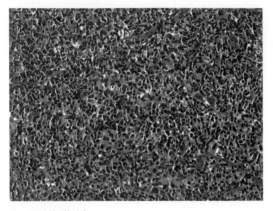

A. Epithelioid
B. Giant cell
C. Gliosarcoma
D. Granular cell
E. Small cell

106.

The lesion biopsy shown in this image, taken from the left temporal lobe in a 42-year-old man, best represent a(n):

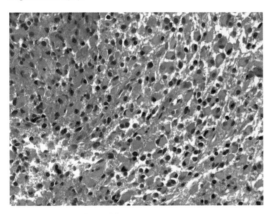

A. Epithelioid glioblastoma
B. Gemistocytic astrocytoma
C. Giant cell glioblastoma
D. Gliosis
E. Subependymal giant cell astrocytoma

107.

The optic nerve mass shown in this image presented in a 4-year-old girl. The tumor is best classified as a:

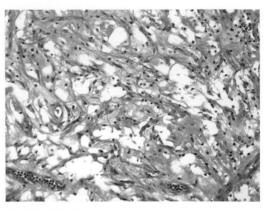

A. Ganglioglioma
B. Low-grade fibrillary astrocytoma
C. Neurofibroma
D. Pilocytic astrocytoma
E. Schwannoma

108.

The findings shown in this peripheral nerve specimen image are most likely secondary to what pathological process?

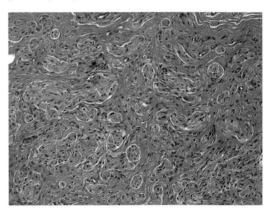

A. Amyloid deposition
B. Prior Guillain-Barré disease
C. Prior infection
D. Prior surgery
E. Prior vasculitis

109.

A 36-year-old woman developed rapidly progressive cognitive impairment. At autopsy, a section from her right frontal lobe demonstrated the findings shown in this image. What is her most likely diagnosis?

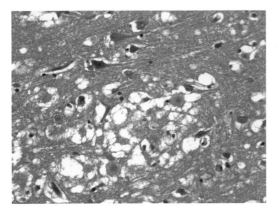

A. Bacterial infection
B. Fulminant demyelinating disease
C. Fungal infection
D. Infarct
E. Prion disease

110.

A 62-year-old cardiac transplant patient developed multiple enhancing brain lesions 6 months after surgery. What are the black-staining organisms highlighted on the Gomori methenamine silver stain shown in this image?

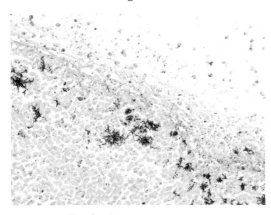

A. *Aspergillus fumigatus*
B. *Clostridium difficile*
C. *Streptococcus pneumoniae*
D. *Mycobacterium* species
E. *Nocardia asteroides*

111.

A 36-year-old liver transplant patient presented with symptoms suggestive of encephalitis. At autopsy, a section from his right temporal lobe was taken and is shown in this image. What was the cause of his symptoms?

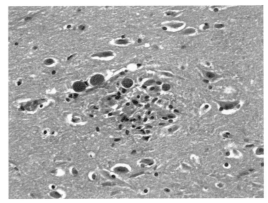

A. *Coccidioides*
B. Histoplasmosis
C. Leishmaniasis
D. Malaria
E. Toxoplasmosis

112.

How do the organisms shown in this pathology slide gain access to the body?

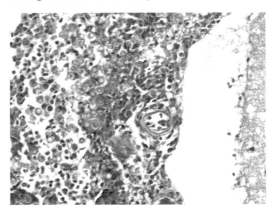

A. Blood
B. Eye
C. Gastrointestinal tract
D. Genitourinary tract
E. Respiratory tract

113.
A 53-year-old man presents to the emergency room with altered mental status and left hemiparesis. CT reveals a large right frontal hematoma. The patient is taken emergently to the operating room for hematoma evacuation. During the operation, the dura is noted to be very dark and discolored. The hematoma and accompanying tissue are sent to pathology, and a representative slide is shown in this image. What is the patient's most likely diagnosis?

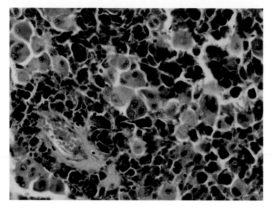

A. Normal neuronal tissue
B. Hematoma with neural tissue
C. Metastatic renal cell carcinoma
D. Metastatic melanoma
E. Melanocytoma

114.
What is the best diagnosis for the pathological findings shown in this image from a 46-year-old woman?

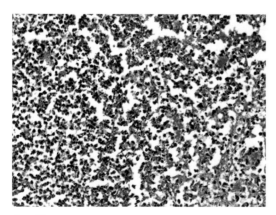

A. Abscess
B. Demyelinating disease
C. Glioblastoma
D. Infarct
E. Lymphoma

115.
A diabetic patient initially presented with a periorbital infection that subsequently spread to involve the brain. The pathology is shown in this image. What is the most likely cause of this patient's infection?

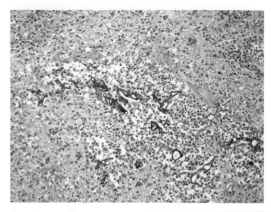

A. *Aspergillus*
B. *Candida*
C. Fusarium
D. *Mucor*
E. *Nocardia*

116.
Holoprosencephaly is associated with what disease/syndrome?

A. Diprosopus
B. Maternal diabetes
C. Smith-Lemli-Opitz syndrome
D. Trisomy of chromosome 5
E. Turner syndrome

117.

The findings shown in this image from the subdural compartment represent a(n):

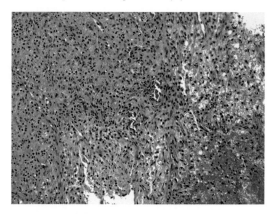

A. Acute subdural hemorrhage
B. Empyema
C. Leptomeningeal carcinomatosis
D. Leptomeningeal extension of a glioma
E. Organizing subdural hemorrhage

118.

The palisaded structure seen in the tumor shown in this image is characteristic of what pathology?

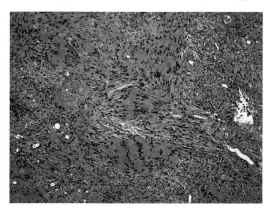

A. Fibroma
B. Fibrous meningioma
C. Neurofibroma
D. Schwannoma
E. Solitary fibrous tumor

119.

The malignant tumor shown in this image arose in the thigh region of a 38-year-old with neurofibromatosis type 1. The tumor most likely arose from what precursor lesion?

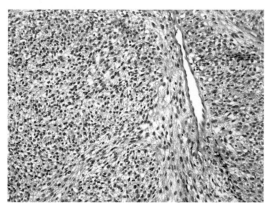

A. Leiomyoma
B. Neurofibroma
C. Perineurioma
D. Schwannoma
E. Traumatic neuroma

120.

What is the most likely etiology of the inflammation in the peripheral nerve shown in this image?

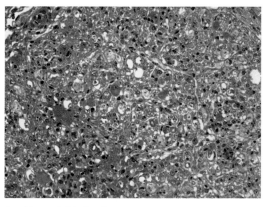

A. Bacterial infection
B. Fungal infection
C. Immune mediated process
D. Parasitic infection
E. Viral infection

121.

What are the organisms seen in the meninges that stain with mucicarmine, as shown in this image?

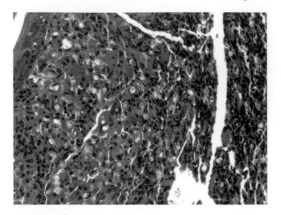

A. Amoebas
B. *Blastomyces*
C. *Candida*
D. *Coccidioides*
E. *Cryptococcus*

122.

The cerebellar lesion shown in this image is associated with what syndrome or disease?

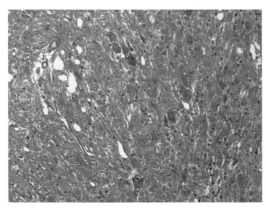

A. Cowden disease
B. Sturge-Weber syndrome
C. Tuberous sclerosis
D. Von Hippel–Lindau syndrome

123.

What tumor most commonly is encountered in the setting of medically intractable seizures?

A. Dysembryoplastic neuroepithelial tumor
B. Ganglioglioma
C. Low-grade fibrillary astrocytoma
D. Pilocytic astrocytoma
E. Pleomorphic xanthoastrocytoma

124.

The biopsy shown in this image is from a 12-year-old girl. What is the likely pathology?

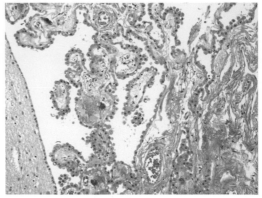

A. Choroid plexus epithelium
B. Choroid plexus papilloma
C. Papillary ependymoma
D. Papillary meningioma
E. Papillary thyroid carcinoma (metastasis)

125.

What immunostain is most useful in differentiating the lesion shown in this image from other tumors in its differential diagnosis?

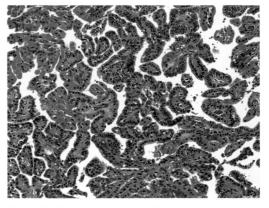

A. Epithelial membrane antigen
B. Glial fibrillary acidic protein
C. S-100 protein
D. Transthyretin
E. Vimentin

126.

The stereotactic biopsy shown in this image was taken from a 62-year-old man. From what location was the biopsy taken?

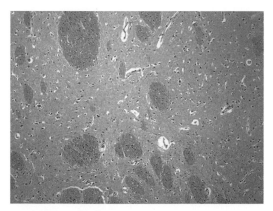

A. Caudate nucleus
B. End plate of the hippocampus
C. Hypothalamus
D. Periventricular white matter
E. Thalamus

127.

The falcine mass shown in this image is classified best as a:

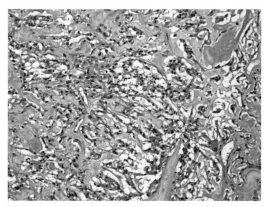

A. Chordoid meningioma
B. Clear cell meningioma
C. Metaplastic meningioma
D. Rhabdoid meningioma
E. Secretory meningioma

128.

What features warrant a WHO grade II designation for the meningioma shown in this image?

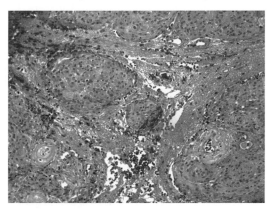

A. Angiomatous features
B. Brain invasion
C. Hypercellularity
D. Necrosis
E. Papillary features

129.

What is the classification of the changes found in the meningioma shown in this image?

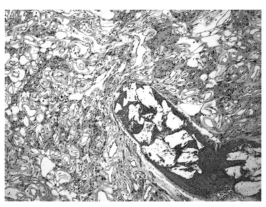

A. Angiomatous change
B. Chemotherapy effect
C. Embolization effect
D. Metastasis to a meningioma
E. Radiation effect

130.

A combination of antibodies to what proteins would stain the tumor shown in this image and allow for its distinction from a solitary fibrous tumor of the meninges?

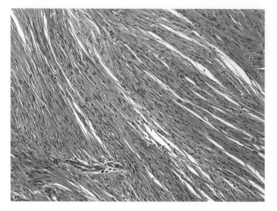

A. CD34 and epithelial membrane antigen (EMA)
B. CD34 and estrogen receptors
C. Estrogen receptors and EMA
D. Progesterone receptors and EMA
E. Progesterone and estrogen receptors

131.

The lesion shown in this image presented in a 48-year-old man along his right frontal convexity. The best diagnosis for this tumor is:

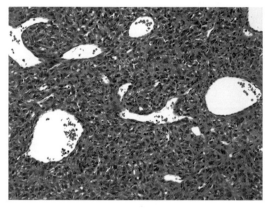

A. Angiomatous meningioma
B. Fibrous meningioma
C. Hemangioblastoma
D. Hemangiopericytoma (solitary fibrous tumor)
E. Meningothelial meningioma

132.

Antibodies against what protein most likely would stain the cerebellar mass shown in this image and allow for its distinction from a metastatic renal cell carcinoma?

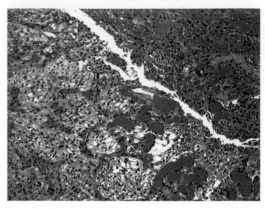

A. Cytokeratin AE1/3
B. Epithelial membrane antigen
C. Inhibin
D. PAX8
E. RCC

133.

What is the best diagnosis for the CD20 positive staining lesion shown in this image?

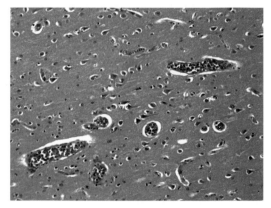

A. Breast carcinoma tumor emboli
B. Diffuse large B cell lymphoma
C. Intravascular lymphoma
D. Leukemia (acute lymphocytic)
E. Leukemia (acute myelogenous)

134.

The patient who presented with the CD20-positive lesion shown in this image most likely has which of the following?

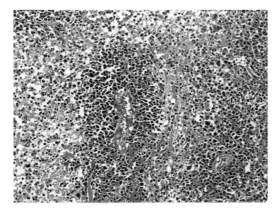

A. Alzheimer disease
B. Alexander disease
C. HIV infection
D. Neurofibromatosis type 1
E. Tuberous sclerosis

135.

A 3-year-old boy presents with a newly discovered mass in the right cerebellar hemisphere. There is no evidence of tumor elsewhere in the brain or body. The lesion is resected and is shown in this image. It stains with synaptophysin antibody. The best diagnosis is:

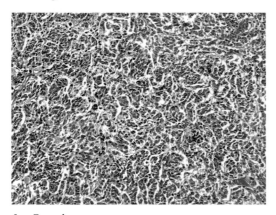

A. Ependymoma
B. Medulloblastoma
C. Neuroblastoma
D. Pilocytic astrocytoma
E. Primary central nervous system lymphoma

Use the following answers for questions 136 and 137:

A. Germinoma
B. Pineal parenchymal tumor of intermediate differentiation
C. Pineoblastoma
D. Pineocytoma
E. Yolk sac tumor

136.

The pineal gland mass shown in this image presented in an 18-year-old man. What is the best diagnosis for this mass?

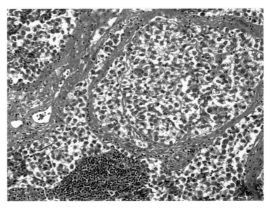

137.

The pineal gland mass shown in this image presented in an 18-year-old woman. What is the best diagnosis for this mass?

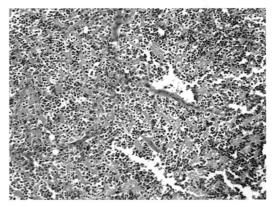

138.

Multiple meningiomas are most likely encountered in the setting of what disease?

A. Gorlin syndrome
B. Li-Fraumeni syndrome
C. Neurofibromatosis type 1
D. Neurofibromatosis type 2
E. Turcot syndrome

139.

A 45-year-old man presented with a mass in the vermis, shown in this image. What is the best diagnosis for the patient's tumor?

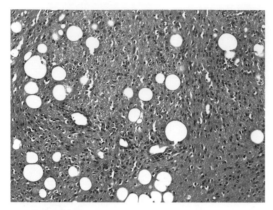

A. Ependymoma
B. Liponeurocytoma
C. Medulloblastoma
D. Oligodendroglioma
E. Pleomorphic xanthoastrocytoma

140.

A 21-year-old woman presents with headaches, ataxia, and a circumscribed mass in the posterior fossa. The tumor is marked by neurocytic type rosettes. What is the most likely diagnosis?

A. Clear cell ependymoma
B. Dysembryoplastic neuroepithelial tumor
C. Oligodendroglioma
D. Rosette-forming glioneuronal tumor of the fourth ventricle
E. Pilocytic astrocytoma

141.

What is a characteristic of hypothalamic hamartomas?

A. Associated with gelastic epilepsy
B. Consists of multinucleated neuronal cells
C. Mostly arises in females
D. More than 90% arise in the setting of Pallister-Hall syndrome
E. Typically greater than 5 cm in size

142.

The tumor shown in this image was removed from the frontal lobe of a 2-year-old and most likely demonstrates what cytogenetic alteration?

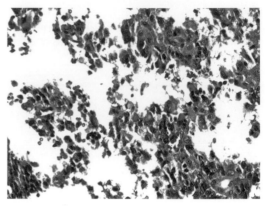

A. C-myc amplification
B. INI-1 loss
C. N-myc amplification
D. PTCH 1 mutation
E. WNT activation

143.

The tumor shown in this image presented as an enhancing mass in the anterior portion of the third ventricle in a 53-year-old woman with headaches. The best diagnosis for this tumor is:

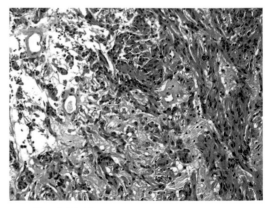

A. Chordoid glioma
B. Chordoid meningioma
C. Ependymoma
D. Pilocytic astrocytoma
E. Pituitary adenoma

144.

What syndrome is characterized by a disorder in peroxisomal biogenesis resulting in dysmorphic features, abnormal neural migration, reduction in myelination, hepatomegaly, and renal cysts?

A. Behçet syndrome
B. Apert syndrome
C. Dejerine-Roussy syndrome
D. Gerstmann syndrome
E. Zellweger syndrome

145.
The tumor shown in this image was diagnosed as a psammomatous melanotic schwannoma. What lesion is associated with this rare variant of schwannoma?

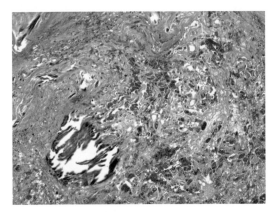

A. Cardiac myxoma
B. Neurofibroma
C. Paraganglioma
D. Pheochromocytoma
E. Thyroid-stimulating hormone–secreting pituitary adenoma

146.
What type of inclusion/mutation is typical for frontotemporal lobar atrophy with ubiquinated inclusions?

A. α-synuclein positive inclusions
B. CHMP2B protein mutation
C. Tau positive inclusions
D. TDP-43 positive inclusions
E. Prion positive inclusions

147.
What is the most likely diagnosis for argyrophilic intracytoplasmic inclusions in dentate granular cell neurons accompanied by ballooned neurons in a 79-year-old with dementia?

A. Argyrophilic grain disease
B. Corticobasal degeneration
C. Multisystem atrophy
D. Pick disease
E. Progressive supranuclear palsy

148.
A 65-year-old man presents with spasticity of the lower extremities, hand weakness and atrophy, and tongue fasciculations. The patient has no cognitive or other neurologic deficits. The patient's brother presented with the same symptoms years earlier, and died 5 years after diagnosis. What is the patient's pathological examination at autopsy expected to reveal?

A. Degeneration of the pars compacta of the substantia nigra
B. Lewy bodies throughout the cortex and hippocampus
C. Atrophy of the caudate nucleus
D. Degeneration of anterior horn cells and corticospinal tracts
E. Normal neural tissue

149.
A man recently came to the United States from Brazil. He presents with lower extremity weakness, fever, chills, and vomiting. Imaging shows multiple ring-enhancing brain lesions. A biopsy is taken of one of the lesions, shown in this image. What is the etiology of this patient's lesion?

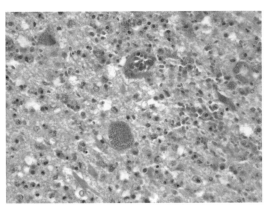

A. Histoplasmosis
B. Leishmaniasis
C. Sarcocystis
D. Trypanosomiasis
E. Toxoplasmosis

150.
What is the most common hereditary ataxia caused by a GAA triplet nucleotide expansion?

A. Charcot-Marie-Tooth disease
B. Dentatorubral-pallidoluysian atrophy
C. Friedreich ataxia
D. Spinocerebellar atrophy type 1
E. Spinocerebellar atrophy type 2

151.
Hinge skull fractures most commonly are associated with what mechanism of injury?

A. Falling down a flight of stairs
B. Gunshot
C. Hanging
D. Motor vehicle accident
E. Strangulation

152.
What muscle biopsy finding is suggestive of a mitochondrial disorder?

A. Nemaline rods
B. Nuclear chains
C. Ragged red fibers
D. Rimmed vacuoles
E. Ring fibers

153.
An accumulation of long unbranched molecules of repeating disaccharides (GAGs) in various organs of the body is characteristic of what group of disorders?

A. Demyelinating diseases
B. Glycogen storage diseases
C. Lysosomal storage diseases
D. Mitochondrial disorders
E. Mucopolysaccharidoses

154.
Devic disease is characterized pathologically by demyelination preferentially involving the:

A. Corpus callosum
B. Medulla
C. Optic nerves and chiasm
D. Pons
E. Temporal lobes

155.
What is the most common of the lysosomal storage diseases?

A. Fabry disease
B. Gaucher disease
C. Globoid cell leukodystrophy
D. Neuronal ceroid lipofuscinosis
E. Pompe disease

156.
What is the enzyme deficiency in Niemann-Pick disease, and what metabolite accumulates?

A. Sphingomyelinase; sphingomyelin
B. Sphingomyelinase; glucocerebroside
C. Hexosaminidase A; GM2 ganglioside
D. Hexosaminidase A; glucocerebroside
E. Glucocerebrosidase; glucocerebroside

157.
Curvilinear and fingerprint bodies are characteristic ultrastructural (electron microscopic) findings occurring in what disorder?

A. Fucosidosis
B. Neuronal ceroid lipofuscinosis
C. Schindler disease
D. Sialidosis
E. Wolman disease

158.
Alzheimer type 2 astrocyte changes marked by astrocytes with large, clear nuclei and marginated chromatin are encountered most commonly with what pathological process?

A. Acute tubular necrosis of the kidney
B. Central pontine myelinolysis
C. Crohn disease
D. Progressive multifocal leukoencephalopathy
E. Wilson disease

159.
A young patient has a marfanoid habitus, dislocated right eye lens, kyphoscoliosis, mental retardation, and a right leg intra-arterial thrombus. The patient most likely has what disorder?

A. Urea cycle disorder
B. Homocystinuria
C. Maple syrup urine disease
D. Menkes disease
E. Phenylketonuria

160.
What autosomal recessive disease is characterized by a deficiency of α-galactosidase A and manifests with angiokeratomas, cardiac disease, renal failure, and neuropathy?

A. Fabry disease
B. Tay-Sachs disease
C. Gaucher disease
D. Krabbe disease
E. Pompe disease

161.

Partial agenesis of the cerebellar vermis with cystic dilatation of the fourth ventricle defines what malformation/syndrome?

A. Chiari type 2 malformation
B. Dandy-Walker malformation
C. Joubert syndrome
D. Lhermitte-Duclos disease
E. Rhombencephalosynapsis

162.

Chalky spots of necrosis in the white matter at the angle of the lateral ventricle of a premature infant are characteristic of what disease process:

A. Germinal matrix hemorrhage
B. Hydranencephaly
C. Periventricular leukomalacia
D. Schizencephaly
E. Ulegyria

163.

What syndrome is characterized by an autosomal recessive pattern of inheritance with defects in peroxin protein, leading to accumulation of long chain fatty acids that causes cortical dysgenesis, white matter degeneration, hepatorenal dysfunction, and death within a few months?

A. Menkes disease
B. Leigh disease
C. Lowe syndrome
D. Lesch-Nyhan disease
E. Zellweger syndrome

164.

Miller-Dieker syndrome is associated with what gross cerebral finding?

A. Lissencephaly
B. Nodular gray matter heterotopia
C. Pachygyria
D. Polymicrogyria
E. Porencephaly

165.

A 32-year-old man with a history of alcohol abuse presents with muscle pain, weakness, and a markedly elevated serum creatinine kinase level. The findings in the muscle biopsy shown in this image are consistent with what pathological process?

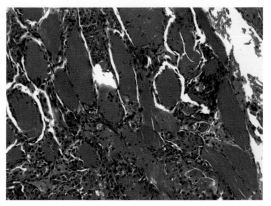

A. Infarct
B. Polymyositis
C. Rhabdomyolysis
D. Scleroderma
E. Vasculitis

166.

A 30-year-old man presents to clinic for routine follow-up. He is now wheelchair bound, which is new since his last visit 2 years ago. The patient has a long history of slowly progressive muscle weakness and pseudohypertrophy of the calves. What would a muscle biopsy demonstrate?

A. Abnormal dystrophin, fatty/fibrous infiltration, and no necrosis
B. Absent dystrophin, fatty/fibrous infiltration, and muscle fiber necrosis and regeneration
C. Chronic inflammatory cells within the muscle and no fiber necrosis or regeneration
D. Accumulation of basophilic bodies with dark centers within the muscle cells
E. Normal muscle tissue

167.

A gunshot wound is marked by stippling around the wound. At what range/position was the gun likely fired?

A. Close range
B. In contact with the patient
C. Distant range
D. On the opposite side of the patient (exit wound)
E. Medium range

168.
The lesion shown in this image from the sacral region most likely represents what pathology?

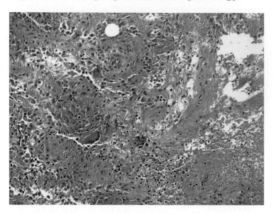

A. Blastomycosis
B. Cysticercosis
C. Nocardial infection
D. Sarcoidosis
E. Tuberculosis

8 Ophthalmology

1.

A patient presents with a central scotoma in the left eye and a superior temporal visual defect in the right eye. Where is the patient's lesion?

A. In the left inferior optic radiations
B. In the right occipital pole
C. In the orbital portion of the left optic nerve
D. At the junction of the left optic nerve and chiasm
E. In the optic chiasm

2.

A 10-month-old girl presents to clinic after her parents noticed that her eyes do not follow a moving object when her head is held in place. She is diagnosed with congenital oculomotor apraxia. What mechanism does she utilize to track objects?

A. Optokinetic reflex
B. Preserved convergence ability
C. Vestibuloocular reflex
D. Tonic labyrinthine reflex
E. Ability to turn head

3.

A man presents with a ptosis of the right eye, anisocoria with the right pupil being smaller than the left, and a history of the right upper half of his face no longer sweating. Intraocular cocaine administration bilaterally dilates only the left eye, and Paredrine (amphetamine) administration has no effect on the right pupil. Where is the lesion causing the Horner syndrome?

A. Brainstem
B. Cervical spinal cord
C. Sympathetic chain proximal to the superior cervical ganglion
D. Sympathetic chain distal to the superior cervical ganglion but proximal to the off-take of the vasomotor fibers
E. Sympathetic chain distal to the superior cervical ganglion and distal to the off-take of the vasomotor fibers

4.

A conjugate horizontal gaze palsy combined with an internuclear ophthalmoplegia (one-and-a-half syndrome) can be caused by a lesion involving the:

A. Contralateral abducens nerve and the ipsilateral medial longitudinal fasciculus

B. Bilateral paramedian pontine reticular formations
C. Ipsilateral paramedian pontine reticular formation and the ipsilateral medial longitudinal fasciculus
D. Contralateral paramedian pontine reticular formation and the ipsilateral medial longitudinal fasciculus
E. Bilateral medial longitudinal fasciculi

5.

Optic nerve sheath meningiomas present with what characteristics?

A. Arising from the dural layer of the meninges lining the intraorbital or intracanalicular optic nerve
B. Painless, slowly progressive monocular vision loss
C. Optociliary shunt vessels without optic atrophy
D. Best treated with surgical resection while there is stability of the vision defect
E. Most commonly affecting young women with an incidence three times that in men

6.

A patient incurs an infarction of the midbrain and develops a right trochlear nerve deficit as manifested on clinical exam. For what should the examiner look in the contralateral eye to localize the extent of the lesion?

A. Mydriatic pupil
B. Abducens nerve deficit
C. Horner syndrome
D. Oculomotor palsy

7.

A patient presents with a pupil that is tonically dilated with a very slow reaction to light. During accommodative testing, there is a more pronounced constriction. Syphilis and dorsal midbrain syndrome are ruled out through workup. Between what two neurons in the pupillary reflex pathway is the lesion?

A. Prior to the first neuron
B. Between the first and second neurons
C. Between the second and third neurons
D. Between the third and fourth neurons
E. After the fourth neuron

8.

A 60-year-old woman presents with a 1-year history of progressive irritability, right-sided anosmia, and decreased right-sided vision. A funduscopic exam shows left-sided papilledema. What is the most likely lesion?

A. A large, left parasagittal meningioma
B. A right olfactory groove meningioma
C. A suprasellar glioma
D. A left sphenoid wing meningioma

9.

What factor predicts the occurrence of Terson syndrome following aneurysmal subarachnoid hemorrhage?

A. Hunt-Hess score
B. Ventriculomegaly
C. Fisher grade
D. Anterior communicating artery aneurysm

10.

A patient closes his eye forcefully, and it is noted that his eye slowly opens after several seconds despite his efforts to keep it closed. What is the likely diagnosis?

A. Myasthenia gravis
B. Hemifacial spasm
C. Hemifacial paresis due to stroke
D. Disinsertion of the levator palpebrae
E. Botulinum toxin injection into the orbicularis oculi

11.

A 13-year-old girl presents to the emergency room for the third time in a year with an acute occurrence of a severe, bifrontal headache (worse on the right) with right orbital pain. She endorses photophobia, nausea, and diplopia. Exam reveals a right oculomotor nerve palsy that the patient states has occurred with past headaches. MRI and MR angiography of the brain are done and are unremarkable. What is the likely diagnosis?

A. Multiple sclerosis
B. Ophthalmoplegic migraine
C. Myasthenia gravis
D. Classic migraine
E. Orbital cellulitis

12.

Which of the following is a characteristic of optic nerve gliomas?

A. They most commonly are pilocytic astrocytomas, WHO grade IV.
B. Seventy percent occur in the third decade of life.
C. They present with optic atrophy and disk edema with an afferent pupillary defect.
D. Surgical resection is the first-line treatment.
E. They are associated with neurofibromatosis type 2.

13.

Where does the Goldman visual field test result shown in this image localize the patient's lesion?

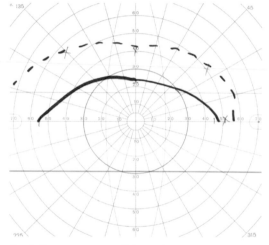

A. Inferior arcuates of the retina
B. Superior arcuates of the retina
C. Optic nerve
D. Optic tract
E. Occipital lobe

14.

A 65-year-old man presents with a severe headache and painful ophthalmoplegia unilaterally that has occurred previously with spontaneous remission each time. An MRI of the body is done, revealing only inflammatory changes in the cavernous sinus, and cerebrospinal fluid studies only reveal a mild lymphocytic pleocytosis. Serum angiotensin-converting enzyme levels are within normal limits. What is the patient's likely diagnosis?

A. Ramsay Hunt syndrome
B. Tolosa-Hunt syndrome
C. Sarcoidosis
D. Multiple sclerosis
E. Tuberculosis meningitis

15.

A 23-year-old woman is referred to the ophthalmologist for unilateral optic disk edema and a painless decrease in visual acuity in the same eye. She endorses headaches and has a body mass index of 38. Funduscopic examination reveals macular exudates in a "star" pattern. What is the most likely cause of her findings?

A. Pseudotumor cerebri
B. Optic nerve glioma
C. Infectious neuroretinitis
D. Glaucoma
E. Nonarteritic anterior ischemic optic neuropathy

16.

A woman presents to the neurosurgery clinic complaining of unilateral diplopia after a 5-cm right convexity meningioma was found on MRI. She has been started on phenytoin. What is the most likely cause of the patient's diplopia?

A. Cranial nerve palsy secondary to the meningioma
B. Cranial nerve palsy secondary to unreported trauma
C. Congenital strabismus
D. Phenytoin side effect
E. Refractive error

17.

What is the prognosis for a patient undergoing a 12-hour spinal surgery with extensive blood loss who wakes up with bilateral loss of vision (light perception only)?

A. Complete recovery of vision in the acute period
B. Complete recovery of vision in a delayed fashion
C. Partial recovery of vision
D. Variable prognosis with some patients having good and others having poor vision outcomes
E. Poor prognosis with little recovery of vision

18.

A 70-year-old man presents with 2 weeks of a tender right scalp and profound vision loss in the right eye. Cotton-wool spots are seen on funduscopic exam. C-reactive protein is elevated, and the patient has been on low-dose steroids for 1 week as prescribed by another physician. What is the next step in management?

A. Start high-dose steroids
B. Plasmapheresis
C. Schedule fluorescein angiography
D. Schedule temporal artery biopsy
E. Observation

19.

What are considered the maximal safe doses of radiation to the visual pathways and optic apparatuses?

A. < 25 Gy total and < 1 Gy fractionated
B. < 50 Gy total and < 2 Gy fractionated
C. < 75 Gy total and < 4 Gy fractionated
D. < 100 Gy total and < 8 Gy fractionated
E. < 8 Gy total

20.

How is isolated optic neuritis associated with multiple sclerosis (MS) during 15-year follow-up?

A. MS will not occur if MRI is negative for lesions at the time of the optic neuritis.
B. More than one demyelinating plaque at the time of optic neuritis indicates an almost 100% chance of developing MS.
C. Severe optic disk swelling and optic disk hemorrhage are associated with an increased risk for developing MS.
D. There is a 50% risk of developing MS across all patients with optic neuritis.

21.

A 38-year-old obese woman presents to the neuro-ophthalmology clinic with symptoms suggestive of pseudotumor cerebri. After mass lesions are ruled out, what is the next disease process that must be ruled out using neuroimaging?

A. Empty sella syndrome
B. Flattening of the posterior aspect of the globes
C. Dural venous sinus thrombosis
D. Thyroid disease
E. Vitamin A deficiency

22.

What investigation is expected to have the highest chance of yielding positive results in a 41-year-old obese patient who presents with bilateral acute optic neuropathy following rapid weight loss?

A. Methylmalonic acid and homocysteine levels
B. Thorough family/genetic history
C. MRI of the orbits
D. History of homemade alcohol consumption

23.

A 55-year-old man presents with a third nerve palsy. MRI of the brain is unremarkable. What is the most likely diagnosis?

A.   Posterior communicating artery aneurysm
B.   Trauma
C.   Myasthenia gravis
D.   Vaso-occlusive disease
E.   Multiple sclerosis

24.

A patient with anisocoria has a reversal of his anisocoria with apraclonidine administered in the eyes bilaterally. He notes in his history a lack of sweating one side of his face only. Amphetamine administration causes dilation of the originally miotic pupil. Given the likely diagnosis, what is the next step in the workup?

A.   No further imaging is indicated
B.   Orbital imaging
C.   Imaging of the medulla with MRI
D.   Chest imaging
E.   CT angiography of the neck looking for internal carotid artery dissection

25.

A patient complains of headaches and declining visual acuity. The fundus is shown in this image. What is the next diagnostic test the physician should perform?

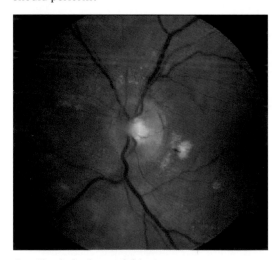

A.   Check the hemoglobin A$_{1c}$.
B.   Order a CT of the brain.
C.   Check the intraocular pressure.
D.   Check the blood pressure.

26.

A 15-year old woman is referred to the neuro-ophthalmologist due to a left esotropia with abduction limitation. On exam, the patient maintains a constant head turn to the left and squints with the left eye. She denies trauma, and photographs over the past 10 years show similar head turns and squinting. What is the most likely diagnosis?

A.   Left abducens nerve palsy
B.   Intracranial mass
C.   Duane syndrome
D.   Multiple sclerosis
E.   Unreported trauma

27.

In general, when localizing a pathology resulting in a bilateral visual cut, how does symmetry of the deficit assist in the localizing?

A.   More symmetrical visual field deficits tend to localize lesions closer to the occipital lobes.
B.   More symmetrical visual field deficits tend to localize lesions closer to the optic chiasm.
C.   More symmetrical visual field deficits tend to localize lesions closer to the lateral geniculate nucleus.
D.   Symmetry of visual field deficits has no relevance when localizing lesions.

28.

A patient is referred to his physician due to bilateral exophthalmos. Without any other clinical information being provided, what structure or system should be the most likely focus of the next step in the patient's workup?

A.   Thymus
B.   Brain
C.   Eye
D.   Thyroid
E.   Bone marrow

29.

A patient with a ventriculoperitoneal shunt is seen in the emergency room and is described as having Parinaud (dorsal midbrain) syndrome secondary to hydrocephalus. There is eyelid retraction when the patient is asked to look upward and good convergence when looking downward. What function of upgaze is expected to be the most conserved?

A.   Voluntary upgaze
B.   Upgaze with "doll's eyes" test
C.   Upgaze with accommodation
D.   Upgaze when lying supine

30.
What is seen in the Goldman visual field of the left eye shown in this image?

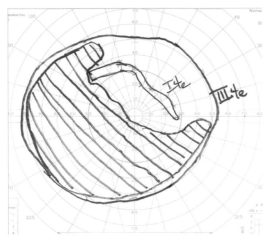

A. Quadrantanopsia
B. Disk edema and enlargement of the blind spot
C. Visual field occlusion due to ptosis
D. Unreliable visual field due to feigning of symptoms

31.
A patient presents with bilateral extorted eyes. What is the etiology most considered until proven otherwise?

A. Demyelination
B. Tumor
C. Congenital
D. Trauma
E. Infarction

32.
Cold water is injected simultaneously into a patient's ears. What will be the direction of the fast phase of nystagmus?

A. Inferiorly
B. Superiorly
C. Left
D. Right
E. Equally to the right and left

33.
What pathology is shown in this image of the visual field in the right eye?

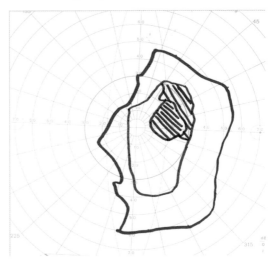

A. Pituitary tumor
B. Methyl alcohol poisoning
C. Optic neuritis
D. Left middle cerebral artery territory infarction

34.
Up to what age can strabismic amblyopia be improved with treatment?

A. 6 years old
B. 8 years old
C. 10 years old
D. 12 years old
E. 14 years old

35.
A patient with severe acne and fever presents with a rapidly developing right eye proptosis, chemosis, slowly reactive pupil, and ophthalmoplegia. In what direction is the right eye most likely unable to look?

A. Laterally
B. Medially
C. Superiorly and medially
D. Inferiorly and medially
E. Superiorly and laterally

9 Critical Care

1.
Dimercaprol, when used as a chelation agent, can increase the brain concentrations of which metal?

A. Lead
B. Arsenic
C. Cadmium
D. Chromium
E. Mercury

2.
A patient was diagnosed with epilepsy over 30 years ago and has been on antiepileptic medications since diagnosis. The patient complains of a lupus-like syndrome and progressive ataxia and is found to have gingival hypertrophy on exam. What antiepileptic drug has the patient likely been taking?

A. Levetiracetam
B. Phenytoin
C. Primidone
D. Valproic acid
E. Lamotrigine

3.
A 69-year-old man on aspirin and warfarin underwent a craniectomy for a traumatic subdural hematoma. Surgery was uneventful except for high-volume blood loss, and a blood transfusion was ordered postoperatively. Ten minutes after the transfusion was started, the patient started having tremors. His temperature was 102.8°F, blood pressure was 130/85 mm Hg, pulse was 100 bpm, and respiratory rate was 22 bpm. Per blood bank policies, the transfusion was stopped, and the patient was given acetaminophen. The blood products and a fresh type and screen sample were sent back to the blood bank. What was the patient's most likely type of blood reaction?

A. Acute hemolytic
B. Delayed hemolytic
C. Febrile nonhemolytic
D. Allergic
E. Transfusion-related acute lung injury (TRALI)

4.
What vitamin should be coadministered with isoniazid to prevent neuropathy?

A. Vitamin A
B. Vitamin B12
C. Vitamin C
D. Vitamin B6
E. Vitamin E

5.
A 35-year-old patient admitted to the neurology ICU following polytrauma becomes hypotensive. What hemodynamic parameters are compatible with hypovolemic shock?

A. Decreased right atrial pressure, decreased pulmonary capillary wedge pressure, decreased cardiac output, and increased systemic vascular resistance
B. Normal or increased right atrial pressure, increased pulmonary capillary wedge pressure, decreased cardiac output, and increased systemic vascular resistance
C. Variable right atrial pressure, variable pulmonary capillary wedge pressure, increased cardiac output, and decreased systemic vascular resistance
D. Increased right atrial pressure, normal or decreased pulmonary capillary wedge pressure, decreased cardiac output, and increased systemic vascular resistance
E. Increased right atrial pressure, increased pulmonary capillary wedge pressure, decreased cardiac output, and increased systemic vascular resistance

6.
A 10-year-old boy with von Willebrand disease is scheduled to undergo a craniotomy for tumor resection. Besides having blood products readily available, what can be administered preoperatively to ready the patient for surgery?

A. Desmopressin
B. Von Willebrand factor
C. Factor VII
D. Intravenous crystalloids
E. Factor IX

7.

In the conjunction with absence of brainstem reflexes, absent motor response, and the absence of complicating conditions (e.g., hypothermia, intoxication, etc.), what apnea test $PaCO_2$ finding is consistent with brain death?

A. $PaCO_2$ of 40 mm Hg after 10 minutes of testing with no spontaneous respirations
B. $PaCO_2$ of 65 mm Hg with a 20 mm Hg rise over the patient's baseline after 12 minutes of testing with no spontaneous respirations
C. $PaCO_2$ of 60 mm Hg with a 10 mm Hg rise over the patient's baseline after 6 minutes of testing with no spontaneous respirations
D. $PaCO_2$ of 50 mm Hg after 10 minutes of testing with no spontaneous respirations

Use the following answers for questions 8 and 9:

A. Opening pressure 15, 2 WBC without an abnormal differential, protein 30, glucose 60
B. Opening pressure 22, 250 WBC with more than 80% being lymphocytes, protein 500, glucose 25
C. Opening pressure 30, 1,500 WBC with more than 80% PMN, protein 400, glucose 10
D. Opening pressure 21, 110 WBC with more than 50% lymphocytes, protein 80, glucose 50

Abbreviations: WBC, white blood cells; PMN, polymorphonuclear leukocytes

8.

What lumbar puncture cerebrospinal fluid study profile is consistent with bacterial meningitis?

9.

What lumbar puncture cerebrospinal study profile is consistent with viral meningitis?

10.

What aspect of propofol requires the use of an additional intravenous agent when propofol is used as a sedative in the acute trauma setting?

A. Its lack of analgesia
B. Its lack of hypnotic effects
C. Its poor ability to lower intracranial pressure and offer cerebral protection
D. Its poor induction properties in the setting of rapid intubation

11.

A woman with a family history of unknown but reportedly "significant" reactions to anesthesia is undergoing induction of anesthesia with a halogenated agent. She is noted to have a sudden increase in end-tidal PCO_2 and tachycardia. The arterial blood gas reading indicates a metabolic acidosis. The patient had a previous surgery without any complications. What is the next step in the management of this patient?

A. Stop the anesthetic agent.
B. Administer dantrolene.
C. Hyperventilate the patient to 100% FiO_2.
D. Administer calcium chloride.
E. Administer glucose and insulin.

12.

What inhalational neuroanesthetic does not reduce cerebral metabolism?

A. Halothane
B. Enflurane
C. Nitrous oxide
D. Isoflurane
E. Desflurane

13.

What is a major advantage of halogenated inhalational anesthetic agents?

A. They suppress EEG activity.
B. They decrease cerebral blood flow.
C. They increase cerebral metabolism.
D. They decrease intracranial pressure.
E. They are relatively nonhepatotoxic at high doses.

14.

Propofol has what analgesic effect?

A. Complete analgesia reversal
B. No analgesic effect
C. Strong analgesic effect
D. Blunting of the effects of other analgesics

15.

What is the major side effect of nitroglycerin and nitroprusside when used for hypertension control in neurosurgical patients?

A. Nitroglycerin and nitroprusside lower the seizure threshold.
B. Nitroglycerin and nitroprusside can cause paralysis in acute use.
C. Nitroglycerin and nitroprusside cause vasoconstriction.
D. Nitroglycerin and nitroprusside raise intracranial pressure.
E. Nitroglycerin and nitroprusside increase cerebral perfusion pressure.

16.

A patient with various intraparenchymal hemorrhages following trauma has been resuscitated fully except for a continued coagulopathy. As the coagulopathy is corrected, what fluids should be avoided for prolonged administration with regard to the coagulopathy?

A.   Nonhypertonic crystalloids (e.g., normal saline)
B.   Colloids (e.g., dextran, hetastarch)
C.   Hypertonic crystalloids (e.g., 3% normal saline)
D.   Osmotic agents (e.g., mannitol)
E.   Isotonic solutions (e.g., Isolyte)

17.

What is the definitive way to identify a patient at risk for malignant hyperthermia?

A.   Obtaining a muscle biopsy for in vitro testing
B.   Performing genetic testing
C.   Obtaining an adequate family history
D.   Assessing serum potassium levels
E.   Assessing serum creatine kinase levels

18.

What pressor agent should be avoided in spinal shock?

A.   Dopamine
B.   Phenylephrine
C.   Isoproterenol
D.   Levophed
E.   Dobutamine

19.

How do the steroid replacement requirements differ between primary and secondary adrenal insufficiency?

A.   In primary adrenal insufficiency, only glucocorticoids need to be replaced.
B.   In secondary adrenal insufficiency, only mineralocorticoids need to be replaced.
C.   In secondary adrenal insufficiency, both glucocorticoids and mineralocorticoids need to be replaced.
D.   In primary adrenal insufficiency, both glucocorticoids and mineralocorticoids need to be replaced.
E.   In primary adrenal insufficiency, only mineralocorticoids need to be replaced.

20.

What are the side effects associated with using a long-term, properly dosed, cortisone regimen for a patient with panhypopituitarism secondary to a pituitary adenoma?

A.   Hypertension and hypokalemia
B.   Hyperglycemia and salt wasting
C.   Hyperglycemia and volume depletion through dieresis
D.   Hypertension and hyperglycemia
E.   Salt wasting and volume depletion

21.

What anesthetic is ideal for a patient experiencing elevated intracranial pressure?

A.   Thiopental
B.   Enflurane
C.   Halothane
D.   Isoflurane

22.

A 45-year-old woman developed marked pallor and a petechial rash following a craniotomy for tumor resection. Her temperature is 101.2°F, blood pressure is 105/75 mm Hg, heart rate is 90 bpm, and respiratory rate is 18 bmp. Lab work reveals a serum creatinine of 2, hemoglobin of 8, platelet count of 36,000, prolonged bleeding time of 5 minutes, prothrombin time of 12.1 seconds, and partial thromboplastin time of 30 seconds. A peripheral blood smear shows fragmented red blood cells. There is no elevation in the serum d-dimer level. What is the most likely diagnosis?

A.   Idiopathic thrombocytopenic purpura
B.   Disseminated intravascular coagulation
C.   Thrombotic thrombocytopenic purpura
D.   Hemolytic uremic syndrome
E.   Sepsis

23.

What is the most reliable indicator that a patient is experiencing cerebral salt wasting and not the syndrome of inappropriate antidiuretic hormone secretion?

A.   The patient has a high plasma volume.
B.   The patient has a low serum sodium concentration.
C.   The patient has a low urine output.
D.   The patient is volume depleted.
E.   The patient has increasing cerebral edema.

24.
A man with chronic alcoholism is recovering after an alcohol-induced traumatic cerebral contusion. He is neurologically intact awaiting discharge after eating several full meals when he suddenly develops quadriplegia, confusion, difficulty speaking, and trouble swallowing. Serum sodium is 139 mEq/L. What is the most likely diagnosis?

A. Beriberi
B. Central pontine myelinolysis
C. Pseudohyponatremia
D. Cerebral edema
E. Cervical spinal cord contusion

25.
When/how should hyperventilation be used in the setting of a severe head injury and with what goals?

A. It should never be used.
B. Prophylactic hyperventilation to achieve a $PaCO_2$ of 30 mm Hg for 48 to 72 hours is safe and effective in reducing intracranial pressure (ICP).
C. Hyperventilation to achieve a $PaCO_2$ of 30 to 35 mm Hg is appropriate to use as a temporizing measure for patients with signs of progressive neurologic deterioration when ICP monitoring is not yet established.
D. In the case of transtentorial herniation, hyperventilation to achieve a $PaCO_2$ less than 25 mm Hg may be more effective in reducing ICP than achieving a $PaCO_2$ less than 30 mm Hg.

26.
In the event of failed maximal medical management of increased intracranial pressure, what is the dosing regimen for pentobarbital for instituting a pentobarbital coma?

A. 20 mg/kg intravenous bolus followed by 100 mg every 8 hours
B. 100 mg intravenously every 4 hours
C. 20 to 75 µg/kg/min intravenous continuous drip
D. 10 mg/kg intravenous bolus over 30 minutes followed by a 1 mg/kg/h infusion

27.
What antipsychotic medication can lead to agranulocytosis?

A. Clozapine
B. Thioridazine
C. Chlorpromazine
D. Aripiprazole
E. Quetiapine

28.
In patients with low albumin, what equation can be used to convert observed phenytoin levels to equivalent/corrected phenytoin levels?

A. Equivalent level = Observed level/(0.1(Albumin level) + 0.1)
B. Equivalent level = Observed level – 2(Albumin level)
C. Equivalent level = Observed level/(2(Albumin level) + 3)
D. Equivalent level = Observed level/Albumin level
E. Equivalent level = Observed level – 3(Albumin level)

29.
What anesthetic agent can lead to the development of tension pneumocephalus following surgery in the supine position?

A. Halothane
B. Sevoflurane
C. Nitrous oxide
D. Propofol
E. Remifentanil

30.
What are the two main factors that should be present for an air embolism to occur?

A. Noncollapsible vein and negative pressure in the vein
B. Collapsible vein and positive pressure in the vein
C. Noncollapsible vein and positive pressure in the vein
D. Collapsible vein and patent foramen ovale
E. Patent foramen ovale and negative pressure in the vein

31.
Following traumatic skull base fractures, if patients are placed on empiric antibiotic coverage, what organism should be targeted with this coverage?

A. *Staphylococcus aureus*
B. *Staphylococcus epidermidis*
C. *Streptococcus pneumoniae*
D. *Hemophilus influenza*
E. *Neisseria meningitis*

32.

A postoperative patient has a potassium level of 6.7, and an electrocardiogram shows peaked T waves. What should be administered next in this patient's management?

A. Calcium gluconate
B. Kayexalate
C. Insulin and glucose
D. Lasix
E. Albuterol

Use the following answers for questions 33 to 36:

A. Atropine
B. Physostigmine
C. Flumazenil
D. Glucagon
E. Phentolamine
F. Naloxone
G. Protamine
H. Dimercaprol

33.

What is the reversal agent for benzodiazepines?

34.

What is the reversal agent for morphine?

35.

What is the antidote agent for anticholinergic poisoning?

36.

What is the reversal agent for dopamine overdose?

37.

What is the mechanism of action of isoproterenol?

A. Selective β-adrenergic agonism
B. Nonselective β-adrenergic agonism
C. Selective β-adrenergic blockade
D. Nonselective β-adrenergic blockade
E. Trace amine–associated receptor 1 (TAAR1) antagonism

38.

How does assist control ventilation work?

A. Breaths are patient- or time-triggered with a constant tidal volume for each breath.
B. Breaths are patient- or time-triggered, flow limited, and volume cycled; breaths taken by patients are not assisted.

C. Breaths are patient-triggered, and inspiratory pressure is added to patient-initiated breaths.
D. Breaths are not triggered, and continuous pressure is applied to the ventilation circuit throughout the breathing cycle.

Use the following answers for questions 39 and 40:

A. Respiratory alkalosis
B. Metabolic acidosis
C. Combined respiratory and metabolic alkalosis
D. Partially compensated respiratory acidosis

39.

What pathology is represented by the following arterial blood gas values?

pH: 7.30
PCO_2: 43 mm Hg
HCO_3^-: 20 mEq/L

40.

What pathology is represented by the following arterial blood gas values?

pH: 7.56
PCO_2: 28 mm Hg
HCO_3^-: 25 mEq/L

41.

In an adult patient with a normal head CT following a concussion, what risk factors increase the likelihood for intracranial hypertension?

A. Age greater than 60 years, systolic blood pressure less than 100 mm Hg, and posturing on motor exam
B. Age greater than 40 years, systolic blood pressure less than 90 mm Hg, and posturing on motor exam
C. Age greater than 65 years, systolic blood pressure less than 110 mm Hg, and posturing on motor exam
D. Age greater than 35 years, systolic blood pressure less than 80 mm Hg, and posturing on motor exam

42.

What is the conversion factor between mm Hg and cm H_2O?

A. 1 mm Hg = 1.36 cm H_2O
B. 1 mm Hg = 1.63 cm H_2O
C. 1 mm Hg = 0.735 cm H_2O
D. 1 mm Hg = 0.375 cm H_2O

43.
A 22-year-old patient with a traumatic brain injury is admitted to the intensive care unit with a Glasgow Coma Scale score of 7. What is the recommended goal for the body temperature state for this patient?

A. Induced hypothermia
B. Permissive hypothermia
C. Normothermia
D. Permissive hyperthermia
E. Induced hyperthermia

44.
What intravenous anesthetic may cause adrenal insufficiency?

A. Propofol
B. Dexmedetomidine
C. Etomidate
D. Ketamine

45.
A 55-year-old woman remains comatose for 4 days following resuscitation from a heart attack. She is off sedation and shows absence of brainstem reflexes. The patient is unable to complete the apnea test portion of the brain death examination. Median nerve somatosensory evoked potentials (SSEPs) are obtained. What finding would be predictive of a poor neurologic outcome?

A. Bilateral absence of the N20 waveform
B. Bilateral absence of the N9 waveform
C. Bilateral absence of the N13 waveform
D. Unilateral absence of the N13 waveform

46.
How does pressure support ventilation work?

A. Breaths are patient- or time-triggered with a constant tidal volume for each breath.
B. Breaths are patient- or time-triggered, flow limited, and volume cycled; breaths taken by patients are not assisted.
C. Breaths are patient-triggered, and inspiratory pressure is added to patient-initiated breaths.
D. Breaths are not triggered, and continuous pressure is applied to the ventilation circuit throughout the breathing cycle.

Use the following answers for questions 47 to 49:
A. *Tenia solium*
B. *Herpes simplex*
C. *Cryptococcus*
D. Toxoplasmosis
E. West Nile virus
F. JC virus

47.
A 35-year-old man with HIV has a multiple ring-enhancing lesions on MRI. What is the most likely diagnosis?

48.
A 70-year-old woman with HIV and noncompliance with HAART has 3 weeks of progressively worsening mental status along with a left visual field deficit and right-sided weakness. MRI reveals nonenhancing white matter lesions without surrounding edema. The lesions appear hyperintense on T2 and hypointense on T1 sequences. What is the most likely diagnosis?

49.
A 73-year-old woman with neck stiffness, headache, left leg weakness, and fever rapidly progressed to having flaccid paralysis and areflexia. Cerebrospinal fluid studies show a white blood cell count over 200, a normal red blood cell count, protein of 87, and a normal glucose level. Cerebrospinal fluid Gram stain shows no organisms, and the culture is negative. What is the most likely diagnosis?

50.
A 65-year-old man with a history of chronic obstructive pulmonary disease is admitted for a lobar intracranial hemorrhage. The patient is intubated and sedated. He suddenly develops pulseless electrical activity. Auscultation of the lungs reveals absent breath sounds on the right. The trachea is deviated to the left. What is the best next step in the patient's management?

A. Chest tube placement
B. Chest radiograph
C. Needle thoracotomy
D. Ultrasound of the lungs
E. Decrease the tidal volume on the ventilator

51.

A 28-year-old man is admitted to the intensive care unit after being hit by a car. He has a 5-mm subdural hematoma on the right and a right femur fracture. Two days after admission, he develops tachypnea, tachycardia, and hypotension and becomes disoriented. On exam, he has new petechiae across his chest. An electrocardiogram is obtained and is unremarkable. A chest radiograph is normal except for two rib fractures. What is the patient's most likely diagnosis?

A. Subdural hematoma expansion
B. Pulmonary embolism
C. Fat embolism
D. Cardiac contusion
E. Pulmonary contusion

Use the following answers for questions 52 to 54:

A. Benign intracranial hypertension
B. Aseptic meningitis
C. Cerebellar ataxia
D. Cochlear and vestibular damage
E. Unpleasant taste

52.

What are the major potential side effects of penicillin and cephalosporins?

53.

What are the major potential side effects of amphotericin B?

54.

What are the major potential side effects of ethambutol?

55.

How will the urine osmolalities of a patient with central diabetes insipidus (DI) and of a normal individual respond to the injection of DDAVP?

A. In a patient with central DI, DDAVP will cause a 50% increase in urine osmolality, whereas it will cause an increase of 5% in a normal individual.
B. In a patient with central DI and in a normal individual, DDAVP will cause a 50% increase in urine osmolality.
C. In a patient with central DI and in a normal individual, DDAVP will cause a 25% increase in urine osmolality.

D. In a patient with central DI, DDAVP will cause a 50% increase in urine osmolality, whereas it will cause a decrease of 5% in a normal individual.
E. In a patient with central DI, DDAVP will cause a 25% increase in urine osmolality, whereas it will cause a decrease of 5% in a normal individual.

Use the following answers for questions 56 to 59:

A. Hodgkin lymphoma
B. Neuroblastoma
C. Small cell lung cancer
D. Thymoma
E. Carcinoid tumor

56.

What clinical syndrome/condition is associated with opsoclonus-myoclonus in a child?

57.

What clinical syndrome/condition is associated with cerebellar dysfunction in an adolescent?

58.

What clinical syndrome/condition is associated with limbic encephalitis and myasthenia gravis?

59.

What clinical syndrome/condition is associated with Lambert-Eaton myasthenia syndrome?

60.

During hyperventilation therapy, a PCO_2 below what level could worsen cerebral ischemia?

A. 35 mm Hg
B. 32 mm Hg
C. 28 mm Hg
D. 25 mm Hg
E. 20 mm Hg

61.

What is the main anticipated outcome in proceeding with donation after cardiac death?

A. Asystole or pulselessness will occur within 1 hour of withdrawal of care.
B. The patient needs to undergo brain death examination after withdrawal of care.
C. The transplant surgeon will have to declare the patient deceased.
D. The heart will be removed for donation.

62.
What is the total blood volume of a 1-year-old boy weighting 10 kg?

A. 200 mL
B. 400 mL
C. 800 mL
D. 1.4 L
E. 1.6 L

63.
A patient develops leukopenia after starting a new drug therapy regimen for trigeminal neuralgia. What medication likely is the cause of the leukopenia?

A. Gabapentin
B. Baclofen
C. Carbamazepine
D. Levetiracetam
E. Lamotrigine

64.
A 45-year-old homeless man is admitted to the hospital after being hit by a car. Thirty-six hours after admission, he becomes agitated and starts complaining of hearing people cursing him and feeling people touching him. His vitals are stable. The patient has a history of alcohol intake and smokes one pack of cigarettes per day. He does not use any drugs and has no significant psychiatric history. What is his most likely diagnosis?

A. Alcoholic hallucinosis
B. Intensive care unit delirium
C. Schizophrenia
D. Brief psychotic episode
E. Delirium tremens

65.
The lower limit of a normal systolic blood pressure for a given age in children may be estimated by what formula?

A. 70 mm Hg + 2(Age in years)
B. 70 mm Hg + 3(Age in years)
C. 50 mm Hg + 2(Age in years)
D. 40 mm Hg + 2(Age in years)
E. 40 mm Hg + 3(Age in years)

66.
Pulmonary capillary wedge pressure is reflective of:

A. Pulmonary artery pressure
B. Central venous pressure
C. Left atrial pressure
D. Right atrial pressure
E. Left ventricular pressure

67.
In the setting of liver failure, an ammonia level of greater than what value is associated with cerebral herniation due to cerebral edema?

A. 100 μmol/L
B. 150 μmol/L
C. 200 μmol/L
D. 250 μmol/L
E. No ammonia level is predictive of cerebral herniation.

68.
Where does antidiuretic hormone (ADH) act in the kidneys?

A. Glomerulus
B. Proximal renal tubule
C. Distal renal tubule
D. Loop of Henle
E. Collecting duct

69.
What is the mechanism of action of ketamine when used as an intravenous sedative?

A. GABA-A agonist
B. GABA-B agonist
C. NMDA receptor antagonist
D. Decreases the extent of gap junction cell coupling
E. Unknown mechanism of action

70.
What is the crystalloid of choice to be administered along with a blood transfusion?

A. Lactated Ringer's solution
B. 0.9% normal saline
C. D5 water
D. 0.225% normal saline

71.
A patient presents to the emergency room in status epilepticus. According to the standard treatment algorithm for status epilepticus, after securing the patient's airway, breathing, and circulation, what medication should be given first?

A. Lorazepam 0.1 mg/kg intravenously
B. Phenytoin/fosphenytoin 20 mg/kg intravenous load
C. Phenytoin/fosphenytoin 125 mg/kg intravenous load
D. Dextrose 50 mL of D50 intravenous bolus
E. Thiamine 100 mg intravenously

72.

Deficiency of what nutrient is associated with ophthalmoplegia, ataxia, and confusion?

A. Cyanocobalamin
B. Thiamine
C. Pyridoxine
D. Folate
E. Niacin

73.

A patient is in coma with the respiratory pattern shown in this image. Where is the patient's lesion?

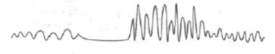

A. Diencephalon or bilateral cerebral hemispheres
B. Nonorganic (psychogenic origin)
C. Superior medulla or inferior pons
D. Superior pons
E. Medulla

74.

A 45-year-old man with a recent diagnosis of von Hippel–Lindau disease is admitted to the hospital with a blood pressure of 199/110. He has been complaining of recurrent headaches for the past few days. What is his most likely diagnosis?

A. Pheochromocytoma
B. Hyperaldosteronism
C. Renal artery stenosis
D. Renal cell carcinoma
E. Primary hypertension

75.

Following resection of a brain tumor, a patient is maintained on minimal intravenous fluids. The next morning, he has an elevated creatinine. A fractional excretion of sodium (FENa) is obtained and is 0.7. What is the most likely etiology of his elevated creatinine?

A. Dehydration
B. Acute kidney injury
C. Kidney stones
D. Drug toxicity

76.

What is the most sensitive monitoring method to detect a venous air embolism during surgery?

A. Right atrial central venous pressure catheter
B. Transesophageal echocardiogram
C. Precordial Doppler probe
D. Radial arterial line
E. End-tidal PCO_2 detector

77.

A 78-year-old man develops a pulmonary embolus on day 3 following tumor resection. He is not started on anticoagulation and is scheduled for an inferior vena cava filter placement. While waiting for filter placement, he develops acute abdominal pain with bloody diarrhea. His abdomen is soft. What is the next best step in his management?

A. *Clostridium difficile* studies
B. Stool parasitic studies
C. Stool for fecal occult blood testing
D. Emergent vascular consultation and abdominal CT angiogram
E. Abdominal ultrasound

78.

The rapid shallow breathing index (RSBI) is a weaning assessment tool measured during 1 minute of spontaneous breathing. A value of more than 105 determines a poor chance of ventilator weaning success. How is the RSBI calculated?

A. RSBI = Breath frequency/Tidal volume
B. RSBI = Tidal volume/Breath frequency
C. RSBI = PaO_2/Breath frequency
D. RSBI = PCO_2/Tidal volume
E. RSBI = Tidal volume/PaO_2

79.

Although controversial, a negative inspiratory force (NIF) of –25 or less is considered a criterion for readiness for extubation. What is the NIF?

A. Pressure generated by a patient during forced expiration
B. Pressure generated by a patient during forced inspiration
C. Pressure generated by a patient during regular expiration
D. Volume circulated by a patient during one breath
E. Volume circulated by a patient during 1 minute of spontaneous ventilation

80.

A 78-year-old man is admitted to the intensive care unit with an intracranial hemorrhage. His systolic blood pressure is 190 mm Hg. What are the current guidelines regarding acute blood pressure lowering in the setting of intracranial hemorrhage for a patient with a presentation systolic blood pressure between 150 and 220 mm Hg?

A. Acute lowering of the systolic blood pressure to 140 mm Hg is safe and can be effective in improving functional outcome.
B. Acute lowering of the systolic blood pressure to 140 mm Hg is dangerous and should be avoided.
C. Acute lowering of the systolic blood pressure to 170 mm Hg is safe and can be effective in reducing mortality.
D. Acute lowering of the systolic blood pressure to two thirds of the presentation blood pressure is safe and can be effective in improving functional outcome.
E. Acute lowering of systolic BP to 120 mm Hg is probably safe.

81.

Emergency administration of what medication is indicated in the setting of symptomatic acute alcohol withdrawal with ataxia and confusion?

A. Glucose
B. Magnesium
C. Beta-blockers
D. Nicotine
E. Thiamine

82.

How does polymyositis compare with dermatomyositis regarding associations with malignancy and B- and T-cell infiltration?

A. Polymyositis more often is associated with malignancy and T-cell infiltration more than B-cell infiltration.
B. Polymyositis more often is associated with malignancy and B-cell infiltration more than T-cell infiltration.
C. Polymyositis more often is associated with malignancy and T-cell infiltration more than B-cell infiltration.
D. Polymyositis more often is associated with malignancy and B-cell infiltration more than T-cell infiltration.
E. Polymyositis and dermatomyositis are associated equally with malignancy and B- and T-cell infiltration.

83.

While doing a myelogram, the radiology resident realizes that he just injected an ionic contrast agent intrathecally. What is the best next step in management of the patient?

A. Do nothing, as this should not be a problem.
B. Withdraw fluid through a myelogram needle.
C. Start intravenous steroids.
D. Start antiepileptic drugs.
E. Administer antihistamines.

84.

What is the effect of nimodipine on a patient with an aneurysmal subarachnoid hemorrhage?

A. Decreases the risk of vasospasm and mortality rate
B. Decreases the risk of vasospasm but not the mortality rate
C. Increases the risk of vasospasm and mortality rate
D. Does not affect the risk of vasospasm but decreases the mortality rate
E. Increases the risk of vasospasm but decreases the mortality rate

85.

A man has an allergic reaction to receiving a blood transfusion. A direct Coombs test is negative, no free hemoglobin was found in the blood, and the urinalysis was normal. The allergic reaction stopped spontaneously during the workup of its cause. What could have been done to prevent the described reaction?

A. Warming the transfused blood products
B. Transfusing whole blood
C. Administering better clerical training
D. Premedication with acetaminophen
E. Washing the transfused cells

86.

A 26-year-old patient with a history of a selective IgA-deficiency syndrome requires a blood transfusion following a traumatic injury. What is the major risk of transfusing regular packed red blood cells to this patient?

A. Anaphylactic transfusion reaction
B. Rejection of donor blood due to incompatibility
C. Sepsis
D. Chemical meningitis
E. Disseminated intravascular coagulation

87.
A 60-year-old man with a glomerular filtration rate of 30 mL/min secondary to chronic diabetes mellitus type 2 is being evaluated for a newly discovered brain mass. Three days after he is discharged from the hospital, he develops large areas of indurated skin with fibrotic nodules and plaques. What might have prevented the development of his symptoms?

A. Avoiding contrasted MRI studies
B. Stopping metformin during hospitalization
C. Immediate dialysis following contrast-enhanced CT head scans
D. Better management of the blood glucose during hospitalization
E. Antihistamine use prior to contrast-enhanced studies

88.
A 22-year-old man admitted with a traumatic brain injury develops a pulmonary embolism 4 days following a craniectomy. What is the most sensitive clinical sign for detecting a pulmonary embolism?

A. Tachycardia
B. Hypotension
C. Tachypnea
D. Oxygen desaturation
E. Low-grade fever

10 Competencies/Health Care/Biostatistics

1.
An HIV test result is positive. The patient asks how likely he is to have HIV, given this positive result. The patient is asking about what aspect of the test?

A. Sensitivity
B. Specificity
C. Positive predictive value
D. Negative predictive value

2.
In clinical trials, what biases do randomization and single blinding minimize?

A. Selection and placebo effect biases
B. Selection and observer biases
C. Design and placebo effect biases
D. Definition and observer biases
E. Selection and observer biases

3.
Which of the following factors is most predictive of subsequent disciplinary actions during a career as a physician?

A. Undergraduate science class grades
B. MCAT score
C. Medical school grades
D. USMLE Step 1 score
E. Unprofessional behavior during medical school

4.
In the setting of a mass casualties, the Centers for Disease Control and Prevention recommends following the SALT algorithm for triage. For what does the acronym SALT stand?

A. Sort, Assess, Lifesaving interventions, and Treatment/Transport
B. Separate, Assess, Lifesaving interventions, and Transport
C. Save, Alert, Lifesaving interventions, and Transport
D. Save, Alert, Limit damage, and Treatment/Transport
E. Save, Assess/Alert, Lifesaving intervention, and Treatment

5.
In the setting of mass causalities, to what do the conventional triage colors red, yellow, green, and black refer?

A. Immediate, delayed, minimal, expectant
B. Delayed, immediate, minimal, expectant
C. Minimal, delayed, immediate, expectant
D. Expectant, immediate, delayed, minimal
E. Expectant, minimal, immediate, delayed

6.
The focus on positive deviance is an essential component for process improvement as defined by the international health-care institution. What is the major focus of this component?

A. Identifying the characteristics of bad performance
B. Identifying the characteristics of successful performance
C. Identifying opportunities for improvement
D. Expressing appreciation for hard work
E. Rejecting lazy behaviors

7.
Closing films following a posterior spinal decompression and fusion show that you have performed surgery at the wrong level. What is the best next course of action?

A. Inform the family of the mistake, complete the procedure at the correct level, and inform the risk management team.
B. Complete the procedure at the correct level, and do not inform the family.
C. Finish closing, and do not disclose the wrong-level surgery.
D. Finish closing, and inform the risk management team.
E. Finish closing, and inform the patient that he might need revision surgery at a later date.

8.

In the 2010 guidelines for the management of intracranial hemorrhage, there is a class 2b, level B recommendation in favor of minimally invasive clot evacuation with or without thrombolytic usage. What is the interpretation of this level of recommendation?

A. The benefits largely outweigh the risks of procedure, but there are very limited data to endorse it.
B. It is reasonable to perform the procedure, but there are very limited data to endorse it.
C. It is not unreasonable to perform the procedure, and there are multiple population-based studies to endorse it.
D. It is not unreasonable to perform the procedure, but there are limited data to endorse it.
E. The procedure is contraindicated because of a lack of data to endorse it.

9.

The wife of a spine surgeon owns a rehabilitation facility. Her husband frequently refers patients to her institute for postoperative rehabilitation. Which of the following laws is the spine surgeon violating?

A. Stark law
B. Federal anti-kickback statute
C. Antitrust law
D. False claim act

10.

A 30-year-old man sustained a massive neurologic injury following a motor vehicle collision. Despite all medical efforts, he is declared brain dead, and the regional organ procurement organization is contacted. The patient is confirmed to have listed himself as an organ donor; however, his wife refuses to proceed with donation. What is the best course of action?

A. Proceed with the donation.
B. Stop the donation, as the wife is the patient's medical decision maker.
C. Proceed with the donation after obtaining consent from the patient's brother.
D. Proceed with the donation after obtaining consent from the patient's mother.
E. Obtain a court order to proceed with the donation.

11.

One hundred new cases of craniopharyngiomas are diagnosed every year in the United States (population 320 million), and there are currently 6,400 people known to be living with craniopharyngiomas. What is the incidence and prevalence of craniopharyngiomas?

A. Incidence: 1/3,200,000; prevalence: 1/50,000
B. Incidence: 1/1,600,000; prevalence: 1/100,000
C. Incidence: 1/3,200,000; prevalence: 1/100,000
D. Incidence: 1/1,600,000; prevalence: 1/50,000
E. Incidence: 1/1,000,000; prevalence: 1/25,000

12.

The investigators of the HEAT (Hydrogel Endovascular Aneurysms Treatment) trial wanted to compare the effectiveness of hydrogel coils to the effectiveness of bare platinum coils. They designed a study in which patients were allocated to the hydrogel group or the bare platinum group on a random basis just prior to undergoing the procedure. Patients were not told which type of coils was being used. What was the design of this study?

A. Randomized, double-blinded, prospective clinical study
B. Randomized, single-blinded, prospective clinical study
C. Nonrandomized, single-blinded, prospective clinical study
D. Nonrandomized, single-blinded, retrospective clinical study
E. Randomized, double-blinded, retrospective clinical study

13.

What ACGME Core Competency is demonstrated when residents present and discuss their research with colleagues at national meetings?

A. Patient care
B. Medical knowledge
C. Interpersonal skills and communication
D. Practice-based learning and improvement
E. System-based practice

14.

A medical device manufacturer is rewarding spine surgeons who use its devices with free vacations. What law is violated by this arrangement?

A. Stark law
B. Federal anti-kickback statute
C. Antitrust law
D. False claim act

15.
A group of undergraduate students develops image processing software that automatically assesses the degree of midline shift in a head CT scan as soon as the images are acquired and before the images are sent to the radiologist. The test is repeated four times on the first volunteer, and the obtained values are 0, 3, 5, and 2 mm of midline shift. This study can be considered NOT:

A. Reliable
B. Valid
C. Accurate
D. Sensitive
E. Specific

16.
Two studies were conducted on the same population to assess the association between smoking and the development of carotid artery atherosclerosis. The first study showed a relative risk of 5.0 and a 95% confidence interval of 3.8 to 5.2. The second study showed a relative risk of 4.9 and a 95% confidence interval of 0.9 to 5. What is the most likely explanation of the observed results?

A. The first study is not statistically significant.
B. The first study is biased.
C. The second study is inaccurate.
D. The sample size in the second study is small.
E. The sample size in the first study is small.

17.
What statistical test would be the most appropriate to compare a quantitative variable in four groups?

A. ANOVA
B. Student t-test
C. Paired t-test
D. Chi-square test
E. Fisher exact test

18.
A group of medical students was asked to design a study to assess the efficacy of intracranial hemorrhage evacuation versus nonsurgical management. The students decided to enroll patients with large posterior fossa hemorrhages in their study and randomly assign them to one of the two study arms. What major ethical principle of clinical trials did the students most violate?

A. Equipoise
B. Autonomy
C. Nonmaleficence
D. Justice
E. Disclosure

19.
What ACGME core competency is demonstrated when residents present errors at a morbidity and mortality conference?

A. Patient care
B. Medical knowledge
C. Practice-based learning and improvement
D. Systems-based practice
E. Professionalism

20.
A pharmaceutical company has developed a test to predict the eventual development of Alzheimer disease in currently asymptomatic patients. This test has an 85% sensitivity and 80% specificity. For asymptomatic patients between the ages of 40 and 55, the test's positive predictive value is 25%, and its negative predictive value is 96%. A 50-year-old asymptomatic patient has a negative test. What is the probability that the patient develops Alzheimer disease?

A. 30%
B. 20%
C. 15%
D. 4%
E. 0%

21.
A pharmaceutical company develops a test to screen for glioblastomas. A study run by the company showed that this new test prolongs the survival of patients with glioblastomas by several months. The researchers conclude that use of the test improves the outcome of glioblastoma patients. What is the most likely bias of this study?

A. Observer bias
B. Measurement bias
C. Lead-time bias
D. Confounding bias
E. Sampling bias

22.
What is the size of treatment effect classification if a procedure is reasonable to perform in the setting of a certain pathology?

A. Class 1
B. Class 2A
C. Class 2B
D. Class 3
E. Class 4

23.

Following a motor vehicle collision, a 3-year-old child is diagnosed with an intracranial hemorrhage and is taken emergently to the operating room. While there, a blood transfusion becomes indicated. The patient's parents are informed and refuse transfusion on religious grounds. They threaten to sue the surgeon if blood is transfused. What is the next best course of action?

A. Do not transfuse the patient.
B. Try to reason with the family and obtain permission to transfuse.
C. Contact the hospital legal counsel and proceed with transfusion.
D. Proceed with transfusion after documenting the indication in the chart.
E. Obtain a court order to proceed with transfusion.

Use the following information to answer questions 24 and 25:

The box plot in this image reports the time in minutes required by a surgeon to perform an aneurysm clipping procedure.

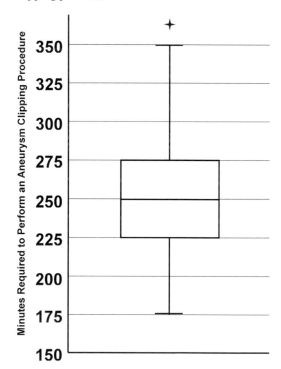

24.

What is the upper limit of the first quartile?

A. 175
B. 225
C. 250
D. 275
E. 350

25.

What is indicated by the upper whisker of the box plot?

A. The greatest outlier
B. The greatest non-outlier
C. The lower limit of the fourth quartile
D. The ninth decile
E. The 95% confidence interval

26.

A study is being conducted to evaluate daily variations in intracranial pressure in head trauma patients. The following values (in mm Hg) are obtained every 5 minutes over a 1-hour period:

13, 14, 13, 15, 16, 14, 15, 13, 16, 14, 16, 14

What are the median, mode, and mean of this distribution?

A. 14, 14, 14.4
B. 15, 14, 14.4
C. 14, 15, 16
D. 15, 14, 14.9
E. 14, 15, 14.4

Use the following information to answer questions 27 and 28:

In a recent trial comparing observation to interventional therapy for unruptured brain arteriovenous malformations, the risk of death or stroke from an arteriovenous malformation was significantly lower in the observation group compared with the interventional therapy group, with a hazard ratio (HR) of 0.27.

27.

How is the HR defined in this study?

OBS = number of deaths or strokes in the observation group

INTER = number of deaths or strokes in the interventional group

A. HR = OBS/INTER
B. HR = INTER/OBS
C. HR = (OBS + INTER)/(Total number of patients)
D. HR = INTER/(Total number of patients)
E. HR = OBS/(Total number of patients)

28.
The 95% confidence interval for the above HR of 0.27 was 0.14–0.54. What is the 95% confidence interval?

A. 95% of the calculated HRs for this study lie within the interval 0.14–0.54.
B. There is a 95% probability that the real HR for the above study lies within the interval 0.14–0.54.
C. If the study is repeated 100 times, the HR will be between 0.14 and 0.54 at least 95 times.
D. There is only a 5% chance that the obtained HR is incorrect.
E. The interval of 0.14–0.54 represents the values of the HRs for which the difference between the real population HR and the calculated HR is not statistically significant.

29.
An unconscious patient brought into the emergency room following a car crash is found to have a large epidural hematoma. The patient's identity is unknown, and he has no family available. The neurosurgeon on call believes that a craniotomy would save the patient's life. What should be done regarding an emergent procedure?

A. No procedure should be done as it is illegal to operate on a patient without informed consent.
B. The neurosurgeon should document the need for surgery in the chart and then proceed with surgery.
C. At least two doctors should document the need for surgery in the chart prior to the surgeon's proceeding with surgery.
D. A court order for surgery should be obtained prior to surgery.
E. The ethics committee of the hospital should be consulted prior to surgery.

30.
A new test is developed to screen for gliomas. The blood level of the biomarker has been demonstrated to correlate with the presence of a glioma in a positive population, and the blood level is minimal in a healthy population. A cutoff point was chosen at point A in the graph shown in this figure. If the cutoff is moved from point A to B, the positive predictive value of the test:

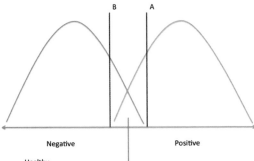

A. Will decrease
B. Will increase
C. Will remain the same
D. Will randomly change
E. Cannot be determined

31.
In the STASCIS trial (early versus delayed decompression for traumatic cervical spinal cord injury), 30% of patients were lost to follow-up at 6 months. Although this is typical for a trauma study, what type of bias could this represent?

A. Selection bias
B. Recall bias
C. Confounding bias
D. Observer bias
E. Ascertainment bias

32.

A study is conducted to assess how the initial blood flow through a graft determines the duration for which the graft will remain patent. The plot shown in this figure was obtained. What type of relationship is demonstrated?

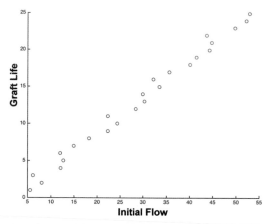

A. Linear with a positive correlation coefficient
B. Linear with a null correlation coefficient
C. Linear with a negative correlation coefficient
D. Logarithmic with a positive correlation coefficient
E. Logarithmic with a negative correlation coefficient

33.

A group of vascular neurosurgeons wants to study the relationship between smoking and the development of carotid atherosclerosis. They enroll the first 1,500 patients aged between 40 and 60 years that present to clinic, checked their smoking statuses, and obtained carotid ultrasounds to assess for atherosclerosis. What is the design of this study?

A. Prospective cohort
B. Retrospective cohort
C. Case-control
D. Cross-sectional
E. Randomized clinical trial

34.

In enhancing quality of care, what is a process change?

A. Change in how a task is performed
B. Change in the way the team perceives a task
C. Change in the outcome
D. Change in the work culture/environment
E. Change in the amount of work

35.

A neurosurgical resident does not remember how to renally dose levetiracetam. He performs a search in an electronic pharmacological database. This scenario best represents which ACGME Core Competency?

A. Medical knowledge
B. Professionalism
C. Systems-based practice
D. Patient care
E. Interpersonal skills and communication

II Answers

11 Physiology

1.

C Activation of S2-S4 α-motor neurons causing contraction of the external urethral sphincter striated muscle fibers.

The external urethral sphincter is under voluntary (somatic) control, and muscle fiber contraction causes closure of the sphincter. A full bladder sends afferent signals causing inhibition of sympathetic tone and an increase in parasympathetic activity to the bladder through the pelvic splanchnic nerves. The parasympathetic activity relaxes the internal urethral sphincter and induces bladder contraction.

2.

D Acetylcholine

Acetylcholine acts through nicotinic receptors at the ganglionic synapse. (A) Norepinephrine is the neurotransmitter used in most postganglionic sympathetic fibers.

3.

A Botulism toxin

4.

C Diphtheria toxin

(B) Tetanus toxin inhibits the release of GABA and glycine in the spinal cord. (D) Alpha bungarotoxin inhibits acetylcholine from binding to its receptors at the neuromuscular junction. (E) Tetrodotoxin blocks action potentials by binding to and inhibiting fast, voltage-gated sodium channels.

5.

C Increasing axonal membrane resistance

The length constant (λ) describes the distance over which a passively conducted electrical signal decays to 37% of its initial voltage. A larger length constant means a slower rate of degradation. The equation is:

$$\lambda = \sqrt{(r_m/(r_i+r_o))}$$

where r_m is the membrane resistance, r_i is the internal axonal resistance, and r_o is the extracellular resistance. Increasing myelination increases membrane resistance, and internal axonal resistance is decreased with increasing axonal cross-sectional area (i.e., diameter).

6.

E Thrombin

Factor VIII is bound to von Willebrand factor (vWF) and inactive in circulation. Under the action of thrombin, factor VIII is released form vWF and thus activated. When not bound to vWF, factor VIII quickly degrades.

7.

C The lack of cerebral autoregulation causes an increase in ICP.

With brain death, there is a loss of cerebral autoregulation, so the brain's normal response of maintaining a vascular tone sufficient to counteract increases in mean arterial pressure (MAP) is lost. The brain experiences the increases in MAP, which translate to increases in intracranial pressure.

8.

A Unipolar

Sensory neurons are classified as unipolar with an axon and dendrites on each end and a cell body branching from some point along the axon. (B) Bipolar neurons have an axon with dendrites on each end with a cell body along the axon. They are found as interneurons, like in the retina. (C) Multipolar neurons have dendrites surrounding a cell body from which a single axon originates. They are found as motor neurons. (D) Pyramidal neurons appear as bipolar neurons with numerous arboretic dendritic processes extending from the cell body and axons. Prime examples are found in the cerebellum as Purkinje cells. (E) Multiaxonic neurons do not exist.

9.

C Stopping at a stop sign in a motor vehicle

Both the utricle and saccule respond to changes in linear acceleration with the utricle being oriented horizontally and the saccule vertically. Deceleration in a motor vehicle traveling straight or a head tilt downward each causes anterior displacement of the otoliths in the macula of the utricle and excites hair cells that respond to movement in that direction. In contrast, the act of jump roping mainly would be sensed by action in the saccule. (A, D) Both of these activities cause a shift of endolymph in the semicircular canals that is detected in the ampulla of each canal. The ampullae respond to angular acceleration. (B, E) The vestibular system only responds to changes in acceleration and will adapt with no or constant motion in the same direction.

10.

B Growth hormone

Excess growth hormone in adults results in arthropathy, paresthesias, polyneuropathy, cardiomyopathy, arrhythmias, upper airway obstruction due to palatal/pharyngeal tissue overgrowth, increased risk for malignancies and colon polyps, and diabetes. (A) Excess adrenocorticotropic hormone (ACTH) secretion results in Cushing disease, characterized by weight gain, hypertension, mood changes, hypertelorism, fatigue, and "moon face." (C) High prolactin levels are associated with infertility, spontaneous lactation, loss of libido, erectile dysfunction, and abnormal menstrual cycles. (D) Excess thyroid-stimulating hormone results in hyperthyroidism with symptoms of tremors, anxiety, weight loss, heat intolerance, brittle hair, and insomnia. (E) Excess follicle-stimulating hormone results in infertility.

11.

B IL-1 and TNF-α

The major proinflammatory cytokines are the interleukins (IL) IL-1, IL-6, IL-8, TNF-α (tumor necrosis factor-alpha), and IFN-γ (interferon-gamma). These produce fever, tissue destruction, and inflammation. The major anti-inflammatory cytokines include IL-4, IL-6, IL-10, IL-11, and IL-13. Of note, IL-6 can be anti- or proinflammatory depending on how it is used in a signaling cascade. (A) TGF-α and VEGF are examples of growth factors.

12.

C Response of the postsynaptic terminal caused by the release of a single vesicle into the synaptic cleft

MEPs summate in the postsynaptic terminal to induce a response of either hyperpolarization or depolarization. (A, B) Miniature end-plate potentials (MEPs) can be excitatory or inhibitory.

13.

B Between the resting and threshold potentials

Found initially in cardiac smooth muscle cells, T-type calcium channels are unique voltage-gated calcium channels that open at around –55 mV, which is slightly higher than the resting potential in cardiac cells of –60 mV. T-type calcium channels open to allow a large calcium flux into the cell to aid in the depolarization required to reach the triggering threshold for an action potential.

14.

D Prolong action potential duration and maintain normal conduction velocity

By blocking only potassium channels (notably the inward rectifier channels), hyperpolarization (returning to a negative resting potential) is inhibited, and cardiac cells remain depolarized longer. This prolongs the action potential and the refractory period. Conduction velocity is unaffected, as there is no prevention of the opening of subsequent sodium channels and depolarizing adjacent membrane segments.

15.

E All neurotransmitters can be used to upregulate downstream neural network activation

Although neurotransmitters are labeled as excitatory or inhibitory, this refers only to the effect of a neurotransmitter on a specific type of receptor at a specific synapse. It is how the various receptors and neurons containing the receptors are organized that causes a downstream effect. For example, the basal ganglia circuitry is full of circuits that inhibit inhibitory circuits so that an inhibitory synapse/receptor on an inhibitory neuron could result in the activation of a downstream neuron.

16.

B Phosphodiesterase inhibition

By inhibiting phosphodiesterase, cAMP degradation is reduced. All of the actions of caffeine serve to upregulate the nervous system in a stimulatory manner. (A) Caffeine competitively inhibits glycine receptors. (C) Caffeine competitively inhibits adenosine receptors. Activation of adenosine receptors leads to the sensation of drowsiness. (D) Caffeine competitively inhibits acetylcholinesterase. (E) Caffeine is an agonist for the ryanodine receptor.

17.

A Inhibition of the presynaptic uptake of monoamines

Cocaine blocks the monoamine transporter proteins on the presynaptic cleft, thus preventing monoamine reuptake and vesicular storage in the presynaptic terminal. (B) Amphetamines both block the reuptake of monoamines into the presynaptic terminal and induce the release of monoamines into the synaptic cleft.

18.

D Choline and acetate

Following the breakdown of acetylcholine by acetylcholinesterase in the extracellular space, acetate is transported into the intracellular space, where it is converted to acetyl CoA, which then can combine with choline to reform acetylcholine.

19.

C Caspases typically are not part of necrosis

Caspases are proteases necessary for apoptosis. They signal and regulate the controlled process by which DNA and cellular components are fragmented and degraded. In contrast, necrosis is uncontrolled cell death and results in inflammation. Caspases typically play little to no role in necrosis.

20.

A Glutamate and glycine

Two molecules of either glutamate or aspartate and two molecules of either glycine or serine need to bind to an NMDA receptor in order to activate it. The receptor also has a voltage-gated component requiring depolarization of the neuron on which it is located. The voltage-gated component of the receptor is controlled by the calcium channel being blocked by either a zinc or magnesium ion when the receptor is inactive.

21.

D Inhibition of osteoclasts

Bisphosphonates bind to calcium and are taken up by osteoclasts. Bisphosphonates then induce apoptosis of these bone-reabsorbing cells. These are useful agents in osteopenia and osteoporosis. (A) Bisphosphonates have no effect on the body total stores of calcium. (B) Osteocytes are osteoblasts that have entrapped themselves in their secretory bony matrix. They do not divide, but they do play a role in the turnover and maintenance of the bony matrix. They express TGF-β to suppress bone resorption. (C) Inhibition of osteocytes would lead to increased bone resorption. (E) Osteoblasts form new, nonmineralized bony matrix on the surface of mature, mineralized bone. They are regulated and recruited in part by osteocytes.

22.

C Between the α and β subunits

(E) The benzodiazepine binding site on the $GABA_A$ receptor is between the α and γ subunits.

23.

C Cell bodies in the lumbar prominence of the spinal cord

The patellar reflex occurs independently of input from the brain; however, the brain does work to suppress the reflex when all spinal circuitry is intact. This is why hyperreflexia and clonus can be seen with significant spinal cord compression. The actual reflex only requires the sensory nerves from the patellar tendon to be intact and synapse on cell bodies within the lumbar spinal cord. The reflex arc then stimulates motor neurons at that same level to provide the motor component of the reflex.

24.

D DNA alkylation

Temozolomide and procarbazine are DNA alkylating (methylating) agents that interfere with protein synthesis. (A) Microtubule function inhibitors include vincristine and vinblastine. (B) DNA cross-links by carbamylation of amino groups are formed by the nitrosoureas such as BCNU and CCNU. (C) Bevacizumab (Avastin) is an anti-VEGF antibody. (E) Tamoxifen is a topoisomerase inhibitor.

25.

D ACTH, β-lipotrophin, and γ-MSH

Following the initial cleavage of pro-opiomelanocortin into ACTH, β-lipotrophin, and γ-MSH, ACTH can be processed further to α-MSH and CLIP. β-lipotrophin can be processed into β-endorphin and γ-lipotrophin with the latter eventually becoming β-MSH.

26.

A The H-wave disappears

The H-wave is the electrophysiological equivalent of the stretch reflex and represents the muscle's electrical response to a square wave stimulus to the skin that first propagates in the antidromic direction (away from the muscle) to the cell bodies. The reflex arc continues with an electrical signal sent in the orthodromic direction (toward the muscle) to elicit a response. This response is the H-wave. As stimulation amplitude increases, the H-wave diminishes and disappears with supramaximal stimulation. It is most useful for evaluating the Ia sensory afferents. (B, D) The M-wave is the orthodromic response recorded in the muscle to electrical stimulation of the skin overlying the muscle. It bypasses the reflex arc and increases with increasing stimulation amplitude. (E) The F-wave increases with increases in amplitude but not to the extent seen in the M-wave. The F-wave is the result of alpha-fiber stimulation and is useful to evaluate proximal (near the spinal cord) nerve conduction velocities.

27.

D Arginine

Arginine along with cofactors NADPH and oxygen react in the presence of nitric oxide synthetase to produce nitric oxide, NADP, and citrulline. (A, E) Tyrosine and asparagine are not involved in nitric oxide synthesis. (B, C) NADP and citrulline are products in the reaction creating nitric oxide.

28.
B The curve is wider with smooth muscle, as shown in this image.

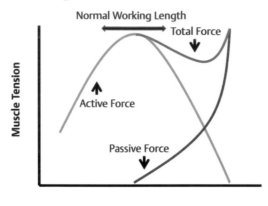

(A) Tension equals the force of the muscle. (C) Tension increases to its maximum as the muscle is stretched beyond its ideal working length (at the point of maximal myosin and actin overlap). Tension will increase indefinitely at the far right of the tension–length curve until muscle tissues begin to tear. (D) When the single peak of active muscle tension versus length is added to the exponential relationship of tension to length in resting muscle, there is a tension peak, followed by a trough, followed by a continued rise in tension with both smooth and skeletal muscle.

29.
B Glutamate

Glutamate triggers the activation of NMDA receptors. When the magnesium ion is displaced from its channel-blocking site, there is calcium influx into the cytosol. Elevated calcium levels trigger apoptotic changes in the affected cells.

30.
C Pericytes

Pericytes are the cells surrounding the endothelial cells of capillaries and venules throughout the body. In the brain, pericytes create and maintain the tight junctions between endothelial cells and regulate vesicle trafficking between endothelial cells. It is this role that creates the selectivity of the blood–brain barrier. Pericytes also inhibit the expression of endothelial markers that increase vascular permeability. (A) Astrocytic foot processes historically were thought to be the key component creating the blood–brain barrier; however, their role is to provide biochemical support to the endothelial cells creating the barrier. (B) Arachnoid "cap" cells are cells of the arachnoid villi from which meningiomas originate. (D) The endothelial cells themselves are not the key component to the blood–brain barrier. Instead, the highly selective tight junctions between endothelial cells allow for the specialized function of the blood–brain barrier.

31.
A Irreversible binding to and inhibition of acetylcholinesterase

Organophosphates irreversibly bind to acetylcholinesterase and inactivate this acetylcholine-degrading enzyme. Pralidoxime can be used as an antidote in organophosphate poisoning, as it is able to reactivate the enzyme prior to degradation.

32.
B The affinity of hemoglobin for oxygen decreases, and the oxygen-hemoglobin dissociation curve shifts to the right, as shown in this image.

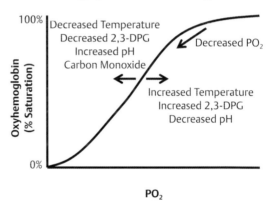

Increasing temperature, carbon dioxide, and 2,3-DPG along with decreasing pH all decrease the binding affinity of hemoglobin for oxygen and thus shift the hemoglobin-oxygen dissociation curve to the right. Conditions opposite to these will increase binding affinity and shift the curve to the left. As blood passes through a capillary, metabolically active tissues release 2,3-DPG, which induces an allosteric change in hemoglobin and leads to oxygen unbinding. Oxygen is taken up by tissues, and carbon dioxide enters the blood. The partial pressure of oxygen thus is reduced as is the pH causing subsequent oxygen unbinding from hemoglobin. A decrease in the partial pressure of oxygen causes a shift along the curve to the left.

33.

A –65 mV; potassium

All ions considered, the actual resting membrane potential for a neuron is between –60 and –70 mV. This is due in large part to the flux of potassium ions from inside to outside the neuron through open channels along the concentration gradient. The equilibrium potential for potassium is around –90 mV. (B) Sodium flux is from the extracellular to the intracellular space when a membrane is at rest, but there are far fewer sodium than potassium channels open when a neuron is at rest. (C) The equilibrium potential for sodium is around +60 mV, whereas it is around –60 mV for chloride. (D) Although the resting membrane potential is based largely on potassium conductance, it is more positive than the equilibrium potential for potassium alone. (E) The equilibrium potential for calcium is around +20 mV, but the ion plays little role in the membrane resting potential.

34.

C Sonic hedgehog proteins

Sonic hedgehog proteins are secreted from the notochord and signal the development of the floor plate and motor neurons in a concentration-dependent fashion. (A, B) Bone morphogenic proteins from the ectoderm overlying the notochord and Wnt family proteins establish the dorsal axis. (D) The patched gene (*Ptc*) expresses the ligand-binding domain for the sonic hedgehog proteins. (E) The Ras family proteins are GTPases involved cell signal transduction and can signal aberrantly in cancers.

35.

B Increased postsynaptic activity

Myasthenia gravis is a condition characterized by antibodies that bind to postsynaptic acetylcholine receptors and inhibit acetylcholine binding. This reduces the postsynaptic activity. Medications for myasthenia gravis act by competitively inhibiting acetylcholinesterase, thus decreasing acetylcholine breakdown and increasing acetylcholine in the synaptic cleft. Organophosphates irreversibly bind to and inhibit acetylcholinesterase and have a similar end result on the postsynaptic activity.

36.

A Its resting state would become more positive.

Due to its high potassium relative to sodium concentration compared with perilymph and normal neuronal extracellular fluid, endolymph has a

potential of 80 to 120 mV. The normal resting concentration of potassium in a neuron is about 150 mmol, which is the same concentration of potassium in endolymph. This means that there essentially would be almost no passive flow of potassium ions in this situation, and according to the Nernst equation, the resting potential due to potassium flux would be about 0 mV.

37.

D Inhibition of glycine receptors

Strychnine is a rodenticide that works by binding to, and thus blocking, glycine and acetylcholine receptors on motor neurons in the spinal cord. This leads to a hyperactivation of skeletal musculature and death by asphyxiation due to tonic contraction of the respiratory muscles.

38.

C 18 mL/h

Cerebrospinal fluid (CSF) is produced at an average rate of 18 mL/h, yielding a total daily production of 400 to 500 mL. The total CSF volume in an adult is approximately 140 mL at any given time. Seventy percent of CSF is produced by the choroid plexus.

39.

A Shorten the muscle spindles with skeletal muscle fiber contraction

The cells bodies of gamma motor neurons are located in the anterior horns of the spinal cord. They are activated along with their corresponding alpha motor neurons and contract the intrafusal muscle fibers to keep the muscle spindles taut regardless of extrafusal muscle fiber length. (B) Beta motor neurons activate both extrafusal and intrafusal muscle fibers, thus shortening muscle length and keeping muscle spindles taut. They greatly are outnumbered by gamma motor neurons. (C) Gamma and alpha motor neurons are activated simultaneously in a given muscle. (D) Type 2 afferents are highly myelinated stretch receptors in the muscle that, unlike type 1a afferents, are non-adapting and thus fire continuously with a stable muscle length. (E) The Golgi tendon organs are proprioceptive sensory receptors oriented in series with skeletal muscle fibers. They are located where skeletal muscles join their tendons and sense the force on the muscles. With signaling through 1b afferents, the Golgi tendon reflex can be initiated, which inhibits further contraction of the muscle involved through inhibitory interneurons in the spinal cord.

40.

B Aromatic amino acid decarboxylase

Aromatic amino acid decarboxylase uses activated B6 as a cofactor. (A) Tyramine β-hydroxylase converts tyramine to octopamine (an amine that acts in place of norepinephrine in sympathetic neurons with chronic monoamine oxidase inhibitors). (C) Tryptophan hydroxylase converts tryptophan to 5-hydroxy-tryptophan during serotonin synthesis. (D) Tyrosine hydroxylase converts tyrosine to levodopa during dopamine synthesis. (E) Catechol-O-methyl transferase inactivates catecholamine neurotransmitters including dopamine, levodopa, norepinephrine, and epinephrine.

41.

D It allows for more precise spatial resolution.

Presynaptic inhibition has an advantage over postsynaptic inhibition in that presynaptic inhibition downregulates only one synapse acting on the postsynaptic cell. The entire neuronal chain thus does not simply become inhibited based on one postsynaptic action. In addition, the multiple miniature end-plate potentials (MEPPs) from several presynaptic terminals (whether inhibitory or excitatory) can be grouped together at the postsynaptic cell to induce or inhibit an action potential (spatial resolution). (B) Temporal summation involves the grouping of MEPPs together in a temporal fashion to induce an action potential postsynaptically. (C) With presynaptic inhibition, there are fewer quanta of neurotransmitters entering the synaptic cleft.

42.

D Respond to depolarization and activate calcium channels on the sarcoplasmic reticulum

As the action potential at the neuromuscular junction occurs, depolarization propagates through the T-tubules in the muscle fiber. L-type voltage-dependent calcium channels are activated, and they open ryanodine receptors in the adjacent sarcoplasmic reticulum. The calcium that then is released binds to troponin C on the myofibrils to start sarcomere contraction. (A) Once activated, calcium-release channels (ryanodine receptors) on the sarcoplasmic reticulum allow for stored calcium to be released within the muscle cells' cytoplasm. (E) This is the role of calcium and not a channel.

43.

B Inhibits osteoblasts

By inhibiting osteoblasts, parathyroid hormone (PTH) is not able to inhibit osteoclasts and reduce bone reabsorption. As bone is reabsorbed, calcium is released into the circulation. (A) Calcitonin is secreted by the thyroid and inhibits intestinal calcium absorption of calcium, inhibits osteoclast activity, stimulates osteoblast activity, and promotes renal secretion of calcium. All of these effects work to reduce the serum calcium concentration. Calcitonin can be thought of as having the opposite activity of PTH. (C) PTH promotes the reabsorption of calcium from the distal tubules and thick ascending limbs in the kidneys and reduces phosphate reabsorption. This leads to an increase in the calcium/phosphate ratio, meaning that more calcium is free in the serum. Increasing renal phosphate reabsorption would have the opposite effect. (D) PTH upregulates the enzyme responsible for activating vitamin D, which in turn increases the intestinal reabsorption of calcium. (E) Osteoclast inhibition would reduce bone turnover and calcium release from the bony matrix.

44.

C Uncompetitive inhibitor

An uncompetitive inhibitor binds to an enzyme/substrate complex to reduce or inhibit its activity. The enzyme/substrate must first form for this type of inhibition to take place. (A) In a simple form, a competitive inhibitor binds to an enzyme and, when bound, prevents the enzyme from binding to its substrate. In other words, the enzyme may either be bound to its inhibitor or substrate but not both at the same time. (B) A noncompetitive inhibitor binds to and acts on an enzyme to reduce its activity and interaction with its substrate. A noncompetitive inhibitor binds to an enzyme equally well whether or not the enzyme is bound to its substrate. The substrate does not have to be present for a noncompetitive inhibitor to act. (D) A mixed inhibitor is a type of noncompetitive inhibitor that has a higher affinity for the enzyme in a particular state (e.g., bound to its substrate).

45.

D Vesicles and corresponding receptors each on only one side of the synaptic cleft

Excitatory synapses have vesicles and corresponding receptors each on only one side of the synaptic cleft; thus, there always is a "signaling" end and a "receiving" end for vesicular traffic. (A) The absolute refractory period forces axons to propagate action potentials in only one direction. (C) Presynaptic neurotransmitter reuptake receptors exist but do not play a role in signal direction across a synapse.

46.

E Increase CBF and increase ICP

When the brain detects a rising carbon dioxide level in the blood, the cerebrovasculature dilates to increase cerebral blood flow (CBF) and thus increase the clearance of carbon dioxide. In turn, this raises intracranial pressure. With the increase in CBF, the PO_2 the brain experiences also increases. This mechanism is impaired in brain death and severe stroke.

47.

A Absolute refractory period

The absolute refractory period is determined by the inability of voltage-gated sodium channels to open for a period of time once they have opened and closed during an action potential. Without a large sodium flux from outside to inside the axon, there can be no depolarization and thus no subsequent action potential. The action potential thus must propagate in an anterograde fashion to a portion of the axon where the sodium channels have not been activated and closed recently. (B) Protein transport goes in both an anterograde and retrograde fashion in axons but is not the mechanism behind action potential direction. (C) Saltatory conduction describes the process by which the action potential "leaps" between nodes of Ranvier in a design that speeds signal conduction along axons. Action potentials are triggered only in the unmyelinated nodes, and the voltage differential produced at one node must be transmitted at a sufficient level to the next node to trigger another action potential. (D) The relative refractory period promotes an action potential to propagate in one direction but is not the absolute mechanism. The relative refractory period refers to the point at which a neuron is hyperpolarized by potassium flux with voltage-gated sodium channels that are not inactivated. The neuron is resistant to depolarization, but a sufficient depolarization would trigger an action potential. If the relative refractory period was the only mechanism present, a large depolarization would send an action potential propagating in two directions along an axon. (E) Temporal summation refers to the summation of multiple small depolarizations in the postsynaptic terminal over a given period of time with each small depolarization alone not being sufficient to trigger an action potential. It requires the summation of signal to initiate the action potential.

48.

D No postsynaptic blockade

Hexamethonium is an antagonist of nicotinic acetylcholine receptors and thus is a ganglionic blocker in the autonomic nervous system. It binds to the nicotinic acetylcholine receptors but not in the binding site for acetylcholine. Hexamethonium has no effect on the postsynaptic muscarinic acetylcholine receptors. (C) Hexamethonium administration will decrease signaling in both the sympathetic and parasympathetic nervous systems.

49.

B By simple diffusion

Steroids are lipophilic and thus can pass through lipophilic cell membranes without the use of channels or receptors. (A) Membrane channels for steroids do not exist. (C) Facilitated diffusion relies on membrane channels to allow molecules to pass through cell membranes along their electrochemical and/or osmotic gradients. (D) G proteins allow extracellular molecules to induce cell signaling within cells, without signaling molecules passing through the membranes. (E) Active transport requires the use of energy (usually in the form of ATP) for molecules to pass through membrane channels against a gradient.

50.

D Hyperpolarization of the retinal cells results in phototransduction.

As in the auditory and vestibular systems, the stimulus (light) induces hyperpolarization of the retinal cells, which is due to the closure of sodium channels and reduction of the inward sodium flux of sodium in the case of phototransduction. (A) Phosphodiesterases are essential for continuing the phototransduction cascade. (B) Rhodopsin contains retinal in the 11-cis conformation until light evokes a configuration change to the all-trans form. This change makes rhodopsin no longer fit into the opsin-binding site, and upon disengagement, opsin changes forms, continuing the phototransduction cascade. (C) Molecules of cGMP are hydrolyzed, which causes the closure of cGMP dependent sodium channels.

51.

A G1 phase

The G1 (growth 1) phase is characterized by cell growth and synthesis of mRNA and proteins in preparation for DNA replication in S phase. Various checkpoint systems like the p53 tumor-suppressor protein prevent progression to S phase and DNA replication if errors are present. (B) During the S (synthetic) phase, cells replicate their DNA and are resistant to radiation due to the numerous DNA proofreading and repair mechanisms at play. (C) The G2 (growth 2) phase is characterized by cell growth and protein synthesis after cell DNA has replicated. Some rapidly dividing cells (e.g., cancer cells) may skip the G2 phase. There exist checkpoints in the G2 phase that induce cell arrest if errors are detected. (D) The M (mitotic) phase is characterized by division and separation of the cellular nuclear material and division of cells into two daughter cells. Cells are very sensitive to radiation during the M phase. (E) The G0 (resting) phase occurs when cells are in a quiescent state. Cells can enter the G0 phase due to a variety of conditions including nutrient deficiency and lack of growth factors. Most neurons in the central nervous system are in the G0 phase of the cell cycle.

52.

A A motor neuron and all of the muscle fibers innervated by that neuron

Each motor neuron innervates several muscle fibers. There are numerous motor neurons in each peripheral nerve.

53.

D Synaptic vesicle

During the process of conversion of dopamine to norepinephrine, the latter is transported into synaptic vesicles by the vesicular monoamine transporter. The actual synthesis of norepinephrine mostly takes place in the synaptic vesicle. (A) Dopamine synthesis from tyrosine takes place in the neuronal cytoplasm. (E) The synaptic cleft is where acetylcholine is degraded by acetylcholinesterase.

54.

B The blood–brain barrier is closed in cytotoxic edema and disrupted in vasogenic edema.

The blood–brain barrier (BBB) becomes disrupted in vasogenic edema, as breakdown of the endothelial tight junctions occurs. In addition, gliomas and certain brain tumors can secrete vascular endothelial growth factors that increase permeability. Proteins and molecules leave the intravascular space and create an oncotic force driving fluid into the extracellular space. Fluid spreads along white matter tracts, creating a large area of edema. In cytotoxic edema, alteration of cellular metabolism leads to a failure of ion pumps (notably the sodium-potassium pumps), which in turn creates an osmotic gradient and increased fluid in the intracellular space. (A) Vasogenic edema responds better to steroids, in that steroids decrease endothelial permeability by various means. (C) Cytotoxic edema is characterized by cell swelling, whereas cells remain of similar size in pure vasogenic edema. (D) Although ischemic injury initially is characterized by cytotoxic edema, when cells die and the BBB breaks down, elements of vasogenic edema arise. (E) Proteins expand the extracellular space in vasogenic edema due to disruption of the BBB.

55.

B Myosin heads are bound to actin following the power stroke.

The power stroke occurs as phosphate is released from the cocked myosin heads, and they change conformation to move relative to the actin thin filaments. Without the addition of ATP, the myosin heads cannot unbind actin. This accounts for the rigid muscles and tonic sarcomere length seen in rigor mortis. (A) The myosin heads are able to unbind from actin thin filaments with the addition of ATP and return to their resting (uncocked) positions. (C) Once cocked, myosin heads bind actin. (D) Myosin heads cock in a high-energy, ready position as ATP is hydrolyzed into ADP and phosphate.

56.

E Phenylethanolamine N-methyltransferase

Phenylethanolamine N-methyltransferase converts norepinephrine to epinephrine creating homocysteine in the process. (A) Monoamine oxidase degrades monoamines like dopamine. (B) Tyrosine hydroxylase converts tyrosine to L-dopa in dopamine synthesis. It is the rate-limiting factor in dopamine synthesis. (C) Aromatic L-amino acid decarboxylase converts L-dopa to dopamine in dopamine synthesis. (D) Dopamine β-hydroxylase converts dopamine to norepinephrine.

57.

C Inhibition of synthesis of proteins C, S, and Z

Vitamin K is required for the complete synthesis of the coagulation factors prothrombin (factor II), factor VII, factor IX, factor X, protein C, protein S, and protein Z. These factors are present (in the classic coagulation model) in the intrinsic, extrinsic, and common pathways. (A) Antithrombin inhibits several factors in the clotting cascade, and its effects on factors II and X are inhibited by heparin. (B) Factor XII acts on factor XI to begin the clotting cascade in the intrinsic pathway. (D) Bleeding time and platelet function are unaffected by a vitamin K deficiency. (E) With a vitamin K deficiency, prothrombin time (a measure of the extrinsic pathway) and partial thromboplastin time (a measure of the intrinsic pathway) both are prolonged, with the former being affected to a greater extent.

58.

B Astrocytic scarring

Astrocytic scarring disrupts the axonal tracts following wallerian degeneration, and astrocytes secrete axonal growth inhibitory proteins in the central nervous system. (A) There is a relative paucity of axonal growth–promoting factors in the central nervous system, but this is not due to, nor does it change relative to, the presence of axonal injury. (C) There is a lack of progenitor cells in the central nervous system, but axons in the peripheral nervous system regenerate without such progenitor cells. (D) Directional markers and signaling molecules do degrade following neurogenesis, but axons still can regenerate in the peripheral nervous system along axon tracts following the supporting matrix (e.g., endoneurium and other such components) after wallerian degeneration.

59.

D Membrane repolarization

As the sodium channels close, the open potassium channels are able to keep the net flux of positive ions out of the cell, resulting in membrane repolarization toward the resting membrane potential of potassium. (B) Potassium channels are open at this point, which allows for cellular repolarization and eventual hyperpolarization as the sodium channels close. (C) The relative refractory period is the time at which the cell is hyperpolarized so that the membrane depolarization required to trigger a subsequent action potential is greater than it is when the cell is at its resting membrane potential. (E) Voltage-gated calcium channels open with depolarization and not repolarization.

60.

E Inhibition of the sodium-chloride cotransporters in the distal tubules

By competing for the chloride-binding site and blocking the sodium-chloride transporters, hydrochlorothiazide prevents the reabsorption of sodium in the distal convoluted tubules. This maintains the osmotic gradient in the tubules, thus promoting natriuresis. In addition, hydrochlorothiazide increases calcium reabsorption in the tubules through an unrelated mechanism. (A) One mechanism by which vasopressin acts is by promoting the insertion of aquaporin channels in the apical membrane of the distal convoluted tubules and collecting ducts, allowing water to be reabsorbed into the blood along its osmotic gradient. This creates an antidiuretic effect. (B) Spironolactone acts on the distal nephron on the distal convoluted tubules where it inhibits the sodium-potassium exchangers. This prevents the exchangers from reabsorbing sodium and excreting potassium, resulting in a diuretic effect. It is considered a potassium-sparing diuretic. (C) Furosemide is a loop diuretic that works by inhibiting the sodium-potassium-chloride symporters in the thick ascending limb of the loops of Henle. Blockade of the transporter prevents reabsorption of sodium, chloride, and potassium. (D) Carbonic anhydrase inhibitors reduce sodium chloride and bicarbonate reabsorption in the proximal tubules by blocking the luminal conversion of bicarbonate to carbon dioxide. Without the inhibitors, carbon dioxide diffuses passively back into the cells of the proximal tubules. Without the conversion, sodium remains with the bicarbonate ions in the lumen due to their electrochemical attraction.

61.

A Large size and negative charge

The basement membrane and podocytic epithelium in the glomerulus have a positive charge and thus resist passage of negatively charged molecules. In addition, the effective pore size in the glomerular wall is about 8 nm, preventing passage of most proteins and other large molecules. The oncotic pressure in the glomerular capillaries increases as blood passes through as proteins are retained while ions and small molecules are filtered through the wall. This causes a gradient of flow back into the capillaries at their distal ends as oncotic pressure builds. Finally, the hydrostatic pressure in the glomerular capillaries is low relative to capillaries elsewhere in the body. This resists filtration through the capillary walls.

62.

A Concentric

Lateral geniculate nucleus cells have concentric (center-surround) receptive fields that are either on-center or off-center, with the surrounding region being antagonistic. Similar receptive fields are seen in retinal ganglion cells. (B) Rectangular receptive fields are seen in simple cells of the visual cortex. (C, D) Motion, direction, and orientation receptive fields are seen in complex cells of the visual cortex. Cells are dedicated and specialized to respond to certain aspects of visual stimuli.

63.

D Calcium

During the secondary (delayed) phase of traumatic brain injury, neurons spill the neurotransmitter glutamate that in turn causes a large calcium flux into neurons. Excess intracellular calcium can initiate apoptosis and open mitochondrial pores, leading to metabolic dysfunction. (A) Glutamate is the neurotransmitter involved in excitotoxic brain injury, but the molecule only activates the receptor that opens calcium channels. (B, C) During the primary phase of traumatic brain injury, there is cell damage and cellular membrane damage due to the direct forces involved. Cellular membrane damage can allow numerous ions and molecules to pass freely along their concentration and electrochemical gradients.

64.

E Retrograde transport

Retrograde transport of vesicles using dynein is an ATP-dependent process. (A) There are two types of slow anterograde transport. The slower mode carries microtubules and neurofilaments, whereas the faster slow transport mechanism carries actin and a variety of other proteins. (B) There is no single carrier protein that serves bidirectional axoplasmic transport. (C) Both slow and fast anterograde transport of molecules in vesicles are mediated by kinesins along microtubules.

65.

A C-band

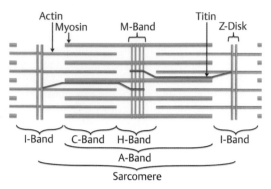

Sarcomere

The C-band enlarges with sarcomere shortening, as shown in this image. It is the region of the A-band not including the H-band. (B) The A-band is the region of the sarcomere containing myosin thick filaments with actin thin filament overlaps at the ends of the band. The A-band remains the same size during sarcomere contraction. (C) The I-band is the portion of the sarcomere with actin thin filaments that are not overlapping with myosin thick filaments. It decreases in size with sarcomere contraction. (D) The H-band is the portion of the sarcomere containing myosin thick filaments that are not overlapping actin thin filaments. It shortens with contraction. (E) The M-band is the center anchoring point of the myosin thick filaments and does not change in size as sarcomere length changes.

66.

C Reverse transcriptases

Reverse transcriptases create cDNA from RNA templates in the very error-prone process of reverse transcription. (A) RNA polymerases are involved in RNA translation from DNA. (B) DNA polymerases are involved in transcription and DNA replication. (D) Integrases allow the DNA created from retroviruses to be incorporated into host cell genomes. (E) Helicases separate two annealed strands of DNA, RNA, or DNA-RNA hybrids, and are involved in the processes of transcription and translation among other roles that they play.

67.

B Tyrosine hydroxylase

Tyrosine hydroxylase converts tyrosine to L-dopa. (A) Tyrosine is abundant and does not limit the rate of dopamine synthesis. (C) Dopa decarboxylase converts L-dopa to dopamine. (D) Dopamine β-hydroxylase converts dopamine to norepinephrine. (E) Tetrahydrobiopterin is a cofactor for the conversion of tyrosine to L-dopa, but being widely available, it does not limit the reaction.

68.

B Exogenous administration that mimics the endogenous activity

To prove that the action seen in a neuronal chain is due to signaling by a neurotransmitter, the effect from exogenous administration must be the same as endogenous activity. (A) Neurotransmitters are present in the presynaptic terminal and only released in a controlled amount and fashion to exert a particular effect. (C) Some neurotransmitters can be seen throughout the nervous system, whereas others are found in only a few select locations. (D) Although a neurotransmitter may be excitatory or inhibitory at a particular synapse, the downstream effects can vary depending on the arrangement of the neural network. (E) An effect distant from the site of production/release is part of the definition of a hormone.

69.

A Promoting arousal

Orexin/hypocretin is a neurotransmitter that promotes arousal and wakefulness along with appetite. Despite decreased levels of production in the brains of narcoleptics, narcoleptics tend to have higher body mass indices, highlighting that the chemical plays more of a role in arousal and thermogenesis than in promoting that appetite. The weight gain effect is due to the lowered metabolic rate in orexin-deficient individuals.

70.

C Resting membrane potential would increase, and the threshold to trigger an action potential would be reached with fewer MEPPs.

The equilibrium potential for an ion is determined by the relative concentration of the ion outside compared with inside the neuron. If the extracellular concentration of potassium increases and the intracellular concentration remains constant, the equilibrium potential would become more positive. Because the resting membrane potential for a neuron is determined mainly by potassium ions, it also would increase. The threshold for trigging an action potential would remain the same but now would be closer to the resting potential.

12 Anatomy

1.

A Neglect syndromes

Neglect syndromes and attentional deficits can occur with pulvinar nuclear lesions. The pulvinar nucleus is the largest nucleus in the thalamus; it is located most posteriorly, and is associated with visual pathways. (E) Memory difficulties may occur with lesions of the anterior nucleus of the thalamus, which is considered part of the limbic system.

2.

C Rubro-olivary tract/central tegmental tract (triangle of Mollaret)

The triangle of Mollaret is a functional circuit connecting the dentate nucleus of the cerebellum to the contralateral red nucleus through the superior cerebellar peduncle, the red nucleus to the ipsilateral inferior olivary nucleus through the central tegmental tract, the inferior olivary nucleus to the contralateral cerebellar cortex through the inferior cerebellar peduncle, and the cerebellar cortex to the ipsilateral dentate nucleus. Lesions of the triangle of Mollaret produce palatal myoclonus, which is one of the few movement disorders that do not disappear during sleep. Palatal myoclonus appears in a delayed fashion following such lesions. Ocular myoclonus can accompany palatal myoclonus due to lesions in the central tegmental tract.

3.

A Medial forebrain bundle

The medial forebrain bundle carries information from the ventral tegmental area to the nucleus accumbens in the ventral striatum. The nucleus accumbens also receives input from the hippocampus, amygdala, and prefrontal cortex with output to the ventral pallidum.

4.

B Nucleus tractus solitarius

The nucleus tractus solitarius is a medullary nucleus also receiving afferents from chemoreceptors in the aortic and carotid bodies.

5.

A Area postrema

The area postrema is located in the medulla and is the only paired circumventricular organ. (C) The nucleus prepositus hypoglossi is a medullary struc-ture and neural integrator responsible for horizontal gaze control during smooth-pursuit eye movements. (D) The nucleus ambiguus is located in the lateral and rostral medulla and supplies the efferent motor fibers for the glossopharyngeal and vagus nerves. (E) The inferior salivary nucleus is a medullary structure responsible for the parasympathetic efferents to the parotid gland to induce salivation.

6.

D Pacinian corpuscles

Pacinian corpuscles detect rapid vibrations and have peak sensitivity with vibrations around 250 Hz. They also are keen at detecting surface texture, which makes their localization in the skin ideal. Additionally, they are found in internal organs. (A) Ruffini endings are slowly adapting receptors found in subcutaneous tissues and respond to sustained pressure. (B) Meissner corpuscles are very sensitive to light touch and function best with vibrations less than 50 Hz. They rapidly adapt and are found in areas very sensitive to light touch, such as the finger pads. (C) Merkel disks occur in the superficial skin layers and mucosa, and provide information about pressure and texture. They are slowly adapting. (E) Free nerve endings are unencapsulated receptors in the skin that detect painful stimuli.

7.

B Floor of the third ventricle

There is no choroid plexus along the floor of the third ventricle. Choroid plexus is present at the other locations and is responsible for the bulk of cerebrospinal fluid production. Cerebrospinal fluid is produced by bulk transependymal flow along the floor of the third ventricle.

8.

C Sympathetic nerve that unites with the greater superficial petrosal nerve to form the Vidian nerve

The deep petrosal nerve emerges from the internal carotid plexus and traverses the carotid canal to join the superficial petrosal nerve to form the Vidian nerve (also known as the nerve of the pterygoid canal). The deep petrosal nerve carries the sympathetics that innervate the pterygopalatine ganglion.

9.

D Deep peroneal nerve

The deep peroneal nerve innervates the tibialis anterior, extensor digitorum longus, extensor hallucis longus, extensor digitorum brevis, and extensor hallucis brevis, and provides cutaneous innervation to the webbing between the first and second toes. (A) The superficial peroneal nerve innervates the peroneus longus and brevis, and provides cutaneous innervation over the anterolateral leg and the dorsum of the foot, except for the first web space. (B) The medial dorsal cutaneous nerve divides into three branches, and provides sensation to the medial side of the hallux and adjacent sides of the second and third toes. (C) The intermediate dorsal cutaneous nerve divides into four branches, and supplies sensation to the medial and lateral sides of the third, fourth, and fifth toes. (E) The tibial nerve innervates the gastrocnemius, popliteus, soleus, and plantaris, and contributes to the sural nerve. It also innervates the tibialis posterior, flexor digitorum longus, flexor hallucis longus, sole of the foot, and posterior lower leg.

10.

D Recurrent artery of Heubner

The recurrent artery of Heubner is the most proximal branch of the A2 segment distal to the anterior communicating artery. It runs in a retrograde fashion and enters the anterior perforating substance. (A) The tentorial artery is a branch of the meningohypophyseal trunk that runs posteriorly to supply blood to the tentorium. (B) The McConnell capsular artery/arteries arise from the medial trunk of the intracavernous internal carotid artery and supply blood to the pituitary gland. They are present in only 28% of the population. (C) The frontopolar artery is a branch of the A2 segment that supplies blood to the medial frontal lobe and the lateral surface of the superior frontal gyrus. (E) The medial lenticulostriate arteries arise from the A1 segment and supply blood to the globus pallidus and medial putamen.

11.

E Periaqueductal gray matter

The periaqueductal gray matter suppresses and modulates pain in the descending pathways within the midbrain tegmentum. (A) The superior colliculus functions to modulate gaze shifts. (B) The sub-

stantia nigra contains high levels of dopamine, and the loss of neurons in the pars compacta region characterizes Parkinson disease. (C) The crus cerebri is the anterior white matter portion of the cerebral peduncle that contains the motor tracts. (D) The red nucleus controls tone and gait.

12.

C Internal maxillary artery

Epistaxis after transsphenoidal surgery can be immediate or delayed. Injury to the internal carotid artery can cause life-threatening epistaxis, and pseudoaneurysm formation can lead to delayed hemorrhage, illustrating the need for an angiogram after suspected injury. In the external carotid system, the sphenopalatine artery, originating from the internal maxillary artery, is the most common branch injured during transsphenoidal surgeries. The artery is found in the inferolateral corner of the sphenoid ostium, and if it is injured, it can retract toward the maxilla and be difficult to coagulate.

13.

B Spinal accessory nerve

The long thoracic nerve provides innervation to the serratus anterior and is the most common cause of scapular winging. Its origin is the C5-C7 nerve roots. The dorsal scapular nerve (arising from the C5 root) innervates the rhomboids and levator scapulae. The spinal accessory nerve innervates the trapezius and sternocleidomastoid. Injury to any of these three nerves can cause a winged scapula. (A) The suprascapular nerve innervates the supraspinatus and infraspinatus. It is a branch of the upper trunk of the brachial plexus. (C) The thoracodorsal nerve emerges from the posterior cord and innervates the latissimus dorsi. (D) The lateral thoracic nerve does not exist.

14.

B Spinal dura

15.

C C

C is the location of the lateral component of the spinothalamic tracts. (A) A is the location of the dorsal columns. (B) B is the location of the anterior portion of the corticospinal tracts. (D) D is the location of the lateral corticospinal tracts. (E) E is the location of the reticulospinal tracts.

16.

A Along the midline surface of the cerebral hemisphere just anterior to the primary motor cortex leg area

Injury or irritation of the supplementary motor area produces a paucity of volitional movements along with a contralateral hemineglect and apraxias. Typically these symptoms resolve in a week or two when they are due to supplementary motor area damage, whereas the symptoms tend to be long standing when they are due to damage of the motor cortex. (B) The secondary somatosensory area is found in the parietal operculum. (C) The premotor cortex is in Brodmann area 6 on the lateral surface of the cerebral hemisphere. The medical extension of this area is the supplementary motor area. (D) The Broca area is within the pars opercularis and pars triangularis of the inferior frontal gyrus. (E) The paracentral lobule of the parietal lobule lies along the medial surface of the cerebral hemisphere and is continuous with the postcentral gyrus of the parietal lobe. The anterior component of this (the medial surface of the precentral gyrus) is the supplementary motor area.

17.

C Chorda tympani

The petrotympanic fissure is located between the temporomandibular joint and the middle ear to enable communication between these structures. It opens just anterior and superior to the tympanic membrane, and houses the anterior malleus ligament, anterior tympanic branch of the internal maxillary artery, and chorda tympani. (A) The pterygoid artery is a branch of the second part of the internal maxillary artery and supplies blood to the medial and lateral pterygoid muscles. (B) The posterior deep temporal artery is a branch of the second part of the internal maxillary artery and supplies blood to the temporalis muscle. (D) The chorda tympani does not join with the lingual nerve until after it emerges from the skull through the infratemporal fossa. (E) The greater superficial petrosal nerve travels over the surface of the foramen lacerum and joins the deep petrosal nerve to form the nerve of the pterygoid canal (Vidian nerve).

18.

A Frontal bone

The orbit is made up of seven bones: pars orbitalis of the frontal, lacrimal, lamina papyracea of the ethmoid, zygomatic, maxillary, palatine, and greater and lesser wings of the sphenoid. The nasal septum is composed of five bones and structures: perpendicular plate of the ethmoid, vomer, septum cartilage, maxillary, and palatine.

19.

A Abductor pollicis brevis

The median nerve originates from the C5-T1 roots. In the hand, the median nerve innervates the "LOAF" muscles (lumbricals 1 and 2, opponens pollicis, abductor pollicis brevis, and flexor pollicis brevis). The ulnar nerve innervates the opponens digiti minimi, flexor digiti minimi brevis, abductor digiti minimi, lumbricals 3 and 4, interossei, and adductor pollicis. The radial nerve innervates the extensors (digitorum, digiti minimi, carpi ulnaris, pollicis brevis, pollicis longus, and pollicis indicis) as well as the abductor pollicis longus.

20.

A Ectoderm

The pituitary is derived from the dual ectoderm. Around day 28 of embryogenesis, the Rathke pouch arises from a diverticulum from the stomodeum, which is derived from the ectoderm. The infundibulum arises from the neuroectoderm and grows inferiorly, where it eventually contacts the Rathke pouch. By the fifth week of embryogenesis, the neck of the Rathke pouch contacts the infundibulum and separates from the oral epithelium. The residual lumen of the Rathke pouch narrows to form a cleft and regresses. Persistence of the pouch is considered to be the cause of a Rathke cleft cyst.

21.

E Calcarine sulcus

The cuneus (Brodmann area 17) is the primary visual cortex and is bounded anteriorly by the parieto-occipital sulcus and inferiorly by the calcarine sulcus. (C) The lingual gyrus lies between the calcarine sulcus and posterior part of the collateral sulcus and contributes to Brodmann area 19. (D) The collateral eminence is found in the lateral aspect of the occipital horn and is a result of invagination of the collateral sulcus.

22.

A Fornix, tela choroidea, velum interpositum, tela choroidea, and choroid plexus

The tela choroidea is composed of pia that sits on the velum interpositum (the potential space containing the internal cerebral veins). Failure of closure of the posterior end of this potential space results in a cavum velum interpositum that communicates with the quadrigeminal cistern.

23.

B Inferior petrosal sinus

The inferior petrosal sinus drains into the sigmoid sinus/jugular vein. (A) The superior petrosal sinus runs along edge of the tentorium and drains into the transverse sinus. (C) The vein of Labbé is a superficial vein that anastomoses the middle cerebral vein with the transverse sinus. (D) The basal vein of Rosenthal begins in the anterior perforated substance and receives contributions from the anterior cerebral vein, deep sylvian vein, and inferior striate veins. The basal vein of Rosenthal then passes around the cerebral peduncle to drain blood into the vein of Galen. (E) The straight sinus is the union of the vein of Galen and inferior sagittal sinus and drains into the torcular/transverse sinus.

24.

B Middle cerebellar peduncle

Corticopontine fibers project through the middle cerebellar peduncle (brachium pontis) along pontocerebellar fibers. (A) The inferior cerebellar peduncle (restiform and juxtarestiform bodies) receives signals from the spinocerebellar tract, olivary nucleus, and vestibular nuclei. (C) Most fibers emerging from the cerebellum do so through the superior cerebellar peduncle (brachium conjunctivum) and then synapse on the red nucleus or motor nuclei of the thalamus.

25.

E Cingulate gyrus

The medial limbic circuit also is known as the Papez circuit. It essentially is the limbic system circuitry. The Papez circuit begins in the hippocampus (subiculum) and then projects to the fornix followed by the mammillary bodies. The mammillary bodies project along the mammillothalamic tract to the anterior thalamic nucleus and then to the cingulum followed by the entorhinal cortex. The circuit is completed as the entorhinal cortex projects back to the hippocampus.

26.

C Anterior to and between the anterior and posterior cerebellar lobes

The flocculonodular lobe is part of the vestibulocerebellum and is involved with maintenance of posture. (A) The anterior lobe is rostral to the primary fissure. (B) The posterior lobe is caudal to the primary fissure. (D) The vermis is located in a midsagittal position. (E) The tectum of the midbrain is rostral to the anterior lobe and posterior to the sylvian aqueduct.

27.

C Globus pallidus

The globus pallidus sends afferents to the subthalamic nucleus, which also receives fewer afferents from the substantia nigra pars compacta and pedunculopontine nucleus.

28.

A Anterior divisions of the upper and middle trunks

The lateral cord is derived from the anterior divisions of the superior and middle trunks. (C) The posterior cord is formed from the posterior divisions of the superior, middle, and inferior trunks. (D) The medial cord is formed from the anterior division of the inferior trunk.

29.

A Areas 1, 2, and 3

The ventral posterior nucleus is subdivided into the ventral posterior lateral nucleus and the ventral posterior medial nucleus, which receive afferent sensory information from the medial lemniscus/spinothalamic tract and trigeminothalamic tract, respectively. These nuclei then send projections to the primary somatosensory cortex in the postcentral gyrus (Brodmann areas 1, 2, and 3). (B) Brodmann area 4 is the primary motor cortex in the precentral gyrus. (C) Brodmann area 17 is the primary visual cortex in the occipital lobe. (D) Brodmann areas 39 and 40 are the angular gyrus and supramarginal gyrus, respectively, and represent the Wernicke area. (E) Brodmann area 44 is the pars opercularis of the inferior frontal gyrus and represents the Broca area.

30.

C Tibial and common peroneal nerves

The sural nerve is composed of contributions from the medial cutaneous branch arising from the tibial nerve and the lateral cutaneous branch arising from the common peroneal nerve.

31.

B Decreased taste in the anterior two thirds of the tongue

Facial nerve branches distal to the nerve to the stapedius include the chorda tympani, which serves to provide taste to the anterior two thirds of the tongue. (A) The greater petrosal nerve is the first branch of the facial nerve distal to the geniculate ganglion (proximal to the emergence of the nerve to the stapedius). The greater petrosal nerve innervates the lacrimal gland after sending fibers through the zygomatic nerve. (C) Decreased salivation would be expected as the facial nerve innervates the submandibular and sublingual glands through the chorda tympani. (D) The nervus intermedius provides the sensory and parasympathetic components for cranial nerve VII. It joins the motor root of the nerve at the geniculate ganglion and provides minor sensory innervation to the oropharynx and auricle.

32.

D Pronator quadratus

The anterior interosseous nerve is a branch of the median nerve and classically innervates two and a half muscles: the flexor pollicis longus, pronator quadratus, and radial half of flexor digitorum profundus. It contains no sensory fibers. (A–C) The median nerve proper innervates the flexor pollicis brevis, abductor pollicis brevis, and flexor carpi radialis. (E) The abductor pollicis longus is innervated by the posterior interosseous nerve from the radial nerve.

33.

D Wernicke area

The Wernicke area often is localized to the angular gyrus on the banks of the superior temporal sulcus and the supramarginal gyrus found on the banks of the sylvian fissure (Brodmann areas 39 and 40, respectively). Some neuroanatomists also consider the posterior part of Brodmann area 22 (the superior temporal gyrus) to be a part of the Wernicke area. (A) The Broca area is Brodmann area 44 and consists of the pars opercularis of the inferior frontal gyrus and, included by some neuroanatomists, the pars triangularis (Brodmann area 45). (B) The primary visual cortex is Brodmann area 17, whereas Brodmann area 18 is the secondary visual cortex. (C) The somatosensory association cortex is Brodmann area 7. (E) Brodmann area 22 along with the more medially located Brodmann area 41 (the Heschl gyrus) are the primary auditory cortex.

34.

C Interpeduncular and chiasmatic cisterns

The Liliequist membrane separates the interpeduncular from the chiasmatic cistern medially and the carotid cistern laterally. Blood in the chiasmatic cistern should raise concern for aneurysmal rupture.

35.

C Medial branch of the dorsal ramus

The medial branch of the dorsal (posterior) ramus innervates the facet capsule, synovium, multifidus, ligaments, and periosteum of the vertebral arches. (A) The lateral branch of the dorsal ramus innervates the paraspinous musculature and proximal sensory dermatomes. (B) The ventral ramus innervates the musculature and dermatomes of the limbs and truck. The meningeal branch (the sinuvertebral nerve) arises from the spinal nerve root and reenters the intervertebral foramen. (D) The ramus communicans contains autonomic nerves. (E) The dorsal/posterior root contains the afferent (sensory) nerves that contribute to the spinal nerve.

36.

C It is a crossed tract arising from the dentate nucleus that passes through the superior cerebellar peduncle and terminates in the ventral anterior nucleus of the thalamus.

37.

E Spinal nucleus of cranial nerve V

Pain and temperature signals from the face travel through the spinal tract of cranial nerve V to terminate in the spinal nucleus of cranial nerve V, which extends into the cervical spinal cord. (A) Proprioceptive fibers travel to the mesencephalic nucleus of cranial nerve V. (B) Sensory fibers travel to the ventral posterior medial nucleus of the thalamus. (C) Pressure and vibration signals terminate in the chief (principal) nucleus of cranial nerve V. (D) The solitary nucleus receives gustatory signals and regulates cardiorespiratory and gastrointestinal processes.

38.

C Superior hypophyseal artery

The supraclinoidal internal carotid artery branches are, from proximal to distal, the ophthalmic, superior hypophyseal, posterior communicating, and anterior choroidal. (D) The inferior hypophyseal artery originates from the intercavernous meningohypophyseal artery, as does the tentorial artery of Bernasconi and Cassinari and the dorsal meningeal artery.

39.

B V3

The vertebral artery is divided into four segments. The V1 segment runs from the subclavian artery to the foramen transversarium (usually of the sixth cervical vertebra). The V3 segment runs from the foramen transversarium of C2 to the foramen magnum. (A) The V2 segment runs from C6 to C2. (D) The V4 segment is intradural. (E) There is no V5 segment.

40.

C Merkel disk

Merkel disks are found in glabrous and hairy skin, hair follicles, and oral mucosa. They are most sensitive to vibrations and they are slowly adapting. (A) Meissner corpuscles are found in skin sensitive to light touch and are rapidly adapting. (B) Pacinian corpuscles are sensitive to vibration and pressure and are rapidly adapting. (D, E) Hair follicle receptors and A-delta free nerve endings are rapidly adapting, whereas C fiber free nerve endings are slowly adapting.

41.

D Junction of the coronal suture and superior temporal line

(A) The pterion is at the junction of the frontal, parietal, temporal, and sphenoid bones. (B) The asterion is at the junction of the lambdoid, occipitomastoid, and parietomastoid sutures and often approximates the junction of the transverse and sigmoid sinus. (C) Bregma occurs at the junction of the coronal and sagittal sutures.

42.

B Septal nuclei and the habenular nuclei

The stria medullaris thalami (epithalamic structures) connect the septal nuclei along with the anterior thalamic nuclei to the habenula. (A) The ansa lenticularis connects the ventral globus pallidus to the field of Forel H by passing around the posterior limb of the internal capsule. It then joins the lenticular fasciculus to form the thalamic fasciculus. (C) The lenticular fasciculus (field of Forel H2) connects to the thalamic fasciculus in the field of Forel H by passing through the posterior limb of the internal capsule. (D) The anterior commissure connects the amygdalae to one another. (E) The dopaminergic mesolimbic tracts connect the ventral tegmental area to the nucleus accumbens as part of the "reward" circuitry.

43.

D Spinal gray interneurons in Rexed lamina VII

Corticospinal tracts arise in the cerebral cortex and terminate on the spinal gray interneurons (second-order neurons) that are located in the Rexed lamina VII in the ventral horns. (E) Rexed lamina IX contains alpha and gamma motor neurons.

44.

D Ventral spinocerebellar tract

The ventral spinocerebellar tract is composed of sensory afferents and carries information about proprioception to the cerebellum. It decussates in the anterior white commissure of the spinal cord and enters the cerebellum through the superior cerebellar peduncle. The fibers then cross within the cerebellum to synapse ipsilateral to the tract origin. (A) The spinothalamic tract is composed of sensory afferents and carries information about pain, temperature, and crude touch. (B) The posterior columns are composed of sensory afferents and carry information about fine touch and proprioception. They are composed of the fasciculi gracilis and fasciculi cuneatus, providing sensory information from the middle thoracic to the lower extremity dermatomes and the cervical (including the upper extremities) to the midthoracic dermatomes, respectively. (C) The dorsal spinocerebellar tract is composed of sensory afferents and carries information about proprioception to the cerebellum. It enters the cerebellum through the inferior cerebellar peduncle without decussating. (E) The corticobulbar tract is composed of motor efferents to the cranial nerve nuclei.

45.

D Cranial nerve V to the tensor tympani muscle and cranial nerve VII to the stapedius muscle

The tensor veli palatini muscle is also innervated by cranial nerve V, whereas the levator palatini muscle is innervated by cranial nerve X. The acoustic reflex is initiated by the superior olivary complex.

46.

B Medial surface of the lateral mass of C1

The transverse ligament attaches to the odontoid process and lateral masses of the atlas. (A) The alar ligament connects the dens to the medial surface of the occipital condyles. (D) A portion of the cruciate ligament attaches superiorly to the occipital bone near the tectorial membrane and inferiorly to the posterior aspect of the C2 body. (E) The posterior atlanto-occipital membrane attaches to the posterior arch of C1.

47.

E Hyperthermia

The anterior hypothalamus is involved with thermoregulation (cooling) and parasympathetic regulation. Lesions can produce hyperthermia. (A) The ventral medial nucleus is the satiety center. Lesions here will cause obesity. (B) Lesions of the lateral hypothalamus may cause reduced food intake and cachexia. (C) The posterior nucleus is involved in thermoregulation (heating) and sympathetic regulation. Lesions can produce hypothermia and loss of sympathetic tone. (D) Lesions of the mammillary bodies can cause memory deficits and amnestic syndromes.

48.

B Anterior short gyri

The insula is composed of an anterior part subdivided into three or four short gyri that receive information from the ventral medial nucleus of the thalamus and amygdala. (A) The frontal, parietal, and temporal opercula surround the insula. (C) The posterior insula is formed by a long gyrus that receives information from the secondary somatosensory cortex and ventral posterior inferior thalamic nucleus. (D) The cingulate is not part of the insula. (E) The claustrum is deep to the insula.

49.

A Dentate

(B) The globose nucleus is lateral to the fastigial nucleus. (C) The fastigial nucleus is the most medially located. (D) The emboliform nucleus is lateral to the globose nucleus. (E) The inferior olivary nucleus is not a deep cerebellar nucleus. It is part of the medulla.

50.

B 20%

51.

E Notochord

(B) The closure of the anterior neuropore results in the creation of the lamina terminalis. Failure to close results in anencephaly. (C) Failure of posterior neuropore closure results in spina bifida.

52.

C Posterior communicating, posterior cerebral, and anterior choroidal arteries

(A) The ophthalmic artery supplies the retina with blood. (B) The anterior communicating, posterior communicating, and posterior cerebral arteries supply the optic chiasm with blood. (D) The lateral posterior choroidal artery supplies the medial lateral geniculate with blood.

53.

C Area 17

The primary visual cortex resides in Brodmann area 17. (A) Brodmann areas 41 and 42 contain the auditory cortex. (B) Brodmann areas 18 and 19 are the secondary and associative visual cortices. (D) Brodmann area 39 represents the angular gyrus.

54.

C Three and five

The C3 through L5 vertebrae have an ossification center in each vertebral body in addition to a center in each half of each neural arch (a total of three for each vertebra). The C1 vertebra has three primary ossification centers: one in the anterior arch and one in each of the lateral posterior arches. The C2 vertebra has five primary ossification centers: the three typical of the other vertebrae in addition to a center on each side of the odontoid process. Secondary ossification centers for the C3 though L5 vertebrae occur at the tip of each spinous process and each transverse process in addition to one at the ring epiphyses at the upper/lower surfaces of each vertebral body (a total of five for each vertebra). The C1 vertebra has no secondary centers, whereas the C2 vertebra has one at the tip of the dens. Failure of this secondary center to fuse results in an os odontoideum.

55.

D Inferior colliculus; auditory cortex

(A) The superior colliculus and visual cortex are the afferent and efferent projections, respectively, to the pulvinar nucleus. (B) The retina and visual cortex are the afferent and efferent projections, respectively, to the lateral geniculate nucleus. (C) The reticular formation and dorsal thalamic nuclei are the afferent and efferent projections, respectively, to the thalamic reticular nucleus. The thalamic reticular nucleus receives input from the cortex, globus pallidus, reticular formation, and dorsal thalamic nuclei. It is the only thalamic nucleus that does not project to the cerebral cortex. (E) The mammillary bodies and cingulum are the afferent and efferent projections, respectively, to the anterior thalamic nucleus (part of the Papez circuit).

56.

C Tonsillomedullary segment of the posterior inferior cerebellar artery

The arteries at risk during a Chiari decompression include the vertebral artery (V3 segment as it courses around C1) and the caudal loop of the posterior inferior cerebellar artery (tonsillomedullary segment).

57.

C Pars triangularis

The inferior frontal gyrus is composed of, from anterior to posterior, the pars orbitalis (1), pars triangularis (2), and pars opercularis (3). The precentral gyrus (4) is found just posterior to the pars opercularis. The sylvian fissure ends posteriorly in the supramarginal gyrus (7). The central sulcus (5) terminates at a gyral bridge near the sylvian fissure. The angular gyrus (8) usually wraps around the superior temporal sulcus. The postcentral gyrus (6) is also shown.

58.

A On the left side between the T9 and L2 levels

The artery of Adamkiewicz is found on the left side in 80% and between the T9 and L2 levels in 85% of individuals. In 15% of individuals, the artery is found between the T5 and T8 levels. It is the main arterial supply to the spinal cord from T8 to the conus medullaris.

59.

C Posteromedial middle cranial fossa triangle

The Kawase triangle is the posteromedial middle cranial fossa triangle. It is bounded by the mandibular nerve (V3), the greater superficial petrosal nerve, the arcuate eminence, and the superior petrosal sinus. It contains the petrous apex, internal auditory canal, vertebrobasilar junction, and cochlea. (A) The Mullan triangle is the anteromedial middle cranial fossa triangle. It is bounded by the ophthalmic nerve (V1), the maxillary nerve (V2), and a line connecting the superior orbital fissure and the foramen rotundum. It contains the sphenoid sinus, ophthalmic vein, and abducens nerve. (B) The anterolateral middle cranial fossa triangle is bounded by the maxillary nerve (V2), the mandibular nerve (V3), and a line connecting the foramen rotundum and the foramen ovale. It contains the lateral sphenoid wing, sphenoid emissary vein, and cavernous to pterygoid venous anastomosis. (D) The Glasscock triangle is the posterolateral middle cranial fossa triangle. It is bounded by the mandibular nerve (V3), the greater superficial petrosal nerve, and a line from the foramen spinosum to the arcuate eminence. It contains the foramen spinosum, horizontal petrous internal carotid artery, and infratemporal fossa. (E) The Parkinson triangle is the infratrochlear middle cranial fossa triangle. It is bounded by a line from the dural entries of the trochlear and abducens nerves, a line from the dural entries of the abducens nerve and the petrosal vein, and the petrous apex. It contains the dural opening to the Meckel cave.

60.

D Two centimeters above the carotid bifurcation without involvement of the carotid bulb

Typically, the internal carotid artery dissects without involving the carotid bulb. Dissection may cause a Horner syndrome, ipsilateral head or neck pain, and lower cranial nerve neuropathies due to arterial occlusion. (E) The supraclinoidal segment of the internal carotid artery is a less frequent area of dissection.

61.

B Myelomeningocele

(A) Spina bifida occulta is a defect in the vertebral arch without disruption of the underlying meninges. (C) The cystic distention of the meninges without spinal cord/cauda equina involvement is a meningocele. (D) A lipomyelomeningocele is a form of closed spinal dysraphism resulting from a defect in primary neurulation. It is formed by mesenchymal tissue entering a neural placode and forming lipomatous tissue. (E) Diastematomyelia is a postneurulation defect and involves a split spinal cord.

62.

B Mossy

(A) Climbing fibers synapse directly on Purkinje cells and originate in the inferior olive. (C) Parallel fibers are the axons to granule cells. (D) Purkinje fibers are conducting fibers of the heart. (E) Association fibers are bundles of axons within the cerebral cortex that unite different parts of the same cerebral hemisphere.

63.

D Trochlear nerve

The mnemonic for remembering the structures that pass through the superior orbital fissure (in order from superior to inferior) is "Little frosty treats sit near icy appetizers." The lacrimal, frontal, and trochlear nerves all do not pass through the annulus of Zinn, whereas the superior division of the oculomotor, nasociliary, inferior division of the oculomotor, and abducens nerves do. (A–C) These nerves all pass through the cavernous sinus, the superior orbital fissure, and the annulus of Zinn. (E) The optic nerve passes through the annulus of Zinn but is separated from the other nerves by a strut. The optic nerve does not pass through the cavernosus sinus or superior orbital fissure.

64.

A Dorsal interossei

The mnemonic here is "PAD DAB": *palmar interossei adduct, dorsal interossei abduct.*" (B) The lumbricals flex the metacarpophalangeal joints while extending the interphalangeal joints, resulting in a "tabletop" action. (C) The palmar interossei adduct the fingers. (D, E) The actions of the extensor digitorum and flexor digitorum superficialis are explained by their names. They do not result in either abduction or adduction of the fingers.

65.

C Vertebral artery

The anterior spinal artery arises from the junction of two arterial branches, one from each vertebral artery.

66.

B Middle scalene

The long thoracic nerve from nerve roots C5, C6, and C7 travels deep to the proximal brachial plexus and between the anterior and middle scalene muscles. It then courses over the posterolateral part of the first rib and innervates the serratus anterior. (A) The phrenic nerve passes over the surface of the anterior scalene as it enters the thorax to innervate the diaphragm.

67.

A First

Pharyngeal/branchial arches develop during the fourth week of embryogenesis as a series of mesodermal outpouchings on both sides of the pharynx. The first arch develops into the muscles of mastication and is related to the trigeminal nerve. (B) The second branchial arch is related to the facial nerve and muscles of facial expression. (C) The third branchial arch is related to the glossopharyngeal nerve and gives rise to the stylopharyngeus. (D) The fourth branchial arch is related to the vagus and superior laryngeal nerves and gives rise to the cricothyroid and all of the intrinsic muscles of the soft palate except for the tensor veli palatini. (E) There is no fifth branchial arch. The sixth branchial arch gives rise to all of the intrinsic muscles of the larynx except for the cricothyroid and is related to the vagus and recurrent laryngeal nerves.

68.

A Ligament of Struthers

The ligament of Struthers is a common site of compression of the median nerve. (B) The arcade of Struthers is a fascial arcade of the intermuscular septum and a potential compression site of the

ulnar nerve. It often is released during a cubital tunnel release procedure. (C) The arcade of Frohse is the fibrous proximal border of the supinator muscle and is the most common site of compression of the posterior interosseous nerve. (D) The Osborne ligament connects the two heads of the flexor carpi ulnaris and passes between the olecranon and medial epicondyle, forming the cubital tunnel, which is the most common site of compression of the ulnar nerve. (E) The Guyon canal (near the wrist) forms a distal site of potential ulnar nerve compression. Compression at the Guyon canal can be differentiated from compression at the cubital tunnel, as preservation of the dorsal sensation dermatomes of the ulnar nerve is seen in the latter compression site.

69.

C Cranial nerve IX, Jacobson nerve, and inferior petrosal sinus

The anteromedial compartment (pars nervosa) is smaller and consists of cranial nerve IX, the Jacobson nerve (tympanic nerve of cranial nerve IX, providing sensation to the middle ear and parasympathetics through the lesser petrosal nerve to the otic ganglion and parotid gland), and the inferior petrosal sinus. The mnemonic is "nervous nine" to remember the relationship of the pars nervosa to the cranial nerve IX components. (D) The larger, posterolateral compartment (pars vascularis) contains cranial nerves X and XI, the Arnold nerve (involved in sensation of the skin of the ear canal and in the ear–cough reflex), the jugular bulb, and a branch of the ascending pharyngeal artery.

70.

E Subcommissural organ

Circumventricular organs are characterized by their proximity to the ventricles and their lack of a blood–brain barrier. They include the area postrema, subfornical organ, organ of the lamina terminalis, subcommissural organ, posterior pituitary gland, pineal gland, median eminence, and intermediate lobe of the pituitary gland. The subcommissural organ has an intact blood–brain barrier but is considered a circumventricular organ, given its role in the neuroendocrine system. Overall, its function largely is unknown. (D) The area postrema is the only paired circumventricular organ.

71.

B Internal granular

Layer 1 is the molecular layer and is the most superficial. Layer 4 is the internal granular layer and receives afferent fibers from the thalamus. (A,

C) Layers 2 and 3 are the external granular and external pyramidal layers, respectively, and contain commissural/association fibers. (D) Layer 5 is the internal pyramidal layer and contains Betz cells that are the main efferents to the brainstem and spinal cord. (E) Layer 6 is the multiform layer that sends fibers to the thalamus.

72.

B Caudate, putamen, and globus pallidus

(A) Striatum refers to the caudate and putamen. (C) Lentiform nuclei refer to the putamen and globus pallidus. (D) Neostriatum refers to the caudate.

73.

E Crural

(A) The ambient cistern contains the anterior choroidal artery, basal vein of Rosenthal, and posterior cerebral artery. (B) The quadrigeminal cistern contains the superior cerebellar artery, cranial nerve IV, precentral vein, vein of Galen, and posterior cerebral artery. (C) The interpeduncular cistern contains the basilar artery, cranial nerve III, posterior cerebral artery, and superior cerebellar artery. (D) The carotid cistern contains the internal carotid artery, anterior choroidal artery, and posterior communicating artery.

74.

D Oxytocin and antidiuretic hormone

The posterior pituitary (neurohypophysis) releases oxytocin and vasopressin (antidiuretic hormone) derived from supraoptic and paraventricular neurons in the hypothalamus. The anterior pituitary (adenohypophysis) contains releasing factors and inhibitory hormones such as corticotrophin-releasing, thyrotropin-releasing, gonadotropin-releasing, growth hormone–releasing/inhibiting, and prolactin-releasing/inhibiting hormones that release adrenocorticotropic, thyroid-stimulating, luteinizing, follicle-stimulating, growth, and prolactin hormones, respectively.

75.

C Tapetum

The roof and lateral wall of the temporal horn are composed primarily of the tapetum of the corpus callosum and are enveloped by optic radiations. (A) The anterior wall of the temporal horn is formed by the amygdala. (B) The floor of the temporal horn is formed largely by the hippocampus. (D) The choroidal fissure is located along the medial wall of the temporal horn. (E) The collateral eminence forms part of the floor of the temporal horn and lies lateral and parallel to the hippocampus.

76.

A Fibers from the ventral SCT often cross contralaterally in the spinal cord and cross again contralaterally in the superior cerebellar peduncle to reach the cerebellum.

The dorsal spinocerebellar tract (SCT) synapses in the Clarke nuclei (Rexed lamina VII) and then ascends ipsilaterally to reach the cerebellum through the inferior cerebellar peduncle. It is an ipsilateral tract. In contrast, the ventral SCT synapses in Rexed laminae V, VI, and VII before crossing contralaterally through the anterior commissure to continue its ascent. Most fibers cross contralaterally (although some fibers continue ipsilaterally) through the superior cerebellar peduncle to reach the cerebellum. It is an ipsilateral tract with a double crossing.

77.

E Inferior olivary nucleus

Climbing fibers synapse on Purkinje cells after originating in the inferior olivary nucleus of the medulla and are among the most excitatory fibers in the central nervous system. (A) Pontine and vestibular nuclei form mossy fibers. (C) The spinal cord and reticular formation send projections that end in cerebellar glomeruli.

78.

C Superior rectus

There are three extraocular muscles that are innervated by contralateral nuclei. The superior oblique is innervated by the trochlear nerve, which crosses within the midbrain and emerges contralaterally from its nucleus from the dorsal surface of the brainstem. The levator palpebrae superioris is innervated bilaterally by the caudal subnucleus. In addition, the medial subnucleus of cranial nerve III provides innervation to the contralateral superior rectus muscle.

79.

C Basal nucleus of Meynert

The basal nucleus of Meynert is found in the basal forebrain (substantia innominata) and is rich in acetylcholine. The nucleus is important in visual attention. (A) The locus coeruleus is a pontine structure rich in norepinephrine. (B) The raphe nucleus is found in the brainstem and is rich in serotonin. (D) The substantia nigra is found in the midbrain and is rich in dopamine. (E) The suprachiasmatic nucleus is involved in the production of cortisol and melatonin for mediation of circadian rhythms.

80.

D IX

The gray matter of the spinal cord is divided into 10 Rexed laminae. The sensory areas are the most dorsal, whereas the motor areas are the most ventral. Laminae VIII and IX contain medial and lateral motor neuron columns (flexor muscle neurons are located more medially than extensor muscle neurons). (A) Lamina II is known as the substantia gelatinosa and responds to noxious pain. There is a high concentration of substance P in lamina II. (B) Lamina IV is known as the nucleus proprius and is involved in proprioception and light touch. (C) Lamina VII is a large zone that contains a group of interneurons known as the dorsal nucleus (Clarke column) that give rise to the posterior spinocerebellar tract and the intermediolateral nucleus (levels T1 through L2), with the latter containing preganglionic sympathetic neurons. (E) Lamina X is the gray matter surrounding the central canal.

81.

B Inhibitory interneurons found in the spinal cord that release glycine

Renshaw cells are interneurons located in the ventral horn of the spinal cord that project to alpha motor neurons. They are stimulated by acetylcholine and release inhibitory glycine.

82.

A Fibers projecting from CA3 to CA1

In addition to projecting to the fornix, CA3 neurons project to CA1 (the Sommer sector) as Schaffer collaterals. (B) The CA3 neurons transmit information to the fornix, which is the major efferent pathway for the hippocampus. (C) Fibers enter the hippocampus from the dentate gyrus and project to neurons in CA3. (D) Fibers projecting from the cingulate gyrus to the parahippocampus are part of the Papez circuit (parahippocampus to the hippocampus to the fornix to the mammillary bodies to the anterior thalamus to the cingulate to the parahippocampus). (E) The pyriform cortex, entorhinal cortex, and amygdala are part of the olfactory projection area. The pyriform cortex projects to the thalamus and frontal lobe.

83.

D Basal vein of Rosenthal and internal cerebral vein

The two internal cerebral veins join with their respective basal veins of Rosenthal to form the great cerebral vein (of Galen). The vein of Galen also receives drainage from callosal, superior cerebellar, and inferior cerebral veins. (A) The thalamostriate and septal veins join to form the internal cerebral vein. (B) The vein of Galen and the inferior sagittal sinus merge to form the straight sinus. (E) The straight and superior sagittal sinuses form the torcular.

84.

B Congruent homonymous hemianopsia with sparing of central vision

The most caudal area of the visual cortex represents central vision. Lesions affecting the visual cortex with macular sparing can be seen in some cases of posterior cerebral artery infarction due to the middle cerebral artery collaterals supplying the most caudal areas that concern central vision. With diffuse anoxic states, central vision can be affected before or along with the rest of the visual cortex due to the central visual cortex being so far distal in the circulation. A visual cortex lesion produces a homonymous hemianopsia that tends to be much more congruent than optic tract lesions. (C) Incongruent homonymous hemianopsias are due to unilateral optic tract compressions proximal to the thalamus. (D, E) Bitemporal hemianopsia and junctional scotomas are seen with chiasmal compression, with the latter attributed to compression of the Wilbrand knee in the anterior chiasm. A more contemporary theory about the etiology of junctional scotomas is that they are the result of an asymmetric anterior chiasm compression causing an optic neuropathy and scotoma in one eye and a contralateral superotemporal deficit in the other eye.

85.

D Facial nerve and superior vestibular nerve

The facial, cochlear, and inferior and superior vestibular nerves are found in the lateral internal auditory canal. In the lateral portion of the canal, the horizontal (falciform) crest separates the facial and superior vestibular nerves superiorly from the cochlear and inferior vestibular nerves inferiorly. Vertically, the vertical crest (Bill's bar) separates the facial nerve (anterior/superior) from the superior vestibular nerve (posterior/superior). The mnemonic is "7 Up," indicating that cranial nerve VII is in the superior portion of the canal. The "superior" in superior vestibular nerve describes its position in the canal relative to the inferior vestibular nerve. (A, B) The facial and cochlear nerves are separated by the horizontal crest as are the superior and inferior vestibular nerves.

86.

B Ethmoid sinuses

The ethmoid sinuses are innervated by the nasociliary nerve through the posterior ethmoidal nerve. (A) The lacrimal gland is innervated by the lacrimal nerve. (C) The forehead and frontal sinuses are innervated by the frontal nerve. (D) The iris dilator muscle is innervated by sympathetic nerves following the ciliary nerves. (E) The cornea is innervated by the ophthalmic division of the trigeminal nerve through the ciliary nerves.

87.

C Epineurium

The epineurium surrounds multiple fascicles and the vessels supplying the fascicles with blood. (A) The perineurium surrounds each fascicle (a bundle of individual nerve fibers). (B) The endoneurium is the connective tissue that surrounds each myelinated nerve fiber.

13 Adult Neurosurgery

1.

A Colloid cyst

Colloid cysts represent 0.5 to 2% of all brain tumors and occur in the anterior part of the third ventricle near the foramen of Monro. These lesions can be associated with the development of hydrocephalus and rapid clinical deterioration. Sudden death has been reported but is rare, and likely involves the colloid cyst acting as a ball valve and suddenly shifting and occluding cerebrospinal fluid outflow.

2.

A Burning pain, autonomic dysfunction, and trophic changes following obvious nerve damage

Complex regional pain syndrome (CRPS) type 2 follows nerve injury and originally was described following high-velocity missile injuries. CRPS type 1 (also known as reflex sympathetic dystrophy) is similar to CRPS type 2 in symptoms but does not demonstrate obvious nerve damage. (B) Increased perspiration in excess of what is required for regulation of body temperature suggests hyperhidrosis. (C) CRPS type 2 requires nerve damage for the diagnosis. (D) Dejerine-Roussy syndrome follows a thalamic stroke and is characterized by an initial lack of sensation and tingling on one side of the body followed later by severe, chronic dysesthesias or allodynia. (E) Munchausen syndrome is characterized by recurrent hospitalizations with dramatic, untrue, and extremely improbable tales of past experiences.

3.

C Intraventricular hemorrhage (IVH), position of ICH, patient age

The intracranial hemorrhage (ICH) score is calculated from four factors: Glasgow Coma Scale (GCS) score, ICH volume, whether or not the ICH is infratentorial, and patient age. A GCS score of 3–4 yields two points, 5–12 yields one point, and 13–15 yields no points. One point is given to an ICH at least 30 cm³ in size, and an additional point is given to an ICH with an infratentorial origin. Finally, one point is given if the patient is at least 80 years old. The ICH score thus ranges from 0 to 6.

4.

C Obtain blood cultures

The likely diagnosis is diskitis, and the next step is to obtain blood cultures to confirm the hematog-enous source and obtain an organism to treat. If blood cultures are negative, guided needle biopsy of the disk space should be done. Obtaining a serum erythrocyte sedimentation rate and C-reactive protein concentration also can be helpful. (A) A lumbar puncture is contraindicated due to the possibility of seeding the intrathecal space with an infectious agent.

5.

A Improves with activity

Although some patients with severe back pain and muscle spasms may improve with no more than 48 hours of bed rest, patients with mild to moderate back pain should return to near-normal work schedules and have improvement in back pain with activity, as this increases flexibility.

6.

C Through the bulk of the psoas major

The transpsoas approach to the lumbar spine places the entire lumbosacral plexus at risk for injury. The risk can be minimized by staying in the bulk of the psoas major muscle and with close neuromonitoring.

7.

C Ocular neuromyotonia

Although rare, ocular neuromyotonia can occur after skull base radiation, with a reported mean time of 3.5 years following radiation. It is characterized by episodic, tonic contractions of one or more extraocular muscles, resulting in episodic diplopia. Varying success has been reported with membrane stabilizing agents (antiepileptics) or strabismus surgery.

8.

E L5 nerve root and common peroneal nerve at the fibular head

This patient has an injury to the L5 nerve root and the common peroneal nerve as explained. The peroneal nerve must be affected after it has given off its motor innervation to the short head of the biceps femoris, as this muscle is unaffected. The common peroneal nerve is most commonly injured as it crosses the fibular head, resulting in the symptoms seen in this clinical scenario. The fibrillations present on electromyography can indicate an axonal injury and uncontrolled and spontaneous firing of muscle cells. Present but reduced motor unit potentials indicate reduced motor unit recruitment and can indicate impeded nerve conduction. (A) With an L4 nerve root abnormality, abnormalities of the tibialis anterior would be expected. (B) An L5 nerve root abnormality explains the abnormalities in the extensor digitorum longus and gluteus medius but fails to address the abnormalities seen in the common peroneal nerve. Abnormalities in the gluteus minimus also would be seen with an L5 nerve root abnormality. (C) The S1 nerve root innervates the peroneus longus and brevis. (D) The common peroneal nerve supplies the short head of the biceps femoris before passing around the fibular head and branching into a superficial and deep branch. The superficial branch supplies motor innervations to the muscles of the lateral compartment of the leg (the peroneus longus and brevis, which evert the foot) along with sensory innervation to the lateral leg. The deep branch supplies motor innervation to the muscles of the anterior compartment of the leg (the tibialis anterior, extensor hallucis longus, extensor digitorum longus, and peroneus tertius) along with muscles in the foot. It supplies sensory innervation to the dorsum of the foot in the first web space.

9.

D Lungs

When malignant peripheral nerve sheath tumors (MPNSTs) are discovered, a chest CT (fine cut) should be ordered to look for metastatic disease, as this is the most common location of metastatic spread. (E) Metastases of MPNSTs rarely occur in locations like the lymph nodes or the heart.

10.

A Dural

The American/English/French arteriovenous malformation (AVM) classification divides spinal vascular malformations into four types. Type 1 (dural AVM) is the most common; a radicular artery feeds into an engorged spinal vein along the posterior cord. This type is low flow. Type 2 (spinal glomus AVM) is a true AVM of the spinal cord. Type 3 (juvenile spinal AVM) is an enlarged glomus AVM that occupies the entire cross section of the cord and invades the vertebral body. This type may cause scoliosis. Type 4 (perimedullary AVM) forms a direct fistula between arteries supplying the spinal cord and draining veins. (C) Extramedullary/intradural is not an AVM type and instead refers to an anatomic location typically used when describing spinal neoplasms.

11.

A Microvascular decompression

Although multiple sclerosis patients have a poorer response than patients without the disease to any treatment for trigeminal neuralgia, patients with multiple sclerosis respond very poorly to microvascular decompression.

12.

D Diplopia

Diplopia can occur following a stereotactic mesencephalotomy secondary to lesioning near the inferior colliculus. The diplopia is due to a defect in vertical eye movements and often resolves. (A) No motor tracts are encountered during a stereotactic mesencephalotomy. Weakness in the extremities is more likely to occur during a cordotomy.

13.

C 75%

Although the definition of serviceable hearing varies, most sources require a speech discrimination score of at least 50 to 70%. For preoperative counseling, a speech discrimination score under 75% significantly raises the risk of not having serviceable hearing following a vestibular schwannoma resection.

14.

E Preparation for transsphenoidal decompression immediately

The patient displays symptoms of pituitary apoplexy caused by a rapid expansion of her known pituitary adenoma secondary to necrosis or hemorrhage. This can lead to headache, nausea, somnolence, and other neurologic changes due to elevations in intracranial pressure along with exacerbated visual field cuts and ophthalmoplegia due to local mass effect. Treatment is emergent decompression of the sella turcica and pituitary lesion. Immediate administration of a stress dose of steroids also is important. Subarachnoid hemorrhage can be seen with pituitary apoplexy, and an angiogram can be useful to rule out an aneurysm as a cause. (A) The patient likely is not having a migraine due to the new ophthalmoplegia with a known pituitary tumor. (B, D) This patient needs treatment soon to avoid permanent ophthalmic injury and neurologic damage associated with elevated intracranial pressures. (C) Lab work is unlikely to aid in the treatment of this patient as the pituitary lesion is unlikely to have grown suddenly. Outpatient lab work and waiting for inpatient labs to return will not affect the need for definitive treatment.

15.
C 4

House-Brackmann facial nerve function classification grading ranges from 1 (normal) to 6 (total paralysis). Grade 2 is mild dysfunction. Grade 3 is obvious but not disfiguring facial asymmetry. Grade 4 dysfunction entails the inability to close the eye. Grade 5 is barely perceptible motion.

16.
E No form of nicotine avoids the risk of decreased spinal fusion rates.

Nicotine in all its forms has been shown to affect adversely spinal fusion rates.

17.
B 8 in-lbs

(E) The recommended torque for the screws on many halo vests is 30 in-lbs.

18.
B Hemiballism

Hemiballism is a unilateral, involuntary jerking of the proximal limb due to a lesion of the suthalamic nucleus. (A) Myoclonus describes shock-like contractions that are irregular and asymmetric and can have numerous etiologies. (C) A pill-rolling tremor is characteristic of parkinsonism and pathology involving the substantia nigra pars compacta. (D) Dystonias leading to fixed limb postures may be due to putaminal destruction. (E) Chorea is seen in Huntington disease and is a result of striatum atrophy.

19.
B Balance

Patients with Parkinson disease who have undergone deep brain stimulation surgery experience a brief period of improvement in balance followed by a return of balance difficulties. The procedure is more effective at relived symptoms of dyskinesia, tremors, and rigidity.

20.
A Paraspinal muscle fibrillations

Electromyography is not sensitive for radiculopathy; however, when it is abnormal, it is very specific. Paraspinal muscles are innervated by dorsal rami, which exit proximally to the dorsal root ganglion. Paraspinal muscle fibrillations can indicate irritation of these dorsal rami. (B) Sensory nerve action potentials (SNAPs) are normal in lesions proximal to the dorsal root ganglia; therefore, most disk herniations do not affect SNAPs. (C) Increased

motor fiber recruitment indicates a myopathic process. (D) Spontaneous nerve activity (including positive sharp waves and fibrillation potentials) can be seen after denervation.

21.
B Initiate a heparin drip if there are no contra-indications

Blunt cerebrovascular injuries of the internal carotid artery are common following motor vehicle collisions and are thought to be related to neck hyperextension with lateral rotation. The injuries most often occur 2 cm from the origin of the internal carotid artery. The blunt cerebrovascular injury (BCVI) classification is as follows: grade 1, luminal irregularity with ≤ 25% stenosis; grade 2, luminal irregularity with > 25% stenosis or an intraluminal thrombus/raised intimal flap; grade 3, pseudo-aneurysm; grade 4, complete occlusion; grade 5, transection with extravasation. The incidence of stroke increases with the grade. Although outcomes are not entirely known, the data suggest that anticoagulation may reduce the risk of injury progression with grade 1 injuries.

22.
C Midcervical spine fractures

Because of "snaking," which may occur between the halo fixation points and the vest, a halo brace is best suited for upper and lower cervical spinal fractures but is poor at maintaining distraction.

23.
B Anterior inferior cerebellar artery

The anterior inferior cerebellar artery can compress cranial nerve VII to produce hemifacial spasm. (A) The posterior inferior cerebellar artery is associated with glossopharyngeal neuralgia. (C) The superior cerebellar artery is associated with trigeminal neuralgia.

24.
C 1.4

In clinical studies, an INR of 1.4 is considered safe for performing a percutaneous needle liver biopsy. Extrapolated from this, an INR of 1.4 is considered safe for performing neurosurgical procedures. The prothrombin time should be 13.5 seconds or less.

25.
B Postfixed chiasm

A pituitary tumor with a postfixed chiasm (located posterior to its normal position over the dorsum sellae) has an increased likelihood of compressing the optic nerves and causing a "pie in the sky" deficit (superotemporal quadrantanopsia) through compression of the knee of Wilbrand. Postfixed chiasms also can result in chiasmatic compression and a bitemporal hemianopsia. (A) A prefixed chiasm (located anterior to its normal position over the tuberculum sellae) is associated with optic tract compression and a homonymous hemianopsia. (C, D) The optic chiasm normally lies superior to the sella turcica.

26.

D Pure tone audiogram of 40 dB or less; speech discrimination score of at least 60%

Hearing is considered serviceable if the pure tone audiogram is less than or equal to 50 dB and speech discrimination is 50% of more (the "50/50" rule). American Academy of Otolaryngology-Head and Neck Surgery classifications A (30/70) and B (50/50) are considered serviceable and preservable.

27.

A Rapid administration of corticosteroids

Pituitary apoplexy can be considered a surgical emergency if it is rapidly progressive. In addition, given the compromise of the pituitary gland, prompt treatment with corticosteroids is necessary. (B, C) The rapid onset of a headache may suggest an aneurysmal subarachnoid hemorrhage aneurysm, and a posterior communicating artery aneurysm may produce a cranial nerve III palsy. Subarachnoid hemorrhage is not associated with bitemporal hemianopsia, however. (D) Cavernous-carotid fistulae often are associated with a pulsatile proptosis. Infectious etiologies (e.g., Tolosa-Hunt and Gradenigo syndromes) often include a painful ophthalmoplegia. (E) Increased intracranial pressure and uncal herniation could produce a cranial nerve III palsy, but bitemporal hemianopsia in an awake patient likely would not occur.

28.

D D

The American Spinal Injury Association (ASIA) impairment scale indicates the completeness of a spinal cord injury and is different from the ASIA motor scale. ASIA A represents a complete injury without motor or sensory function below the injury level. ASIA E represents normal motor and sensory function. ASIA B is an incomplete injury with preservation of sensory but not motor function below the level of injury. ASIA C is an incomplete injury with preservation of motor function in

at least half of the key muscles below the level of injury graded at less than 3/5, whereas, in ASIA D, half of the key muscles below the level of injury have at least 3/5 strength. Of note, sensory preservation requires that the S4 and S5 segments also be intact. The ASIA impairment scale only applies to patients who have sustained spinal cord injuries and should not be used to describe a neurologic exam otherwise.

29.

B Anterior cord syndrome

Anterior cord syndrome (anterior spinal artery syndrome) presents with paraplegia and dissociated sensory loss, with loss of pain and temperature sensation but with preservation of posterior column function (positional and fine touch sensation). It can result from an infarct involving the anterior spinal artery. (A) Central cord syndrome presents with a greater motor deficit in the upper extremities relative to the lower extremities. It often results from a hyperextension injury in the presence of degenerative osteophytes. The overall prognosis is that half of affected patients eventually will be able to ambulate independently. (C) Brown-Séquard syndrome presents with dissociated sensory loss (loss of pain and temperature sensation with preserved light touch sensation), with ipsilateral paresis and posterior column dysfunction. Of the listed syndromes, Brown-Séquard syndrome has the best prognosis, with 90% of affected patients regaining ambulatory status. (D) Posterior cord syndrome is rare. Symptoms include pain and paresthesias with minimal long tract findings. (E) Cauda equina syndrome is compressions of the cauda equina (not the spinal cord), resulting in urinary retention, saddle anesthesia, motor weakness, and low back pain due to the involvement of multiple nerve roots.

30.

A Superior and medial

The pars interarticularis and pedicle of the C2 vertebral body, from posterior to anterior, are oriented superiorly and medially. The entry point for C2 pedicle screw placement is 3 to 4 mm superior to the inferior margin of the C2 inferior facet and at the midpoint mediolaterally with a trajectory of 20 to 30 degrees medially and 25 degrees superiorly. The vertebral artery courses laterally as it passes through the C2 transverse foramen so that the more superior the screw is placed, the farther away from the vertebral artery the screw is located.

31.

E Barrel chest

Relative contraindications for odontoid screw placement include a type 3 odontoid fracture, large fracture gaps, irreducible fractures, chronic fractures, pathological fractures, and fracture lines that are oblique to the frontal plane. Odontoid screws are useful for acute, type 2 fractures with intact ligaments but can be difficult to place in patients with short, thick necks or barrel chests. This relative contraindication sometimes can be circumvented with appropriate instrumentation. (B) The most significant absolute contraindication for odontoid screw placement is the disruption of the transverse atlantal ligament as seen on MRI or indirectly if the sum of the overhang of the lateral masses of C1 on C2 exceeds 7 mm. This latter assessment is known as the rule of Spence.

32.

D Teardrop fracture

Teardrop fractures are compression/flexion injuries that often are unstable. They usually present with chip fractures and retrolisthesis, sagittally oriented fractures, a kyphotic deformity, facet/disk space disruption, and soft tissue swelling. (A) Avulsion fractures present with chip fractures as a result of anterior longitudinal ligament traction on the fractured bone (a hyperextension injury). There often is no misalignment, body fracture, or posterior element or disk disruption. (B) A clay-shoveler fracture is an avulsion of the C7 spinous process. (C) Jefferson fractures are four-point burst fractures of the C1 ring. They are classified as unstable but often are treated with orthosis; they typically present without neurologic deficits. (E) Locked facets result from distraction/flexion injuries and often present with anterolisthesis.

33.

B Distracting pedicle screws to reduce indirectly the retropulsed segment by putting tension on the posterior longitudinal ligament

Ligamentotaxis is the theory for the practice that is used by some physicians to "pull" bony fragments that are in the central canal back to their normal positions (assuming the posterior longitudinal ligament is intact). Typically, this technique is used with a distraction technique such as with pedicle screws. (A, C–E) These techniques are utilized in deformity and spinal trauma surgery but are not considered ligamentotaxis.

34.

B Zone 2

Sacral zone 2 fractures occur vertically, ascend the sacral foramina, and may cause unilateral L5, S1, or S2 root injuries (including sciatica). (A) Sacral zone 1 fractures occur at the sacral ala and may be associated with an L5 root injury. (C) Sacral zone 3 fractures occur within the sacral canal and can cause sphincter dysfunction with bilateral nerve root injuries and saddle anesthesia. Fractures extending vertically in zone 3 are associated with pelvic ring fractures. (D) Transverse sacral fractures sometimes are classified as zone 4 injuries and occur from falls. They can produce severe neurologic deficits. (E) There is no zone 5.

35.

A Greater than 1 mm of blood

The Fisher grading system is effective in determining the risk of vasospasm associated with aneurysmal subarachnoid hemorrhage according to the amount of blood seen on CT. Grade 1 is without subarachnoid hemorrhage. Grade 2 indicates subarachnoid hemorrhage less than 1 mm in thickness. Grade 3 indicates a localized clot or layer of subarachnoid hemorrhage at least 1 mm in thickness. (C) Grade 4 indicates intraparenchymal or intraventricular hemorrhage.

36.

D Anterior communicating artery

Anterior communicating artery aneurysms often present with blood in the anterior interhemispheric fissure, a hematoma in the gyrus rectus, and intraventricular hemorrhage in the third ventricle, which is thought to reach the ventricles through the lamina terminalis.

37.

C Antibiotics and serial imaging

Mycotic aneurysms are common in bacterial endocarditis and occur in 3 to 15% of patients with this diagnosis. The aneurysms are found most commonly in the distal middle cerebral artery branches. At least 20% of patients have multiple aneurysms, and there is an association with immunocompromised and intravenous drug abuse patients. Treatment consists of antibiotic therapy, as these aneurysms are friable and not easily amenable to surgical or endovascular treatments. Serial angiograms are used to follow the resolution of mycotic aneurysms. Surgical clipping may be indicated in patients with subarachnoid hemorrhage, increasing aneurysm size despite antibiotic treatment, failure of antibiotics to resolve the aneurysm, and focal deficits.

38.

C Brachytherapy has no role as an adjuvant to whole brain radiation

Brachytherapy provides no significant overall survival or quality-of-life benefits when compared with whole brain radiation and should not be used alone or as an adjuvant therapy for high-grade gliomas. This is due to the diffuse nature of gliomas and the side effects of brachytherapy.

39.

A Intravenous chemotherapy

Following resection of a low-grade oligodendroglioma, chemotherapy is the mainstay of adjuvant therapy, with radiation reserved for higher grade lesions due to their aggressiveness and more diffuse characteristics. The typical chemotherapy protocol of procarbazine, CCNU, and vincristine is given intravenously and not intrathecally.

40.

C 25 to 40%

Complications rates are high when shunting patients with normal pressure hydrocephalus, likely in part due to the advanced average age of the patients with the condition. Complications include subdural hematomas, shunt infections, intracranial hemorrhages, seizures, and shunt malfunctions. As for the symptoms of normal pressure hydrocephalus, incontinence followed by gait abnormalities is the symptom most likely to improve with shunting. Dementia is the symptom least likely to improve.

41.

C Presence of a Martin-Gruber anastomosis

A Martin-Gruber median to ulnar nerve anastomosis occurs in 15 to 30% of individuals and consists of a communicating nerve branch between median and ulnar nerves. A clue to the presence of a Martin-Gruber anastomosis with carpal tunnel syndrome is a faster than expected conduction velocity in the median nerve in the forearm. In severe carpal tunnel syndrome, because nerve fibers are passing around the carpal ligament through the ulnar nerve, antecubital fossa stimulation may result in thenar stimulation faster than with stimulation at the wrist (there also will be a positive deflection). (D) Marinacci syndrome is a "reverse" Martin-Gruber anastomosis characterized by an ulnar to median nerve anastomosis that can cause carpal tunnel syndrome from an ulnar nerve compression at the elbow.

42.

A Radiographs are not indicated

There are five NEXUS criteria to indicate the need for cervical spine imaging: midline cervical tenderness, focal neurologic deficits, altered level of consciousness, intoxication, and painful distracting injuries. If these are all negative, radiographic studies are not indicated. In trauma patients who are symptomatic, obtunded, or have an unreliable neurologic exam, a thin-cut axial CT scan is indicated with reconstructions.

43.

D Admit to the floor, obtain blood cultures, and consult interventional radiology for biopsy of the psoas abscess prior to administering antibiotics (if the biopsy can be done in a timely manner)

Medical management of patients with epidural abscesses is preferred when there are long-standing symptoms without progressive neurologic deficits, when imaging is not worrisome for severe compression, in patients with prohibitive operative risk factors, and in patients with complete paralysis for longer than 3 days. Epidural biopsy is not recommended; however, disk space/vertebral body biopsy is a reasonable option.

44.

A Absence of atypical pain

Absence of atypical pain is a favorable prognosticator in surgical and radiosurgical candidates for trigeminal neuralgia treatment. Other favorable factors include using higher radiation doses, a lack of previous trigeminal neuralgia operations, and normal pretreatment sensory function.

45.

C Cranial nerve IX rhizotomy with sectioning the upper one third of cranial nerve X

When an offending vessel (classically the posterior inferior cerebellar artery) is seen compressing cranial nerve IX, microvascular decompression (MVD) is the preferred treatment choice. During an exploration that fails to reveal vascular compression of the nerve, the most effective treatment includes sectioning of cranial nerve IX and the upper rootlets of cranial nerve X. Studies suggested that there is a higher rate of pain recurrence when both nerves are not sectioned simultaneously. The risks of sectioning cranial nerve X may include significant bradycardia, dysphagia, and voice hoarseness.

46.

B Isthmic

There are five types of spondylolisthesis: type 1, dysplastic, is congenital and related to spina bifida; type 2, isthmic (spondylolytic), is a result of pars insufficiency fractures, an elongated pars from repetitive fractures/healing, or acute fractures; type 3, degenerative, usually occurs at L4/L5 without a break in the pars interarticularis; type 4, traumatic, is due to a posterior element fracture (other than the pars); type 5, pathological, is secondary to a tumor or bone disorder.

47.

D Elevate the head of bed, decrease the blood pressure, and irrigate the cannula

The main complication related to a blind, stereotactic-guided biopsy is hemorrhage. Most bleeding is capillary or venous, and can be managed by conventional methods of cannula irrigation, head elevation, and induced hypotension with a systolic blood pressure around 90 mm Hg. Nevertheless, craniotomy and clot evacuation may be necessary to obtain hemostasis in refractory bleeding.

48.

A Distal middle cerebral artery branches

Mycotic aneurysms occur in distal middle cerebral artery branches 75 to 80% of the time. They also occur in distal anterior cerebral artery branches less often. Twenty percent of patients with mycotic aneurysms have multiple aneurysms, and mycotic aneurysms may occur in up to 15% of patients with subacute bacterial endocarditis. The most common pathogen is *Streptococcus viridans.*

49.

C Immediate surgery or endovascular treatment

Vertebral dissections can lead to pain, transient ischemic attacks, strokes, and subarachnoid hemorrhage. Rebleeding is common and occurs in 30% of those with subarachnoid hemorrhage. In dissections without hemorrhage or large ischemic strokes, heparin followed by oral anticoagulation should be started immediately. Surgery (hunterian ligation following a balloon test occlusion study), clipping with or without bypass, graft placement or wrapping, and endovascular treatment (stents/occlusion/angioplasty) are the treatments of choice for patients presenting with subarachnoid hemorrhage, extradural lesions that progress, or symptoms that persist despite medical therapy.

50.

E Condyle fracture

Condyle fractures are not common but can present with delayed cranial nerve palsies, especially a hypoglossal palsy due to the fact that the hypoglossal canals are intimate with the occipital condyles. Brainstem findings also occasionally occur. Treatment is with a rigid collar unless the occipital to C1 interval is more than 2 mm, at which point surgical stabilization is required.

51.

E Cervical spine radiographs with oblique and apical lordotic views

Neurologic thoracic outlet syndrome is rare and usually affects women. One cause is a constricting band that originates from the first rib or an elongated C7 transverse process that causes compression of the C8 and T1 nerve roots, proximal trunk of the brachial plexus, or median cord. Sensory changes often spare the median nerve (which passes through the upper and middle trunks of the brachial plexus) but are seen in the lower trunk (C8 and T1 nerve roots). Electromyography in thoracic outlet syndrome is unreliable but may have positive findings if sensory nerve action potentials are analyzed in the medial antebrachial cutaneous nerve. (D) MRIs of the cervical spine are poor for detecting bony abnormalities in thoracic outlet syndrome but may rule out pathologies that mimic thoracic outlet syndrome such as cervical disk herniation.

52.

E Medulloblastoma

Medulloblastomas often arise from the cerebellar vermis close to the fastigium near the posterior medullary velum (the roof of the fourth ventricle). (A) Ependymomas often arise from the floor of the fourth ventricle. (B) Juvenile pilocytic astrocytomas (JPAs) can occur in the optic/hypothalamic areas, brainstem, cerebellum, and spinal cord. Cerebellar JPAs often are hemispheric. (C) Brainstem gliomas can be diffuse, cervicomedullary, and focal or dorsally exophytic. They do not arise from the roof of the fourth ventricle. (D) Choroid plexus papillomas commonly are found in the lateral ventricles and arise from the choroid plexus.

53.

D Observation

The Spetzler-Martin arteriovenous malformation (AVM) grading system is based on AVM size

(1 to 3 points allocated for an < 3 cm, 3 to 6 cm, and > 6 cm, respectively), eloquence of adjacent brain (eloquent, 1 point; non-eloquent, 0 points), and venous drainage (deep, 1 point; superficial, 0 points). The natural history of the disease process (3 to 4% risk of hemorrhage yearly) must be considered with the risk of treatment. Grade 4 and 5 AVMs often are treated with serial scans and observation. The described AVM is grade 5.

54.
B Recurrent artery of Heubner

The Recurrent artery of Heubner typically originates from the proximal A2 segment of the anterior cerebral artery. It supplies the head of the caudate nucleus, anterior limb of the internal capsule, anterior putamen, and globus pallidus. Unilateral injury results in contralateral face and arm weakness. Bilateral injury results in akinetic mutism. (A) The anterior choroidal artery supplies the posterior limb of the internal capsule and the lateral geniculate body of the thalamus. Occlusion results in contralateral hemiplegia, hemianesthesia, and homonymous visual field deficits. (C) Injury to the middle cerebral artery results in an infarct causing contralateral hemiparesis and neglect. (D) Distal anterior cerebral artery compromise results in infarcts in the paramedian cortex.

55.
D Tumor suppressor gene inactivation on chromosome 3p25

The most common posterior fossa tumor in adults is metastases (most often from lung cancer); however, the most common primary, intraaxial posterior fossa tumor is hemangioblastoma. Von Hippel–Lindau syndrome is associated with 30% of cerebellar hemangioblastomas and is an autosomal dominant, inherited disease found on chromosome 3p25. (A) Smoking is most associated with metastatic lesions. (B) Tumor suppressor gene inactivation on chromosome 9q34 is associated with tuberous sclerosis. (C) Tumor suppressor gene inactivation on chromosome 7q21 is associated with a familial form of cavernomas.

56.
A Periodic electromyography/nerve conduction studies starting 3 to 12 weeks following the injury with consideration of surgical neurotization at 3 to 6 months if there is no improvement

Surgical treatment of peripheral nerve injuries can be defined by the "rule of 3's." Sharp lacerations are explored within 3 days, penetrating injuries are explored in 2 to 3 weeks, and gunshot wounds and traction injuries are explored in 3 to 6 months. An avulsion (traction injury) occurs when a root is pulled from the spinal cord with no chance of reinnervation. Because this injury happens proximal to the dorsal root ganglia, synaptic action potentials are characteristically normal. Neurolysis (lysis of scar tissue) is not successful for lesions that are not in continuity. A dorsal root entry zone (DREZ) lesioning procedure is the procedure of choice for chronic pain for plexus avulsion injuries. Only neurotization (nerve transfers) can restore downstream nerve/muscle/sensory function.

57.
D Clival fracture

Clival fractures can be longitudinal, transverse, or oblique and are highly fatal due to associated injuries and to an elevated risk of meningitis. (A) Longitudinal temporal bone fractures are common and usually run parallel to the external auditory canal. They often spare the facial and vestibulocochlear nerves but may involve ossicular chain. (B) Transverse temporal bone fractures often pass through the cochlea and may stretch the geniculate ganglion, causing facial and vestibulocochlear nerve palsies. (C) Fractures of the anterior fossa (planum sphenoidale) can injure the optic nerves if the fractures extend into the optic canals. Severe fractures may produce shearing injuries of the pituitary gland.

58.
E Between the two heads of the flexor carpi ulnaris

The ulnar nerve enters the forearm by passing between and then deep to the two heads of the flexor carpi ulnaris. (A) For transpositions of the ulnar nerve, the pronator teres is sectioned. (C) The ulnar nerve lies on the surface of flexor digitorum profundus. (D) The ulnar nerve lies medial to the ulnar artery in the forearm.

59.
B Internal, common, and then external carotid artery

The goal of vessel occlusion is to force any embolus/thrombus, if present, into the external carotid artery. The mnemonic for the clamping order is "ICE": internal, common, external carotid artery. The order for releasing the vessels is the reverse.

60.

E 4

Fisher grading correlates the amount of blood on CT scan with the risk of vasospasm and is graded from 1 to 4: grade 1, no subarachnoid hemorrhage; grade 2, diffuse/vertical layer of subarachnoid hemorrhage less than 1 mm in thickness; grade 3, hemorrhage of 1 mm or more; grade 4, intracranial or intraventricular hemorrhage regardless of subarachnoid hemorrhage thickness. Thick, cisternal subarachnoid hemorrhage has the highest risk for vasospasm (grade 3 or 4).

61.

A Suboccipital craniotomy including opening of the foramen magnum and drilling of the occipital condyle

The far lateral approach and its associated craniotomies (transcondylar, transjugular, etc.) often involve removing the subocciput extending down into the foramen magnum as well as trying to achieve a more lateral exposure by drilling the occipital condyle.

62.

D Periventricular location; 2.0 cm in diameter

Surgical management of a cerebral abscess should be considered for large lesions with mass effect, in order to establish a diagnosis, and in the following situations: increased intracranial pressure, poor neurologic condition, association with foreign material, abscesses that are fungal in origin, multiloculated abscesses, and abscesses in close proximity to the ventricular system. The latter finding is due to the poor outcome following intraventricular abscess rupture. Often, an abscess 3 cm or larger is deemed more appropriate for surgical management, whereas smaller abscesses may be responsive to medical therapy alone.

63.

C 15 to 20%

Although many factors play a role in prognosticating re-rupture risk, overall, the risk of aneurysm re-rupture is 4% on the first day and then 1 to 1.5% per day for the next 13 days. This equates to an approximately 15 to 20% risk of re-rupture over the first 14 days. There is a 50% risk of re-rupture over the first 6 months, and a 3% risk per year after that.

64.

E Corpus callosotomy

A corpus callosotomy may be most effective as a treatment for generalized major motor seizures and is used for atonic seizures where the loss of postural tone can result in falls/injuries (70% reduction in seizures expected with the procedure), unilateral hemispheric damage resulting in generalized seizures, Lennox-Gastaut syndrome, and, in some patients, generalized seizures without a resectable focus. (A) Ethosuximide is used for absence seizures. (B) Adrenocorticotropic hormone can be used for West syndrome in which electroencephalography reveals hypsarrhythmias. (C) Subpial transections are used for partial seizure originating in cortical areas. (D) Hemispherectomy is used for unilateral seizures with widespread hemispheric lesions and profound contralateral deficits (e.g., Rasmussen syndrome).

65.

B Ventralis intermedius nucleus

The ventrolateral nucleus is composed of the ventralis intermedius and ventralis oralis nuclei. This also is an effective target when attempting to control essential tremor. (A) The medial nucleus is a target for obsessive compulsive disorder as are the bilateral internal capsules. (C) The nucleus accumbens is an investigational target for treatment of depression, obesity, and anorexia. (D) The anterior nucleus is a potential target for epilepsy. (E) The pedunculopontine nucleus has been used as a target for movement disorders that are primarily posture and gait related.

66.

C Originates at the mid-vertebral body of C7 and is measured from the posterior superior corner of S1

The C7 plumb line is created by dropping a vertical line from the mid-C7 vertebral body. The distance between the C7 plumb line and the posterior superior corner of the S1 vertebral body is measured, and helps to determine the sagittal balance of the patient. The ideal measurement is < 5 cm on either side of the plumb line, as this facilitates a level gaze and prevents falling. Of note, the C7 plumb line approximates the clivus.

67.

C Grade 3

Grade 3 spondylolisthesis is 50 to < 75% anterolisthesis. (A) Grade 1 spondylolisthesis is < 25%

anterolisthesis. (B) Grade 2 spondylolisthesis is 25 to < 50% anterolisthesis. (D) Grade 4 spondylolisthesis is 75% or more anterolisthesis. (E) There is no grade 5 spondylolisthesis. Anterolisthesis of 100% or more is termed spondyloptosis.

68.
C Obtain a lumbar puncture.

A head CT can detect subarachnoid hemorrhage in more than 95% of cases; however, a lumbar puncture is the most sensitive test for subarachnoid hemorrhage. Although traumatic taps can result in false positives, non-clotting bloody fluid that does not clear with sequential tubes (usually RBC more than 100,000) and xanthochromia (the yellow coloration of cerebrospinal fluid supernatant after centrifuging) suggest subarachnoid hemorrhage. Spectrophotometry is more sensitive than visual inspection of cerebrospinal fluid for xanthochromia, but xanthochromia typically does not become apparent until 2 to 4 hours following subarachnoid hemorrhage and is seen in almost 100% of patients 12 hours after subarachnoid hemorrhage. (A) Given the clinical symptomatology, it is important to rule out completely the suspected aneurysm. (E) MRI is not sensitive for the first 24 to 48 hours after subarachnoid hemorrhage but is good for revealing subacute blood. If there is a high degree of clinical suspicion for an aneurysm, a cerebral angiogram may be a reasonable imaging modality.

69.
B Pelvic tilt

Pelvic tilt is the angle measurement between a line drawn from the midpoint of the S1 end plate to the midpoint of the femoral head and a vertical line from the femoral axis. It represents a "compensatory mechanism"; thus, patients with kyphotic deformities may use retropulsion to keep their head aligned with the horizon. Increasing retroversion to accommodate for increasing kyphosis will increase the pelvic tilt. (A) Sacral slope is the measurement of the sacral slant, and is the angle between a line parallel to the sacral end plate and the horizon. (C) Pelvic incidence = Pelvic tilt + Sacral slope. Sacral slope approximates the pelvic incidence. Pelvic incidence is the angle measurement between the line from the mid-femoral head to the midpoint of the sacral end plate and a line perpendicular to the sacral end plate. This parameter does not change.

70.
B Autologous sural nerve

The ideal donor nerve provides a suitable environment for regeneration and results in acceptable donor morbidity. It should be of sufficient length, easy to locate, surgically accessible, and have well developed fascicles. Although sural nerve harvesting does result in a sensory deficit in the lateral leg, it generally is well tolerated. In addition, its length allows for bridging of large gaps. (A) Although motor nerves make better grafts than sensory nerves, there typically would be significant morbidity with a harvest of the anterior interosseous nerve. The anterior interosseous nerve typically is not used, given its motor function, although the terminal branch of the posterior interosseous nerve has been used for distal digital nerve grafts. (D) Allograft (acellularized) nerve material can bridge sensory but not motor nerve gaps up to 4 cm. (E) Vein grafts utilize the concept of hollow tubes, but superiority over conventional nerve grafting has not been established.

71.
B Toward a point on a line intersecting 3 cm anterior to the external auditory meatus and medial aspect of the pupil

During a percutaneous trigeminal radiofrequency rhizotomy, the electrode is placed in a plane intersecting a point 3 cm anterior to the external auditory meatus and medial aspect of the pupil when the eye is directed forward. The tip is advanced toward the intersection of the petrous bone and clivus (5 to 10 mm inferior to the sella) keeping the needle < 8 mm from the clival line to avoid cranial nerve II or VI complications.

72.
D More chance of vertebral artery injury and less C2 neuralgia with transarticular screw fixation compared with the C1 lateral mass–C2 pedicle/pars screw approach

Some advantages of a C1 lateral mass–C2 pedicle/pars screw fixation approach include the fact that anatomic alignment during screw placement is not necessary, in that manipulation can be performed after screw placement and before rod insertion. In addition, the method is associated with a reduced risk of vertebral artery injury compared with the transarticular approach. This is due to the ability to place screws despite aberrant vertebral artery anomalies partially due to the more superior and medial trajectories of C2 pedicle screws. Unfortunately, there tends to be more C2 neuralgia with the C1 lateral mass–C2 pedicle/pars screw approach.

73.

D Injury to the spinal accessory nerve

Injury to the spinal accessory nerve during dissection of the posterior triangle of the neck is a well-known complication of lymph node biopsy. (B) A carotid injury and stroke would manifest with additional symptoms, and the carotid artery is not found in the posterior triangle of the neck. (C) Injury to the C5 nerve root and deltoid weakness can cause an inability to abduct the shoulder, but the C5 root is not found in the posterior triangle of the neck. (E) Damage to the long thoracic nerve causes a serratus anterior weakness and winged scapula and can occur with blunt trauma, over-stretching, and lifting excessive weight over the shoulder. It does not occur with dissection of the posterior triangle of the neck.

74.

E At the junction of the basilar and superior cerebellar arteries

Cranial nerve III palsies often are associated with posterior communicating artery aneurysms, but oculomotor nerve palsy is one of the most frequent complications following surgical treatment of distal basilar artery aneurysms. The incidence of cranial nerve III palsies following surgery ranges from 25 to 80%, although many spontaneously resolve. There is a higher incidence of such a palsy with superior cerebellar artery aneurysms. (B) Lower cranial nerve palsies as well as lateral medullary syndrome (depending on surgical approach) can be seen following surgery for posterior inferior cerebellar artery aneurysms. (C) Complications of middle cerebral artery aneurysm surgery can include contralateral weakness. (D) A concern during anterior cerebral artery aneurysm surgery is the accidental sacrifice of perforators to the optic apparatus, which would cause visual loss but not an oculomotor palsy.

75.

D Speech irregularities

Speech irregularities including mutism can occur with sectioning of the corpus callosum. Other complications include "alien hand" and supplemental motor area syndromes. Most disconnection deficits are not present as long as the splenium is spared. If there is injury to the anterior cerebral arteries, strokes and lower extremity weakness can occur. Retraction during a corpus callosotomy also can lead to postoperative sensory and motor

deficits. (C) Memory problems can occur during transcallosal approaches and are attributable to injuries to the fornix.

76.

C Surgical decompression with or without fixation

Indications for surgical intervention in patients with central cord syndrome include persistent stenosis/cord compression with significant fixed motor deficits or progressive dysfunction, spinal instability, or potentially intractable pain. (A) The high-dose steroid protocol utilized in the NASCIS trial consisted of a 30 mg/kg bolus of methylprednisolone followed by 5.4 mg/kg/h for 24 or 48 hours. This treatment is controversial. (D) Although an unstable cervical spine may lead to the development of central cord syndrome and require surgical fixation, decompression is the mainstay of treatment options with central cord syndrome.

77.

B Second or third degree

With a second- or third-degree injury, there is axonal discontinuity. A third-degree injury also has disruption of the endoneurium. Fibrillations are seen with both degrees of injury, and motor unit potentials (MUPs) are present but abnormal. Surgery may be indicated for successful repair, and this is an axonotmesis. Axonal regeneration occurs at a rate of about 1 mm per day. (A) A first-degree injury results in segmental demyelination. Fibrillations are not seen, and MUPs are normal. Surgery is not indicated, as this is only a neurapraxia. (C) A fourth-degree injury results in a loss of axon continuity and endoneurial tubes, along with the endoneurium and perineurium. The epineurium remains intact. Fibrillations and MUPs are not seen. Surgery is indicated for successful repair, and this is an axonotmesis. (D) A fifth-degree injury equates to nerve transection with all structures including the epineurium losing continuity. Fibrillations and MUPs are not seen. Surgery is indicated for successful repair, as this is a neurotmesis.

78.

C T8

A punctate midline myelotomy (5-mm depth) at the T8 level generally is successful in the management of intractable pain associated with malignancy in the abdominal or pelvic regions. This level is remote from the spinal segments innervated by afferents of the lower abdomen.

79.
A Oriented superiorly/superolaterally

80.
C Anterior one third

Only the anterior one third of the superior sagittal sinus can be sacrificed without risk of venous infarctions. The risk increases greatly if any amount of the sinus is sacrificed distal to the anterior one third along with extensive sacrifice of the cortical bridging veins.

81.
A Obtundation, coma, variable degrees of hemiplegia or hemisensory loss, a vertical gaze palsy, and memory impairment

The artery of Percheron arises from the proximal segment of the posterior cerebral artery and supplies blood to the paramedian thalamus and rostral midbrain bilaterally. The triad of bilateral paramedian thalamic infarcts consists of altered mental status, a vertical gaze palsy, and memory impairment. (B) Hemiparesis, hemisensory loss, and a homonymous hemianopsia are seen with an anterior choroidal artery infarct. (C) Hemiparesis of the upper extremity and face, dysarthria, and hemichorea are seen with a recurrent artery of Heubner (medial striate artery) stroke. (D) A cranial nerve III palsy, Parinaud syndrome, abulia, and somnolence are seen in mesencephalothalamic syndrome or "top of the basilar artery" syndrome. (E) Ipsilateral sensory loss in the face and contralateral sensory loss in the body without pyramidal findings or a change in sensorium are seen with lateral medullary syndrome. Patients also experience vertigo, nausea, vomiting, nystagmus, diplopia, ataxia, Horner syndrome, and dysphagia.

82.
E Midline myelotomy

Visceral cancer pain in the pelvic and rectal area is relayed through a midline pathway in the dorsal columns. Punctate midline myelotomies have been shown to alleviate visceral cancer pain.

83.
B C1-C2 cordotomy

The spinothalamic tract is divided at the level of C1-C2.

A cordotomy at this level is reserved for intractable severe upper extremity pain due to cancer. Side effects include dysesthesia, urinary retention, sleep apnea, and weakness.

84.
D Selective dorsal rhizotomy

A selective dorsal rhizotomy is performed on the lower spinal cord and is best for diplegic spasticity. It is used primarily in treating children with cerebral palsy with lower extremity spasticity who have borderline ambulation abilities. (A) Dorsal root entry zone lesioning is most beneficial in nerve avulsion pain such as that of the brachial plexus or in transitional zone pain following spinal cord injury. The procedure should be reserved for patients who have shown no evidence of functional recovery of the affected nerve. (C) Spinal cord stimulation is useful in treating neuropathic leg pain following failed back surgery, mainly in cases where imaging does not show a compressive lesion impinging on any neural structures. The most appropriate level for implantation is at T10-T11.

85.
E Fornix, superior layer of the tela choroidea, vascular layer, inferior layer of the tela choroidea, choroid plexus of the third ventricle

The correct layers of the roof of the third ventricle, from superficial to deep, are the body of the fornix, superior layer of the tela choroidea, vascular layer, inferior layer of the tela choroidea, and choroid plexus of the third ventricle.

86.
B Temporary decreased spontaneous and voluntary movements of the left upper and lower extremities with spontaneous recovery

Supplementary motor area (SMA) syndrome characteristically causes a contralateral apraxia and loss of spontaneous/voluntary movements, with preservation of muscle tone and strength. It can result in mutism occurring more often when the dominant SMA is involved. Reflexes often are preserved. Classically, there is spontaneous recovery over weeks to months, leaving only a long-term deficit in alternating bimanual movements.

87.

A Retractor placement

Injury to the cervical sympathetic trunk (CST) can lead to Horner syndrome. The CST is located in the fascia over the longus colli muscle 10 to 15 mm lateral from the medial edge of the muscle. It is most medial at C6; therefore, it is more prone to injury during lower cervical surgery. During retractor placement, if the tip of the retractor blade slips out from between the medial edge of the longus colli muscle and the vertebral body, injury can occur to the CST. (B) During the exposure for an anterior cervical diskectomy and fusion, the carotid sheath is encountered; however, careful attention and ensuring that the dissection is medial to the carotid sheath prevents injuries. (C) Injury to the recurrent laryngeal nerve results in hoarseness, and not Horner syndrome. (D) A vertebral artery injury would result in Wallenberg syndrome or lateral medullary stroke symptoms, and not Horner syndrome.

88.

E Linear temporal fracture

(A–E) All of these findings can be seen on skull radiographs and can indicate trauma and the need for possible surgical intervention. Nevertheless, a temporal skull fracture can cause injury to the middle meningeal artery with the subsequent development of an epidural hematoma. A skull fracture is present in about 80 to 95% of all epidural hematomas, and about 24% of all skull fractures are associated with an epidural hematoma. (A) A fluid level in the sphenoid sinus may indicate a basal skull fracture. (B) A pneumocele may be indicative of a fracture with a dural tear. (C) The presence of a double density sign (if confirmed on AP and lateral imaging) may indicate a depressed skull fracture. (D) A fluid level in the frontal sinus may indicate a frontal sinus fracture.

89.

E In patients with good health and asymptomatic carotid stenosis > 60%, a CEA is beneficial if the surgeon maintains perioperative morbidity/mortality rates less than 3%.

(A) This conclusion is derived from the Asymptomatic Carotid Surgery Trial (ACST). This trial did not substantiate what was found previously in terms of benefiting women with asymptomatic carotid stenosis by performing a carotid endarterectomy (CEA). (B) This conclusion is derived from the North American Symptomatic Carotid Endarterectomy Trial (NASCET). (C) This conclusion is derived

from the Carotid Revascularization Endarterectomy versus Stenting Trial (CREST) that demonstrated that stenting may be an option for carotid stenosis but is not superior to a CEA. This finding makes stenting attractive for patients with advanced age, poor surgical anatomy, previous radiation, or significant comorbidities. (D) This finding is from the Stenting and Angioplasty with Protection in Patients at High Risk for Endarterectomy (Sapphire) trial, which is a noninferiority trial for patients with carotid stenosis and who have a high surgical risk.

90.

C Decreased tearing

The greater superficial petrosal nerve (GSPN) emerges from the facial nerve distal to the geniculate ganglion and carries preganglionic parasympathetic fibers. It innervates the nasal and palatine mucosa and the lacrimal gland of the eye; thus, sectioning of the GSPN may cause decreased tearing when it is sectioned. (A) The otic and submandibular ganglia innervate the parotid/submandibular glands for salivation. (B, D) The facial nerve does not control pupillary diameter. (E) Hyperacusis can develop after damage to the tympanic branch of the facial nerve, which innervates the stapedius muscle.

91.

A Atlanto-occipital dislocation and a type 2A hangman fracture

Traction may worsen a deficit with an atlanto-occipital dislocation. It also may cause increased angulation and widening of the disk space in a type 2A hangman fracture (an angulated and distracted fracture). Traction often is used in an attempt to reduce locked facets in neurologically intact patients able to participate in neurologic testing.

92.

A 18 years old

93.

B Compression of the left midbrain

A mass lesion and uncal herniation often cause an ipsilateral cranial nerve III palsy with a contralateral hemiparesis due to compression of the ipsilateral midbrain. The brainstem can continue to be compressed against the contralateral incisura, affecting the ipsilateral cranial nerve III and the contralateral midbrain causing an ipsilateral hemiparesis. This is known as the Kernohan phenomenon, which is a false localizing sign.

94.

E Steam autoclaving for 1 hour at 132°C

Creutzfeldt-Jakob disease is resistant to all routine sterilization/disinfection procedures commonly used. The two reported effective methods for providing sterilization are steam autoclaving for 1 hour at 132°C and immersion in 1 N NaOH for 1 hour. The other listed options are ineffective at fully sterilizing for equipment contaminated with Creutzfeldt-Jakob disease prions.

95.

B Junction of the transverse and sigmoid sinus

96.

A Anterior

The hypothalamus is anterior to the subthalamic nucleus (STN), and current spread to the hypothalamus causes flushing and sweating. (B) The medial lemniscus is posterior to the STN, and stimulation results in the adverse effect of paresthesia. (C) The corticobulbar tract is lateral to the STN, and stimulation results in the adverse effect of dysarthria. (D) The red nucleus is medial to the STN, and stimulation results in the adverse effect of ataxia. (E) The corticospinal tract is anterolateral to the STN, and stimulation results in the adverse effect of tonic contraction.

97.

C Grade 3 or 4 spondylolisthesis

In high-grade spondylolisthesis, the nerve roots are stretched. Increasing disk space height without first decompressing the nerve roots with some realignment would place the patient at a high risk for nerve root injury.

98.

A Blindness

The patient's case is suggestive of temporal (giant cell) arteritis. It is found in women over 50 years of age and is associated with polymyalgia rheumatic. Involvement of the ophthalmic artery can lead to blindness if the condition is untreated. Diagnosis is by biopsy of the temporal artery and elevated erythrocyte sedimentation rate. Steroid treatment should begin immediately when the diagnosis is suspected. (B) Aneurysm rupture is associated with an acute, "thunderclap" headache, although prodromal headaches can occur. (C) Contiguous spread of a periodontal abscess is rare, and usually is associated with dental procedures or poor dentition. (D) Cerebral herniation from trauma or a large brain tumor would manifest with signs of increased intracranial pressure (nausea, vomiting, hemiparesis, and decreased mental status). (E) Corneal abrasions can be the result of herpes zoster involving the ophthalmic division of the trigeminal nerve.

99.

B 16

The American Spinal Injury Association (ASIA) motor score is based on key muscles representing root levels. There are 50 points available for testing in the upper extremities (25 right and 25 left) and 50 points in the lower extremities (25 right and 25 left). Key muscles include the biceps, wrist extensors, flexor digitorum profundus, hand intrinsics, iliopsoas, quadriceps, tibialis anterior, extensor hallucis longus, and gastrocnemius.

100.

A Epidermoid cyst

Epidermoid tumors are thin walled, with a characteristic smooth, pearly white appearance on gross examination. (B) Dermoid cysts are thick walled, with greasy pilosebaceous contents. (C) Lipomas have a yellow, fatty gross appearance. (D) Adamantinomatous craniopharyngiomas are partly cystic with white speckled keratin nodules.

101.

B L4 exiting nerve root

Most L4/L5 disk herniations affect the traversing nerve root (L5 in this example). Far lateral herniations affect the exiting nerve root (L4 in this example).

102.

D Gymnasts, football linemen, and weight lifters

Isthmic spondylolisthesis is thought to have a higher incidence in sports and activities that involve repetitive hyperextension. (A) HLA-B27 positivity is seen in ankylosing spondylitis. (C) Rheumatoid arthritis causes atlantoaxial subluxation, subaxial subluxation, and basilar invagination. (E) Being black, having diabetes, and being a woman over 40 years of age are risk factors for degenerative spondylolisthesis. The occurrence in women is thought to be due to ligamentous laxity related to hormonal changes.

103.

B Epidermoid cyst

Epidermoid cysts appear as well-defined, often relatively round masses with thin, pearly white walls. The cysts contain a dense, keratinous substance. (A) Arachnoid cysts are thin walled (often translucent), and contain clear fluid similar to the makeup of cerebrospinal fluid. (C) Dermoid cysts (mature teratomas) are thick walled, and contain a variety of mature tissues, including hair, sebaceous glands, and skin. (E) Neurenteric cysts are thick walled, and often have variable contents but typically contain a thick, creamy, mucin-like substance.

104.

C 50

The Karnofsky Performance Scale classifies patients based on their functional impairments. The lower the score, the worse the survival is for most serious illnesses. Scores of 0 to 40 indicate that patients are unable to care for themselves. Score of 50 to 70 indicate that patients are unable to work but otherwise are able to live at home with varying amounts of assistance needed. Scores of 80 to 100 indicate that patients are able to carry on normal activities and work with no special care needed.

105.

C HLA-B27

(A) HLA-DQA1 is associated with diabetes type 1 and celiac disease. (B) HLA-DRB1 is associated with rheumatoid arthritis and multiple sclerosis. (D) HLA-DR2 is associated with lupus. (E) HLA-B47 is associated with 21-hydroxylase deficiency.

106.

E Inferomedial

The nuclei of cranial nerves III and IV are inferomedial to the STN. Current spread to this area causes diplopia and miosis. (A) The hypothalamus is anterior to the subthalamic nucleus (STN), and stimulation results in the adverse effect of flushing and sweating. (B) The medial lemniscus is posterior to the STN, and stimulation results in the adverse effect of paresthesia. (C) The corticobulbar tract is lateral to the STN, and stimulation results in the adverse effect of dysarthria. (D) The red nucleus is medial to the STN, and stimulation results in the adverse effect of ataxia.

107.

B Superior thyroid artery arising from the ECA

The superior thyroid artery is the first branch arising from the external carotid artery. The remaining branches (in ascending order) are the ascending pharyngeal, lingual, facial, occipital, posterior auricular, and superficial temporal and internal maxillary arteries. (E) The internal carotid artery has no extracranial branches.

108.

D At the arterial branch from the superior extent (cranial loop) of the telovelotonsillar segment of the posterior inferior cerebellar artery

The choroid point is located at the point where the choroidal artery emerges from the telovelotonsillar segment of the posterior inferior cerebellar artery. (A) The venous angle occurs at the convergence of the septal and thalamostriate vein at the foramen of Monro. These two veins join to form the internal cerebral vein. (B) The copular point is where the inferior vermian artery forms the inferior inflection point of the posterior inferior cerebellar artery on cerebral angiogram. (E) The plexal point is where the anterior choroidal artery enters the lateral ventricle and can be seen on cerebral angiogram.

109.

A Opticocarotid cistern

The image accompanying the question illustrates a left-sided approach that may be seen with a pterional craniotomy. The carotid artery is seen lateral to the optic nerve. The internal carotid artery bifurcation is seen as the anterior cerebral artery A1 segment crosses the optic nerve in the five o'clock position of the image. The middle cerebral artery M1 segment is found at the seven o'clock position. The arrow points to the opticocarotid recess. (B) The carotico-oculomotor membrane is bound superiorly by the superior dural ring and inferiorly by the inferior dural ring and is intimately related to cranial nerve III.

110.

D *Haemophilus influenzae* meningitis

Subdural effusions are rare complications of bacterial meningitis (most commonly caused by *Haemophilus influenzae*). Chronic subdural hematomas are referred to as hygromas.

111.

B 2

The Borden classification system grades dAVFs 1 to 3. In addition, each type is subclassified further into type A (single-hole fistula) or B (multiple-hole fistula). Cortical venous reflux (types 2 and 3) is the most important prognostic factor for dAVFs regarding their hemorrhage and nonhemorrhage neurologic deficit rates. A type 2 dAVF has drainage into normal veins/sinuses, with high pressure causing retrograde flow into normal subarachnoid veins (equivalent to a 2B and 2A+B dAVF in the Cognard classification). (A) A Borden type 1 dAVF has normal anterograde flow through the fistula (equivalent to a Cognard type 1 and 2A dAVF). (C) A Borden type 3 dAVF has direct drainage into subarachnoid veins or an isolated segment of a sinus (from thrombosis on either side of the fistula) and is equivalent to a Cognard type 3, 4, or 5 dAVF. (D, E) The Borden classification system only grades dAVFs as 1 to 3.

112.

C Diaphragm

The attachment of the diaphragm at the T12 to L1 levels increases the difficulty of transthoracic access to the thoracic spine around the T10 level and inferiorly.

113.

B Administer bethanechol.

Postoperative urinary retention (POUR) due to anesthesia is a common phenomenon. Bethanechol is a parasympathomimetic agent that facilitates detrusor contraction and relaxes the bladder sphincter. (A) The patient's surgery was for a proximal (ventricular catheter) shunt revision only. The distal shunt catheter was not touched, and the abdomen was not entered; therefore, it is unlikely the bladder was injured. (C) Diazepam is an anxiolytic agent that binds to benzodiazepine receptors. It acts as a muscle relaxant. Studies show that diazepam is not effective in treating POUR. (D) Oxybutynin antagonizes acetylcholine at muscarinic receptors and relaxes bladder smooth muscles. Due to its anticholinergic affect, it inhibits involuntary detrusor muscle contractions and is used to treat overactive bladder and not urinary retention. (E) Morphine is an opioid narcotic and only will make the urinary retention worse.

114.

A Transvenous coil embolization

Transvenous coil embolization to occlude the proximal draining veins just distal to the point of the fistula is the most effective endovascular technique in treating a dAVF. (B) Transarterial embolization with Onyx glue is an option in treating a dAVF, but using a liquid embolic agent can risk occluding perforating vessels. (C) Direct surgical clip ligation should be done on the draining veins and not the arteries in a dAVF. (D) Stereotactic radiosurgery is an option for treating a dAVF, but it can require multiple treatments.

115.

B Middle turbinate

The middle turbinate provides the most obstruction in the working space during the endonasal transsphenoidal approach. The middle turbinate on one side can be removed, whereas the one in the opposite nostril can be lateralized for more working space. (D) The posterior portion of the nasal septum, not the anterior portion, often is removed to create an optimal working space.

116.

D Tension pneumocephalus

In theory, because of pressure changes and the decreased atmospheric pressure maintained within the pressurized cabins of commercial aircraft (about 0.75 atm), the brain following craniotomy may be at an increased risk for tension pneumocephalus. Patients also may be at an increased risk for developing deep venous thromboses due to the prolonged immobility associated with air travel.

117.

B Cubital tunnel

The cubital tunnel is the most common site of ulnar nerve compression. The second most common site is the Guyon canal at the wrist. Decompression of the arcade of Struthers (not the Struthers ligament) occurs when freeing the ulnar nerve during a cubital tunnel release.

118.

D Diffusion-weighted imaging

Both CT and MR with contrast sequences are helpful to view abscesses with high sensitivity, but it can be difficult to differentiate between an abscess and a tumor. Classically, abscesses show diffusion restriction (dark on apparent diffusion coefficient [ADC] sequences), suggesting viscous fluid, whereas tumors most often will be dark on diffusion-weighted imaging (DWI) sequences. Positive diffusion restriction is seen more often with pyogenic abscesses, and becomes less reliable with fungal or tuberculosis abscesses.

119.

D Near-infrared light source with an optical filter to block ambient and excitation light

(A) This describes the modern microscope. (B) Arc lamps often are used for black-and-white photomicrography. (C) This describes true confocal scanning microscopy. (E) This describes high-speed specimen image capturing.

120.

B Dysarthria and cognitive impairment

Dysarthria and cognitive impairment are complications of bilateral thalamotomy. (A) Hemiparesis and homonymous hemianopsia are complications of pallidotomy due to injury to the internal capsule and optic tract. (C) Horner syndrome, characterized by myosis and anhydrosis, is a complication of sympathectomy. (D) Quadriparesis and respiratory depression (Ondine curse) are associated with bilateral cordotomy complications. (E) Hemiparesis and bladder dysfunction are complications of midline myelotomy in the treatment of pelvic pain due to cancer.

121.

B Prophylactic antibiotics must be received within 1 hour prior to the surgical incision

(A) There are specific algorithms for prophylactic antibiotic selection for surgical patients depending on the surgical site and infection risks; therefore, not every surgical patient should receive cefazolin as the prophylactic antibiotic. (C, D) Prophylactic antibiotics are discontinued within 24 hours after the surgery end time.

122.

C Dorsal root entry zone lesioning

Dorsal root entry zone lesioning is most beneficial for symptom relief with nerve avulsion pain such as that of the brachial plexus or in transitional zone pain following a spinal cord injury. The procedure should be reserved for patients who have shown no evidence of functional recovery of the nerve. (A) Cordotomies are used for cancer-related pain of the upper extremity, chest, or peritoneum. (B) Midline myelotomies are used for relieving midline visceral cancer pain in the pelvic and rectal regions. (D) Anterior cingulotomies are used for chronic, noncancer pain. (E) Rhizotomies destroy nerve roots and are used for spastic cerebral palsy. Selective dorsal rhizotomies are performed in the lower spinal cord and are best for diplegic spasticity. The procedures are used primarily in treating children with cerebral palsy with lower extremity spasticity who have borderline ambulatory abilities.

123.

C Oriented inferolaterally

124.

B Melanoma is mostly radiation insensitive, but radiation may be somewhat effective.

125.

D Upper gastrointestinal imaging

Esophageal perforation can present in an immediate or delayed fashion after anterior cervical diskectomy and fusion surgery. Occasionally, if the plating is high profile or if the screws are proud, they can irritate and erode through the esophagus over time, especially when the patient is swallowing. Imaging should include an esophagoscopy, barium swallow study, or esophagogastroduodenoscopy. (A) Dental abscesses are unlikely to be the source of the infection at the surgical site. (B) An echocardiogram can assess the presence of endocarditis from vegetations on the cardiac valves. Although this is a possible explanation for the patient's infection, a cardiac source is unlikely unless esophageal perforation has been completely ruled out. (C) Blood cultures help determine if the patient has a systemic infection/sepsis but are not helpful in determining the direct source. (E) A nuclear bone scan only confirms the MRI finding of osteomyelitis and is not helpful in elucidating the infectious source.

126.

B Bone morphogenic protein

Optimal success of a bone growth provides structural support, fills voids, and improves healing through osteoconductive (matrix for bone growth), osteoinductive (growth factors to encourage cells to differentiate into osteoblastic cells), and osteogenic (directly transplanted osteoblasts/periosteal cells) properties. Autograft is the gold standard to induce bone growth. Bone morphogenic protein is primarily an osteogenic material. Cortical bone grafts are less biologically active than cancellous bone grafts, but they provide more structural support and may provide an osteoconductive scaffold. Demineralized bone matrix is prepared from cadaveric bone, and although it has some low osteoinductive potential, demineralized bone matrix is considered mainly an osteoconductive agent. (D, E) Tricalcium phosphate and hydroxyapatite are components of bone and bone growth and are considered osteoconductive

127.

D 2.5 cm

In general, giant aneurysms are thought to have a lower annual rate of rupture compared to non-giant aneurysms.

128.
D Oriented superiorly and arising from the superior wall

Ophthalmic artery aneurysms tend to point toward the optic nerve.

129.
E Directed contralaterally and arising from the branch point of the dominant A1 segment and the ACOM

130.
B Cerebellopontine angle

Epidermoid cysts occur in the cerebellopontine angle in 40 to 50% of cases and are the third most common cerebellopontine angle tumor. They also are found in the fourth ventricle and sellar region. Less common locations are the cerebral hemispheres, brainstem, and extradural spine/skull.

131.
A Common peroneal nerve

Iatrogenic common peroneal nerve injuries can result from improperly placing the patient in the supine position. These injuries result in foot drop and weakness with foot eversion. To avoid this, pillows are placed under the knee with the leg midline and not externally rotated. (B) Deep peroneal nerve injuries result in vague pain and dysesthesia over the dorsum of the foot. (C) Superficial peroneal nerve injuries result in pain and numbness over the lateral malleolus and occasionally in the lateral leg. (D) The obturator nerve is prone to injury during obstetric and gynecologic procedures. (E) Injury to the lateral femoral cutaneous nerve results in "meralgia paresthetica."

132.
C Olfactory groove meningioma

The patient has Foster-Kennedy syndrome with ipsilateral anosmia, ipsilateral optic nerve atrophy, and contralateral papilledema. This classically is seen with olfactory groove meningiomas. Neurologic localization would place this lesion at the inferior surface of the left inferior frontal lobe.

133.
D Five

The roof of the third ventricle contains five layers; from rostral to caudal, they are the body of the fornix, the superior layer of the tela chorioidea, the velum interpositum (vascular layer), the inferior layer of the tela chorioidea, and the choroid plexus.

134.
C Small saphenous vein

The small saphenous vein originates in the dorsolateral foot and courses around the lateral foot and then between the heads of the gastrocnemii to drain into the popliteal vein in the popliteal fossa.

135.
B Morbidity may be associated with positioning.

The major disadvantage of the infratentorial supracerebellar approach concerns positioning difficulties and morbidity. This approach often involves a patient in the sitting position (or a variation thereof) and utilizes gravity to allow the cerebellum to fall away from the surgical corridor. The sitting position is notorious for being associated with an elevated risk for developing an air embolism and with surgeon discomfort and fatigue. (A) The deep venous system typically is superior to pineal region tumors. (C) Visual deficits occur with occipital transtentorial procedures. (D) Seizures are more common with transcortical approaches. (E) Disconnection syndromes are more prevalent with interhemispheric approaches that are more posteriorly based.

136.
D Prophylactic anticonvulsants are indicated to decrease the incidence of early posttraumatic seizures.

In the setting of a traumatic brain injury, anticonvulsants typically are used for no more than 1 week as early post-traumatic seizure prophylaxis.

137.
E Incorporation of the anterior choroidal artery into the aneurysm clip

When clipping a posterior communicating artery aneurysm, it is important to identify the anterior choroidal artery as it is in close proximity to the posterior communicating artery and can be incorporated into an aneurysm clip. The anterior choroidal artery supplies the blood to the posterior limb of the internal capsule and can lead to the classic "triple H" syndrome consisting of hemiparesis, hemisensory loss, and a homonymous hemianopsia. If the posterior cerebral artery is fetal, incorporation into an aneurysm clip may cause an occipital stroke and consequential visual loss.

138.

D 4 to 5 cm; 6 to 7 cm

Some neurosurgical centers spare the superior temporal gyrus during resections, if possible. A resection of more than 5 cm in the dominant temporal lobe risks injuries to the speech centers. A resection of more than 7 cm in the nondominant temporal lobe risks a partial quadrantanopsia, whereas an 8- to 9-cm resection leads to a complete quadrantanopsia.

139.

D Baclofen withdrawal

Baclofen is used to treat spasticity. Withdrawal can lead to hyperthermia, hyperreflexia, spasticity, seizures, and delirium. Immediate treatment includes baclofen administration. (A, C) Unless the patient has constitutional signs of infection, these symptoms are more similar to neuroleptic malignant syndrome-like findings associated with baclofen withdrawal. (B) Baclofen toxicity causes hyporeflexia, bradycardia, hypothermia, and even respiratory arrest.

140.

A Nontraumatic anterior wedging of at least 5 degrees in at least three adjacent thoracic vertebral bodies

Scheuermann disease is due to an uneven growth of the vertebrae in the sagittal plane resulting in a kyphotic spine. (C) Klippel-Feil syndrome is described as the congenital fusion of two or more cervical vertebrae. (D) Grisel syndrome is described as the nontraumatic subluxation of the atlanto-axial joint caused by inflammation or infection. (E) Forestier disease is defined as the compression of the esophagus and dysphagia resulting from a cervical osteophyte.

14 Pediatric Neurosurgery

1.

E Mammillary bodies, as shown in this image.

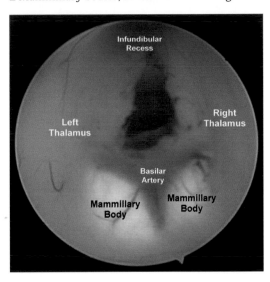

2.

D Precentral cerebellar vein

The vein of the cerebellomesencephalic fissure (also called the precentral cerebellar vein) is formed by the union of the paired veins of the superior cerebellar peduncles, and ascends through the quadrigeminal cistern to drain into the vein of Galen, either directly or through the superior vermian vein.

3.

C Grade 3

A grade 3 hemorrhage also extends into the ventricles, and there is ventricular dilation. (A) A grade 1 hemorrhage does not extend beyond the subependyma. (B) A grade 2 hemorrhage extends into the ventricles, but they are not dilated. (D) A grade 4 hemorrhage includes intraventricular hemorrhage with intraparenchymal extension.

4.

D Dermoid tumor

Congenital dermal sinus tracts are a type of closed spinal dysraphism in which an epithelium-lined sinus tract from the dorsal skin surface extends inward for a variable distance. Thoracic and cervical regions, where the neural folds fuse first, are the rarest sites for dorsal dermal sinus tracts, whereas lumbosacral and occipital dermal sinus tracts are relatively frequent. Spinal canal dermoid tumors can be seen in association with dorsal dermal sinus tracts. Surgical excision can lead to cure of these lesions and can de-tether the spinal cord.

5.

B Occipital encephalocele

A Chiari type 3 malformation includes a suboccipital encephalocele with herniation of all brainstem structures into the foramen magnum as well as through a defect in the posterior fossa wall (posterior fossa encephalocele). A Chiari type 4 malformation typically refers to an extreme hypoplasia or frank aplasia of the cerebellum. (A) Cervical cord syringes can occur with any type of Chiari malformation. (C) Chiari type 2 malformations occur in more than 95% of patients with myelomeningoceles, which are exclusive to this population of Chiari malformation patients. (D) Cerebellar vermian agenesis occurs in Dandy-Walker malformation. (E) Platybasia is "flat clivus" and is seen in Paget disease.

6.

A Chemotherapy alone

Children with medulloblastoma who are at least 3 years of age should receive radiation to the tumor site and the complete craniospinal axis, as well as chemotherapy. Children younger than 3 years of age typically are managed with chemotherapy until they reach the age of 3, at which time radiation is considered. This delay is due to the severe detrimental effects of radiation on the immature, developing nervous system.

7.

A Syringomyelia secondary to a tethered spinal cord

Tethered spinal cord syndrome is a neurologic disorder caused by tissue attachments that limit the movement of the spinal cord within the spinal column during growth. These attachments cause an abnormal stretching of the spinal cord. This syndrome is associated closely with spina bifida. It is estimated that 30% of children with spina bifida defects repaired shortly after birth will require surgery at some point to untether the spinal cord later during childhood.

8.

A Dermoid cyst

Dermoid and epidermoid cysts are the most common lesions of the scalp and calvarium encountered in the pediatric population. They account for 15 to 60% of masses in this region. Dermoid cysts and dermal tracts are more likely to involve the scalp and skull in young children, whereas epidermoid cysts tend to occur intracranially in older children and young adults. In addition, dermoid cysts typically are in the midline, whereas epidermoid cysts tend to occur off the midline.

9.

C Pfeiffer syndrome

Fusion of both coronal sutures leads to a head shape called brachycephaly. This causes restriction of the growth of the anterior fossa, resulting in a shorter and wider than normal skull. Compensatory vertical growth also occurs, which is called turricephaly. Bicoronal synostosis often is seen in patients with associated syndromes, such as Crouzon, Apert, Saethre-Chotzen, Muenke, and Pfeiffer syndromes. (A) Pierre Robin syndrome is a sequence of developmental events that result from a small mandible and tongue abnormalities and involve airway obstruction. (B) Treacher Collins syndrome is an autosomal dominant condition resulting in craniofacial abnormalities. (D) Goldenhar syndrome involves the incomplete development of the nose, lips, soft palate, jaw, and ears. (E) Moebius syndrome is characterized by congenital facial weakness.

10.

A L1-L2

Embryologically, ascent of the conus medullaris results in the tip of the conus lying most commonly opposite the L1-L2 disk space. A conus medullaris below the mid-body of L2 is considered to be tethered radiographically.

11.

E Lower extremity hyperesthesia

The major (although uncommon) complications of selective dorsal rhizotomy include paraplegia, sensory loss, cerebrospinal leak, bladder and bowel incontinence, and infection. Many patients may experience hyperesthesia in the legs for several months.

12.

C Injury to the basilar artery bifurcation

Overall, the complication rate after an endoscopic third ventriculostomy is about 2 to 15%, with most of the complications resulting only in temporary morbidities. Complications include fever, bleeding, hemiparesis, gaze palsies, memory disorders, altered consciousness, diabetes insipidus, weight gain, and precocious puberty. Intraoperative neural injuries such as thalamic, forniceal, hypothalamic, and midbrain injuries also are observed. Intraoperative fatal hemorrhage due to basilar artery injury and rupture has been reported. Forniceal and other neural injuries can be avoided with proper bur hole planning and placement.

13.

C Posterior fossa

Central nervous system atypical teratoid/rhabdoid tumors (ATRTs) are rare, clinically aggressive tumors that most often affect children aged 3 years or younger but can also occur in older children and adults. About one half of ATRTs arise in the posterior fossa.

14.

E Corpus callosotomy

Corpus callosotomy (typically involving the resection of the anterior two thirds of the corpus callosum) should be considered as a treatment option in pediatric patients with disabling drop attacks and generalized seizures. Although vagal nerve stimulation (VNS) has comparable results in controlling drop attacks, corpus callosotomy is a viable option in patients who do not respond well to VNS.

15.

A Arteriovenous malformation (AVM)

Arteriovenous malformations are the most common symptomatic intracranial vascular abnormality in children. They consist of direct artery-to-venous connections without intervening capillaries, and they occur in the cerebral hemispheres, brainstem, and spinal cord. Hemorrhagic events from AVMs in childhood have been associated with a 25% mortality rate.

16.

C Foramen magnum stenosis

Foramen magnum stenosis is a common finding in children with achondroplasia, resulting in severe compromise of cerebrospinal fluid flow at the cervicomedullary junction and brainstem compression in severe cases. Surgical decompression is recommended for patients with brainstem dysfunction.

17.

C Obstructive hydrocephalus secondary to aqueductal stenosis

Idiopathic aqueductal stenosis is the most common cause of noninfectious obstructive hydrocephalus during infancy. Endoscopic third ventriculostomy commonly is recommended as surgical treatment, although success rates decrease when the procedure is performed in children younger than 1 year of age.

18.

A Lead

Lead intoxication often results in progressive weakness of the bilateral wrist and finger extensors (wrist drop). Other symptoms include seizures, psychiatric changes, abdominal pain, and anemia (with basophilic stippling of red blood cells). Patients with lead poisoning exhibit increased urinary excretion of lead and porphobilinogen. Treatment with chelators, including EDTA, penicillamine, and BAL, results in a gradual improvement of the neuropathy.

19.

A Wnt subgroup

Prognosis differs markedly across medulloblastoma tumor subgroups. The Wnt subtype has a high 5-year overall survival rate that can exceed 90%, with the current standard therapy consisting of maximal safe surgical resection of the tumor, risk-adapted radiation therapy, and adjuvant chemotherapy. (C) By contrast, group 3 tumors have a substantially worse prognosis, with a 5-year overall survival rate ranging from 40 to 60%. (B, D) The other two subgroups of medulloblastoma (the SHH subtype and group 4 tumors) have an intermediate overall survival rate at 5 years after treatment of around 75%, which varies depending on the presence or absence of metastatic disease and molecular abnormalities, and on the histological category.

20.

E Pineoblastoma

Trilateral retinoblastoma is a malignant midline primitive neuroectodermal tumor (PNET) occurring in patients with inherited uni- or bilateral retinoblastoma. In most cases, trilateral retinoblastoma presents as pineoblastoma.

21.

B 19 through 26 weeks

Results of the MOMs trial (published in 2011) suggest a 50% reduction in shunted hydrocephalus at 12 months of age and improved Chiari 2 malformations when fetuses underwent in-utero repair of myelomeningoceles between 19 and 26 weeks of gestational age.

22.

B Os odontoideum

Os odontoideum is an uncommon craniovertebral junction abnormality characterized by a separate ossicle superior to the dens. On CT, a smooth, well-corticated ossicle is seen at the superior ossicle of a hypoplastic dens. The condition is hypothesized to be a result of previous trauma in some cases.

23.

E *Streptococci*

Gram-negative bacilli and group B *Streptococci* are the most common pathogens implicated in neonatal meningitis.

24.

A Pleural effusion

Ventriculopleural shunts are considered safe alternatives to ventriculoperitoneal or ventriculoatrial shunts. Asymptomatic, mild pleural effusions frequently are encountered with shunting to the pleural space; however, symptomatic pleural effusions are abnormal. In most cases, the effusion resolves spontaneously, seldom requiring specific treatment. The risk of pleural effusion seems to be highest in infants, but can occur at any age.

25.

C A Chiari malformation

A syrinx associated with a Chiari 1 malformation (tonsillar herniation below level of foramen magnum) is treated with posterior fossa decompression.

26.

D Hemangioblastoma

Hemangioblastomas are grade I tumors; they are more common in males than in females, and are associated with Von Hippel–Lindau (VHL) syndrome. Microscopically, these tumors exhibit a dense network of vascular channels and a large population of lipid-containing interstitial cells with nuclear pleomorphism. They are vimentin positive and EMA negative. Patients with VHL are at risk for the development of renal cell carcinoma, which interestingly is EMA positive.

27.

E 90%

Approximately 90% of patients with agenesis of the corpus callosum have evidence of developmental delays, and 60% have concomitant seizures.

28.

D Moyamoya disease

Moyamoya disease is a progressive cerebrovascular disorder caused by occluded cerebral arteries, resulting in recurrent transient ischemic attacks or strokes. The name *moyamoya* means "puff of smoke" in Japanese and describes the angiographic appearance of this disease: tangled, tiny vessels formed to compensate for the occlusions.

29.

C Right lambdoid suture

Acquired post-shunt craniosynostosis is a relatively uncommon complication, with over-drainage in young or premature infants with open fontanelles being the main risk factor. A CT scan with 3D reconstruction is helpful to diagnose it. Surgical treatment is required in severe cases with abnormal head shapes.

30.

A Choriocarcinoma

Cerebrospinal fluid levels of α-fetoprotein and β-HCG are most useful for diagnosing yolk sac tumors and choriocarcinomas, respectively. Levels also may be used to assess treatment response and recurrence. (C, D) Pure germinomas and teratomas usually present with negative markers (α-fetoprotein and β-HCG), although low levels of β-HCG sometimes can be detected.

31.

A 100%

Chiari II malformations are encountered relatively commonly, with an incidence of about 1:1,000 live births. When a child is born with a myelomeningocele, the vast majority (95 to 100%) have an associated Chiari II malformation.

32.

D 35 and 55 cm

Males have slightly larger head circumferences than females.

33.

D Perform an angiogram

There should be a high suspicion for a vein of Galen malformation in this scenario. In fact, a vein of Galen malformation should be considered in any newborn with heart failure that is not linked to congenital heart anomaly. An angiogram and confirmation of this pathology is the next step in correctly diagnosing and subsequently devising a treatment plan for this etiology. Treatment typically involves a staged endovascular embolization while treating heart failure with medical agents. (C) Biopsy or surgical resection of this lesion potentially would be fatal.

34.

A Spastic diplegia

Selective dorsal rhizotomy is suited best for the treatment of children with primarily lower extremity spasticity (spastic diplegia). (B–E) These conditions are managed best with intrathecal baclofen pump therapy.

35.

D Neurofibromatosis type 2

Meningiomas are common primary brain tumors accounting for up to 25% of all primary brain tumors, with a peak incidence in the fifth decade of life. However, meningiomas are rare in the pediatric population, representing less than 5% of all supratentorial brain tumors in children. Risk factors for developing pediatric meningiomas include prior irradiation or a history of neurofibromatosis type 2. In some series, 50% of pediatric intracranial meningiomas have been associated with these risk factors.

36.

D Metopic suture

In single-suture craniosynostosis, premature closure of the metopic suture results in a triangular shaped head (trigonocephaly). (A) Premature closure of the coronal suture results in flattening of the forehead (anterior plagiocephaly or brachycephaly). (B) Premature closure of the sagittal suture results in an elongated and narrow head (scaphocephaly). (C) Premature closure of the lambdoid suture results in flattening at the back of the skull (posterior plagiocephaly).

37.

B Infantile spasms

Infantile spasms (also known as West syndrome) are a form of generalized epilepsy, and they usually begin before the age of 6 months. They commonly are associated with tuberous sclerosis in 20% of cases. The electroencephalogram (EEG) is characteristic, and consists of high-amplitude, irregular, asynchronous, sharp and slow waves with a slowed background rhythm. This gives the EEG a chaotic appearance known as hypsarrhythmia.

38.

C Sacral agenesis

Caudal regression syndrome is a generic term that refers to a continuum of neural tube defects ranging from coccygeal agenesis to complete agenesis of the entire lumbosacral spine. Sacral agenesis is sporadic, and commonly is associated with maternal hyperglycemia.

39.

E Folic acid

The U.S. Public Health Service (USPHS) recommends that all women capable of becoming pregnant consume 400 µg of folic acid daily to prevent neural tube defects (NTDs). Studies have demonstrated that peri-conceptional folic acid supplementation can prevent 50% or more of NTDs, such as spina bifida and anencephaly. For women who previously have had an NTD-affected pregnancy, the Centers for Disease Control and Prevention (CDC) recommends increasing the intake of folic acid to 4,000 µg per day beginning at least 1 month before conception and continuing through the first trimester.

40.

D Six months

Early surgery, preferably in the first 3 months of life, yields the best outcomes with the endoscope-assisted craniectomy technique for sagittal craniosynostosis. Postcorrection helmet therapy for 12 months is used commonly prescribed.

41.

E IX and X

Symptoms of moderate to severe Chiari 2 malformation commonly include dysfunction of cranial nerves IX and X, which may lead to dysphagia and respiratory distress.

42.

D Older than 12 years

Although vagal nerve stimulation (VNS) may be used "off label" in patients 12 years old and younger, it is important to counsel patients on the risks and unknowns of doing so. VNS is considered as a palliative treatment for intractable epilepsy.

43.

A 50 mcg

Intrathecal baclofen at 50 µg generally is used during the baclofen screening trial. This dose will cause at least a 1-point decrease in the mean Ash-worth score in the lower extremities of children with spasticity but not with dystonia or athetosis.

44.

C Eosinophilic granuloma

Eosinophilic granuloma is the most common type of Langerhans cell histiocytosis. It is characterized by the proliferation of pathogenic Langerhans cells and cytokine overproduction, and causes inflammation, infiltration, and destruction of many tissues in the body, most commonly bones.

45.

A Fourth ventricle outlet obstruction

As cerebrospinal fluid (CSF) is produced by the choroid plexus in the fourth ventricle and CSF flows in a rostral-to-caudal fashion, an endoscopic third ventriculostomy (ETV) would relieve hydrocephalus in the lateral and third ventricles but not in the fourth ventricle. (B-E) These all represent relative contraindications and risk factors for ETV failures.

46.

C Astrocytoma

Intrinsic tumors of the spinal cord comprise up to 55% of all intradural neoplasms in children. The most common are astrocytomas. In adults, intramedullary ependymomas are the most common intramedullary spinal cord tumor.

47.

B 3 to 9 months

Premature closure of the metopic suture results in trigonocephaly. (A) The posterior fontanelle typically closes at 1 to 2 months of age. (C) The anterior fontanelle typically closes at 9 and 18 months of age. (D) The coronal suture fuses at around 24 months of age.

48.

D Idiopathic aqueductal stenosis

Pediatric patients over 1 year of age with idiopathic aqueductal stenosis are considered the ideal candidates to receive endoscopic third ventriculostomies. Five-year success rates are 80 to 90%.

49.

C Germinoma

Pineal germ cell tumors are more common than pineal parenchymal tumors. Germinomas are the most common pineal region tumors in children, accounting for up to 60% of intracranial germ cell tumors.

50.

A Low-lying conus and fatty filum terminale

Tethered cord syndrome should be ruled out as the cause of newly diagnosed neurogenic hyper-reflexic bladder during childhood, even in the presence of the conus medullaris in a normal position.

51.

C Intradural and extramedullary

Neurenteric cysts more commonly occur intraspinal (90% of cases) than intracranial (10% of cases), and they usually present in the first or second decades of life. The majority of spinal neurenteric cysts are intradural and extramedullary, and they typically occur at the cervicothoracic junction or near the conus medullaris.

52.

B Two hemicords in two separate dural sacs

Split cord malformation (SCM) is a new term used for diastematomyelia and diplomyelia. SCMs are a form of occult spinal dysraphism, which is defined as a skin-covered lesion that has no exposed neural tissues and no visible cystic masses. SCMs are of two types: type 1 consists of two hemicords, each contained within its own dural tube and separated by a median bony spur, whereas type 2 consists of two hemicords housed in a single dural tube separated by a fibrous median septum.

53.

A Flexion-extension X-rays of the cervical spine if there are no other cervical spine injuries or fractures

Pseudosubluxation of C2 on C3 is common in children up to 10 years old due to ligamentous laxity. This finding often is seen on X-rays showing slight flexion, which often will reduce in a neutral or extended position. If a line is drawn between the spinolaminar junctions of C1 to C3 (the Swischuk line), the anterior C2 spinous process should be within 2 mm of this line. Anything beyond 2 mm is suggestive of pathological subluxation. Lack of soft tissue swelling also would be consistent with pseudosubluxation.

54.

A Visual accommodation paralysis

A symmetric neuropathy develops in 20% of patients who become infected with diphtheria (*Corynebacterium diphtheriae*). Patients initially develop visual accommodation (ciliary) paralysis followed by facial and oropharyngeal paralysis. Typically, there is preservation of extraocular movements. Distal sensorimotor polyneuropathy then follows in the fifth to eighth week of illness and results in mild to severe ascending paralysis.

55.

C Ganglioglioma

Gangliogliomas are WHO grade 1 circumscribed tumors that often have a solid, mural, contrast-enhancing nodule with a small cystic component. These lesions often are located in the temporal lobe, and they usually present with epilepsy in children of 5 to 6 years of age.

56.

C Cerebrospinal fluid leak and infection

The single most common complication of lipomyelomeningocele resection and de-tethering of the spinal cord is cerebrospinal fluid leak and subsequent infection. This complication occurs in less than 15% of patients in most series. A watertight dural closure and careful postoperative patient positioning are critical steps to reduce this complication.

57.

A *Staphylococcus epidermidis*

Pediatric patients with ventricular shunt catheters are at risk of developing ventriculitis, which most commonly is caused by infections with Staphylococcus epidermidis. In ventriculitis, the ventricles become covered by a prominent exudate, and the inflammatory infiltrates extend into the adjacent periventricular white matter.

15 Neurology

1.

D Agenesis of the corpus callosum

Agenesis of the corpus callosum is seen along with mental retardation, epilepsy, and patches of retinal pigmentation in Aicardi syndrome. The syndrome is inherited in an X-linked dominant fashion and is lethal in most males. (A) Absence of the septum pellucidum has many etiologies and is seen in Morsier syndrome (septo-optic dysplasia). (B) A Dandy-Walker malformation is a partial or complete absence of the cerebellar vermis. (C) Fusion of any two of the cervical vertebrae is associated with Klippel-Feil syndrome. (E) A Chiari type 3 malformation is characterized by an occipital encephalocele containing neuroectodermal tissues from the posterior fossa and is associated with hydrocephalus.

2.

A Posterior columns

A positive Romberg test is not a test of cerebellar function. Patients with cerebellar ataxia are not able to balance even with their eyes open. The cerebellum is responsible for unconscious proprioception and receives input from the dorsal nucleus of Clarke, with information traveling through the ipsilateral dorsal spinocerebellar tract. Vestibular disorders can have a positive Romberg sign; however, the sign most commonly is seen in patients with loss of conscious proprioception or dorsal column–medial longitudinal fasciculus system dysfunction.

3.

C Herpes simplex encephalitis; begin intravenous acyclovir

Herpes simplex virus (HSV) encephalitis presents acutely and most commonly with fever and an altered level of consciousness often accompanied by seizures. There is a predilection for the temporal and orbitofrontal lobes with edema in these areas visualized on MRI (bilateral lesions raise the suspicion for HSV encephalitis). Treatment should be initiated quickly if a patient has fever, encephalopathy, supporting cerebrospinal fluid studies, and another supporting study. (A, B) Varicella zoster encephalitis more commonly affects immunocompromised individuals and typically follows cutaneous herpes zoster.

4.

C Mental retardation

Both Apert and Crouzon syndromes are associated with craniosynostosis and a high incidence of hydrocephalus, and are inherited in an autosomal dominant manner. Individuals with Crouzon syndrome usually are of normal intelligence once the hydrocephalus is treated. On the other hand, individuals with Apert syndrome have with mental retardation, complex syndactyly, short thumbs, and cleft palates.

5.

A Mid-fusiform gyrus and inferior occipital gyrus

Damage to or inappropriate development of the mid-fusiform and inferior occipital gyri independently and with either unilateral or bilateral defects are associated with prosopagnosia (difficulty with face recognition). (B) Kluver-Bucy syndrome occurs in bilateral amygdala lesions. It is associated with hyperoral and hypersexual behaviors, visual agnosia, and hypomotility. (C) Mesial temporal lobe lesions result in long-term memory deficits. (D) Damage to the dominant angular gyrus results in dysgraphia (writing apraxia). (E) The superior parietal lobule and supramarginal gyrus are part of the association cortex. Damage to these areas can cause contralateral astereognosis, resulting in failure to recognize objects when felt with the contralateral hand but not when visualized.

6.

C Progressive supranuclear palsy

The progressive supranuclear palsy (Steele-Richardson-Olszewski syndrome) triad is progressive supranuclear ophthalmoplegia (paresis of voluntary eye movements with down-gaze palsy and frequent falls as a result), pseudobulbar palsy (masked facies with dysarthria, dysphagia, and a hyperactive jaw jerk), and axial dystonia. Patient with this condition do not walk bent forward and do not have a tremor despite progressive supranuclear palsy being characterized as pseudo-parkinsonism. Progressive supranuclear palsy can be differentiated from Parkinson disease by a poor response to levodopa in the former. (A) Triad of parkinsonism is resting tremor, cogwheel rigidity, and bradykinesia. (B) Olivopontocerebellar degeneration is related to multiple system atrophy and often presents with cerebellar ataxia, dysarthria, and dysphagia without paresis. (D) Multiple system atrophy (Shy-Drager syndrome) is a Parkinson plus syndrome. It is a progressive disorder of the central and autonomic nervous systems with idiopathic orthostatic hypotension.

7.

C Herpes simplex encephalitis

Bilateral periodic lateralizing epileptiform discharges (PLEDs) are seen with acute focal insults and in 85% of cases of herpes simplex encephalitis. (A) Subacute sclerosing panencephalitis has a pathognomonic pattern of periodic high-amplitude complexes with accompanying myoclonic jerks that does not change with painful stimulation. (B) PLEDs are defined as spikes occurring at regular intervals. The electroencephalogram in sporadic Creutzfeldt-Jakob disease often shows bilateral sharp waves that may resemble PLEDs but are reactive to painful stimulation. (D) Hepatic encephalopathy may show nonspecific triphasic waves on electroencephalography.

8.

B Measuring the middle cerebral to internal carotid artery velocity ratio

A Lindegaard ratio (V_{MCA}/V_{ICA}) greater than 3 is seen in vasospasm. In a hyperemic state, velocities in both the middle cerebral and internal carotid arteries are elevated equally, so the ratio is near 1. (A) Multiple factors can influence cerebral artery flow velocity, including systemic blood pressure, cerebral blood flow, and cerebral perfusion. Transcranial Doppler measures the cervical carotid and intracranial artery velocities. Elevated flow velocity more than 100 cm/s can be seen in both hyper-

emic and vasospastic states. (C) Vasospasm can affect the circulation bilaterally, so symmetry is not a key differentiating factor. (D) Vessel diameter is not a determining factor in either state. (E) Antegrade versus retrograde flow is not used to differentiate between hyperemia and vasospasm.

9.

A Hemifacial spasm

Hemifacial spasm and palatal myoclonus are involuntary movement disorders that persist during sleep. (B) Blepharospasm is sustained, abnormal blinking. It involves the orbicularis oculi muscle only (in contrast to hemifacial spasm, which involves various muscles on one side of the face). Blepharospasm typically ceases during sleep. (C) Athetosis is slow, writhing movements of the distal muscles (fingers, hands, toes, feet, and even face). (D) Facial myokymia is continuous facial spasms secondary to multiple sclerosis or a brainstem glioma. One of the treatments is rest.

10.

D Loss of consciousness, posttraumatic amnesia, and symptom duration

The Cantu concussion grading system is a three-grade system based on posttraumatic amnesia (PTA), loss of consciousness (LOC), and symptom duration. The scoring system is as follows: grade 1: no LOC, PTA less than 30 minutes, and postconcussion symptoms lasting no more than 15 to 30 minutes; grade 2: LOC less than 1 minute and PTA and symptoms lasting 30 minutes to 24 hours; grade 3: LOC of 1 minute or longer, PTA lasting more than 24 hours, and symptoms lasting as long as 1 week. (A) The American Academy of Neurology system uses a progressive three-grade system for concussion grading based on transient confusion, symptom duration, and loss of consciousness. (B) The Ruff Concussion system is a progressive three-grade system based on loss of consciousness, posttraumatic amnesia, and neurologic deficits. (C) The Glasgow Coma Scale ranges from a minimum score of 3 to a maximum score of 15. The score is the sum of the individual scores for eye opening, verbal response, and motor response. The scoring system is as follows: eye opening score: spontaneous (4), to speech (3), to pain (2), no response (1); verbal response score: alert and oriented (5), confused (4), inappropriate words (3), incomprehensible sounds (2), no response (1); motor response score: follows commands (6), localizes to pain (5), withdraws to pain (4), flexor (decorticate) posturing (3), extensor (decerebrate) posturing (2), no response (1).

11.

C Posterior interosseous neuropathy

The posterior interosseous nerve is a continuation of the deep branch of the radial nerve. Entrapment occurs in the forearm at the arcade of Frohse, causing extensor weakness of the thumb and fingers without involvement of the wrist extensors or triceps. This is a motor syndrome, and there is no sensory loss as seen in a radiculopathy. (A) A radial nerve palsy can occur at the axilla, causing triceps and distal weakness or at the mid-upper arm (spiral groove or intramuscular septum), sparing the triceps but causing weakness of wrist and finger extensors. (B) Tennis elbow (also known as lateral epicondylitis) is an inflammatory process of the tendons on the lateral aspect of the elbow. This results in pain of the extensor muscles of the forearm, wrist, and fingers. The tendon of the extensor carpi radialis brevis is usually involved. (D) A C8 radiculopathy results in flexion weakness of the index and middle fingers and paresthesias in the fifth digit. (E) Radial tunnel syndrome (also known as supinator syndrome) causes inflammation and pain in the origin of the extensor muscles at the lateral epicondyle on resisted extension of the middle finger. The condition may mimic lateral epicondylitis, and though the compression site is similar to the compression site in posterior interosseous nerve compression, there is usually no muscle weakness with radial tunnel syndrome.

12.

D Incomplete Horner syndrome with neck pain and delayed contralateral weakness and sensory loss

Spontaneous internal carotid artery dissections usually present with ipsilateral headache. Although difficult to detect clinically, these dissections often present with an incomplete Horner syndrome (oculosympathetic palsy) with ptosis and miosis without anhydrosis. The lack of anhydrosis is because the sympathetic nerves to the facial sweat glands travel on the external carotid artery. Ischemic events can be a complication of carotid artery dissection. (A) Wallenberg (also known as lateral medullary) syndrome is characterized by dissociated sensory loss from vertebral or posterior inferior cerebellar artery occlusion. This results in a complete Horner syndrome, dysphagia, ataxia, vertigo, nystagmus, hoarseness, and loss of pain and temperature sensation in the ipsilateral face and contralateral body. (B) Pancoast tumors cause Horner syndrome with shoulder and arm pain. (E) Weber syndrome results from a stroke of the ventral midbrain and is characterized by ipsilateral mydriasis and contralateral hemiparesis.

13.

D Gradenigo syndrome

The classic triad of symptoms in Gradenigo syndrome is an abducens palsy, retro-orbital pain, and a draining ear from acute otitis media with mastoiditis and involvement of the petrous apex. The abducens palsy occurs when the infection involves the Dorello canal and ophthalmic branch of the trigeminal nerve, given the anatomic proximity of these structures to the petrous apex. (A) Cranial nerve VI palsies can be a false localizing sign, so intracranial hypertension (sinus thrombosis) must be in the differential. This is not the patient's most likely diagnosis, however. (B) Tolosa-Hunt syndrome is inflammation of the superior orbital fissure/cavernous sinus that usually includes painful ophthalmoplegia, multiple cranial nerve palsies with sparing of the pupil, and dramatic improvement with steroids. (C) Raeder paratrigeminal neuralgia consists of Horner syndrome and trigeminal neuralgia-like pain. (E) Ramsay-Hunt syndrome (also known as Herpes zoster oticus) is reactivation of the varicella zoster virus in the geniculate ganglion, causing otalgia, auricular vesicles, and peripheral facial paralysis.

14.

D Spinocerebellum

Common cerebellar syndrome is found in alcoholics and is due to damage to the anterior part of the cerebellar cortex (spinocerebellum). (A) A vestibulocerebellum (flocculonodular lobe and adjacent vermis) lesion impairs the ability to stand upright and maintain gaze direction. Patients have a wide-based stance with small, shuffling movements. (B) Cerebellar tonsil pathology often is seen in patients with Chiari 1 malformations. (C) The cerebrocerebellum (lateral cerebellar hemispheres) is involved in highly skilled, learned movements. (E) Lesions interfering with the triangle of Guillain-Mollaret (olivary nucleus, dentate gyrus, and red nucleus) may result in palatal myoclonus.

15.

D Abduction of fifth digit due to weakness of the third palmar interosseous muscle

The Wartenberg sign is abduction of the fifth digit due to paralysis of the adducting palmar interosseous muscle and unopposed action of the extensor digiti minimi and digitorum communis muscles (innervated by the radial nerve). (A) Wasting of the interossei muscles in the hand is common in ulnar neuropathies. (B) A Froment thumb sign is seen when a patient grasps a sheet of paper resulting in extension of the proximal phalanx and flexion of the distal phalanx. This occurs as the anterior interosseous and flexor pollicis longus substitute for the weakened, ulnar-innervated adductor pollicis. (C) Hyperextension at the metacarpophalangeal joints and flexion at the interphalangeal joints in digits four, five, and partially three describes a "claw hand" deformity (also called "main en griffe"), resulting from an ulnar nerve injury. This condition should not be confused with a median nerve injury resulting in a "hand of benediction" deformity. (E) Ulnar nerve compression at the Guyon canal spares the dorsal cutaneous nerve that branches from the ulnar nerve in the forearm proximal to the wrist. Compression at this site also spares the flexor digitorum profundus medial heads.

16.

B Tumor compression of the stellate ganglion

The stellate ganglion is a sympathetic ganglion implicated in some pain syndromes, and lesions of this ganglion can cause a Horner syndrome. Iatrogenic injuries sometimes occur during injections or blocks for complex regional pain syndrome. A Pancoast tumor also may compress the nerve roots or trunks of the brachial plexus to cause upper extremity weakness.

17.

D Acute disseminated encephalomyelitis

Acute disseminated encephalomyelitis (ADEM) is the most common white matter disease in children. It typically follows an illness or vaccination and is differentiated from multiple sclerosis because multiple sclerosis has a multiphasic presentation. The first-line treatment for ADEM is intravenous steroids followed by a prednisone taper. Cases that do not respond to steroids may require intravenous immunoglobulins.

18.

C Thiamine; irreversible; medial dorsal thalamic nuclei

Korsakoff psychosis/syndrome is present in 80% of individuals who survive the preceding Wernicke encephalopathy, which is triggered by a thiamine deficiency. Korsakoff syndrome is irreversible. The classic triad for Wernicke encephalopathy is encephalopathy, ophthalmoplegia, and ataxia. With either condition, MRI FLAIR sequences typically demonstrate signal in the medial thalamus, floor of the fourth ventricle, and periaqueductal gray matter of the midbrain.

19.

C Intubate the patient.

This question emphasizes the importance of the "ABCs" (airway, breathing, and circulation) in emergency situations. Although quick initiation of treatment for Guillain-Barré syndrome is important, the patient is showing clinical signs of impending respiratory failure, making intubation the correct option.

20.

B Left lateral medulla

Lateral medullary syndrome (also known as Wallenberg syndrome) is due to infarction of the lateral medulla. Structures in this region include the nucleus and descending tract of the fifth cranial nerve, nucleus ambiguus, lateral spinothalamic tracts, inferior cerebellar peduncle, and descending sympathetic fibers of the vagus and glossopharyngeal nerves. Patients with Wallenberg syndrome have a classic constellation of symptoms including (1) ipsilateral Horner syndrome, (2) ipsilateral ataxia, (3) ipsilateral loss of facial pain and temperature perception, (4) ipsilateral loss of the corneal reflex, (5) ipsilateral impairment of corneal reflexes, (6) contralateral loss of pain and temperature sensation, (7) dysphagia, and (8) dysphonia.

21.

D INR of 2.3

An INR over 1.7 is an absolute contraindication to thrombolysis. Other absolute contraindications to thrombolysis include (1) uncertainty about time of stroke onset (e.g., patients awakening from sleep); (2) coma or severe obtundation with fixed eye deviation and complete hemiplegia; (3) hypertension with a systolic blood pressure at least 185 mm Hg or a diastolic blood pressure over 110 mm Hg on repeated measures (if reversed, a patient can be treated); (4) clinical presentation suggestive of subarachnoid hemorrhage, even if the CT scan is unremarkable; (5) presumed septic embolus; (6) patient having received a heparin medication within the last 48 hours, with an elevated activated prothrombin time (APTT) or with a known hereditary or acquired hemorrhagic diathesis; (7) known advanced liver disease, advanced right heart failure, or coagulopathy disorder with an INR over 1.5; (8) platelet count less than 100,000/µL; and (9) serum glucose less than 2.8 mmol/L or greater than 22.0 mmol/L. (A–C) Age over 80 years, major surgery within 2 weeks of presentation, hip replacement within 3 weeks of presentation, and recent myocardial infarction all are relative contraindications to thrombolysis.

22.

A Hartnup disease

Hartnup disease (also known as pellagra-like dermatosis) is an autosomal recessive disease affecting the absorption of nonpolar amino acids, particularly tryptophan, which is a precursor to serotonin, melatonin, and niacin. Niacin is a precursor to nicotinamide, which is a necessary component of NAD. Clinically, the disease is characterized by a childhood presentation, with symptoms ranging from failure to thrive, photosensitivity, intermittent ataxia, nystagmus, and tremor. Supplementation with high doses of nicotinamide usually is sufficient to treat the disease. (B) Phenylketonuria is caused by absent phenylalanine hydroxylase. It usually is treated with a strict phenylalanine-restricted diet. If untreated, patients suffer intellectual disability and seizures and eventually could die. (C) Homocystinuria leads to multisystemic disorders of connective tissue, muscles, and the central nervous and cardiovascular systems. There is no specific cure for homocystinuria; however, many people are treated with high doses of vitamin B6. (D) G6PD deficiency does not affect the central nervous system. Treatment is by preventing exposure to drugs and foods that cause hemolysis. (E) Tetrahydrobiopterin deficiency is a rare metabolic disorder that increases the blood levels of phenylalanine, which leads to low muscle tone and possible difficulty swallowing, seizures, progressive problems with development, and an inability to control body temperature. Treatment consists of tetrahydrobiopterin supplementation and a low phenylalanine diet.

23.

A Multiple sclerosis

Multiple sclerosis is the most common autoimmune disorder affecting the central nervous system, and patients can have a wide range of neurologic symptoms. In this clinical vignette, the patient has symptoms of optic neuritis, which affects up to 50% of multiple sclerosis patients. (B) Guillain-Barré syndrome is characterized by a rapid-onset weakness of the limbs as a result of an acute polyneuropathy affecting the peripheral nervous system. (C) Transient ischemic attacks are characterized by focal neurologic deficits that resolve within 24 hours. (D) Myasthenia gravis is an autoimmune or congenital neuromuscular disease characterized by fluctuating muscle weakens and fatigue. Extraocular muscles often are involved. (E) Amyotrophic lateral sclerosis is characterized by gradually worsening weakness and stiff muscles with fasciculations.

24.

C Angiogram

An angiogram is the most sensitive modality to diagnose sagittal sinus thrombosis. The presence of headache, hemiparesis, and focal epilepsy in a relatively young patient is indicative of sagittal sinus thrombosis. The likelihood of having the pathology is much higher in patients with a history of hypercoagulable disorders such as homocystinuria.

25.

B Proprioception

The tests described are the Romberg and heel-shin tests. Both of these test proprioception. The Romberg test combines vision, proprioception, and vestibular function. The heel-shin test assesses vision, proprioception, and cerebellar function.

26.

D Deposition of β-amyloid plaques

Chronic traumatic encephalopathy often is described in retired boxers, and the risk of developing this condition increases with career length. Patients develop motor, cognitive, and psychiatric disturbances. Pathological examination reveals cerebral and cerebellar atrophy, neurofibrillary tangles, and β-amyloid deposition.

27.

A Inhaled 100% O_2

Inhaled 100% O_2 is the best treatment to abort a cluster headache within minutes. (B) Sublingual nitroglycerin is not recommended for the treatment of headaches. (C) Ergotamine can help abort some vascular type headaches but is not efficient in aborting cluster headaches. (D) Methysergide is the classic drug used to prevent cluster headaches, but it is no longer used due to retroperitoneal and retropulmonary fibrosis.

28.

B West syndrome

West syndrome is a generalized seizure disorder of infants characterized by a triad of recurrent spasms, hypsarrhythmia, and developmental regression. Hypsarrhythmias are abnormal interictal patterns consisting of high amplitude and irregular waves and spikes in a background of chaotic and disorganized activity. (A) Absence seizures are characterized by a brief loss of consciousness without a notable postictal phase. (C) Epilepsia partialis continua is a rare seizure disorder in which the patient experiences recurrent focal motor epileptic seizures that recur every few seconds or minutes for long periods of time (months or years). (D) Complex partial seizures are seizures that are associated with unilateral cerebral hemisphere involvement and cause impairment of awareness or responsiveness. (E) Juvenile myoclonic seizures usually begin around puberty and tend to have a genetic basis. These seizures can be stimulus selective.

29.

B T1; sympathetics

Spinal shock is characterized by hypotension (systolic blood pressure less than 80 mm Hg) following a spinal cord injury. It is mediated by an injury to the spinal cord above T1, which causes an interruption in the sympathetic fibers. This leads to a loss of vascular tone causing hypotension. The loss of sympathetics leads to an unopposed parasympathetic tone, which causes the bradycardia seen in spinal shock.

30.

C Myopathy and neuromuscular junction disease

Myopathy and neuromuscular junction disease both demonstrate decreased amplitudes and durations of motor unit potentials. (A, B) Denervation and reinnervation exhibit decreased motor unit potential amplitudes but increased durations. "Giant units" may form during reinnervation, and polyphasic potentials may be seen during reinnervation with myopathy or neuromuscular junction disease.

31.

A Injection of central nervous system proteins into animal brain parenchyma

Experimental autoimmune encephalomyelitis is an animal model of brain inflammation. It is an inflammatory demyelinating disease of the central nervous system that can be induced by injecting central nervous system proteins, such as spinal cord homogenate and purified myelin, into animal brain parenchyma.

32.

B Diffuse axonal injury

Diffuse axonal injury is a primary lesion of a rotational acceleration/deceleration head injury, which can be associated with petechial hemorrhages in the dorsolateral rostral brain stem and corpus callosum.

33.

B Penicillamine

This patient has Wilson disease, a rare disorder of copper metabolism. Wilson disease also is known as hepatolenticular degeneration and is inherited in an autosomal recessive pattern. Copper accumulates in tissues including the basal ganglia, which leads to parkinsonism as well as cognitive deterioration and clumsiness. Patients can have Kayser-Fleischer rings, which are pathognomonic copper deposits in the cornea. Penicillamine binds accumulated copper and eliminates it in the urine.

34.

E Paroxysmal, lancinating pain in the depth of the ear with loss of taste in the anterior two thirds of the tongue with possible increased salivation

The diagnosis of nervus intermedius (geniculate) neuralgia is rare. The nerve carries general visceral efferents from the superior salivatory nucleus and passes through the geniculate ganglion without synapsing before heading to the pterygopalatine ganglion and lacrimal gland through the greater petrosal nerve. The nervus intermedius also carries special visceral afferents from the chorda tympani to the nucleus solitarius and general special afferents from the inner ear, middle ear, and part of the pinna. (A) Paroxysmal, lancinating pain in the lower one third of the face can be seen in trigeminal neuralgia. (B) The chorda tympani relays taste from the anterior two thirds of the ipsilateral tongue. (C) Herpes zoster ophthalmicus is characterized by a periorbital vesicular rash, conjunctivitis, keratitis, and uveitis with involvement of the tip of the nose.

35.

D Voice change; during device discharge

The most common side effect of vagal nerve stimulation is voice change occurring during device discharge and typically resolving afterward. Bradycardia, neck pain, and gastrointestinal irritation also can occur but are less frequent than voice change.

36.

A Rapid mental deterioration, myoclonus, and 1- to 2-Hz periodic electroencephalography complexes

The definitive diagnosis of Creutzfeldt-Jakob disease is accomplished with a biopsy, but this is used infrequently due to a lack of an effective treatment and a potential for iatrogenic infection. Clinical criteria (clinically proven Creutzfeldt-Jakob disease) for diagnosis include (1) symptoms of less than 12 months' duration and (2) cerebrospinal fluid with proteins 130 and 131 as well as 14-3-3. (D) In Creutzfeldt-Jakob disease, electroencephalography often shows pseudoperiodic sharp wave complexes resembling periodic lateralized epileptiform discharges, but they are responsive to noxious stimuli (unlike with herpes encephalitis). (E) A serum assay positive for S-100 can be found in Creutzfeldt-Jakob disease, but this test is very insensitive and nonspecific.

37.

C Increased interpeak latency in waves I through V

Brainstem auditory evoked potentials measure the auditory pathway, with the most important information being derived from the amplitude and latency of waves I, II, and V. The mnemonic "ACOLIMA" can be used to describe the peaks I through VII, respectively: *a*uditory nerve, *c*ochlear nucleus, superior *o*live, *l*ateral lemniscus, *i*nferior colliculus, *m*edial geniculate, and *a*uditory radiations.

38.

A Cranial neuritis, meningitis, radiculopathy

The neurologic symptoms of Lyme disease can be nonspecific and can mimic many other neurologic conditions. Serological testing aids in the diagnosis, with a false-positive rate under 3% and a false-negative rate that is much higher (especially early in the course of the disease). (B) Neurosyphilis presents with symptoms including tabes dorsalis (loss of motor coordination due to loss of dorsal column proprioception), Argyll-Robertson pupils (constricted pupils that further constrict to near accommodation but do not react to bright lights), and general paresis "of the insane." (C) Encephalopathy, dementia, and myelopathy are neurologic manifestations of AIDS. (D) Dementia, ataxia, and myoclonus classically are seen with Creutzfeldt-Jakob disease.

39.

B Ventriculitis

The differential diagnosis for ependymal lining enhancement includes ependymal spreading of glioblastoma, primary central nervous system lymphoma, metastasis, germinoma, and ventriculitis. Ventriculitis is due to infection of the ependymal lining of the cerebral ventricles, and most commonly is secondary to intraventricular rupture of a brain abscess.

40.

C Hypothalamic hamartoma; poor seizure response to medications

A patient with precocious puberty, gelastic seizures, and a hypothalamic mass likely has a hypothalamic hamartoma. Gelastic seizures typically respond poorly to medications and progress to epileptic encephalopathy. Surgery for these lesions is indicated when the precocious puberty fails medical therapy, seizures fail medical therapy, or if there is a deficit from the tumor's mass effect. Radiosurgery also is a treatment option for smaller lesions.

41.

C Weakness of dorsiflexion and ankle eversion

The common peroneal nerve is derived from the L4 to S2 roots and innervates the short head of the biceps femoris by a motor branch that exits close to the gluteal cleft. The remainder of the common peroneal nerve innervates muscles through the deep and superficial peroneal nerves. The deep peroneal nerve innervates the tibialis anterior, extensor digitorum longus, peroneus tertius, and extensor hallucis longus. Damage to the deep peroneal nerve results in footdrop. The superficial peroneal nerve innervates the peroneus longus and brevis. Injury to this nerve results in an inability to evert the foot and loss of sensation over the dorsum of the foot, with the exception of the first web space. Injury to the common peroneal nerve results in footdrop and weakness of ankle eversion, with loss of sensation along the dorsal surface of the foot as described.

42.

A Weakness of dorsiflexion and ankle inversion

An L5 radiculopathy is characterized by weakness in extension of the hallucis and potentially can result in footdrop as well. Numbness and pain can be felt on the superior aspect of the foot. (B) An S1 radiculopathy causes weakness of plantarflexion and ankle eversion. (D) The tibial nerve is a branch of the sciatic nerve and gives motor branches to the gastrocnemius, popliteus, soleus, and plantaris muscles. It also innervates the tibialis posterior, flexor digitorum longus, and flexor hallucis longus. Injury to the tibial nerve causes weakness of plantarflexion and ankle inversion.

43.

D Methotrexate

Subacute necrotizing leukoencephalitis is characterized by coagulative necrosis with lipid-laden macrophages in the absence of inflammatory cells. There is mineralizing atrophy of astrocytes in the gray matter. This condition occurs when methotrexate is used with radiation. Other side effects include meningitis and encephalitis. (A) Cisplatin's side effects include hearing and vision loss along with other neuropathies. It can cause leukoencephalopathy. (B) Bevacizumab's side effects include inhibition of wound healing, hemorrhage diathesis, and hypertension related to its antiangiogenic mechanism of action. (C) Temozolomide's side effects include nausea, vomiting and, rarely, acute respiratory failure. (E) Vincristine's side effects include axonal degeneration related to the drug's inhibition of microtubule formation. The drug does not cross the blood–brain barrier but can cause respiratory failure with intrathecal injection.

44.

B Niacin

Niacin deficiency results in pellagra, characterized by rashes, posterior column dysfunction, spastic and weak extremities, confusion, and fatigue. It is seen in individuals with corn-heavy diets. (A) Thiamine deficiency causes Wernicke encephalopathy in the subacute setting, and is characterized by lateral recti palsies, nystagmus, confusion, and gait ataxia. It is seen most commonly in alcoholics. Beriberi also is caused by thiamine deficiency, and is characterized by peripheral neuropathies, axonal degeneration, and autonomic dysfunction. It is seen in individuals with rice-heavy diets. (C) B6 deficiency results in lower extremity paresthesias, weakness, and pain. It is associated with isoniazid (a tuberculosis treatment) and hydralazine therapies. (D) B12 deficiency results in a megaloblastic anemia and subacute combined degeneration of the spinal cord, characterized by demyelination of the posterior followed by lateral columns. Cognitive deterioration and peripheral neuropathies also can occur. One cause is pernicious anemia resulting from a decrease in intrinsic factor production (the binding factor for B12). (E) Vitamin A deficiency results in decreased visual acuity.

45.

B Ape hand and benediction sign deformities

The patient has a median nerve injury and has lost his ability to flex his second and third digits at the metacarpophalangeal joints and his ability to flex and extend the proximal and distal inter-

phalangeal joints. The extensor digitorum (left unopposed) acts on the metacarpophalangeal joints of digits two and three to keep them extended when attempts are made to make a fist. This results in a "hand of benediction" deformity. This is in contrast to a "claw hand" deformity, which has a similar appearance when a patient attempts extension of all digits and which is seen with an ulnar nerve injury. Patients with median nerve injuries also develop "ape hand" (also known as simian hand) deformities, referring to the inability to move the thumb away from the rest of the hand.

46.

A Upward gaze paralysis, eyelid retraction, and "setting sun" sign

Dorsal midbrain syndrome (also known as Parinaud syndrome) is characterized by paralysis of upgaze with preservation of downgaze, pseudo–Argyll-Robertson pupils with accommodative paresis and mid-dilated pupils that show light-near dissociation, convergence-retraction nystagmus (on fast upgaze, the globes adduct and retract), eyelid retraction, and conjugate downgaze in the primary position (also known as the "setting sun" sign).

47.

A Niemann-Pick disease

Vertical supranuclear ophthalmoplegia is a clinical feature of Niemann-Pick type C (NP-C) disease and is present in approximately 65% of patients with the disease. Along with gelastic cataplexy, vertical supranuclear ophthalmoplegia is an important indicator of NP-C disease. Vertical supranuclear ophthalmoplegia in NP-C disease is characterized by paralysis of vertical saccades with sparing of the slow, vertical eye movement systems in the early phase of the disease secondary to selective vulnerability of neurons in the rostral interstitial nuclei of the medial longitudinal fasciculus. Other metabolic diseases that can cause vertical supranuclear ophthalmoplegia are Wilson disease, kernicterus, and barbiturate overdose.

48.

C Spasmodic torticollis

Spasmodic torticollis is a common form of focal dystonia. It begins in early adulthood and consists of spasms affecting the sternocleidomastoid and trapezius muscles typically in a unilateral fashion. (A) Meigs syndrome entails focal dystonia characterized by blepharospasms, forceful jaw opening, lip and neck retractions, and tongue thrusting. (B) Tardive dyskinesia is a disorder of involuntary, repetitive movements usually related to long-term antipsychotic use.

49.

D Carotid endarterectomy

The North American Symptomatic Carotid Endarterectomy Trial (NASCET) found that carotid endarterectomy can reduce the risk of stroke in patients with 70% or more carotid artery stenosis. The risk of ipsilateral stroke was found to be 26% in the medically treated group versus 9% in the surgically treated group. (A) Combined warfarin and aspirin therapy has been shown to be equivalent to aspirin therapy alone in the management of carotid artery stenosis; therefore, there currently is no role for warfarin in the management of carotid artery stenosis. (B) Carotid angioplasty (with stenting) is a valid alternative to a carotid endarterectomy for selected patients who have an indication for revascularization but are high-risk surgical candidates. (C) Statins currently are considered a standard of care in the treatment of carotid artery stenosis. They have been shown to decrease the risk of stroke by 25%; however, surgery still is indicated for patients with high grade or symptomatic carotid artery stenosis. (E) Antiplatelet drug therapy and aggressive correction of stroke risk factors are the mainstays of medical therapy in carotid artery stenosis.

50.

B Oxcarbamazepine

Surgical management usually is reserved for patients with trigeminal neuralgia refractory to medical treatment. The first-line medical treatment for trigeminal neuralgia is oxcarbamazepine; however, there have been several randomized trials comparing oxcarbamazepine to carbamazepine, and both medications were found to be equally effective. Oxcarbamazepine has the advantage of being taken once daily and thus increases compliance.

51.

B HLA-B*1502 allele

The HLA-B*1502 allele is a genetic susceptibility marker in Asians that is associated with an increased risk of developing Stevens-Johnson syndrome and toxic epidermal necrolysis. Patients with Asian ancestry should be screened for this allele before they are started on carbamazepine, oxcarbamazepine, or phenytoin.

52.

E Hemiparesis of the contralateral upper extremity and face with dysarthria

The recurrent artery of Heubner is a medial striate artery that often arises from the proximal A2 (less often distal A1) segment of the anterior cerebral artery. The artery supplies blood to the head of the caudate, part of the lentiform nucleus, and anterior limb of the internal capsule. Injury to these areas results in weakness of the contralateral upper extremity and face with speech deficits. (A) Anterior choroidal infarcts cause the classic "triple H" syndrome of hemisensory changes, hemiparesis, and a homonymous hemianopsia. (B) The triad of altered mental status, vertical gaze palsy, and memory impairment is characteristic of bilateral paramedian thalamic infarcts, which may arise after injury to the artery of Percheron.

53.

C 3 to 21 days

Following initial complete spinal cord injury, the predominant symptoms are related to spinal shock and include flaccid quadriplegia and areflexia. Spasticity and hyperreflexia develop within days of the initial injury and are thought to represent exaggeration of the normal stretch reflexes secondary to loss of cortical inhibition.

54.

A GABA agonism

Baclofen is a $GABA_B$ receptor agonist that works as an inhibitory neurotransmitter and blocks mono- and polysynaptic reflexes. (E) Cyclobenzaprine is a muscle relaxant with an unknown mechanism of action. It is thought to increase norepinephrine release from the locus coeruleus through γ fibers, which innervate and inhibit α motor neurons in the ventral horn of the spinal cord.

55.

B Anterior hypothalamus

The patient is suffering from diencephalic syndrome in its classic sense, which generally results from tumor involvement of the anterior hypothalamus (despite both the hypothalamus and thalamus residing in the diencephalon).

56.

B Multiple sclerosis

Multiple sclerosis is found in approximately 18% of patients experiencing bilateral trigeminal neuralgia. Usually, a pontine plaque is the culprit. Only a very small percentage of multiple sclerosis patients have trigeminal neuralgia, however. Heat can cause a sudden flare or emergence of multiple sclerosis symptoms. When symptoms of trigeminal neuralgia occur unilaterally, they most often occur on the right and in females.

57.

B Long thoracic

The long thoracic nerve derives from the C5 through C7 nerve roots and is particularly vulnerable to iatrogenic injury because it runs superficially along the serratus muscle. Injuries to the long thoracic nerve denervate the serratus anterior muscle, which usually protracts the scapula and counteracts the action of the trapezius and rhomboids. Serratus anterior dysfunction leads to posterior protraction of the scapula. (A) The axillary nerve innervates the teres minor and the deltoid muscles. It courses around the surgical neck of the humerus and is prone to injury secondary to humeral fractures. In axillary nerve injuries, patients typically are unable to abduct their upper limbs beyond 15 to 20 degrees. (C) The musculocutaneous nerve innervates the biceps brachii, coracobrachialis, and brachialis. If this nerve is disrupted, patients typically develop weakness with elbow flexion. (D) The radial nerve innervates the extensors of the forearm and triceps brachii. In the setting of a radial nerve injury, patients are unable to extend their forearms and have slightly weakened arm extension. (E) The lower subscapular nerve usually innervates the teres major muscle and lower part of the subscapularis muscle. Injuries to this nerve lead to weakness with arm adduction.

58.

C Right anterior spinal

The anterior spinal artery supplies the medial part of the medulla. Occlusion of this artery leads to a medial medullary stroke (Dejerine syndrome). The affected structures are the medullary pyramid, medial lemniscus, and hypoglossal nerve fibers passing through the medulla. Usually, the spinothalamic tract is spared because it is located more laterally in the brainstem. The trigeminal nucleus also is spared because it is situated higher in the pons, and its spinal part is lateral to the affected region. Presentation includes tongue deviation to the side of infarct, contralateral limb weakness or hemiplegia, and loss of discriminative touch, conscious proprioception, and vibration sensation contralateral to the infarct. (A) Hallmarks of basilar artery occlusion include decreased consciousness, quadriparesis, pupillary and oculomotor abnormalities, dysarthria, and dysphagia. (D, E) Occlusion of the posterior inferior cerebellar artery leads to a lateral medullary syndrome (also known as Wallenberg syndrome). Symptoms include vertigo, nystagmus, ipsilateral cerebellar signs (ataxia and dysmetria), contralateral loss of pain and temperature sensation in the body, ipsilateral loss of pain and temperature sensation in the face, ipsilateral laryngeal and pharyngeal hemiparesis (diminished gag reflex), and ipsilateral Horner syndrome.

59.

A Anticoagulation

Anticoagulation is the mainstay treatment for cerebral venous thrombosis (CVT). The rationale for using it is to prevent thrombus growth, facilitate recanalization of the sinus, and prevent a pulmonary embolism. Multiple trials have demonstrated the efficacy of using anticoagulation in the management of CVT. (B) There are no controlled trials or observational studies that assess the role of aspirin or clopidogrel in the management of CVT. (C, D) The use of intra-sinus thrombolytic therapy and mechanical clot aspiration is supported only by small case series. The major inconvenience of these therapies is that they only are available at select centers and cannot be performed on a routine basis. If clinical deterioration occurs despite adequate anticoagulation or if the patient develops venous infarction or intracranial hemorrhage, these interventional techniques should be considered strongly. (E) Steroids may have a role in CVT by decreasing vasogenic edema; however, steroids may enhance hypercoagulability and are not usually indicated in the management of CVT.

60.

A Continuous intravenous fosphenytoin

Status epilepticus is defined as a seizure persisting for more than 5 minutes (30 minutes was the previous definition) or more than one seizure occurring within a 5-minute interval without the person returning to baseline between the seizures. Treatment begins with administration of intravenous lorazepam at 0.1 mg/kg or 4 mg once, not exceeding 2 mg/minute. Alternatively, diazepam and midazolam may be used. After the initial benzodiazepines infusion, fosphenytoin (or alternatively phenytoin or valproic acid) should be infused. Of note, benzodiazepines and antiepileptics are not compatible chemically and cannot be infused through the same IV; therefore, a second IV should be available. The use of intravenous propofol, continuous midazolam, and phenobarbital is indicated for refractory status epilepticus resistant to the above-cited treatments. (E) Continuous electroencephalogram monitoring is indicated for refractory status epilepticus.

61.

A Bell palsy

The diagnosis of Bell palsy is based on two criteria: (1) acute onset of symptoms over a day or two, with a progressive course reaching a maximum within 3 weeks and recovery within 6 months, and (2) diffuse facial nerve involvement/weakness. Bell palsy usually is a diagnosis of exclusion of more serious pathologies such as stroke and brain tumor. (B, C) Stroke or transient ischemic attack are possible etiologies of facial nerve palsy; however, they are unlikely to be the cause in the this young woman with a normal MRI. (D, E) Sarcoidosis is a possible cause of Bell palsy; however, it is unlikely in the above patient. The mnemonic "*A*lexander gra*H*am *B*ell had *STD*s" is used to remember the possible diseases associated with Bell palsy: *A*IDS, *L*yme disease, *H*erpes simplex, *s*arcoidosis, *t*umors, and *d*iabetes.

62.

C Serum angiotensin-converting enzyme level

Bilateral cranial nerve VII and VIII palsies are suggestive of neurosarcoidosis. When suspected, evidence of systemic disease should be investigated. Chest radiographs are abnormal in 90% of patients with sarcoidosis, and serum angiotensin-converting enzyme levels are elevated in many patients. Sarcoidosis affects blacks more than whites at a 10:1 ratio. (A) Neurologic manifestations of Lyme disease (caused by infection by *Borrelia burgdorferi*) include meningitis, radiculopathy, and facial nerve palsy. It is the most common cause of bilateral Bell palsy. ELISA for IgM or IgG antibodies to *Borrelia burgdorferi* is indicated when this disease is suspected. (B) Optic neuritis and internuclear ophthalmoplegia are common in multiple sclerosis along with trigeminal neuralgia-like symptoms; however, other cranial nerve involvement is rare. Performing a cerebrospinal fluid analysis for oligoclonal bands is indicated when multiple sclerosis is suspected.

63.

D Deviation of both eyes toward a hemiparetic limb

Deviation of both eyes toward a hemiparetic limb indicates a lesion in the pons contralateral to the direction of the eyes due to damage to the paramedian pontine reticular formation. (A) Deviation of both eyes toward a jerking limb often is seen with seizure of the frontal lobe. (B) Deviation of both eyes away from a hemiparetic limb often is seen with a frontal lobe stroke. (C) Each eye abducted (wall eyes) is known as wall-eyed bilateral internuclear ophthalmoplegia (WEBINO) syndrome resulting from midbrain infarction. (E) A cranial nerve III palsy with a contralateral hemiparetic limb is seen in Weber syndrome, resulting from an infarct of the midbrain in the distribution of the paramedian branches of the posterior cerebral or basilar artery.

64.

C Inability to perform rapid, alternating movements

Ataxia, dysmetria, and dysdiadochokinesia are symptoms of cerebellar dysfunction. (A) Ataxia is the lack of voluntary coordination of muscle movements. (B) Dysmetria is the breakdown of movements with "overshooting" when performing specific motor tasks such as the finger-to-nose test. (D) Dolichoectasia is the dilation and elongation of an artery often resulting in tortuosity. (E) Bradykinesia is slowness in the execution of movements.

65.

E Posterior column dysfunction

Classically, the Romberg sign is indicative of proprioception (dorsal column) dysfunction. It is positive when patients are able to stand with their feet together and their eyes open, but fall when they closes their eyes. The Romberg sign often is misinterpreted to represent cerebellar dysfunction; however, it can be positive with vestibular dysfunction but not for the other types of ataxias listed.

66.

C Left paramedian pontine reticular formation

A stroke in the paramedian pontine reticular formation causes a gaze preference away from the lesion (toward the hemiparesis). (A, B) A frontal lobe stroke causes the eyes to deviate toward the lesion, whereas seizures cause the eyes to deviate away from the lesion. With frontal lobe infarcts, patients look away from their motor deficits. (E) The thalamus often causes vertical gaze limitations but also can cause gaze deviation contralateral to the hemiplegia (as in frontal lobe infarcts). Occasionally, thalamic infarcts can cause deviations toward the hemiplegia ("wrong-way eyes").

67.

D Transcortical motor aphasia

There are seven types of aphasia: the four listed in answers A to D as well as global, mixed transcortical, and anomic. Global aphasia results from large left hemispheric insults, whereas conduction aphasia stems from lesions of the arcuate fasciculus. Broca, Wernicke, global, and conduction aphasias have impaired repetition, whereas transcortical and anomic aphasias have preserved repetition.

68.

D Lambert-Eaton syndrome

In Lambert-Eaton syndrome, antibodies are formed against presynaptic voltage-gated calcium channels at the neuromuscular junction. Repeated stimulation increases muscle action potentials. (A) Myasthenia gravis involves weakness due to antibodies to postsynaptic nicotinic acetylcholine receptors. Extraocular muscles generally are involved. Sustained activity leads to increasing weakness. (B) *Clostridium botulinum* causes neuromuscular paralysis by preventing the release of acetylcholine from presynaptic vesicles. (C) Electromyography in polymyalgia rheumatica is normal. (E) Neuralgic amyotrophy (Parsonage-Turner syndrome) usually begins with severe pain followed by significant weakness.

69.

B Absence seizures

Bursts of frontally predominant generalized 3-Hz spike-and-wave complexes lasting more than 2 seconds seen during awake EEG recordings often are pathognomonic for absence seizures. (A) Electroencephalography (EEG) in Creutzfeldt-Jakob disease often shows periodic sharp wave or spike complexes of a 1- to 2-Hz frequency in the frontal lobes during the early stages of the disease. Such EEG findings have a 95% positive predictive value. (C) Lennox-Gastaut syndrome has an EEG pattern characterized by brief (less than 2 seconds) slow spike-and-wave activity during wakefulness. (D) Subacute sclerosing panencephalitis due to chronic infection from the measles virus shows a classic periodic burst of polyphasic sharp and slow wave complexes of 0.5- to 2-second duration on EEG. (E) The EEG in herpes encephalitis may show periodic slow wave complexes from the temporal lobes. Periodic lateralized epileptiform discharges in the correct clinical context is very suggestive of herpes encephalitis.

70.

E Nasal speech, dysphagia, dysphonia, diminished gag reflex, and deviation of the uvula towards the contralateral side

The nucleus ambiguus controls the motor functions of the soft palate, pharynx, larynx, and upper esophagus. (A) A lesion of the lateral medulla may involve the nucleus ambiguus and produces vertigo, nystagmus, ipsilateral ataxia, contralateral loss of pain and temperature from the body, and ipsilateral loss of pain and temperature from the face. (B) A lesion of the vestibular nuclei produces nystagmus to the contralateral side and ipsilateral ataxia. (C) A lesion of the caudal nucleus solitarius produces increased heart rate. (D) A lesion of the rostral nucleus solitarius produces loss of taste from the ipsilateral anterior two thirds of the tongue.

71.

B Anterior inferior cerebellar artery

Anterior inferior cerebellar artery infarcts lead to a lateral pontine syndrome. (A) Vertebral/posterior inferior cerebellar artery infarcts cause a lateral medullary or Wallenberg syndrome characterized by vertigo, ipsilateral hemiataxia, dysarthria, ptosis, and miosis. (C) Superior cerebellar artery infarcts cause ipsilateral ataxia, nausea, vomiting, dysarthria, contralateral loss of pain/temperature sensation, deafness, and a Horner syndrome. (D) A basilar perforator thrombus or embolism can causes a Millard-Gubler syndrome characterized by ipsilateral cranial nerve VI and VII palsies and contralateral hemiparesis. (E) Artery of Percheron infarcts can manifest as bilateral thalamic infarcts causing altered mental status, vertical gaze palsies, and memory impairment. If there are accompanying midbrain infarcts, oculomotor dysfunction, hemiplegia, ataxia, and tremor can occur.

72.

E Festinating gait

Festinating gaits are typical of advanced parkinsonism and are characterized by small strides at an increasing rate as the feet try to keep up with the forward-leaning trunk. (A) Scissor gait often is seen with corticospinal or upper motor neuron lesions (e.g., with cerebral palsy or spinal cord trauma), in which severe bilateral spasticity causes flexed and adducted legs with compensatory trunk movements, resulting in a "scissor-like" movement. (B) In magnetic gait, the feet seem to be attached to the floor. It often is associated with normal pressure hydrocephalus. (C) Antalgic gait develops as a way to avoid pain where the stance phase is abnormally shortened relative to the swing phase. (D) Steppage gait develops either from footdrop or from impaired sensation (e.g., tabes dorsalis, neuropathy, B12 deficiencies).

73.

B Looking right, the left eye will fail to adduct, and the right eye will have nystagmus

A unilateral lesion causes an inability of the ipsilateral eye to adduct upon contralateral gaze. This is because the contralateral gaze center does not communicate with the ipsilateral cranial nerve III nucleus. There also is a nystagmus in the abducting eye.

74.

E Bilateral visual cortices

Anton-Babinski syndrome (also known as visual anosognosia) occurs following injury to both occipital lobes. Patients who suffer from it are cortically blind but affirm they can see. Patients have symptoms of visual anosognosia (lack of awareness) and confabulation.

75.

D Splenium of the corpus callosum and left visual cortex

Patients with alexia without agraphia or pure alexia suffer from severe reading problems, whereas other language-related skills are preserved. The injury usually is secondary to an infarct of the splenium of the corpus callosum and the left visual cortex. In these patients, only the right occipital lobe can process visual information, but it is not able to send this information of the language areas in the left brain because of damage to the splenium.

76.

A Hearing loss and tinnitus

Hearing loss and tinnitus are the injuries endured by patients following sustained and repeated acoustic trauma, with patients typically losing hearing in the frequencies at which the trauma occurs.

77.

C Diminished conduction in air with normal bone conduction

Air conduction usually is enhanced by the middle ear; thus, middle ear pathology decreases air conduction. Bony conduction depends solely on the cochlea and the skull and thus is not affected in middle ear disease.

78.

A Increased body temperature

Patients with demyelinating diseases, in general and in multiple sclerosis in particular, tend to see worsening symptoms with elevated body temperatures, such as when taking a shower or during summer months. This is known as the Uhthoff phenomenon and is secondary to action potentials being blocked or slowed down in demyelinated nerves.

79.

E Suprascapular nerve

The suprascapular nerve from the upper trunk of the brachial plexus innervates the supraspinatus. Patients with damage to the suprascapular

nerve are not able to initiate shoulder abduction. (A) The axillary nerve is intact because the deltoid exam is intact, in that abduction is possible once it is initiated past 45 degrees. (B) The posterior cord gives rise to the axillary nerve and, therefore, is intact as well. (C) Good bilateral inspiratory function indicates a working diaphragm, and, therefore, the phrenic nerves are intact, meaning that the C3 through C5 nerve roots are intact. Because the scapula is not winged, the long thoracic nerve with contributions from the C5 through C7 roots is intact. (D) The upper trunk is intact because it contributes to the posterior cord, which is intact.

80.

A Alcoholism

The described symptoms of a decreased level of consciousness, ataxia, oculomotor disturbances, and dysarthria are classic findings in Wernicke encephalopathy, which is a potentially fatal complication seen in alcoholic patients. (B) Nicotine withdrawal usually is associated with agitation; however, it has not been associated with a decreased level of consciousness, ataxia, oculomotor disturbances, or dysarthria. (C) Withdrawal from heroin typically occurs 6 to 24 hours after discontinuation of the drug. Symptoms include sweating, malaise, anxiety, depression, akathisia, priapism, extra-sensitivity of the genitals in females, general feeling of heaviness, excessive yawning or sneezing, tears, rhinorrhea, insomnia, cold sweats, nausea, vomiting, diarrhea, cramps, and watery eyes. (D) Uncontrolled hypertension does not explain the patient's symptoms. (E) Uncontrolled diabetes can present with altered mental status; however, it does not explain the patient's symptoms.

81.

B Nucleus ambiguus

The nucleus ambiguus is located in the ventrolateral medulla. It contains the motor neurons that contribute to the glossopharyngeal and vagus nerves, which innervate the tongue and larynx, respectively. The vagus nerve also provides parasympathetic innervation of the esophagus; therefore, injury to the nucleus ambiguus leads to dysphagia. (A) The nucleus solitarius receives sensory input from the facial, glossopharyngeal, and vagus nerves. An injury can lead to dysphagia, as seen in medial medullary syndromes. (C) Involvement of the descending tract of cranial nerve V can lead to mastication problems. (E) The middle cerebellar peduncle is not affected in lateral medullary infarction.

82.

B Corticosteroids

Corticosteroids are adequate for the acute management of multiple sclerosis flares. They can reduce the length and intensity of flares. (A) Interferon β-1B is a maintenance medication used to reduce the frequency of multiple sclerosis flares. (C) Intravenous immunoglobulin can be used to reduce the frequency of multiple sclerosis flares. (D) Glatiramer is an immunomodulator used to decrease the frequency of multiple sclerosis flares. (E) Pramipexole is a dopamine agonist used to treat Parkinson disease and restless legs syndrome.

83.

B Vertebral

The lateral medulla is supplied by several small branches of the distal ipsilateral vertebral artery; therefore, most cases of lateral medullary (Wallenberg) syndrome are secondary to occlusion of the vertebral artery. Occasionally, occlusion of the posterior inferior cerebellar artery (PICA) may cause Wallenberg syndrome; however, when the PICA is occluded, patients also suffer infarctions of their inferior cerebellums. (A) Basilar artery occlusion usually presents with dysarthria, pupillary disorders, and lower cranial nerve involvement as well as consciousness disorders. (C) Symptoms of superior cerebellar artery occlusion include ipsilateral cerebellar ataxias, nausea, vomiting, and slurred speech, as well as contralateral loss of pain and temperature sensation. (D) Occlusion of the anterior inferior cerebellar artery leads to lateral pontine syndrome, which includes a sudden-onset vertigo and vomiting, nystagmus, ipsilateral loss of face sensation, ipsilateral facial paralysis, and ipsilateral hearing loss and tinnitus. (E) Occlusion of the anterior spinal artery leads to anterior spinal artery syndrome, characterized by loss of motor function below the level of injury, bilateral loss of pain and temperature sensation, and preservation of fine touch and proprioception.

84.

D Loss of proprioception of the right trunk and upper and lower extremities

The medial lemniscus is formed from crossing fibers (internal arcuate fibers) from the contralateral nucleus gracilis/cuneatus. These fibers carry information helping with two-point discrimination and vibration and proprioception sensation from the contralateral side of the body before synapsing in the ventral posterolateral nucleus of the thalamus.

85.

A Visual evoked potentials

Because optic neuritis is very common in multiple sclerosis patients, visual evoked potentials tend to be the most affected in these patients. (C) Brain auditory evoked responses are less sensitive than visual evoked potentials in the diagnosis of multiple sclerosis. (D) The Jolly test is an evoked response involving peripheral muscles. (E) Sensory nerve conduction tests are used to study peripheral muscles.

86.

A Mycotic aneurysm rupture

This patient's immunosuppression places him at an increased risk for opportunistic infections. Given his young age and his immunosuppression, the most likely cause of his intraparenchymal hemorrhage is bleeding from a mycotic aneurysm. Mycotic aneurysms usually develop from an infected embolus that gets dislodged from an infected heart valve and stuck in the arterial wall of a distal intracranial vessel. The word *mycotic* does not refer to fungal infections but rather is suggestive of the shape of aneurysms that usually are multiple.

87.

A Peripheral neuropathy

In a patient with renal failure, peripheral neuropathy is the most common neurologic complication and usually is a symmetric, mixed sensorimotor neuropathy that starts in the legs and progresses proximally.

16 Radiology

1.

A Radiation necrosis

Radiation necrosis typically presents with higher apparent diffusion coefficient (ADC) values compared with tumor recurrence, which tends to show restricted diffusion and therefore lower signal in the solid enhancing components. On perfusion MRI, radiation necrosis demonstrates decreased relative cerebral blood volume (rCBV) in contrast to high-grade tumors. Finally, this patient is 1 year from his radiation therapy, which is a peak time for radiation necrosis to appear (usually between 12 and 24 months). (B) A recurrent glioblastoma would tend to have a low ADC signal and increased perfusion on rCBV maps. (C) Secondary malignancies following temozolomide (an alkylating agent) have been reported but are a rare occurrence. These malignancies usually are hematologic. Glioblastoma would be much more likely than a secondary malignancy, given its aggressive nature and expected eventual recurrence. (D) Encephalomalacia would be apparent by parenchymal volume loss and should not show nodular enhancement or restricted diffusion. Some (usually nonnodular) enhancement may be present around the resection cavity due to granulation tissue.

2.

D Esthesioneuroblastoma

Esthesioneuroblastomas (olfactory neuroblastomas) are rare, malignant tumors of the superior nasal cavity and anterior skull base. Treatment strategies vary widely and include surgery, radiotherapy, and/or chemotherapy. The ideal treatment modality has yet to be determined. Esthesioneuroblastomas tend to exert mass effect on the orbits, optic nerves, and optic chiasm, and may result in proptosis. They can occur in the frontal sinus and have variable intracranial extension. They homogeneously enhance on contrasted T1 sequences and appear moderately hyperintense on T2 sequences. (A) An optic nerve glioma would infiltrate and expand the optic nerve. As seen in the second image, there is stretching of the optic nerve due to mass effect and proptosis, but the tumor itself does not involve the optic apparatus. (B) Anterior skull base meningiomas also demonstrate avid enhancement and occasionally can extend into the olfactory recess. They may present with a dural tail and hyperostosis; however, the epicenter of the mass in this case is in the sinonasal cavity without a significant intracranial dural component. This makes a meningioma unlikely. Esthesioneuroblastomas often do extend intracranially, in which case a "waist" at the level of the cribriform plate and cysts at the brain–tumor interface are strongly suggestive of such diagnosis. (C) Skull base chordomas usually are located in the anterior clivus but rarely may extend to the nasal cavity. Primary chordomas in the nasal cavity and maxilla without clival involvement are extremely rare. Chordomas usually demonstrate more heterogeneous enhancement than esthesioneuroblastomas on contrasted T1 sequences and are very hyperintense on T2 sequences.

3.

D Long bone fractures

Long bone fractures can result in fat embolism, which appears as tiny foci of susceptibility artifact that preferentially may be located at the gray matter–white matter interface or diffusely distributed as in this case. Fat embolism may be accompanied by scattered foci of restricted diffusion. (A) Diffuse axonal injury is due to shearing forces from rotational acceleration. Areas of hemorrhage can be detected on susceptibility-weighted imaging (SWI) sequences and tend to be located in the gray matter–white matter junction, corpus callosum, and brainstem. Linear SWI signal loss often can be seen along the white matter tracts. (B) β-amyloid peptide deposits are related to cerebral amyloid angiopathy (CAA). SWI may show multiple foci of signal loss located peripherally in a cortical/subcortical distribution rather than diffusely as in this case. Patients also can have superficial siderosis and present with subarachnoid hemorrhage. (C) Mutations in the *CCM1*, *CCM2*, and *CCM3* genes can be seen in familial cavernous malformation syndromes. Lesions usually are more randomly distributed and not as evenly sized as in the current case.

4.

A Astrocytoma

Astrocytomas in the spinal cord are most common in children but also may occur in adults. The majority of them are histologically low grade and slow growing, and may result in bone remodeling. Half of astrocytomas are of the pilocytic subtype and are relatively well defined, whereas the remainder are infiltrative. They commonly present as expansile masses with variable degrees of ill-defined enhancement, although some tumors may not enhance. (B) Ependymomas are more common in adults. Compared with astrocytomas, their enhancement more frequently is well defined, and they more commonly are associated with cystic changes or hemorrhage. They are located more centrally, as they arise from the ependyma, but such distinction becomes difficult in larger tumors. (C) Metastases to the cervical spine typically are more focal than and not as expansile as the demonstrated lesion. It would be highly unusual for a patient of this age to present with a spinal cord metastasis without a known primary malignancy. (D) Tumefactive demyelination is more common in the brain. Demyelinating lesions may be seen in the spinal cord and may be related to acute disseminated encephalomyelitis (more common in the cervical spine), neuromyelitis optica (which may result in longitudinally extensive transverse myelitis), and multiple sclerosis (usually with small lesions centered in the peripheral white matter and only rarely extending over long segments when confluent). The appearance of the lesion in question is too expansile and is not compatible with a demyelinating or inflammatory process.

5.

A Interhemispheric cysts

The image accompanying the question shows dysgenesis of the corpus callosum with incomplete formation of the cingulate gyrus. Dorsal or occasionally anterior interhemispheric cysts are a common finding. (B) Colpocephaly (dilatation of the atria and occipital horns of the lateral ventricles) is a characteristic secondary finding in dysgenesis of the corpus callosum. (C) Patients with dysgenesis of the corpus callosum can have a "high-riding" third ventricle. Additional findings include bundles of Probst (white matter that failed to cross the midline) and incomplete rotation of the hippocampi. (D) Tubulonodular lipomas have a significantly increased incidence of associated anomalies compared with curvilinear ones.

6.

A Results from premature disjunction of the cutaneous ectoderm from the neuroectoderm during neurulation

Postcontrast sagittal T1 and short tau inversion recovery (STIR) images show a large lobulated mass that appears to be intradural and at least partially intramedullary. Although most of the mass is hyperintense on T1, these areas fully suppress on STIR images, indicating that this signal is related to fat rather than contrast enhancement. Spinal lipomas follow fat signal on all sequences, and subcutaneous fat can be used as an internal control. Embryologically, these lesions result from premature disjunction of the cutaneous ectoderm from the neuroectoderm during neurulation, whereby the open neural tube becomes exposed to the ingrowth of mesodermal tissues. Patients may experience slowly progressing paresis, spasticity, or sensory loss depending on the extent and location of the lesion. (B) An infiltrative hypercellular lesion with variable degrees of mitosis/atypia would describe a neoplastic process such as an astrocytoma, which may or may not show enhancement. (C) Clonal transformation of cells of B-cell origin would result in lymphoma (e.g., Hodgkin). These lesions are rare in the spinal cord and usually enhance. (D) Hemangioblastomas are very vascular and avidly enhance. They can occur in the spinal cord or leptomeninges. They may be associated with endolymphatic sac tumors, renal cell carcinomas, retinal angiomas, pheochromocytomas, and cystic lesions.

7.

A Enhancing lesion involving the brainstem

Manifestations of Behçet disease in the central nervous system are varied. The brainstem is the most commonly affected, and lesions can be focal or multifocal. There usually is associated edema and contrast enhancement, particularly in the acute phase. Patients also can present with meningoencephalitis and nonspecific white matter lesions. (B) T2/FLAIR hyperintensity in the brainstem sparing the red nuclei and substantia nigra commonly is described in Wilson disease. (C) A leading edge of restricted diffusion can be seen in large or new lesions in progressive multifocal leukoencephalopathy. (D) Lesions involving the pulvinar and dorsomedial thalamic nuclei are characteristic of variant Creutzfeldt-Jakob disease. (E) Active demyelination can present with an incomplete rim of enhancement.

8.

D Meningioma

The demonstrated homogeneously enhancing dural-based mass along the left ventral aspect of the spinal canal at the level of C2 is most consistent with a meningioma. It is more common in females and, when in the spine, it most frequently occurs in the thoracic region. It nearly always is completely intradural, but also may protrude through the neural foramina, resulting in a "dumbbell" configuration and thus may look similar to schwannomas. (A) Leptomeningeal metastases usually develop along the pial surface of the cord and spinal nerves. The lesion in question is dural based. (B) Neurofibromas may be indistinguishable from schwannomas by imaging. They may show a so-called target sign with central hypointensity on T2-weighted sequences due to a fibrocollagenous core. (C) Schwannomas tend to enhance more avidly and heterogeneously than meningiomas, particularly due to the presence of cystic changes and hemorrhages in larger lesions. They follow the course of the involved nerve and do not show a dural base. Although not entirely specific, they can extrude through and expand the neural foramina, resulting in a "dumbbell" configuration.

9.

A Central tegmental tract

The axial FLAIR image accompanying the question demonstrates hyperintensity of the left inferior olivary nucleus in a patient with hypertrophic olivary degeneration. This can be caused by a lesion involving the triangle of Guillain-Mollaret, a circuit connecting the dentate, red, and inferior olivary nuclei. Efferent fibers from the dentate nucleus ascend via the superior cerebellar peduncle and decussate to the contralateral red nucleus, from which fibers project inferiorly to the ipsilateral inferior olivary nucleus through the central tegmental tract. Patients characteristically present with palatal tremors. (B) The lateral lemniscus is not part of the Guillain-Mollaret triangle. Bilateral lesions are associated with hearing loss. (C) The spinothalamic tract is a sensory pathway that transmits pain and temperature sensation from the spinal cord to the thalami. (D) The reticulospinal tract transmits information from the reticular formation in the pons and medulla to the spinal cord. It is not part of the Guillain-Mollaret triangle.

10.

B Epidural scar

The axial T2 images accompanying the question show hypointense tissue projecting into the right paracentral zone. This tissue shows diffuse enhancement on the postcontrast image, and therefore is most consistent with scar. Note the evidence of a prior right-sided laminotomy. (A, C, E) A disk protrusion or extrusion or a sequestered disk should not enhance. (D) There is no fluid collection with peripheral enhancement to suggest an epidural abscess.

11.

B Deep venous thrombosis

The sagittal noncontrast T1-weighted image *(right)* accompanying the question shows increased signal in the straight sinus, vein of Galen, and internal cerebral veins due to thrombosis. Also note the profound hypointensity of the thalami compared with the brain. The axial FLAIR image *(left)* shows marked swelling of the basal ganglia and thalami bilaterally due to venous infarction. Risk factors for deep venous thrombosis include severe dehydration and other hypercoagulable states such as pregnancy, malignancy, and sepsis. Venous infarction occurs in a nonarterial distribution and may be complicated by hemorrhage. (A) Cortical venous thrombosis may lead to lobar infarctions sparing the deep gray structures. (C) Leigh disease is a mitochondrial encephalopathy that may affect the basal ganglia, periaqueductal gray, and cerebral peduncles. Changes in the putamina seem to be a consistent feature. (D) Hypoxic ischemic encephalopathy can occur following hypoxia, such as in cardiorespiratory arrest, drowning, or various forms of asphyxiation. In older children and adults, the watershed zones initially may be affected after mild insults, with more severe cases involving gray matter structures, particularly the cerebral cortex, basal ganglia, and hippocampi. Perinatal hypoxic ischemic injury preferentially may affect the thalami, brainstem, and perirolandic cortex. There may be white matter involvement in the setting of global ischemia. (E) The imaging abnormalities in this case do not follow an arterial distribution.

12.

C Intracranial hemorrhage

There is a hemispheric subdural hematoma along the right convexity that is isodense to the cortex. This appearance can occur depending on when the patient is imaged, as the density of blood decreases over time and, at some point, will have the same attenuation as cortex. The best way to recognize such hematomas is to identify their associated mass effect and the displacement of the darker white matter, which can be seen medial to the hematoma. (A) An infiltrative tumor would involve the cortex and white matter more diffusely. The demonstrated process is centered in the extra-axial space and is subdural due to its overall crescentic shape and the fact that it crosses sutures. (B) A noncontrast head CT in acute infarct may be normal, particularly in the first 6 hours after ictus. Early findings include a hyperdense middle cerebral artery territory, loss of gray matter–white matter distinction in the basal ganglia or peripheral brain, and loss of the insular ribbon. (D) The majority of noncontrast head CT studies in meningitis are normal, and patients sometimes may present with hydrocephalus as an isolated finding. Areas of edema due to cerebritis or intra- and extra-axial abscesses may be seen in complicated meningitis. Contrast studies, in particular MRI, may be able to show the presence of leptomeningeal disease.

13.

B Rhombencephalosynapsis

Rhombencephalosynapsis is characterized by an absent vermis and midline continuation of the dentate nuclei, cerebellar hemispheres, and superior cerebellar peduncles. It can be seen in isolation or associated with other malformations such as the VACTERL spectrum and Gomez-Lopez-Hernandez syndrome. (A) Pontine tegmental cap dysplasia is a rare hindbrain malformation that includes dysplasia of the cerebellar vermis, lateralized superior cerebellar peduncles, ectopic dorsal transverse pontine fibers (tegmental cap), flattened ventral pons, absence of the inferior olives, and absence or near absence of the middle cerebellar peduncles. (C) Joubert syndrome is characterized by vermian hypoplasia or aplasia and lack of decussation of the superior cerebellar peduncles, resulting in a "molar tooth" appearance. (D) A Dandy-Walker malformation can result in cystic enlargement of the posterior fossa in communication with the fourth ventricle. The vermis is hypoplastic, but there is no continuation of the cerebellar structures.

14.

C Bullet tract crossing the deep midline structures

Various studies consistently have shown that bullet tracts crossing the midline (i.e., bihemispheric involvement) are associated with increased mortality and worse functional outcomes in those patients who survive, although there are recent data suggesting that individuals with isolated bifrontal involvement may have a relatively better prognosis. Other significant negative prognostic factors include brainstem involvement, posterior fossa injuries, transventricular injuries, low Glasgow Coma Scale score, nonreactive pupils, and older age. (A) The presence of both entry and exit wounds is not a significant predictor of worse outcomes. (B) Involvement of the inner and outer tables of the calvaria is not a significant predictor of worse outcomes. (D) The presence of bullet fragments is not a significant predictor of worse outcomes. (E) The presence of an open comminuted fracture is not a significant predictor of worse outcomes.

15.

A Globus pallidus interna

The image accompanying the question shows bilateral deep brain stimulator leads terminating in the globus pallidus interna (GPi) that are used to treat motor fluctuations in advanced medication resistant Parkinson disease or levodopa induced dyskinesia. (B) The subthalamic nuclei are an alternative target for deep brain stimulation in Parkinson disease. They are located at a lower level superior to the substantia nigra, lateral to the red nuclei, and medial to the internal capsule. (C) The ventral intermediate nuclei are located in the ventral thalami just lateral to the red nuclei. They are a common target for the treatment of essential tremors. (D) The red nuclei are paired, round T2 hypointense structures located in the rostral midbrain.

16.

C Fibromuscular dysplasia

The medial type of fibromuscular dysplasia is by far the most common and can show a "string of pearls" appearance on angiography. The same descriptor also is sometimes used for cerebral vasculitis, which can show areas of alternating segmental vascular stenoses and dilatation. (A) A "string sign" sometimes is described with severe carotid artery stenosis due to a very thin column of contrast flowing through the narrowed segment. (B) The "buzz" term for a dural arteriovenous fistula is "retrograde cortical venous drainage" or "cortical venous reflux," which is associated with more aggressive behavior and an indication for emergent treatment.

(D) Arteriovenous malformations display early draining veins and the presence of a nidus sometimes with venous or arterial aneurysms. (E) Carotid artery dissections can show a "string sign" in the narrowed segment; however, dissection of the internal carotid artery typically is associated with a "flame shape" configuration when it occurs just above the level of the carotid bulb.

17.

C Secondary to premature disjunction of the neural ectoderm

Lipomyelomeningoceles, lipomyeloceles, and lipomas are secondary to premature disjunction of the neural ectoderm from the cutaneous ectoderm. (A) Studies have not found a decreased incidence of lipomyelomeningoceles following folic acid supplementation, suggesting that the pathogenesis is different from that of other neural tube defects. (B) Open myelomeningoceles are the sine qua non of Chiari 2 malformations. Closed defects covered by skin such as this one do not result in Chiari 2 malformations. (D) The vast majority of lipomyelomeningoceles are sporadic. A few familial cases have been reported, but they are exceedingly rare.

18.

A Facial nerve

There is an avidly enhancing mass involving the right geniculate ganglion as well as the labyrinthine and canalicular segments of the right facial nerve compatible with a schwannoma. The vast majority of intracranial schwannomas arise from the vestibular nerve followed by the trigeminal and facial nerves. (B) A vestibular schwannoma would not involve the facial nerve canal or geniculate ganglion. (C) An aberrant internal carotid artery is seen more inferiorly as a more lateral extension of the internal carotid artery beyond the cochlear promontory. It may appear as a pulsating "mass" on clinical exam. (D) The inferior petrosal sinus is located along the inferior aspect of the petrous bone. It drains blood from the cavernous sinus into the jugular vein.

19.

A Meningohypophyseal trunk

The tentorial artery (of Bernasconi and Cassinari) is the most constant branch of the meningohypophyseal trunk, which in turn arises from the cavernous internal carotid artery. It is an important structure due to its vascular supply to lesions in the region of the tentorium cerebelli, such as vascular malformations and meningiomas. (B) The inferolateral trunk arises along the lateral aspect of the cavernous internal carotid artery and projects inferiorly. It usually has three or four branches and multiple anastomoses with branches of the external carotid artery. (C) The neuromeningeal trunk is a branch of the ascending pharyngeal artery and consists of jugular and hypoglossal divisions. (D) The posterior cerebral arteries most commonly arise as bifurcations of the basilar artery.

20.

D Flexion-distraction injury

The fracture demonstrated is a classic case of a severe flexion-distraction injury with a teardrop-type fracture of the anteroinferior C4 vertebra as well as distraction of the C4-C5 facets and posterior elements as can be seen on the CT images. The STIR image shows extensive edema in the posterior soft tissues including the interspinous ligaments, which are disrupted. These are highly unstable fractures associated with acute anterior cervical cord syndrome. (A) A hangman (or more correctly "hangee") fracture involves both pedicles or both partes interarticulares of C2 and is secondary to hyperextension and distraction. (B) A clay-shoveler fracture is a stable fracture involving a lower cervical vertebra (usually C7) and sometimes the upper thoracic spine. The fracture is a type of hyperflexion avulsion injury. (C) A Jefferson fracture is a burst fracture of the C1 vertebra. It is considered unstable if the combined offset of the lateral C1 masses measures more than 7 mm or if the atlantodental distance measures more than 3 mm. (E) Locked facets may be a result of a flexion-distraction injury and can result in listhesis. The C4-C5 facets in this case are mildly distracted.

21.

B Convex posterior vertebral margins

Convex posterior vertebral margins are suggestive of metastatic disease. Other features that would support this etiology are epidural or paravertebral masses or the presence of vertebral metastases at other levels. Metastases tend to involve the pedicle and posterior elements more commonly, but these sites also can show edema related to benign fractures. (A) Horizontal low signal intensity bands can be seen on both T1- and T2-weighted images and are more common in benign osteoporotic fractures. (C) Areas of spared vertebral marrow (best seen as high signal on noncontrast T1 images) are seen more commonly in benign compression fractures. (D) Retropulsion of a bone fragment is more suggestive of a benign compression fracture. (E) Both benign and pathological compression fractures can be accompanied by significant enhancement.

22.

A Trinucleotide repeat expansion

The CT shows atrophy of the heads of the caudate nuclei bilaterally, resulting in abnormal ballooning of the frontal horns of the lateral ventricles, which is consistent with Huntington disease, given the patient's clinical presentation. Huntington disease results from trinucleotide (CAG) repeat expansion in the *huntingtin* gene, which is located on chromosome 4. (B) Point mutations are modifications of a single nucleotide base and include substitutions, deletions, and insertions. (C) Frameshift mutations result from insertions, deletions, or duplications that alter the normal trinucleotide reading frame. (D) Deletions indicate of loss of genetic material and can involve individual bases or an entire gene.

23.

E Blood products

Gradient echo (GRE) sequences generate images that particularly are susceptible to magnetic field inhomogeneities such as those produced in the presence of paramagnetic blood degradation products (e.g., hemosiderin and ferritin). The presence of these products manifests as signal loss and can be used to detect hemorrhage. Dynamic susceptibility contrast MRI and functional MRI are different techniques based on GRE sequences. (A) Myelin injury is difficult to demonstrate on conventional MRI unless there is clear disruption of the white matter. Certain metrics based on advanced MRI techniques such as radial diffusivity (RD) in diffusion tensor imaging (DTI) may serve as indicators of primary myelin injury. A different technique called magnetization transfer can provide a measure of the contribution of protons that are bound to macromolecules (e.g., myelin) and has been employed in the evaluation of demyelinating disorders. (B) Diffusion-weighted imaging (DWI) with apparent diffusion coefficient (ADC) maps is very sensitive for the detection of purulence within abscesses, cavities, or the ventricular system. (C) Acute ischemia is best demonstrated with DWI and ADC maps. (D) Glucose metabolism can be assessed with positron emission tomography (PET) by using fluorodeoxyglucose (FDG).

24.

A It may be related to connective tissue disorders.

The image on the left shows somewhat crescentic and nearly circumferential mural thickening of the left vertebral artery in a patient with a sponta-

neous dissection (compare with the normal dark vascular flow void on the right). The image on the right shows cerebellar infarcts. Minor or sometimes unrecalled trauma may account for some cases of "spontaneous" dissection, and there is an increased incidence in patients with connective tissue disorders. (B) Vertebral artery dissection occurs in young and middle age adults with a mean age of presentation of 40 years of age. (C) Extradural vertebral artery dissections are more common than intradural ones. (D) Rupture is more common in intradural vertebral dissections because of a lack of external elastic lamina, fewer elastic fibers in the media, and a thinner adventitial layer.

25.

C It is associated with Morquio syndrome and multiple epiphyseal dysplasia.

An os odontoideum is a rare anomaly of the cervical spine characterized by a deformity of the odontoid process that appears as a smooth and well-corticated ossicle separated from the body of C2. There may be hypertrophy of the anterior C1 arch, as seen in this case. It may be orthotopic where the ossicle is in a relatively anatomic location with a gap between it and the body of C2, or dystopic where the ossicle is located in any other position. An increased frequency of os odontoideum has been reported in patients with multiple epiphyseal dysplasia and in Morquio, Down, and Klippel-Feil syndromes. (A) The ossicle above the body of C2 is round and features smooth, well-corticated margins; therefore, the abnormality shown is not an acute fracture. (B) Failure of fusion of the ossiculum terminale usually results in a much smaller ossicle above an overall normal-appearing odontoid process (except for a small notch at the tip). The ossiculum terminale normally fuses with the body of the dens around age 12. When persistent, it usually is asymptomatic and rarely associated with instability. (D) An os odontoideum usually is asymptomatic and, in many instances, is discovered incidentally; however, it may be associated with instability due to hypermobility of C1 over C2. This immobility may lead to spinal cord or, less frequently, vertebral artery compression. Dystopic lesions are more likely to be unstable than orthotopic lesions.

26.

A Dural venous sinus stenosis

The axial T2 image shows distention of the optic nerve sheaths and prominence of the optic cups bilaterally due to an increased intracranial pressure and papilledema in a patient with idiopathic intracranial hypertension (pseudotumor cerebri). The sagittal CISS image on the right shows an expanded and partially empty sella turcica. Additional findings in these patients include dural venous sinus stenosis, enlargement of the Meckel caves, and cerebrospinal fluid arachnoid pits in the sphenoid bones. (B) Venous sinus engorgement is seen in intracranial hypotension, not hypertension, due to decreased cerebrospinal fluid volumes (and in keeping with the Monro-Kellie doctrine). (C) Brainstem sagging is a feature of intracranial hypotension. (D) Decreased mammillopontine distance is a sign of brainstem sagging in intracranial hypotension.

27.

D Cranial nerve XII

The hypoglossal canals course along the medial and superior aspects of each occipital condyle between the basiocciput and the jugular process. They transmit cranial nerve XII, which is at high risk of injury in the presence of condylar fractures. (A) Cranial nerve IX courses through the pars nervosa of the jugular foramen along with the inferior petrosal sinus. (B, C) Cranial nerves X and XI course through the pars vascularis of the jugular foramen along with the jugular bulb.

28.

A Has a tendency for leptomeningeal spread

The axial T2 image shows a T2 hypointense mass involving the left posterior globe and left optic nerve extending posteriorly to the level of the chiasm. There are foci with even lower signal intensities within the globe consistent with hemorrhage. Although an optic glioma may cause enlargement of the optic nerve, involvement of the eye and deletion of chromosome 13q (which contains the *RB1* gene locus) indicates a diagnosis of retinoblastoma. This is a highly malignant tumor that has a tendency for leptomeningeal spread. (B) Anterior eye segment enhancement generally represents reactive angiogenesis. (C) Retinoblastomas, as with other primitive neuroectodermal tumors, commonly have profoundly low apparent diffusion coefficient values due to high cellularity and restricted diffusion. (D) The lesion shown likely has areas of low signal intensity on susceptibility-weighted imaging due to calcifications and hemorrhage.

29.

A Usually heals well with traction and immobilization

This is a type 3 fracture of the odontoid process extending from its base into the body of C2. These fractures are unstable, as they allow the odontoid process to move with the occiput as a unit; however, they have the best prognosis of all odontoid fracture types. They usually heal well with traction followed by bracing. (B) Although type 3 odontoid fractures have the best prognosis of all odontoid fracture types, they are considered unstable. (C) Type 2 odontoid process fractures are the most common. They occur across the base of the odontoid process at its junction with the body of C2. (D) Type 3 odontoid fractures occur inferior to the level of the transverse band of the cruciform ligament. (E) Type 2 odontoid process fractures are the most likely to progress to nonunion.

30.

B Carotid-cavernous fistula

The axial precontrast T1 image on the left shows a round, mixed signal intensity lesion in the left cavernous sinus. Note a subtle horizontal band at the level of the lesion propagating in the phase-encoding direction compatible with pulsation artifact. The T2 image on the right shows areas of profound hypointensity. Findings are indicative of an aneurysm, which probably is partially thrombosed. Compared with anterior and posterior circulation aneurysms, cavernous carotid aneurysms have the lowest rate of rupture (posterior circulation aneurysms have the highest). Rupture of cavernous carotid aneurysms may result in direct carotid-cavernous fistulae. (A) Malignant transformation may be seen in certain neoplasms. The lesion in this case is an aneurysm. (C) Subarachnoid hemorrhage can occur from rupture of an intradural aneurysm. (D) Posterior circulation infarcts can be the result of embolic phenomena from aneurysms located more proximally in the posterior circulation.

31.

C Deep venous drainage connotes increased surgical risk

With arteriovenous malformations, deep venous drainage, involvement of eloquent cortex, and larger nidal sizes connote an increased surgical risk and are part of the Spetzler-Martin grading system. (A) Cortical venous reflux is associated with an increased bleeding risk in patients with dural arteriovenous fistulas. The patient in this case has a pial arteriovenous malformation with a large nidus supplied from branches of the anterior and middle cerebral arteries. (B) Most arteriovenous malformations (98%) are solitary, but they rarely may be multiple particularly in patients with certain syndromes such as Osler-Weber-Rendu (who also can have microaneurysms), Wyburn-Mason, and craniofacial arteriovenous metameric syndromes (CAMS). Klippel-Trenaunay-Weber syndrome is characterized by capillary, venous, and lymphatic malformations as well as soft tissue and osseous hypertrophy. (D) Most arteriovenous malformations (75%) have a primary pial blood supply from the internal carotid artery; 15% have dual supply from the external carotid artery; 10% receive blood from both the internal and external carotid arteries.

32.

B Frequently associated with diving head first into shallow water

This is a burst fracture of C1 (also known as Jefferson fracture) that develops due to axial loading transmitted through the occipital condyles into the C1 vertebra and is seen frequently after diving head first into shallow water. Jefferson fractures tend to be stable, and neurologic deficits are infrequent unless there is disruption of the transverse ligament, fractures at other levels, or injury to the vertebral arteries. Disruption of the transverse ligament is suspected if there is widening of the atlantodens interval (normally less than 3 mm in adults and 5 mm in children) or if the combined offset of the lateral masses of C1 relative to the lateral C2 pillars measures greater than 6 mm. If the transverse ligament is disrupted, stability depends on the alar ligaments connecting the dens with the medial aspect of the occipital condyles. (A) Combined offset of the lateral C1 masses relative to C2 greater than 6 mm suggests disruption of the transverse ligament and raises concern about an unstable fracture. (C) Jefferson fractures have a low frequency of neurologic injury unless there is disruption of the transverse ligament, fractures at other levels, or injury to the vertebral arteries. (D) Jefferson fractures are extremely rare in infants and young children, probably due to the plasticity of their bones and the presence of soft synchondroses. (E) These fractures usually are managed conservatively unless they are unstable.

33.

C Remote injury

The area of hypoattenuation in the left frontal lobe is consistent with encephalomalacia. It demonstrates very low attenuation and is associated with volume loss, as can be seen by ex vacuo expansion of the frontal horn of the left lateral ventricle. This likely is secondary to remote trauma, infarction, or other injury. This patient also has an acute, right frontal, extra-axial hematoma. (A, B) Acute or subacute infarction or cortical contusion would not be associated with volume loss, and the lesion margins would likely be less well defined. (D) A neoplasm would show some degree of mass effect and may have surrounding edema. (E) There is no fluid collection or evidence of vasogenic edema to suggest an abscess.

34.

C Subacute combined degeneration

Subacute combined degeneration is caused by vitamin B12 deficiency, and leads to demyelination and vacuolization of the dorsal columns of the spinal cord with or without involvement of the lateral columns. It most commonly occurs in the upper thoracic and cervical cord. MRI shows T2 signal hyperintensity with rare contrast enhancement. Subacute combined degeneration can be exacerbated or caused by nitrous oxide toxicity, which temporarily interrupts metabolism of B12. (A) There is no evidence of a space-occupying lesion to suggest a neoplasm. Ependymomas tend to occur centrally within the spinal cord, and cysts, hemorrhage, and calcifications are common findings. (B) Neuromyelitis optica results in greater cord expansion than demonstrated in the image and usually is more central and not confined to the dorsal columns. (D) Infectious myelitis is rare, and imaging may show edema that is not confined to the dorsal columns.

35.

B Invasive fungal infection

The "black turbinate" sign refers to nonenhancing nasal mucosa due to tissue infarction, and has been described in angioinvasive fungal infections.

The skull base findings in this case are secondary to fungal osteomyelitis. (A) Bacterial infection can lead to osteomyelitis of the skull base but does not result in a "black turbinate" sign. (C) Nasopharyngeal carcinoma can invade the skull base but does not produce a "black turbinate" sign. (D) Osseous infarctions can present with mixed signal intensities on T2-weighted MRI sequences due to areas of edema and sclerosis and irregular enhancement. Skull base infarcts are rare but occur more commonly in patients with sickle cell disease, in which case they can be complicated by osteomyelitis.

36.

B Failure of diverticulation

These images show nonseparation of the frontal lobes and an azygous anterior cerebral artery in a patient with lobar holoprosencephaly. These occur secondary to the failure of diverticulation and cleavage of the prosencephalon during embryonic life. Holoprosencephaly represents a spectrum of abnormalities, with the alobar form being the most severe and commonly presenting with a monoventricle, thalamic fusion, and facial anomalies. (A) Failure of closure of the rostral neuropore leads to anencephaly. (C) Nondisjunction of the neural tube can result in open spinal dysraphisms. (D) Premature disjunction of the neural tube can lead to lipomyeloceles, lipomeningoceles, and lipomyelomeningoceles.

37.

A Atypical teratoid rhabdoid tumor

Atypical teratoid rhabdoid tumors and other embryonal tumors as well as medulloblastomas are highly malignant and typically show the lowest apparent diffusion coefficient (ADC) values due to their high cellularity. (B) Juvenile pilocytic astrocytomas are WHO grade I tumors that do not show significant restricted diffusion. (C) Ependymomas may show variable degrees of restricted diffusion, but their ADC values typically are higher than those of embryonal tumors. (D) Dysembryoplastic neuroepithelial tumors are benign glioneuronal neoplasms (WHO grade I) that do not show restricted diffusion; therefore, their ADC values are high. (E) Diffuse astrocytomas are WHO grade II lesions that do not show significant restricted diffusion.

38.

D It is typically a monophasic process.

Acute demyelinating encephalomyelitis (ADEM) usually is a monophasic process, but some patients are at an increased risk of recurrence (defined as a new event after 3 months) or the development of multiple sclerosis. (A) Approximately 75% of cases of ADEM occur after viral and less commonly bacterial (e.g., *Campylobacter*) infections. (B) The deep gray nuclei (particularly the thalami) are involved in 60% of patients with ADEM. These structures are involved less commonly in multiple sclerosis. (C) Only 25% of ADEM lesions show contrast enhancement. There usually is no mass effect except for cases of tumefactive demyelination, which also may be accompanied by a leading edge of restricted diffusion.

39.

A Adrenoleukodystrophy

The presentation and imaging findings are consistent with X-linked adrenoleukodystrophy. This disease typically occurs in 4- to 6-year-old boys and is caused by mutations in the *ABCD1* gene, leading to accumulation of very long chain fatty acids. Death or progression to a vegetative state usually occurs 2 years after symptom onset. (B) Canavan disease is caused by mutations in the *ASPA* gene on chromosome 17. It results in macrocephaly, with imaging showing sequelae of white matter demyelination and signal abnormalities in the globi pallidi and thalami. (C) Alexander disease is caused by mutations in the *GFAP* gene on chromosome 17. It is characterized by demyelination that progresses from anterior to posterior. Patients have astrocytic Rosenthal fibers and macrocephaly. (D Krabbe disease results from mutations in the *GALC* gene on chromosome 14 and leads to the deficiency of galactocerebroside β-galactosidase. The condition most commonly is diagnosed between the third and sixth months of life. Imaging shows abnormalities in the white matter, basal ganglia, cerebellum, and corticospinal tracts. (E) Pelizaeus-Merzbacher disease is an X-linked recessive disorder characterized by oligodendrocyte dysfunction leading to hypomyelination. Patients usually are males and present with nystagmus, seizures, hypotonia, and ataxia. On MRI, there is diffuse T2 signal hyperintensity in the white matter due to hypomyelination (myelinated white matter is dark on T2 and bright on T1 sequences).

40.

D Subacute combined degeneration

Subacute combined degeneration can be caused by vitamin B12, copper, or vitamin E deficiencies. It results in an abnormal signal within the dorsal columns of the spinal cord in an inverse V-shaped configuration with variable involvement of the lateral columns. Abuse of nitrous oxide can produce the same syndrome through inactivation of vitamin B12. Neurosyphilis (tabes dorsalis) is also known to involve the dorsal columns. (A) Poliomyelitis may show an abnormal signal and enhancement of anterior horn cells as well as ventral roots of the cauda equina if accompanied by radiculitis. (B) Amyotrophic lateral sclerosis preferentially involves the anterior and lateral columns of the spinal cord, which may show increased T2 signal. (C) Guillain-Barré syndrome presents with preferential pial enhancement of the conus medullaris and dorsal roots of the cauda equina. It should not be associated with intramedullary signal abnormalities.

41.

D Capillary telangiectasia

The imaging description of this lesion and its location are characteristic of capillary telangiectasias. Low signal on gradient echo (GRE) sequences is thought to be related to slow flow and increased deoxyhemoglobin content. These lesions sometimes can have areas of gliosis, and they nearly always are asymptomatic and found incidentally. (A) A demyelinating plaque does not show the constellation of features described, which are characteristic of capillary telangiectasias. (B) Capillary telangiectasias should be differentiated from metastases. The latter usually have surrounding edema (except for small lesions) and do not show signal loss on GRE sequences unless they are hemorrhagic, melanotic, or calcified. (C) Cavernous malformations may show various signal intensities depending on the stage of their blood products. They typically are described as having a "popcorn" or "berry" appearance with a surrounding rim of hemosiderin.

42.

A Between meningeal branches of the external carotid artery and cavernous sinus

Carotid cavernous fistulas can be direct or indirect. Direct fistulas (Barrow type A) develop between the cavernous internal carotid artery and cavernous sinus and are therefore high flow. They are more frequent in younger males and occur secondary to trauma or rupture of a cavernous internal carotid aneurysm. Types B, C, and D occur between meningeal branches of the internal or external carotid arteries, are slow flow, and are most frequently seen in women older than 50 years of age. A type C carotid cavernous fistula occurs between meningeal branches of the external carotid artery and cavernous sinus. (B) A Barrow type B fistula occurs between meningeal branches of the internal carotid artery and cavernous sinus. (C) A Barrow type A fistula occurs directly between the cavernous internal carotid artery and cavernous sinus. (D) A Barrow type D fistula occurs between meningeal branches of both the external and internal carotid arteries and cavernous sinus.

43.

E Associated with a risk of malignant transformation

T2, FLAIR, and diffusion-weighted imaging (DWI) MRI sequences are presented showing an epidermoid cyst. These lesions are characterized by very bright DWI signal (presumably a combination of restricted diffusion and T2 shine-through effect), lack of contrast enhancement, and nonsuppression on FLAIR. Epidermoid cysts arise from ectodermal inclusions during neural tube closure and rarely can degenerate into squamous cell carcinomas. (A) Arachnoid cysts and not epidermoid cysts are lined by arachnoid cells, resulting in accumulation of cerebrospinal fluid. (B) Up to 50% of epidermoid cysts are located in the cerebellopontine angle, although they uncommonly may arise within the ventricles. (C) Although signal in epidermoid cysts may resemble cerebrospinal fluid on T2, they do not suppress on FLAIR as demonstrated in the second image. The signal of epidermoid cysts on FLAIR sometimes has been described as "dirty" appearing and used to be the main imaging discriminator for diagnosis before DWI was available. This is in contradistinction to arachnoid cysts, which do suppress on FLAIR and follow cerebrospinal fluid signal on all sequences. (D) Although there sometimes can be minimal marginal contrast enhancement, epidermoid cysts should not show patchy or any significant enhancement, which would be suspicious for malignant transformation.

44.

C Pilocytic astrocytoma

A well-circumscribed cystic mass with an avidly enhancing mural nodule in the cerebellum most likely is a juvenile pilocytic astrocytoma in a patient of this age, which has a peak incidence between 5 and 15 years of age. Despite its classification as

WHO grade I, a pilocytic astrocytoma shows avid contrast enhancement of the solid components and paradoxically may exhibit aggressive-appearing imaging characteristics, with a metabolite pattern mimicking a high-grade lesion on MR spectroscopy (increased choline, decreased N-acetylaspartate, and increased lactate) and increased metabolism on 18F-fluorodeoxyglucose PET studies. A pilocytic astrocytoma most commonly occurs in the cerebellum followed by the optic nerve and chiasm (particularly when syndromic in neurofibromatosis type 1) and around the third ventricle and hypothalamus. It is a slow-growing tumor and most commonly presents with manifestations of increased intracranial pressure (such as in this case where there is hydrocephalus) and cerebellar signs. (A) Medulloblastomas usually occur in patients younger than 5 years of age but may be seen in older individuals. They have low apparent diffusion coefficient (ADC) values, and therefore appear dark on the ADC maps (in contrast to this case, where the solid component of the tumor is bright). Medulloblastomas arise from the superior medullary velum and fill the fourth ventricle rather than displace it. (B) Ependymomas arise from the floor of the fourth ventricle and fill it rather than displace it, in contrast to the tumor of this case. Ependymomas characteristically extrude through the ventricular outflow tracts into the foramen magnum and posterior fossa with a "plastic" or "toothpaste" appearance. They also tend to be seen in younger patients with a peak incidence between 1 and 5 years of age, although there is a smaller peak in young adults later in life. Cystic changes would be an unusual finding in ependymomas. (D) Hemangioblastomas more commonly present in adults and are rare in children unless they are syndromic (peak at 40 to 60 years of age). They also can present as a cystic mass with an enhancing mural nodule that typically abuts the pial surface, and they often have prominent flow voids due to hypervascularity. They may be associated with von Hippel–Lindau syndrome, but most are sporadic. (E) Some metastases may present with cystic changes, particularly from squamous cell primaries such as in head and neck, lung, and cervical cancers. Metastases, in general, are the most common cerebellar tumor in adults. They would be unexpected in a patient of this age.

45.

B Acute infarction

Noncontrast CT and diffusion-weighted images are presented, and the distribution of the abnormality and presence of restricted diffusion are most compatible with an acute posterior inferior cerebellar artery (PICA) territory infarct. PICA infarcts may be associated with significant mass effect in the posterior fossa and herniation with rapid deterioration and death. Although they can present with specific neurologic syndromes (such as lateral or medial medullary syndromes), symptoms can be vague and nonspecific, and sometimes may be confused with labyrinthitis or gastroenteritis. (A) Hemorrhagic or high-grade primary neoplasms may result in areas of restricted diffusion due to blood products or high cellularity, respectively; however, they would be expected to be more heterogeneous and would not preserve the cerebellar architecture as in this case (note that some of the folia still can be defined on the diffusion image). Additionally, the vascular distribution of the abnormality and the evolution of symptoms over a few hours are compatible with a PICA territory infarct. (C) Approximately 50% of intracranial metastases may be solitary; however, findings in this case argue against a metastatic lesion. (D) Although the lesion presented is hypodense on CT, it is intra-axial and demonstrates restricted diffusion, both of which rule out an arachnoid cyst. (E) Epidermoid cysts can show restricted diffusion, and some can be intra-axial; however, in this case, the vascular distribution is characteristic of a PICA infarct.

46.

C Global anoxic injury

This is a case of diffuse cerebral edema/global anoxic injury. The noncontrast head CT shows effacement of the cerebral sulci, small ventricles, loss of the gray matter–white matter distinction, lack of definition of the deep gray nuclei, and effacement of the basal cisterns. (A) A ruptured intradural cerebral aneurysm would result in subarachnoid hemorrhage. The hyperdense appearance of the suprasellar cistern in this case often is referred to as "pseudosubarachnoid hemorrhage" and is due to the relative hypodensity of the swollen brain parenchyma and cisternal effacement. (B) Acute arterial infarction would lead to edema and mass effect in a territorial distribution. (D) Venous thrombosis may or may not result in ischemia that sometimes can become hemorrhagic. Findings that can be seen on CT include a hyperdense clot within the dilated vein (cord sign), cortical/subcortical edema (when cortical veins are involved), and deep gray matter edema (when deep draining veins are involved and often occurring bilaterally).

47.

A Glioma

This is a case of neurofibromatosis type 1. The provided images show dysplasia of the left sphenoid bone with ipsilateral proptosis as well as a diffuse, nodular, and trans-spatial lesion involving the left head, face, neck, and parapharyngeal tissues compatible with plexiform neurofibromata. A central T2 dark spot may be seen within some of these lesions (the "target sign") and is considered highly suggestive of neurofibromas. Approximately 15% of children with neurofibromatosis type 1 develop optic nerve gliomas, and they are also at an increased risk of developing gliomas in other regions of the brain. In addition, 4% of patients with neurofibromatosis type 1 develop peripheral malignant nerve sheath tumors. (B, C) Multiple inherited schwannomas, meningiomas, and ependymomas (MISME syndrome) are features of neurofibromatosis type 2 and not type 1. (D) Endolymphatic sac tumors are very rare neoplasms that can occur sporadically and have been reported to develop in 10 to 15% of patients with von Hippel–Lindau syndrome. (E) Almost all subependymal giant cell tumors are seen in the setting of tuberous sclerosis.

48.

D Less common cerebral edema

Epidural empyemas are associated less frequently with cerebral edema due to the presence of thick intervening dura between the collection and the brain. (A) Both epidural and subdural hematomas show restricted diffusion. (B) Similar to subdural hematomas, a crescentic shape is more consistent with a subdural hematoma, whereas epidural collections characteristically have a biconvex or lenticular shape. Note that subdural empyemas and hematomas sometimes can show a lenticular shape particularly if they are loculated. (C) Epidural collections including empyemas and hematomas do not cross sutures due to the firm dural attachments at these sites. (E) Both subdural and epidural empyemas enhance peripherally.

49.

A Extension beyond the lateral intercarotid line

Extension beyond the lateral intercarotid line, as measured on coronal images, is highly suggestive of cavernous sinus invasion by a pituitary adenoma with a positive predictive value of 85%. Other findings include obliteration of the carotid venous sulcus compartment (the space between the sphenoid bone and the ipsilateral cavernous internal carotid artery) with a positive predictive value of 95% and internal carotid artery encasement of ≥ 67% (about 240 degrees) with a positive predictive value of 100%. (B) Carotid encasement of ≥ 67% has been associated with the highest likelihood of ipsilateral cavernous sinus invasion. (C) Obliteration of the superior venous compartment is not significantly associated with cavernous sinus invasion. (D) Obliteration of the inferolateral venous compartment is not significantly associated with cavernous sinus invasion.

50.

A Fibromuscular dysplasia predisposes to an increased risk of direct-type lesions.

The angiogram shows early opacification of the cavernous sinus compatible with a carotid cavernous fistula. This is most evident on the left side, where the ophthalmic vein also can be seen. These lesions result from either a direct communication between the carotid artery and cavernous sinus (direct or high-flow fistulas; Barrow type A) or between the cavernous sinus and dural branches of the internal carotid artery, external carotid artery, or both (indirect, low flow, and dural fistulas; Barrow types B, C, and D, respectively). Other than trauma and aneurysmal rupture, conditions associated with direct carotid cavernous fistulas include fibromuscular dysplasia, Ehlers-Danlos syndrome, and pseudoxanthoma elasticum. (B) Spontaneous parenchymal or subarachnoid hemorrhage can be seen in direct fistulas, particularly when there is retrograde cortical venous flow, and occurs in about 5% of cases. Bruits and visual manifestations are much more common. (C) Direct (not dural type) fistulas commonly present with a subjective bruit (about 85% of cases) that sometimes also may be auscultated. (D) Venous thrombosis is a known mechanism in the development of some carotid cavernous fistulas; however, by far the most common etiologies of direct fistulas are trauma and aneurysm rupture. (E) Dural fistulas most commonly present in middle-aged and elderly women. Traumatic direct fistulas are more common in young males.

51.

E Usually shows minimal to no contrast enhancement

Subependymomas are benign, slow-growing neoplasms classified as WHO grade I. They typically show minimal to no contrast enhancement; however, this is variable, as some subependymomas may enhance more prominently, particularly those located in the fourth ventricle. They may have microcystic changes (both on histological examination and on MRI), are well circumscribed, are noninvasive, and may contain foci of calcification. The classic location in the fourth ventricle is at the obex, although they can occur anywhere in the ventricular system. (A) Subependymomas are highly resectable neoplasms. Recurrence is rare and usually related to incomplete excision. (B) Subependymomas present most commonly in middle-aged and elderly adults, with a peak incidence in the fifth and sixth decades of life. Symptomatic patients may present earlier with signs of intracranial hypertension. (C) Hemorrhage may occur with subependymomas, but it is a rare event. (D) Subependymomas are not associated with *TSC-1* or *TSC-2* mutations, in contrast to the subependymal giant cell astrocytomas of tuberous sclerosis.

52.

A They are most common in basal ganglia and dentate nuclei.

The focal areas of signal intensity (FASI) or unidentified bright objects (UBOs) are thought to represent myelin vacuolization in patients with neurofibromatosis type 1. They are most common in the basal ganglia, dentate nuclei, and brainstem. (B–D) These lesions are not premalignant, and many regress in adulthood. They do not show contrast enhancement or mass effect, the presence of which should raise concern about a glioma.

53.

B Diffusion weighted

The two most important sequences in the evaluation of a cerebral abscess are contrast-enhanced T1-weighted sequences and diffusion-weighted imaging (DWI). An abscess usually shows a relatively smooth and homogeneous enhancing wall that often (but not always) is thicker on the side of the gray matter and thinner toward the ventricles and white matter. Pus within an abscess almost always shows prominent restricted diffusion, which is reflected as bright signal on DWI and corresponding dark signal on apparent diffusion coefficient (ADC) maps. (A) Susceptibility-weighted

imaging (SWI) is a gradient echo–based technique that is exquisitely sensitive for the detection of paramagnetic and diamagnetic substances such as ferritin, calcium, hemosiderin, and deoxyhemoglobin. The capsule of an abscess may appear dark on SWI or T2, presumably due to the presence of paramagnetic free radicals within macrophages. (C) Time of flight is an MR angiography technique that does not routinely require the administration of contrast material and is based on the flow-related enhancement of spins entering an imaging slice in one direction. (D) Constructive interference in steady state (CISS) is an MRI technique that is based on consecutive steady-state free precession (SSFP) sequences. It produces images that have very high T2 signal and therefore excellent contrast between fluid and parenchyma. (E) Fluid-attenuated inversion recovery (FLAIR) is a pulse sequence that uses an inversion recovery technique to null the signal of simple fluid.

54.

C Hemangioma

These CT images show the characteristic imaging features of a vertebral hemangioma with vertical trabeculations on the sagittal image and a corresponding "polka dot" appearance on the axial image. Note the preservation of the cortex despite the presence of the trabeculations; however, also remember that hemangiomas can be aggressive and may present with extraosseous soft tissue extension and mass effect on the spinal cord or nerves. On MRI, they usually are bright on both T1 and T2 sequences due to the presence of a fatty stroma, although atypical (predominantly vascular) hemangiomas may be dark on T1 and simulate metastases. Approximately 30% of hemangiomas are multiple. (A) Metastasis would result in variable degrees of marrow replacement and osseous destruction without the vertical trabecular pattern of a hemangioma. (B) Paget disease is associated with expansion of the bone; in the spine, the involved vertebra often appears larger than the ones above and below it. Paget disease also presents with cortical thickening and would not show a uniform, vertical trabecular pattern. (D) Plasmacytomas cause osseous destruction and do not respect the trabeculae.

55.

B Synovial cyst

The axial T2 image shows a well-circumscribed, cystic-appearing, extradural mass, with its base along a degenerated and hypertrophied left facet joint, which is compatible with a synovial cyst. In this case, the cyst impinges on the left descending nerve roots, which explains the patient's symptoms. The morphology of the cyst and its anatomic relationship with a degenerated facet joint are more important than the signal of its contents, which may vary depending on the presence of hemorrhage or proteinaceous material. Synovial cysts can contain gas, and their walls may show enhancement or calcification. They most commonly develop in patients older than 60 years of age and are more common in females; 90% occur in the lumbar spine. (A) In this case, the open base of the lesion is centered along the facet rather than the disk, and the T2 bright contents also seem to communicate with the facet joint. Additionally, the lesion has a convex, well-circumscribed margin anteriorly. These features make a synovial cyst the right diagnosis; however, note that disk material can separate from the parent disk and migrate virtually anywhere within the epidural space. (C) Cysts also can originate from the ligamenta flava; however, the lesion in this case is centered along the facet joint. (D) The uncovertebral joints form between the uncus and uncinate processes of the cervical spine between C3 and C7. There are no uncovertebral joints in the lumbar spine. Additionally, hypertrophied bone and osteophytes would look dark on T2 and not bright as in this lesion.

56.

B It is composed of radially arranged medullary veins emptying into a dilated draining vein.

This image shows radially arranged medullary veins in a "caput medusae" configuration emptying into a dilated draining vein compatible with a developmental venous anomaly (also known as a venous angioma). These lesions usually are benign and constitute an incidental finding in the majority of cases, although rarely they may thrombose. Some reports have described seizures, headaches, and hemorrhage, but the association of venous angiomas and these manifestations has not been established firmly. Approximately 20 to 30% of these lesions are associated with cavernous malformations, which may explain symptoms in at least some cases. The majority of developmental venous anomalies are isolated, but they also can be multiple particularly when associated with the blue rubber bleb nevus syndrome. Blood oxygen level dependent (BOLD) imaging sequences, such as susceptibility-weighted imaging (SWI), are the preferred modality for their detection, as these lesions may be missed on other sequences due to their slow flow. (A) Developmental venous anomalies have a characteristic appearance on angiography, showing exclusive enhancement in the venous phase, although sometimes a faint blush may be evident in the late arterial phase. Angiographically occult vascular lesions include capillary telangiectasias and cavernous malformations. (C) High flow from shunting may result in flow-related aneurysms in arteriovenous malformations. There is no arteriovenous shunting in developmental venous anomalies. (D) A larger nidus is associated with an increased surgical risk in arteriovenous malformations and upgrades these lesions in the Spetzler–Martin grading system.

57.

D Renal cell carcinoma

The MRI shows a heterogeneously enhancing destructive lesion in the left petrous bone. There are areas of intrinsic T1 hyperintensity secondary to hemorrhage, proteinaceous contents, or cholesterol. The appearance and location are suggestive of an endolymphatic sac tumor, particularly in a patient presenting with spontaneous retinal detachment, which may be seen in von Hippel–Lindau (VHL) syndrome due to hemorrhage from retinal capillary hemangioblastomas; 15% of patients with VHL develop an endolymphatic sac tumor, and 40 to 70% of them ultimately develop renal cell carcinoma, the incidence of which increases with age. (A) Lisch nodules are the most common ocular lesions in neurofibromatosis type 1. They are not associated with VHL syndrome. (B) Bilateral vestibular schwannomas are diagnostic of neurofibromatosis type 2. (C) Subependymal giant cell astrocytomas occur in patients with tuberous sclerosis complex secondary to mutations in the *TSC-1* or *TSC-2* genes, although isolated tumors rarely have been described. These tumors are not associated with VHL. (E) Low levels of serum ceruloplasmin result in an abnormal accumulation of copper in Wilson disease.

58.

B Frequently accompanied by microcephaly and other cerebral anomalies

This is a case of "open lip" (type 2) schizencephaly, which may result from a variety of insults in utero (including infection and ischemia)

that affect the germinal zone during cortical development and lead to abnormal neuronal migration. There also has been an association with *COL4A1* and *COL4A2* mutations. Schizencephaly manifests as a transmantle cleft lined by dysplastic gray matter (not white matter) that connects the subarachnoid space with the ventricular system (pia to ependyma). It has been associated with various anomalies including gray matter heterotopia, polymicrogyria, absence of the septum pellucidum, and frontal lobe dysplasia. Approximately 80% of cases are "open lip" and the rest are "closed-lip." (A) Schizencephaly is lined by dysplastic gray matter and not white matter, as would be the case in porencephalic cysts. (C) Schizencephaly is lined by dysplastic gray matter and not endodermal endothelium, which would be the case in a neurenteric cyst. (D) A schizencephalic cleft openly communicates with the subarachnoid and intraventricular spaces, and therefore follows cerebrospinal fluid signal on all sequences. Cysts with proteinaceous (e.g., neurenteric cysts) or hemorrhagic contents may show variable signal intensities. (E) A bilateral vascular insult to the anterior and middle cerebral arteries in utero would lead to hydranencephaly and destruction of parenchyma in these territories with preservation of the posterior circulation; however, large bilateral schizencephaly with hydrocephalus may be difficult to differentiate from hydranencephaly. Some authors suspect that they may be part of a continuum.

59.

B Chordoma

Skull base chordomas most commonly present in patients between 20 and 40 years of age, but 16% occur in patients younger than 18 years of age. Location in the lower clivus with associated osseous erosion is typical. On MRI, they demonstrate very bright T2 signal, presumably related to mucinous contents along with thin T2 dark fibrous septations. They show moderate to marked enhancement often along the septations in a "honeycomb" configuration. Skull base chordomas carry a poor prognosis, worse than that for chondrosarcomas. (A) Chondrosarcomas have imaging features similar to those for chordomas, but they more often occur off midline and centered at the petroclival fissure, and may be accompanied by calcified chondroid matrix. Chondrosarcomas are unusual at this age. (C) Nasopharyngeal carcinoma is rare at this age; it would have a more infiltrative appearance, and it is not as bright on T2 sequences. Additionally, the nasopharyngeal mucosa is preserved in this case, and the tumor is centered at the skull base, resulting in anterior deviation of the prevertebral muscles as seen on the axial images. (D) Meningiomas can invade bone but tend to do so more diffusely. They also are not as bright on T2 sequences (unless there are areas of degeneration) and tend to show more homogeneous enhancement without the honeycomb appearance of this case. They are rare in children unless associated with a syndrome. (E) Lymphoma can arise from lymphoid tissue in the nasopharynx and extend to the skull base; however, the nasopharyngeal mucosa in this case is preserved. Lymphoma also usually enhances more avidly and homogeneously.

60.

A Cholesterol granuloma

This is a well-circumscribed, expansile lesion centered in the left petrous apex. It does not enhance, and it shows intrinsic T1 brightness as well as T2 dark material within it, corresponding to blood products. There is no restricted diffusion as demonstrated by increased signal on the apparent diffusion coefficient (ADC) map. Findings are compatible with a cholesterol granuloma. These are benign lesions related to repeated middle ear infections. They contain cholesterol crystals, lipids, and fluid and are prone to recurrent hemorrhage. Cholesterol granulomas can occur anywhere in the temporal bone where there are mucosa-lined aerated cells, and rarely have been reported in the paranasal sinuses. (B) Cholesteatomas can occur in this location but show restricted diffusion (they would be dark on ADC and bright on diffusion-weighted imaging) and usually are not bright on T1. (C) Trapped secretions within pneumatized petrous cells sometimes can show intrinsic T1 brightness due to proteinaceous contents, but they would not result in an expansile mass. The normal trabeculae should be preserved, although this is difficult to visualize on MRI. (D) A trigeminal schwannoma would show enhancement and would follow the course of the cranial nerve sometimes with involvement of the Meckel cave.

61.

E Flexion and distraction

The sagittal CT image shows a compression fracture involving a midthoracic vertebra with a fracture line extending posteriorly across the spinous process above. This is consistent with a Chance fracture, which features a horizontal fracture orientation through the entire spinal column and is a result of a flexion and distraction injury. These fractures usually are associated with lap belts. Neurologic injury is rare, but there is an increased frequency of intra-abdominal injuries. Up to 25% of Chance fractures may be purely ligamentous. (A) Extreme lateral bending can result in a lateral compression fracture or, potentially, a fracture of the transverse processes. Avulsion fractures of the transverse processes in the lumbar spine also can occur due to abrupt contraction of the psoas muscles. (B) Axial rotation can lead to facet dislocations, particularly in the cervical spine. (C) Abrupt extension of the neck can disrupt the anterior longitudinal ligament and result in an extension teardrop fracture, which is an unstable injury. (D) Axial loading can lead to burst or compression fractures of the anterior column if the injury occurs during flexion.

62.

A Presence of lactate and amino acids on MR spectroscopy

The images in this case show an intra-axial lesion with peripheral enhancement and increased signal on diffusion-weighted imaging (DWI). Although apparent diffusion coefficient (ADC) maps are not presented, the degree of brightness in the center of the lesion on DWI is high enough that this is expected to represent restricted diffusion and would therefore look dark on ADC maps. These findings essentially are diagnostic of an abscess; a few rare cases of necrotic metastases with central restricted diffusion have been reported. Abscesses can show various amino acids on MR spectroscopy, including alanine, valine, leucine, and succinate as well as lactate and lipid peaks. Of note, necrotic primary or metastatic tumors also may show lactate and lipid peaks. (B) The capsule of a cerebral abscess usually is iso- to hypointense on T2-weighted sequences. This is attributed to the presence of collagen, blood products, or free radicals generated by phagocytosing macrophages. (C) The necrotic center of an abscess demonstrates significant restricted diffusion that manifests as very bright signal on DWI and low ADC values. (D) The capsule of an abscess typically has lower relative cerebral blood volume (rCBV) relative to white matter. Glioblastomas, which may look similar to abscesses, have been associated with high rCBV ratios in the capsule.

63.

D Paget disease

The etiology of Paget disease is not entirely certain. Its hallmark is excessive bone remodeling and overgrowth and is defined by three stages: lytic, mixed, and sclerotic. The spine and skull are the most common sites of involvement followed by the pelvis. The presence of pain or focal destructive lesions on imaging should raise concern for sarcomatous degeneration. (A) Multiple myeloma characteristically shows numerous lucent (lytic) lesions throughout the calvaria that may result in a "punched out" appearance. (B) Bone marrow hyperplasia in β-thalassemia can lead to significant skull thickening often showing a so-called hair-on-end appearance. It would not produce the lucent and sclerotic pattern of this case. (C) Prostate cancer metastases typically are osteoblastic (sclerotic) and can be diffuse; however, they do not result in the mixed lytic/sclerotic geographic pattern of this case. Note on the provided images that, despite the diffuse involvement of the calvaria, the inner and outer tables are relatively preserved.

64.

B Posterior communicating artery aneurysm

The image shown is a lateral projection of a digital subtraction angiogram following a carotid artery injection. It shows a vascular outpouching projecting posteriorly from the dorsal aspect of the C7 (communicating or terminal) segment of the internal carotid artery at the expected origin of the posterior communicating artery. Aneurysms in this location represent about 30% of all ruptured intracranial aneurysms and may result in intraparenchymal hemorrhage, typically in the mesial temporal lobe. Patients may present with subarachnoid hemorrhage or a third cranial nerve palsy due to mass effect. (C) This is a carotid injection and thus does not depict the posterior circulation and basilar tip. (D) The ophthalmic artery arises from the C6 (ophthalmic or supraclinoid) segment of the internal carotid artery and projects anteriorly.

65.

B Increased relative cerebral blood volumes

Studies have shown that recurrent tumor has a higher relative cerebral blood volume (rCBV) normalized to the contralateral white matter compared with radiation necrosis, although there is some overlap. rCBV values greater than 2.6 have been suggested as a cutoff for the presence of recurrent tumor, and values lower than 0.6 suggest pseudoprogression. (A) Several studies show that recurrent tumor tends to have lower apparent diffusion coefficient (ADC) values compared with radiation necrosis. ADC ratios related to the contralateral white matter appear to be more accurate than absolute ADC values. (C) A "cut green pepper," "soap bubble," or "Swiss cheese" appearance has been described in radiation necrosis, although this usually does not allow reliable discrimination between these processes. (D) Decreased FDG uptake on PET favors radiation necrosis. False negatives may occur in the presence of a large area of necrosis.

66.

C HIV encephalopathy

HIV encephalopathy is the most common central nervous system infection related to the HIV virus. Although the incidence of frank dementia has decreased substantially following the advent of highly active antiretroviral therapy, the prevalence of mild to moderate cognitive deficits in this population has increased and probably is at least partially related to longer survival. Note the prominent cerebral volume loss for the patient's age, lack of mass effect, and symmetric confluent white matter signal abnormalities that spare the U fibers. (A) Lymphoma would have some degree of mass effect and would be more focal than the image demonstrates. Lymphoma in patients with HIV/AIDS commonly has central necrosis, whereas lymphoma occurring in the nonimmunocompromised population is diffusely solid and enhances homogeneously. (B) Progressive multifocal leukoencephalopathy usually is bilateral but asymmetric. When there are subcortical signal abnormalities, they virtually always involve the U fibers; note that these are spared in this case and are seen as dark gray bands between the cortex and the bright white matter lesions. (D) Cerebritis would present with variable degrees of gray and white matter edema.

67.

D Flexion/extension sequences

Flexion/extension sequences are important in the evaluation of Hirayama disease (monomelic amyotrophy), as they would demonstrate detachment and anterior displacement of the dura on neck flexion, with resultant spinal cord compression and myelopathy. Hirayama disease is a benign and self-limiting disease that usually occurs in patients between 15 and 25 years of age. (A) Gradient echo sequences in the spine are useful to differentiate disks from osteophytes and to demonstrate foci of hemorrhage within the cord. These sequences also are less prone to cerebrospinal fluid pulsation artifact. (B) Routine postcontrast sequences help delineate the enhancing epidural space in Hirayama disease and may facilitate identification of the dura. Delayed contrast sequences are not particularly helpful. (C) Diffusion-weighted sequences are technically difficult to acquire in the spine. They may be useful in the evaluation of acute spinal cord ischemia and spinal infection.

68.

B Tuberculous spondylitis

Tuberculous spondylitis (also known as Pott disease) originates in the end plates and typically spreads in a subligamentous fashion to involve the adjacent vertebrae, frequently, but not always, sparing the intervertebral disks, as seen in this case. The provided contrast-enhanced T1 image shows a dark lesion (presumably fluid/pus) with peripheral enhancement. There also is enhancement of the adjacent vertebra above with preservation of the intervening disk. Tuberculous spondylitis has a higher incidence of extensive paraspinal abscess formation compared with pyogenic infections. Its onset tends to be insidious and gradual, which not uncommonly leads to a delayed diagnosis. Constitutional symptoms including fever and weight loss are seen in less than 40% of cases. (A) Pyogenic osteomyelitis typically involves the intervertebral disks. In children, infection is thought to start in the disks, with secondary involvement of the adjacent vertebrae. In adults, the disease is thought to start in the end plates, with involvement of the disks in the majority of cases. (C) Degenerative disk disease would be centered in the intervertebral disk spaces and may result in secondary degenerative changes in the adjacent end plates. (D) Osseous metastases usually enhance and tend to involve the pedicles and posterior elements. They would not show the cystic appearance of the larger lesion seen in the provided image.

69.

C Acute extravasation

The "swirl" sign is seen on noncontrast head CT and is defined as areas of low attenuation within an acute intracranial hematoma. It indicates freshly extravasated and unclotted blood and is associated with expansion of the hematoma and a worse prognosis. (A) Thrombosis can present as a hyperdense clot on noncontrast head CT or a filling defect following the intravenous administration of contrast material. (B) Malignant transformation can occur in various neoplasms. It is not associated with a "swirl" sign. (D) An abscess presents as a fluid collection with an enhancing wall and surrounding edema. MRI shows central restricted diffusion. It is not associated with a "swirl" sign.

70.

A Cytokine release and production of mucopolysaccharides

Thyroid orbitopathy can affect any extraocular muscle, but the most typical presentation is that of involvement of the inferior, middle, and superior rectus muscles, which are markedly enlarged in this case. Involvement of the lateral rectus muscle almost never occurs in isolation. The pathophysiology is thought to be related to lymphocytic infiltration and cytokine release, which stimulates fibroblasts to produce mucopolysaccharides and, in turn, leads to soft tissue edema due to a hyperosmolar shift. (B) The most common primary tumors to metastasize to the orbit are breast, lung, prostate, and melanoma. It would be unusual for orbital metastases to result in this symmetric appearance of extraocular muscle enlargement. (C) IgG4-related disease of the orbit is being increasingly recognized as a cause of "idiopathic" inflammatory pseudotumor. It can be bilateral and involve any orbital structure, including the extraocular muscles, lacrimal sac, and optic nerve sheath complex. (D) Lymphoma may present as a soft tissue mass frequently related to the lacrimal gland or conjunctiva (MALT lymphoma). Other orbital structures also may be involved.

71.

D Mediastinal deviation to the contralateral side

A tension pneumothorax is accompanied by shift of the mediastinal structures to the contralateral side due to a progressive mass effect. (A) The diaphragm typically is flattened and depressed on the side of the tension pneumothorax. (B) The ipsilateral (not contralateral) intercostal spaces increase secondary to increased intrathoracic volume and pressure on the side of the tension pneumothorax.

(C) The "deep sulcus" sign may be seen in pneumothoraces on supine radiographs, as air collects basally and anteriorly rather than at the apex in an upright projection. It does not necessarily reflect a tension pneumothorax. (E) As with mediastinal structures, the trachea may be deviated to the contralateral side in tension pneumothorax.

72.

A Paget disease

Paget disease is a disorder of uncertain etiology where there is excessive bone remodeling and overgrowth. It most commonly occurs in the spine, skull, and pelvis. In the osteosclerotic phase, there is cortical thickening and coarsening of the trabeculations, which often lead to expansion of the involved bone. In the spine, the vertebrae become squared, and a thick, sclerotic margin may be seen, resulting in the "picture frame" sign. (B) Vertebral hemangiomas can lead to increased vertical trabeculations that may be seen as dense dots on axial images. (C) Lytic metastases do not cause a "picture frame" appearance. (D) Blastic metastases can produce the "ivory vertebra" sign if they involve the entire vertebral body. Blastic metastases can be seen in various malignancies such as prostate and breast cancer, transitional cell carcinoma, and neuroendocrine tumors.

73.

A Posterior limb of the internal capsule

The arrows point to the anterior choroidal arteries, which originate between the posterior communicating arteries and the carotid termination. The posterior communicating arteries can be seen immediately medial to these on the provided image. The anterior choroidal arteries supply the posterior limbs of the internal capsules, lateral geniculate nuclei, optic tracts and chiasm, hippocampi, amygdalae, and choroid plexus, among other structures. (B) The anterior limb of the internal capsule (lower half) is supplied by the recurrent artery of Heubner, which is a branch of the proximal anterior cerebral artery. The upper half is supplied by the lateral lenticulostriate arteries. (C) The anteromedial caudate nucleus as well as the anterior portion of the lentiform nucleus are supplied by the recurrent artery of Heubner. (D) The external capsule is supplied by the lateral lenticulostriate arteries, which are branches of the proximal middle cerebral artery and also supply the lateral aspect of the putamen and upper half of the internal capsule. (E) The various vascular territories of the thalamus all are supplied by branches of the posterior cerebral and posterior communicating arteries.

74.

B High incidence of neurovascular injury

The sagittal CT image shows too much space between the dens and tip of the clivus (basion–dens interval) consistent with atlanto-occipital dissociation. This is a severe craniocervical injury that results from sudden deceleration, with hyperflexion or hyperextension of the head, which disrupts the alar, cruciate, and apical ligaments and tectorial membrane. The condition is fatal in the great majority of patients secondary to a high incidence of neurovascular injury. (A) Atlanto-occipital dissociations are two to three times as common in children as in adults, presumably due to their relatively large head sizes, small size of their occipital condyles, and near horizontal orientation of the atlanto-occipital joints. (C) Other less severe injuries such as the Jefferson fracture may occur secondary to axial loading. (D) Atlanto-occipital dissociation injuries may be identified by a basion–dens interval greater than 12 mm as originally measured on lateral cervical spine radiographs. One study suggest a lower cutoff value (8.5 mm) with CT imaging, due to the presence of magnification on plain radiography.

75.

B Headache

Leptomeningeal carcinomatosis occurs in about 5% of patients with metastatic cancer and portends a poor prognosis. Half of these patients present with headaches, which represent the most common clinical manifestation. The incidence of leptomeningeal carcinomatosis is four times higher in autopsy studies. (A) Meningismus is present in 13% of patients with leptomeningeal metastases. (C) Ischemia is an uncommon complication of leptomeningeal carcinomatosis. In contrast, tuberculosis can manifest with leptomeningeal disease that characteristically results in cerebral infarcts. (D) Diabetes insipidus can occur in patients with infundibular involvement but is much less common than headache. It also is more frequently seen in leukemic patients rather than in patients with solid tumor leptomeningeal disease. (E) Dysarthria is an uncommon complication that occurs in 7% of patients with leptomeningeal metastases.

76.

D Leptomeningeal cyst

The CT shows a cyst-like structure projecting through a calvarial defect. The T2 image better demonstrates that there is encephalomalacia in that area of the brain, and therefore findings are compatible with a leptomeningeal cyst. These findings develop from fractures with associated dural tears and herniation of the pia-arachnoid through the dural defect, with progressive osseous erosion (also known as a "growing" skull fracture) due to cerebrospinal fluid pulsations. (A) Langerhans cell histiocytosis is an important cause of a lytic calvarial defect in a child. Given the underlying encephalomalacia demonstrated, findings are more likely related to prior trauma. (B) An epidermoid can be primarily calvarial, but there is no evidence of it on the MRI shown in these images, which instead shows underlying encephalomalacia. (C) The T2 image demonstrates encephalomalacia and no evidence of an abscess or parenchymal edema. Additionally, an abscess would not result in a calvarial defect.

77.

A Commonly produces a chondroid matrix

The CT image shows a destructive lesion involving the left petrous apex and petroclival junction, with contrast enhancement on the MRI study. There are small, calcific densities within it that could represent either chondroid matrix or eroded bone. Of the provided options, this lesion is most consistent with a chondrosarcoma, which comprises a heterogeneous group of malignant neoplasms characterized by the production of a chondroid matrix (sometimes seen as "rings" and "arcs" within a lytic lesion). About 1% of chondrosarcomas occurs at the skull base and commonly slightly off midline at synchondroses such as the petroclival and spheno-occipital sutures. (B) Cholesterol granulomas are thought to arise secondary to repeated episodes of hemorrhage within mucosa-lined air cells. They consist of granulation tissue and cholesterol crystals and typically are hyperintense on noncontrast T1-weighted images with areas of T2 hypointensity related to blood products. (C) In trapped secretions, the air cell septations are preserved, and there would not be erosive changes or an expansile enhancing lesion. (D) Aberrant ectoderm within petrous apex cells may result in a cholesteatoma, which does not enhance and usually is very bright on diffusion-weighted sequences due to a combination of restricted diffusion and T2 shine-through effects. (E) The vast majority of chondrosarcomas are slow-growing WHO grade I or II neoplasms that do not show significant restricted diffusion.

78.

C Widening of the spinal canal on a midsagittal image

Anterior listhesis secondary to pars defects (but not due to facet hypertrophy) often results in widening of the spinal canal on a midsagittal image. (A) Small size or hypoplasia of the L5 vertebra may predict the presence of bilateral pars interarticularis defects and should prompt a search for them. (B) Sclerosis of the contralateral pars interarticularis can occur with a chronic unilateral pars interarticularis defect. This patient likely has bilateral defects as indicated by significant listhesis of L5 over S1. (D) There may be variable degrees of neural foraminal narrowing depending on the severity of the listhesis, as can be seen on this image.

79.

D Vasospasm

The reconstruction from the CT angiogram on the left shows marked vasospasm affecting the left greater than right middle cerebral and posterior cerebral arteries and bilateral anterior cerebral arteries. There are accompanying regions of decreased perfusion most evident in the left middle cerebral and bilateral anterior cerebral arteries, where there are acute infarctions. Clinically significant vasospasm after subarachnoid hemorrhage is seen in 30% of patients and is associated with increased mortality. (A) Embolic infarcts are a known complication of angiography, which likely was done in this patient with aneurysmal subarachnoid hemorrhage, but they tend to be small and usually are located peripherally at the gray matter–white matter junction. (B) Vasospasm following subarachnoid hemorrhage is thought to be related to the release of spasmogenic factors during lysis of subarachnoid blood clots and not due to cerebritis. (C) Venous thrombosis may result in ischemia but is not a primary complication of subarachnoid hemorrhage and would not result in the territorial arterial perfusion deficits seen in this case (primarily bilateral anterior cerebral and left middle cerebral arteries).

80.

B It may show abnormal MRI signal in engorged pial vessels.

The MRA (left) demonstrates extensive collateralization in the region of the proximal middle cerebral arteries due to bilateral intracranial carotid artery stenoses in a patient with (true or idiopathic) moyamoya disease. The more distal middle cerebral arteries and visualized anterior cerebral arteries are abnormally narrowed in this case with preservation of the posterior circulation. Moyamoya disease may show abnormal signal in engorged pial vessels due to collateral flow through leptomeningeal anastomoses (the "ivy sign"). Moyamoya syndrome or secondary moyamoya (different from moyamoya disease) is a nonspecific radiographic finding that can show a similar pattern of collateralization and may be seen in various entities including sickle cell disease, neurofibromatosis type 1, Down syndrome, and connective tissue disorders, among others. (A) Moyamoya disease has a bimodal age distribution with peaks between 5 and 9 years of age and 35 and 39 years of age. (C) The most common manifestations of moyamoya disease are ischemia and hemorrhage. There have been rare reports of dystonia and choreoathetosis. (D) Moyamoya disease much more commonly involves the anterior circulation, although the posterior circulation also may be affected.

81.

B Commonly associated with focal cortical dysplasia

Dysembryoplastic neuroepithelial tumors (DNETs) are tumors of children and young adults who usually present with a long-standing history of intractable seizures. The lesions occur most commonly in the temporal followed by the frontal lobes, and these areas account for over 90% of cases. DNETs commonly are associated with focal dysplasia in the adjacent cortex. On imaging, they characteristically show a bubbly appearance, are cortically based, are bright on T2, and usually do not show contrast enhancement. Calcification is relatively common. (A) DNETs are WHO grade I lesions. (C) DNETs do not have restricted diffusion; therefore, they should not show low signal on apparent diffusion coefficient maps. (D) Only about 20% of DNETs show contrast enhancement in a nodular, heterogeneous, or ring-like fashion. (E) DNETs are slow-growing tumors that do not have a propensity for leptomeningeal spread.

82.

C Fornix

The fornix is a white matter structure that connects the hippocampus and mammillary bodies. It features a blood–brain barrier and does not normally show contrast enhancement. (A, B, D, E) The circumventricular organs are small, highly vascularized, midline structures surrounding the third and fourth ventricles. They are devoid of a blood–brain barrier, which enables contrast enhancement to be demonstrated routinely in the larger organs. Enhancement of the smaller structures is more difficult to appreciate but has been documented to variable degrees in studies done on higher field magnets.

83.

C Anterior inferior cerebellar artery

There is increased FLAIR signal along with restricted diffusion involving the anterior aspect of the right cerebellar hemisphere and middle cerebellar peduncle compatible with acute infarction. The abnormality follows the arterial distribution of the anterior inferior cerebellar artery, which also supplies the inferolateral aspect of the pons and flocculus. (A) The superior cerebellar artery supplies the superior cerebellum, superior vermis, dentate nuclei, and part of the midbrain. (B) The cerebellar parenchyma posterior to the infarcted area is supplied by the posterior inferior cerebellar artery (PICA) and is not involved. The PICA is the major artery of the cerebellum and supplies its posteroinferior portion, the inferior cerebellar vermis, and the lateral medulla. (D, E) The superior and inferior cerebellar veins drain their respective regions of the cerebellum and transmit blood to the dural sinuses and deep venous vasculature. The infarct in this case shows an arterial distribution.

84.

D Capillary telangiectasia

The imaging description of the lesion and its location are characteristic of a capillary telangiec-tasia. Low signal on GRE sequences is thought to be related to slow flow and increased deoxyhemoglobin content. Capillary telangiectasias sometimes can have areas of gliosis and are nearly always asymptomatic and found incidentally. (A) A demyelinating plaque does not show the constellation of features described, which are characteristic of capillary telangiectasias. (B) Capillary telangiectasias should be differentiated from metastases. The latter usually have surrounding edema (except for small cortical lesions) and do not show signal loss on gradient echo (GRE) imaging unless they are hemorrhagic, melanotic, or calcified. (C) Cavernous malformations can show various signal intensities depending on the stage of their blood products. They typically are described as having a "popcorn" or "berry" appearance with a surrounding rim of hemosiderin.

85.

E Joubert syndrome

Joubert syndrome is characterized by vermian hypoplasia or aplasia and a lack of decussation of the superior cerebellar peduncles. Thickening and a more horizontal configuration of the superior cerebellar peduncles leads to a "molar tooth" appearance. Diffusion tensor imaging studies show a lack of the expected "red dot" of pyramidal decussation. Most cases are autosomal recessive. (A) Rhombencephalosynapsis is characterized by an absent vermis and midline continuation of the dentate nuclei, cerebellar hemispheres, and superior peduncles. (B) A Dandy-Walker malformation can result in cystic enlargement of the posterior fossa in communication with the fourth ventricle. It does not lead to a "molar tooth" deformity. (C) A Blake pouch cyst develops due to the persistence of the embryonic Blake pouch. It can exert mass effect on the posterior fossa structures. (D) A mega cisterna magna is an incidental finding that presents as an increased subarachnoid retrocerebellar space in the lower posterior fossa. It may be asymmetric and mistaken for an arachnoid cyst.

86.

A Histologically consists of balloon cells with prominent nucleoli

The patient's history and clinical examination are compatible with tuberous sclerosis. The facial rash represents multiple angiofibromas, which tend to occur in the malar region. The nodular plaques on the lower back are Shagreen patches, which are considered highly specific for this entity. MRI shows a mixed cystic and solid mass centered in the left foramen of Monro (location is typical) compatible with a subependymal giant cell astrocytoma (SEGA) in this clinical context. There is resultant obstructive hydrocephalus, which is why the patient presented with signs of increased intracranial pressure. Other MRI findings of tuberous sclerosis include cortical tubers, subependymal nodules, and various white matter lesions. Histologically, SEGAs consist of balloon cells with prominent nucleoli, although spindle cells may be encountered and predominate in some tumors. Pathologically, they are indistinguishable from subependymal nodules, and on imaging, the only reliable differentiating feature is an increase in tumor size over serial studies (both subependymal nodules and SEGAs can enhance). (B) SEGAs are categorized as WHO grade I lesions. (C) SEGAs become symptomatic between 10 and 30 years of age but have been reported in patients as young as 1½ years of age. It is unusually rare for a SEGA to develop after the age of 20, and, in fact, patients without this tumor by age 25 do not need continued surveillance, as per the International Tuberous Sclerosis Complex Consensus recommendations. In contrast, SEGAs diagnosed early may become symptomatic later, and lifetime monitoring may be required for such lesions. (D) Spontaneous malignant transformation of SEGAs has been described but is unusually rare. (E) A bubbly appearance on MRI and attachment to the septum pellucidum is a description that would fit a central neurocytoma.

87.

B Craniopharyngioma

A heterogeneously enhancing suprasellar mass with cystic components and calcifications in a child (note that the spheno-occipital synchondrosis has not yet fused) is a craniopharyngioma until proven otherwise. These tumors most commonly occur in children between 5 and 14 years of age (adamantinomatous type), with a second peak in adults between the ages of 50 and 75 years (papillary type). They arise from remnants of the craniopharyngeal duct and are histologically benign but locally aggressive. These tumors are almost always sellar/suprasellar, although they rarely may present as purely intrasellar or even intrasphenoid, within the third ventricle, or in the optic apparatus without a sellar component. They have solid, enhancing components and show calcifications on CT in 90% of cases. (A) Epidermoid tumors are rare in the pediatric population. Except for FLAIR and diffusion-weighted sequences, they are homogeneous, usually have a cystic appearance, and should not show enhancing solid components. (C) The suprasellar region is the second most common location for germinomas, which also tend to present in the pediatric population. Calcification is rare. (D) Aneurysms, in general, are rare in children. Aside from vascular enhancement of the lumen, they do not show solid enhancing components. They may show a calcified rim corresponding to the aneurysm wall, but they do not demonstrate the coarse, scattered calcifications seen in this case. (E) Pituitary adenomas are rare before puberty. They can be heterogeneous in the presence of cystic or hemorrhagic changes and may resemble craniopharyngiomas; however, calcification is rare in adenomas.

88.

A Absent body of the corpus callosum

Syntelencephaly is also known as the middle interhemispheric variant of the holoprosencephaly spectrum. In this entity, there is nonseparation of the midportion of the cerebral hemispheres (posterior frontal and anterior parietal lobes) and absence or hypoplasia of the body of the corpus callosum. (B) The frontal and occipital poles characteristically are separated in syntelencephaly. (C) The sylvian fissure is present in syntelencephaly but has an abnormally vertical orientation and crosses the midline in the majority of patients. (D) An interhemispheric fissure is present in syntelencephaly, but is interrupted or intercepted by the sylvian fissure crossing the midline.

89.

C It is formed by sheets of small round blue cells.

These images show characteristic features of a medulloblastoma as an enhancing mass in the region of the cerebellar vermis projecting into the fourth ventricle. The lesion demonstrates restricted diffusion, as evidenced by increased signal on diffusion-weighted imaging *(center)* and corresponding low signal on the apparent diffusion coefficient (ADC) map *(right)*. Of the most common posterior fossa tumors, medulloblastomas have the lowest ADC values. They are formed by sheets of small round blue cells with minimal cytoplasm, hyperchromatic nuclei, and are similar to pineoblastomas and retinoblastomas. (A) Ependymal rosettes are characteristic of ependymomas. These are "plastic" tumors that may extrude through the fourth ventricular outflow tracts in a "toothpaste" configuration. They usually show less restricted diffusion than medulloblastomas. (B) Hemangioblastomas are low-grade, capillary-rich neoplasms that can occur sporadically or in the setting of von Hippel–Lindau syndrome. They are very vascular, enhance avidly, and may show vascular flow voids. Two thirds of them may present as a cyst with an enhancing nodule (typically abutting the pial surface), and the rest are entirely solid. (D) Rosenthal fibers are characteristic of juvenile pilocytic astrocytomas. They also may be present in reactive glial tissue surrounding vascular malformations and slow-growing tumors. Rosenthal fibers have been described in pleomorphic xanthoastrocytomas and Alexander disease. The solid enhancing component of pilocytic astrocytomas usually does not demonstrate much restricted diffusion.

90.

A Lesions commonly occur at gray matter–white matter junctions.

Lesions in neurocysticercosis commonly occur at gray matter–white matter junctions due to hematogenous spread. In the racemose form, there is proliferation of lobulated cysts without a scolex, which may spread throughout the subarachnoid space and ventriculoependymal surfaces. (B) Neurocysticercosis is acquired by ingesting *Taenia solium* eggs shed in the feces of carriers infected with the adult tapeworm. Ingestion of undercooked pork does not cause cysticercosis but may result in taeniasis with proliferation of the adult tapeworm in the small intestine. (C) Contrast enhancement is not seen in the vesicular stage, as the organism's membrane still is intact. There also is no surrounding edema, and patients usually are asymptomatic. Once the cyst degenerates and dies, it incites an inflammatory reaction, edema, and contrast enhancement (colloidal vesicular stage) followed by involution in the granular nodular stage, where there may be a nodular or ring enhancing lesion with a thick capsule. In the final stage (nodular calcified), the lesions calcify, and there usually is no contrast enhancement. (D) Neurocysticercosis is the most common parasitic infection of the central nervous system in immunocompetent patients. Its incidence is not increased in AIDS. (E) Spinal cord involvement is rare and occurs in about 1% of cases.

91.

A Can result in vasospasm after rupture

T1-weighted images without intravenous contrast (note that the choroid plexus does not enhance) demonstrate a lesion in the left frontal lobe, which is intrinsically bright due to fat and compatible with a dermoid cyst. A fat–fluid level is seen *(left image)*, which is characteristic. There also are scattered bright subarachnoid fat droplets in the sulci as well as intraventricular extension with fat in the frontal horns. Dermoid cysts derive from the intracranial inclusion of cutaneous ectoderm during closure of the neural tube and may develop after traumatic/iatrogenic implantation. In contrast to epidermoid cysts, they contain dermal appendages (sebaceous and sweat glands and hair follicles). Rupture is a rare event, and may result in chemical meningitis, seizures, vasospasm, and ischemia. Fistulous tracts may lead to recurrent bouts of bacterial meningitis. (B) Dermoid cysts contain dermal appendages (absent in epidermoid cysts). (C) Dermoid cysts may show a lipid peak from 0.9 to 1.3 ppm. Meningiomas (not dermoid cysts) may show increased alanine on MR spectroscopy at short TE values. (D) Chemical meningitis may occur after rupture of a dermoid cyst, which is in itself a rare event. (E) Rarely, dermoid cysts may degenerate into squamous cell carcinomas but not into high-grade glial tumors.

92.

A More common in women

Pineal cysts are more common in women than in men, by a ratio of 3:1. Most pineal cysts measure less than 1 cm but may be larger, with lesions greater than 4 cm reported in the literature. They typically do not enhance, but may show a thin rim of enhancement peripherally. Very rarely, nodular areas of enhancement have been reported, in which case pineal cysts cannot be distinguished from pineal region tumors on the basis of imaging. Gadolinium will diffuse slowly into pineal cysts, and, given enough time, a pineal cyst may show enhancement on delayed imaging. The majority are asymptomatic, but approximately 5% can compress the cerebral aqueduct and result in hydrocephalus. Size tends to be stable in males, but pineal cysts may grow in young females with later regression, suggesting a hormonal role in their development. (B) Pineal cysts usually do not suppress fully on FLAIR sequences. (C) Pineal cysts do not show restricted diffusion. (D) The majority of pineal cysts are asymptomatic. (E) Pineal cysts are lined by a thin layer of glial cells, fibrous tissue, and pineal parenchyma with or without calcifications.

93.

C Flow voids

As with paragangliomas occurring in the neck, lesions are highly vascular, enhance avidly, and may be associated with hemorrhage. Flow voids can be seen in and around the lesion. (A) The "target" sign has been described on T2 images in neurofibromas due to a dark fibrocollagenous core. It may be seen less commonly in schwannomas probably due to the relative distribution of Antoni A and Antoni B tissues. (B) Intrinsic T1 hyperintensity sometimes can be seen in myxopapillary ependymomas, which is the other major differential diagnosis in the lumbar spine. (D) Paragangliomas are extramedullary and usually occur in the region of the filum terminale and cauda equina; therefore, they do not expand the cord, although on occasion, there may be an associated intramedullary cyst.

94.

C Gray matter heterotopia is present in 10 to 30% of cases.

The image accompanying the question shows the typical imaging features of a Chiari type 2 malformation, with descent of the brainstem through the foramen magnum, a small posterior fossa, beaking of the tectum, a flattened and elongated fourth ventricle, and a thinned/dysplastic corpus callosum. Gray matter heterotopia is seen in 10 to 30% of cases, predominantly in a periventricular distribution. (A) Virtually 100% of Chiari type 2 malformations are associated with "open" spinal dysraphism (not "closed" as with a skin-covered defect). The presence of a skin-covered myelomeningocele essentially excludes the development of a Chiari type 2 malformation, and this is the reason why some myelomeningoceles are corrected in utero. (B) This option refers to a Chiari type 1 malformation, which presents with inferior herniation of peg-like cerebellar tonsils and is usually not clinically significant unless the tonsils are displaced more than 5 mm below the foramen magnum. (D) A "monoventricle" may be seen in holoprosencephaly depending on its severity. This is not a feature of a Chiari type 2 malformation.

95.

D Peripheral nerve sheath tumor

The pathology shown in the images accompanying the question is an extramedullary neoplasm that is partially intradural and partially extradural. It extends to the paraspinal soft tissues through the left neural foramen, which is expanded and remodeled, indicating that this is a slow-growing process. Findings are most consistent with a nerve sheath tumor. The presence of a T2 dark center (i.e., the "target sign" due to a fibrocollagenous core) in the lower image suggests a neurofibroma, although schwannomas sometimes can show a similar appearance, depending on the relative distributions of Antoni A and Antoni B tissues. (A) Paragangliomas are rare in the spine. They tend to occur in the conus medullaris and filum terminale. (B) Ependymomas usually are parenchymal except for the myxopapillary type, which occurs exclusively in the filum terminale and sometimes involves the conus medullaris. (C) Meningiomas in the spine are much more common in females and more frequently occur in the thoracic spine. They are dural-based masses, but on occasion may extrude through a neural foramen.

96.

C Increased risk of hemorrhage expansion

The "spot sign" indicates a focus of active extravasation and predicts the expansion of a parenchymal hematoma. It is seen as a single focus or multiple foci of enhancement within the hematoma, and is present in about one third of patients within the first 6 hours after symptom onset. Other factors that have been associated with increasing hemorrhage size include large initial volumes and the use of anticoagulants. (A, B, E) The "spot sign" does not indicate the presence of a neoplasm, arteriovenous malformation, or arteriovenous fistula, although all of these may be associated with parenchymal hemorrhage. (D) The "spot sign" can be seen in, but is not exclusive to, hypertensive hemorrhage.

97.

B Pulmonary edema

This constellation of radiographic findings is most consistent with pulmonary edema. Blunting of the costophrenic angles reflects the presence of pleural effusions. Kerley lines represent thickening of the interlobular septa and pulmonary interstitium, and may be seen with edema, lymphatic engorgement, or carcinomatosis. Potential causes of postoperative pulmonary edema are varied and can be related to over-administration of intravenous fluids, neurogenic edema, acute respiratory distress syndrome (ARDS), hyponatremia, sepsis, and other causes. (A) *Pneumonitis* is a general term with various etiologies indicating alveolar inflammation, which may or may not result in pulmonary edema. (C) Aspiration pneumonia most commonly occurs in the posterior segment of the upper lobes and the superior segment of the lower lobes in postoperative patients who usually are recumbent. (D) Pneumonia usually is focal but may be extensive and bilateral if it is severe.

98.

A Leptomeningeal angiomatosis

The description of this case is consistent with Sturge-Weber syndrome, the hallmark of which is disorganized capillary vascular malformations involving the face, eye, and brain, typically on the same side. Leptomeningeal enhancement reflects the presence of a pial angiomatosis, which more commonly occurs in the parieto-occipital region and is thought to lead to cortical/subcortical calcifications due to a steal phenomenon and chronic ischemia. Patients may develop seizures, hemiplegia, and visual deficits. The pial angiomatosis is bilateral in 20% of cases where the clinical presentation is more severe. (B) In Sturge-Weber syndrome, there is engorgement of the ipsilateral choroid plexus and often recruitment of ependymal collaterals. (C) The facial capillary malformation of Sturge-Weber syndrome ("port-wine" stain) typically involves the ophthalmic division and sometimes the maxillary division of the trigeminal nerve. It virtually never involves the mandibular division in isolation. (D) The ipsilateral frontal sinuses may be enlarged due to the compensatory growth of the calvaria, sometimes resulting in the Dyke-Davidoff-Masson phenomenon (compensatory thickening of the cranial vault with frontal sinus enlargement, elevation of the petrous ridge, ipsilateral falcine displacement, and capillary malformations). (E) There is compensatory thickening of the ipsilateral calvaria in chronic cases of Sturge-Weber syndrome due to the hemiatrophy.

99.

C Pseudocysts

Gelatinous pseudocysts are a characteristic finding of cryptococcal meningoencephalitis and are filled with mucous exudates produced by the fungus. The pseudocysts commonly occur in the basal ganglia and medial cerebellum. Because they are not simple fluid, they do not suppress on FLAIR sequences. Patients also can have enhancing cryptococcomas and dilated perivascular spaces. (A) A concentric T2 FLAIR "target" sign is seen in one third of patients with toxoplasmosis, and represents alternating layers of necrosis, edema, and hemorrhage. (B) The eccentric "target" sign is seen on contrast-enhanced T1-weighted images, and is highly suggestive of toxoplasmosis (seen in about one third of patients with the diagnosis). (D) Low T2 signal intensity can be seen in enhancing granulomas, including cryptococcomas and tuberculomas but is not specific.

100.

B Hand and arm dysesthesia

The coronal CT image shows large cervical ribs arising from the C7 vertebrae bilaterally. They may constitute a cause of thoracic outlet syndrome. By far, the most common clinical manifestations of thoracic outlet syndrome are neurogenic (about 95%), and include pain, dysesthesias, weakness, and cold intolerance in the hands, arms, or shoulders. Most commonly, neurogenic thoracic outlet syndrome involves the C8 and T1 cervical roots, which may result in symptoms along the ulnar nerve distribution. Less commonly, the upper cervical brachial plexus roots may be affected and lead to symptoms in the neck, upper chest, and back. (A) Signs and symptoms of arterial compression with or without thromboembolism, including hand ischemia, are the least common presentations of thoracic outlet syndrome, constituting approximately 1% of cases. (C) Muscle atrophy can be seen in cases of severe and prolonged compression of the brachial plexus, but this is extremely uncommon. (D) Upper extremity swelling may be a manifestation of venous compression and/or thrombosis; however, neurogenic symptoms are more common manifestations of thoracic outlet syndrome. (E) Chronic venous compression can lead to the development of collateral veins, but neurogenic symptoms are more common in thoracic outlet syndrome.

101.

B *TSC1/TSC2*

The constellation of findings presented is compatible with tuberous sclerosis complex (TSC). In particular, the combination of glioneuronal hamartomas (also known as cortical tubers) and subependymal nodules is sufficient to make the diagnosis as per the 2012 TSC Consensus Guidelines. White matter radial migration lines and parenchymal cysts also are characteristic. TSC can develop due to mutations in either the *TSC1* or *TSC2* genes, which code for hamartin and tuberin. (A) Neurofibromatosis type 1 can lead to various lesions in the central nervous system, including gliomas, sphenoid wing dysplasias, and focal areas of high signal intensity (FASI), also known as unidentified bright objects (UBOs). (C) Neurofibromatosis type 2 is characterized by the presence of multiple inherited schwannomas, meningiomas, and ependymomas (MISME). (D) The hallmark central nervous system lesions in von Hippel–Lindau disease are hemangioblastomas, which are very vascular and invariably enhance; two thirds present as typical, cystic masses with mural nodules, and the rest are entirely solid. Patients also can develop endolymphatic sac tumors as well as various extracranial lesions. (E) Mutations in the *SMARCB1* and *LZTR1* genes have been associated with schwannomatosis (neurofibromatosis type 3).

102.

B Dural venous thrombosis

Dural venous thrombosis can lead to the so-called empty delta sign, due to the presence of a nonenhancing thrombus in the dural venous sinus against a background of enhancing blood in the surrounding sinus/dura. (A) Cortical vein thrombosis does not result in an empty delta sign. Depending on bolus timing, it can be seen as a filling defect on a contrast-enhanced study, hyperintensity within the vessel on FLAIR sequences, or associated blooming artifact on gradient echo–based sequences (particularly susceptibility weighted imaging). (C, E) Dense subdural or subarachnoid blood along the posterior falx and dural reflections can cause a "pseudo-delta" sign on a noncontrast CT study. (D) Deep venous thrombosis does not cause an empty delta sign.

103.

D Dorsal arachnoid web

The "scalpel" sign has been described in dorsal thoracic arachnoid webs and refers to the shape of the dorsal subarachnoid space at the level of the lesion. MRI and CT myelography show ventral displacement of the spinal cord due to the presence of an abnormal arachnoid membrane. Dorsal thoracic arachnoid webs can be associated with symptoms of long-standing cord compression. (A) Epidural hematomas can exert mass effect on the intraspinal structures. They are not associated with the "scalpel" sign. (B) Spinal cord herniation is thought to be caused by a dural defect, with resultant communication between the subarachnoid and epidural spaces. The spinal cord progressively herniates through the defect, with subsequent distortion and potential development of myelopathy. (C) An arachnoid cyst can result in variable degrees of mass effect on the spinal cord.

104.

C Antiepileptic drug usage

Antiepileptic drug usage and sudden withdrawal of antiepileptic drugs have been linked to transient splenic lesions. Various infectious, inflammatory, and autoimmune processes have been associated with a transient splenic lesion. The etiopathogenesis is uncertain. (A) A demyelinating plaque can occur in the corpus callosum but more commonly is asymmetric, and follow-up imaging may show the sequela of demyelination. (B) The corpus callosum is relatively resistant to embolic infarcts, due to the perpendicular orientation of its penetrating arteries and a rich blood supply. It would be unusual for an embolic infarct to occur at the midline. (D) Acute disseminated encephalomyelitis can affect the corpus callosum but usually is asymmetric.

105.

C *FGFR*

There is trigonocephaly resulting from premature fusion of the metopic suture, which usually closes at 6 to 12 months of age. This deformity can result in ridging along the forehead, bifrontal and bitemporal narrowing, and hypotelorism. Most cases of trigonocephaly are sporadic, and the majority of nonsyndromic cases may be related to a variety of genetic and environmental factors. Trigonocephaly may be associated with many syndromes such as Jacobsen, Saethre-Chotzen, Opitz C, and Say-Meyer, among others. Most syndromic cases are related to mutations in the *FGFR* genes, but alterations also may be seen in chromosomes 9, 11, and 22. (A) *TSC1* and *TSC2* mutations are the hallmark of tuberous sclerosis complex. (B) *NOTCH3* mutations can result in cerebral autosomal dominant arteriopathy with subcortical infarcts and leukoencephalopathy. (D) Mutations in the *SMARCB1* gene can lead to Coffin-Siris syndrome and an increased risk of developing rhabdoid tumors such as ATRT.

106.

B Arachnoiditis

An "empty sac" sign has been described in arachnoiditis due to peripheral displacement of nerve roots that are adherent to the sac. Nerve roots also can be clumped, and there rarely may be soft tissue masses in patients with fibrosing or ossifying arachnoiditis. Although most cases are postsurgical, arachnoiditis also may be seen after infection, trauma, subarachnoid hemorrhage, and intrathecal steroids. (A) An arachnoid cyst appears as a well-circumscribed filling defect within the thecal sac and can result in displacement of the spinal contents. If there is communication with the subarachnoid space, an arachnoid cyst eventually will fill with contrast and may become invisible on delayed imaging; 80% of spinal arachnoid cysts are thoracic, and only 5% are lumbar. (C) An intradural tumor can displace the spinal nerve roots but does not produce an "empty sac" sign. (D, E) Epidural and subdural collections can result in variable degrees of mass effect on the thecal sac and its contents.

107.

D Auriculotemporal nerve

The auriculotemporal nerve arises from the posterior division of the mandibular branch of the trigeminal nerve. It anastomoses with the temporofacial division of the facial nerve and is a common route of perineural spread, particularly from tumors in the temporal scalp, parotid gland, and external auditory canal. (A) The maxillary nerve is the second division of the trigeminal nerve. Perineural spread along this nerve can occur from malignancies arising in the facial region. (B, C) The greater superficial petrosal nerve is a branch of the facial nerve that arises from the geniculate ganglion. The Vidian nerve is formed by the confluence of the greater superficial petrosal nerve, deep petrosal nerve, and ascending sphenoidal branch from the otic ganglion. These are potential routes of spread in various tumors from the nasopharynx, paranasal sinuses, and orbits.

108.

A Metastasis

The images accompanying the question demonstrate an intra-axial mass in the left cerebellum with peripheral enhancement *(left)* and restricted diffusion of the enhancing component as evidenced by high signal on the diffusion-weighted image *(center)* and dark signal on the apparent diffusion coefficient map (ADC, *right*), which also demonstrates increased surrounding signal due to edema. Metastases constitute the most common cerebellar tumors in adults. (B) Primary cerebellar glioblastomas are rare and constitute less than 1% of all such tumors. Solid components may show restricted diffusion. (C) Tumefactive demyelination may present as an enhancing mass, typically with an incomplete ring of enhancement that may show variable degrees of restricted diffusion. (D) Abscesses show restricted diffusion in the central necrotic component, not in the enhancing peripheral rim. (E) Cerebral toxoplasmosis is an AIDS-defining condition, and most cases are seen in this context. *Toxoplasma* lesions tend to be small (2 to 3 cm) and commonly occur in the gray matter–white matter junction of the supratentorial brain and deep gray nuclei. They may show enhancement with an eccentric nodule (the "eccentric target" sign) or alternating rings of T2/FLAIR hypo- and hyperintensity related to areas of necrosis, edema, and hemorrhage.

109.

A Originates from arachnoid meningothelial cells

1p36 deletions have been found in a variety of human cancers. In the central nervous system, these cancers include meningiomas, oligodendrogliomas, and neuroblastomas. Of these, an avidly enhancing intraventricular mass would be most consistent with a meningioma, which originates from arachnoid meningothelial cells. In meningiomas, *1p* deletions are the second most common genetic abnormality after deletions on chromosome 22, and they have been associated with an increased risk of tumor recurrence and progression. (B) The incidence of meningiomas increases with age. They are very rare in the pediatric population except when they are associated with neurofibromatosis type 2, in which case they more frequently develop at an earlier age or in patients with a history of radiation therapy, although the latency in such cases may be long. (C) Hamartin is a ubiquitous protein encoded by the *TSC1* gene in the tuberous sclerosis complex, where it is associated with the development of hamartomas in various tissues. It is not related to the formation of meningiomas. (D) Ependymomas, not meningiomas, arise from the ependymal lining of the ventricular system. (E) Except for a few isolated reports of papillary and rhabdoid meningiomas, these tumors do not show glial fibrillary acidic protein staining.

110.

D Endocarditis

Mycotic pseudoaneurysms form after infectious disruption of all three layers of the arterial wall and formation of a vascular outpouching. These lesions characteristically arise from distal branches of the middle cerebral artery along the surface of the brain and can develop as a complication of endocarditis and septic emboli, as was the case in this patient. (A) The pathogenesis of intracranial aneurysms is complex and multifactorial. Atherosclerosis may play a role in the formation of at least some fusiform aneurysms. The lesion in this case is very peripheral, almost along the inner table of the skull (note the faint subtraction artifact related to the calvaria), a location that is more often seen in mycotic pseudoaneurysms. (B) The imaging presentation of vasculitis is variable, and in many cases the angiogram may be normal and, therefore, does not rule out the diagnosis. The classic finding in vasculitis is regions of segmental stenosis and dilatation resulting in a "string of beads" appearance. (C) Mycotic pseudoaneurysms are infectious in nature.

111.

B Methanol intoxication

The most characteristic imaging finding of methanol intoxication is bilateral putaminal necrosis with variable degrees of hemorrhage, and this may be accompanied by white matter edema or necrosis in severe cases. Findings are thought to be caused by the direct toxic effects of methanol metabolites and metabolic acidosis. Necrosis of the retinae and optic disks/nerves may lead to blindness. (A) The most common findings in sporadic Creutzfeldt-Jakob disease are cortical and basal ganglia signal abnormalities involving the corpus striatum. The variant form more commonly shows involvement of the pulvinar or dorsomedial thalami ("hockey-stick" sign). (C) Carbon monoxide intoxication typically affects the globus pallidus and also may involve the white matter. (D) Wernicke encephalopathy preferentially affects the mammillary bodies, medial thalami, tectal plate, and periaqueductal gray. Contrast enhancement of the thalamus and mammillary bodies has been associated with alcohol abuse.

112.

A Often respects cranial sutures

The CT image shows a hyperdense, acute epidural hematoma with mass effect on the frontal lobe and mild midline shift. Classically, epidural hematomas are limited by tight dural attachments at the cranial sutures, which results in a lentiform or biconcave shape. They usually do not cross sutures unless there is a fracture or sutural diastasis. (B) Supratentorial subdural (not epidural) hematomas do not cross the midline because they are limited by the reflection of the inner layers of the dura as they form the falx cerebri. Epidural hematomas may cross the midline if there are no intervening sutures or if there is a sutural fracture or diastasis. This is seen, for instance, with vertex epidural hematomas, which usually are venous and associated with a fracture crossing the superior sagittal sinus and, therefore, can be seen across the sagittal suture. (C) Mixed density contents with areas of low attenuation within the dense hematoma (i.e., the "swirl sign") indicate active extravasation and are an indication for emergent surgical evacuation. (D) 90 to 95% of epidural hematomas are due to an arterial injury. Epidural hematomas due to a venous injury are less common and usually are associated with fractures crossing the dural venous sinuses. (E) Epidural hematomas develop between the outer (periosteal) layer of the dura and the inner table of the skull.

113.

B The majority are low-grade lesions.

The majority of tectal gliomas are low-grade lesions, but high-grade histologies also may be seen. (A) The vast majority of tectal gliomas are low-grade, insidious lesions that can be observed for relatively long periods of time without intervention. Shunting with an endoscopic third ventriculostomy or ventriculoperitoneal drainage generally is an accepted initial treatment. Tumors that persistently are symptomatic may require further treatment, such as radiotherapy and/or chemotherapy. (C) Aqueductal stenosis is the most common cause of congenital hydrocephalus and may be secondary to congenital stenosis of the cerebral aqueduct or a sequela of intrauterine infection. (D) Five to seven percent of patients with aqueductal stenosis have a congenital form (X-linked hydrocephalus) seen in males and determined by mutations in the *L1CAM* gene.

114.

D Cerebrospinal fluid IgG and IgM oligoclonal bands

The axial FLAIR images accompanying the question show periventricular white matter lesions in a radial orientation, and two juxtacortical (abutting the cortex) lesions on the left side, characteristic of multiple sclerosis. The presence of both periventricular and juxtacortical lesions satisfies the 2010 modified MacDonald criteria for dissemination in space. The concurrent presence of an enhancing lesion *(right image)* and multiple nonenhancing lesions satisfies the criteria for dissemination in time. Oligoclonal bands are found in the cerebrospinal fluid in 95% of patients with clinically definite multiple sclerosis. (A) Serum aquaporin-4 antibodies are highly specific (between 92% and 99%) for the diagnosis of neuromyelitis optica and are seen in about 60% of patients. Lesions in the brain are not entirely specific, but tend to favor areas of high aquaporin-4 expression. White matter lesions with cloud-like enhancement and ependymal enhancement may be seen. (B) Cryptococcal antigen can be detected in the serum and cerebrospinal fluid of patients with cryptococcal meningoencephalitis. Cryptococcomas and gelatinous pseudocysts preferentially develop in the basal ganglia and medial cerebellum, and patients can have dilated perivascular spaces. (C) Lyme disease is caused by the spirochete *Borrelia burgdorferi.* MRI findings in the brain include nonspecific white matter lesions, which sometimes may enhance, and leptomeningeal and cranial nerve enhancement.

115.

C Fibrous dysplasia

The CT image demonstrates osseous expansion and remodeling of the right maxilla, adjacent zygoma, and pterygoid process with a ground-glass appearance that is most consistent with fibrous dysplasia. This is a benign condition that develops as a result of abnormal osteoblastic differentiation and leads to replacement of normal marrow with immature osseous and fibrous elements. Fibrous dysplasia is a disease of children, adolescents, and young adults. It can be monostotic (80%) or polyostotic. In the head, the most common sites of involvement are the frontal, sphenoid, and ethmoid bones along with the maxilla. Although the majority of cases are sporadic, fibrous dysplasia can be seen as part of McCune-Albright and Mazabraud syndromes. On CT, the appearance is often characteristic with areas of ground-glass texture admixed with sclerotic and sometimes cystic changes. Diagnosis on MRI may be challenging, as the appearance is more variable. (A) Blastic (sclerotic) osseous metastases are seen with many primary malignancies including breast and prostate cancer and neuroendocrine tumors. They do not result in the expansile or ground-glass appearance seen in this case. (B) Paget disease essentially can occur in any bone and also can result in osseous expansion; however, it is a disease of middle-aged and elderly individuals. The ground-glass appearance of this case and the location are typical for fibrous dysplasia. (D) A plasmacytoma would have a destructive, lytic appearance on CT with or without a soft tissue component. It also is a condition seen in older individuals.

116.

B Thin middle cerebellar peduncles

The "hot cross bun" sign is produced by degeneration of transverse pontine fibers and is highly specific for multiple system atrophy (MSA), although it only is seen in about half of the patients with this condition. The middle cerebellar peduncles are significantly thinned in MSA patients with predominant cerebellar ataxia, compared with patients with Parkinson disease and control individuals. (A) A molar tooth configuration is characteristic of Joubert syndrome, in which there is a lack of decussation of the superior cerebellar peduncles, which have a more horizontal trajectory. (C) The "hummingbird" sign is produced by midbrain atrophy with preserved volume of the pons in patients with supranuclear palsy. (D) Nonvisualization of the normal signal hyperintensity of nigrosome-1 has been described in patients with Parkinson disease using high field MR magnets.

117.

D A dysplastic cerebellar gangliocytoma

A "corduroy" appearance is often used in MRI reports to describe the striated pattern that is highly characteristic of dysplastic cerebellar gangliocytoma (Lhermitte-Duclos disease). This is a hamartomatous formation occurring in the cerebellum that is seen in association with Cowden syndrome and loss of *PTEN* gene function. Patients are at an increased risk of developing various malignancies, including thyroid, breast, and endometrial cancer. The lesion may show increased signal on T2/FLAIR sequences and hyperperfusion. It also can be associated with increased mass effect and elevated intracranial pressure, which may necessitate ventricular decompression and/or surgical resection. (A) Cerebellitis typically does not result in a "corduroy" imaging pattern. It has various etiologies, and its presentation is varied. Cerebellitis can be unilateral, bilateral, symmetric, asymmetric, or diffuse. (B) A "corduroy" pattern is not typical of medulloblastoma; however, the desmoplastic variant of medulloblastoma features a multinodular architecture that may be confused with Lhermitte-Duclos disease. (C) Posterior inferior cerebellar infarcts are a known cause of mass effect in the posterior fossa and can be mistaken for tumor. They may enhance in the subacute phase, where striations may be seen related to the cerebellar folia; however, these striations tend to be thinner and more uniform than those of Lhermitte-Duclos disease.

118.

C Increased perfusion on an MR relative cerebral blood flow map

Studies have shown increased relative cerebral blood flow (rCBV) perfusion in lymphoma compared with toxoplasmosis, although lymphomas commonly are hypovascular on perfusion imaging sequences. (A) The concentric T2 FLAIR "target" sign is characteristic of toxoplasmosis, and is produced by alternating rings of hemorrhage, edema, and necrosis within the lesion. It is present in approximately one third of cases. (B) The eccentric "target" sign is seen on contrast-enhanced T1 images and is highly suggestive of toxoplasmosis, although it is present only in about one third of cases. It is produced by a leash of inflamed leaky vessels coursing along a sulcus into the lesion. (D) Lymphomas show increased uptake of thallium-201, but the sensitivity decreases with small lesions, particularly those less than 2 cm. (E) Lipid/lactate peaks on MR spectroscopy previously have been suggested to imply toxoplasmosis; however, further studies have shown various spectral patterns in both lymphoma and toxoplasmosis without significant differences.

119.

B Reversible cerebral vasoconstriction syndrome

The patient's clinical presentation and imaging findings essentially are pathognomonic for reversible cerebral vasoconstriction syndrome. The angiogram was performed following an internal carotid injection and shows segmental multifocal narrowing involving both the anterior and posterior (through a fetal posterior cerebral artery) circulations. Initial CT and cerebrospinal fluid studies commonly are normal, although small-volume subarachnoid hemorrhage is present in 20% of patients with reversible cerebral vasoconstriction syndrome. Ischemic stroke, parenchymal hemorrhage, and areas of edema may be seen. (A) Venous infarction may present with headaches, nausea and vomiting, and altered mental status. It is not associated with recurrent "thunderclap" headaches. Additionally, only the arterial phase is shown on the angiogram. (C) There is no evidence of an aneurysm on the angiogram. (D) Acute vascular occlusion is not seen on this exam.

120.

C Neuroblastoma

Neuroblastomas are tumors derived from primitive sympathetic ganglion cells. They most commonly occur in young children with a mean age of presentation of 22 months; 40% arise from the adrenal glands, and 15% are thoracic. When paravertebral, their growth results in remodeling of the adjacent vertebrae and ribs, and they can extend into the spinal canal through the neural foramina. They show heterogeneous enhancement and may be accompanied by cystic change and necrosis. Due to their adrenergic origin, they show avid uptake of ^{123}I-metaiodobenzylguanidine (^{123}I-MIBG), which has shown high sensitivity and specificity. (A) Giant cell tumors rarely occur in the vertebrae. They do not accumulate ^{123}I-MIBG. (B) Eosinophilic granuloma is the localized and most common form of Langerhans cell histiocytosis. It can occur in the spine, where it usually affects the vertebral body and may result in a vertebra plana. (D) Aneurysmal bone cysts are histologically benign but may be locally aggressive. The presence of an expansile vertebral mass with thin bone rims and fluid–blood levels is nearly pathognomonic. They do not demonstrate ^{123}I-MIBG uptake.

121.

B Intravenous drug use

The sagittal T2 *(left)* and contrast-enhanced T1 *(right)* MR images show the typical findings of diskitis/osteomyelitis with fluid/edema in an intervertebral thoracic disk and formation of an epidural abscess that extends dorsally into the spinal canal and compresses the cord. Note the extensive end-plate destruction and bone marrow edema in the adjacent vertebrae. Diskitis/osteomyelitis is more common in males, and its incidence increases with age. Risk factors include bacteremia (nosocomial or secondary to intravenous drug use), spinal procedures, direct inoculation from trauma, and various causes of immunosuppression including diabetes. (A) Metastatic disease usually spares the intervertebral disks and would not result in a fluid collection. Additionally, the bone marrow abnormality in this case is isolated to the vertebrae contiguous with the infected disk. (C) Fall from a height may result in a fracture, which would not explain the disk-centered inflammatory findings of this case. (D) Anemia, hypercalcemia, and renal failure are findings that would be expected with multiple myeloma, which is characterized by multiple lytic lesions that may have a permeative pattern on CT or radiography. Multiple myeloma can be seen as normal on MRI or may present as multiple hyperintense foci or with a variegated, micronodular pattern. (E) A seronegative (rheumatoid factor negative) spondyloarthropathy may present as inflammatory arthritis involving the spine and sacroiliac joints, with corner erosions in the vertebrae and ankylosis.

122.

C Associated with hemorrhagic necrosis

Hemorrhagic necrosis is the pathological hallmark of HSV-1 encephalitis affecting primarily the limbic system and temporal lobes. The classic lesion distribution includes the mesial temporal lobes, insular cortices, and inferior frontal lobes. The abnormalities usually are bilateral but asymmetric, and MRI diffusion-weighted imaging and FLAIR sequences are the most sensitive to define their extension. Contrast enhancement is rare in the early stages of disease but may be present later along the gyri or leptomeninges. Prognosis is poor, with a high incidence of neurologic sequelae. Mortality is related directly to the time of initiation of acyclovir after disease onset. (A) Herpes simplex virus (HSV) encephalitis beyond the neonatal period is caused by HSV-1 in the majority of cases. Neonates can be infected with either HSV-1 or HSV-2 and usually present with a more diffuse type of encephalitis. (B) HSV-1 encephalitis typically spares the basal ganglia, but may cause middle cerebral artery strokes that could otherwise have a similar appearance to the image shown. (D) The majority of patients with paraneoplastic encephalomyelitis have antineuronal (anti-Hu) nuclear antibodies. The distribution of imaging abnormalities in limbic encephalitis may mimic that of HSV-1 encephalitis, but the clinical picture differs, with a more subacute progression of cognitive and behavioral changes and sometimes seizures in the former. (E) Diffuse infiltration of two or more lobes with neoplastic glial cells is the definition of gliomatosis cerebri. This potentially could mimic some of the signal abnormalities seen in HSV encephalitis but would not explain the acute presentation of symptoms in this patient.

123.

A Fluid-attenuated inversion recovery

The two most relevant differential considerations for a nonenhancing, extra-axial, cystic mass are an arachnoid cyst and an epidermoid cyst. Arachnoid cysts follow cerebrospinal fluid signal intensity on all sequences and fully suppress on fluid-attenuated inversion recovery (FLAIR) sequences. Epidermoid cysts show a "dirty" appearance on FLAIR and very high signal intensity on diffusion-weighted sequences. (B) Susceptibility-weighted imaging (SWI) is a gradient echo MRI sequence that maximizes tissue differences by virtue of their local magnetic fields. SWI is highly sensitive to the presence of ferritin, calcium, deoxyhemoglobin, and hemosiderin, but does not play a role in characterizing arachnoid cysts. (C) Gradient recalled echo sequences generate images that are particularly susceptible to magnetic field inhomogeneities. Dynamic susceptibility contrast MRI and functional MRI are different techniques based on GRE sequences. (D) T2-weighted images would not be helpful, as both epidermoid tumors and arachnoid cysts will show high signal. (E) Dynamic susceptibility contrast perfusion would show only a nonperfusing, space-occupying lesion and would not aid in differentiation.

124.

C Occipital lobe, thalamus, and part of the midbrain

This is a digital subtraction angiogram following an internal carotid injection. It shows a fetal origin of the posterior cerebral artery that supplies the occipital lobe, thalamus, and part of the midbrain. (A) The superior cerebellar artery supplies the superior cerebellum, superior vermis, dentate nuclei, and part of the midbrain. (B) The posterior inferior cerebellar artery supplies the posteroinferior cerebellum, inferior cerebellar vermis, and lateral medulla. (D) The anterior inferior cerebellar artery supplies the anterior aspect of the right cerebellar hemisphere, middle cerebellar peduncle, inferolateral aspect of the pons, and flocculus.

125.

A Aneurysm

This is a well-circumscribed extra-axial lesion with mixed signal intensities and profound peripheral T2 hypointensity along the expected course of the posterior inferior cerebellar artery (PICA). Findings are most concerning for an aneurysm, which probably is partially thrombosed (note the enhancement of a nonthrombosed lumen on the third image). There is a small, old infarct in the left cerebellum seen on the FLAIR image likely related to thromboembolism. PICA aneurysms are rare, and the great majority arises proximally. (B) Although most meningiomas enhance homogeneously, they can calcify and sometimes present with cystic change or, very rarely, hemorrhage, and therefore they also may show variable signal intensities on MRI. Eighty percent of intraventricular meningiomas arise from the atrium of the lateral ventricle, and only 5% are seen in the fourth ventricle. (C) Eighty percent of choroid plexus tumors are benign papillomas. They are rare in adults, where they most commonly occur in the fourth ventricle. Papillomas tend to enhance avidly and diffusely and characteristically show frond-like margins with a texture that is similar to that of the normal choroid plexus. (D) Subependymomas are slow-growing tumors that commonly are seen in adults. They most commonly occur in the fourth ventricle, particularly at the obex followed by the frontal horns of the lateral ventricles. They typically do not enhance, but enhancement may be seen in a minority of them.

126.

A Giant perivascular space

This lesion is formed by a cluster of cystic spaces that follow cerebrospinal fluid signal and fully suppress on FLAIR sequences. There is a small FLAIR hyperintense focus in the intervening parenchyma, consistent with gliosis, but no evidence of mass effect or any contrast enhancement. A somewhat branching pattern is present, which may be easier to appreciate on consecutive slices. Findings are most consistent with a giant or tumefactive perivascular space. Although headache is the most common complaint, its association with the presence of a giant perivascular space is uncertain. (B) Dysembryoplastic neuroepithelial tumors can have a bubbly appearance, and most do not enhance. These lesions are centered in the cortex,

and there usually is some identifiable mass effect. Note that the cortex is thinned but not primarily involved in this case. (C) Metastases almost always have some degree of contrast enhancement. A lesion of this size also should have considerable surrounding edema. (D) A cystic glioma would be associated with enhancing components or with nonenhancing infiltrative tumor, none of which are evident in this case.

127.

A Precocious puberty

A nonenhancing mass that is isointense to gray matter in this location in a patient of this age is suggestive of a hypothalamic (tuber cinereum) hamartoma. These hamartomas are composed of disorganized neural elements, can be sessile or pedunculated, and may be iso- to hyperintense on T2 images (as in this case), depending on the proportion of glial cells within them. These are benign lesions that do not grow and classically are associated with central precocious puberty and uncontrollable laughing spells (gelastic seizures). The main diagnostic consideration is a low-grade glioma. (B–D) Hypothalamic hamartomas do not enhance or grow, and calcifications are rare.

128.

B *CCM1*

Approximately 20% of cavernomas are familial, and these are more commonly multiple. They can be associated with mutations in the *CCM1* (usually in Hispanics), *CCM2*, or *CCM3* genes. (A) Mutations in the *ENG* gene are associated with hereditary hemorrhagic telangiectasia type 1. (C) Mutations in the *ACVRL1* gene are associated with hereditary hemorrhagic telangiectasia type 2. (D) Phenotypic manifestations of *RASA1* gene mutations include capillary and arteriovenous malformations and arteriovenous fistulas.

129.

B Rathke cleft cyst

Rathke cleft cysts are true cysts lined by epithelium that develop from remnants of Rathke's pouch between the pars intermedia and pars distalis of the pituitary gland. Because the pars intermedia is difficult to visualize on imaging, it typically appears as a homogeneous mass separating the adenohypophysis from the neurohypophysis. It almost always is homogeneous, and its signal intensity varies depending on the presence of tri-glycerides, cholesterol, and protein (note intrinsic T1 hyperintensity on this noncontrast scan). It sometimes can occur in the suprasellar compartment and almost never is symptomatic. (A) Craniopharyngiomas are heterogeneous masses that usually arise at the level of the infundibulum. They show areas of enhancement, and the great majority of the adamantinomatous type (seen predominantly in children) have associated calcifications. (C) Lymphocytic hypophysitis is a nonneoplastic inflammatory condition that may affect any part of the pituitary gland and infundibulum. It does not present as a discrete mass, as seen in this case. (D) Granular cell tumors arise from granular cell nests in the neurohypophysis or infundibulum. They most commonly are suprasellar and almost never are purely intrasellar. Note the normal-appearing posterior pituitary bright spot along the posterior aspect of the cyst. (E) Neurosarcoidosis can involve the pituitary gland and infundibulum but would not result in a discrete, well-defined mass with intrinsic T1 hyperintensity, as in this case.

130.

B Solid appearance

Craniopharyngiomas have a bimodal distribution with peaks at 5 to 14 years of age and 50 to 75 years of age. Adamantinomatous craniopharyngiomas tend to occur in children and more commonly are associated with cystic changes (filled with what is described as "motor oil" on gross exam) and calcifications. Adult craniopharyngiomas more commonly are of the papillary subtype and are more solid and devoid of cystic changes. (A) Cystic changes are more common in adamantinomatous craniopharyngiomas, which usually occur in children. (C) Calcifications are more common in adamantinomatous craniopharyngiomas. (D) Heterogeneous contrast enhancement can be present in both types of craniopharyngiomas but may be more commonly homogeneous in the papillary type due to their usually solid appearance. (E) Apparent diffusion coefficient (ADC) values do not discriminate between papillary and adamantinomatous craniopharyngiomas. They may, however, help distinguish solid papillary craniopharyngiomas from germinomas, which show restricted diffusion and therefore lower ADC values by virtue of their high cellularity.

131.

D Semicircular canal

The arrow points to the posterior limb of the posterior semicircular canal. (A) The singular canal transmits nerve fibers from the vestibule to the posterior semicircular canal. It is very small and not shown on this image. (B) The tympanic segment of the facial nerve canal can be seen more anteriorly along the medial aspect of the epitympanum. (C) The normal vestibular aqueduct is seen as a flat line posterior and medial to the posterior semicircular canal.

132.

C Leading edge of high diffusion-weighted imaging signal

A leading edge of high diffusion-weighted imaging signal has been described in larger and new progressive multifocal leukoencephalopathy (PML) lesions and is thought to be related to cytotoxic edema. (A) Signal abnormalities in PML are usually bilateral but asymmetric. (B) There generally is no significant edema in PML, and when it is present, it should raise concern about immune reconstitution inflammatory syndrome (IRIS), particularly when accompanied by contrast enhancement. (D) There usually is no contrast enhancement in PML. (E) Involvement of the U fibers is a characteristic of subcortical PML, which results in a scalloped appearance.

133.

A Low apparent diffusion coefficient values

The lesion's location, imaging characteristics, and pathological description are most consistent with a pineoblastoma. These lesions are primitive neuroectodermal tumors that most commonly occur in children younger than 10 years of age. Like other highly cellular tumors with a similar histology, pineoblastomas commonly have profound restricted diffusion due to very low apparent diffusion coefficient values. (B) "Engulfed" calcifications characteristically are described in germinomas. Calcifications in pineoblastomas tend to be more peripheral ("exploded"). (C) Because of their high cellularity, pineoblastomas usually show high density on CT. They may be heterogeneous due to cystic changes and necrosis. (D) A dural tail is characteristically seen in meningiomas. It should enhance more avidly than the tumor and taper away from it.

134.

A Pituitary apoplexy

Pre- and postcontrast MR images of the pituitary fossa accompany the question. The noncontrast image (*left;* note the lack of enhancement of the nasal mucosa) shows bright foci expanding the pituitary gland consistent with blood products. Pituitary apoplexy is an acute syndrome that can present with severe headaches, diplopia (due to mass effect on the oculomotor nerves), visual deficits (if the optic chiasm or optic nerves are compressed), and hypopituitarism. Sudden deficiency of adrenocorticotropin/cortisol may result in life-threatening hypotension. Hemorrhage usually occurs into a preexisting pituitary adenoma (such as in this case; note how the sella is mildly expanded) and rarely into a healthy gland. (B) Craniopharyngiomas typically are seen in children but have a bimodal age peak and also can present in young and middle-aged adults. They tend to develop around the infundibulum (rather than within the pituitary gland) and have a more insidious course compared with pituitary apoplexy. (C) Epidermoid tumors in this region usually are suprasellar. On T1-weighted sequences, they tend to have signal intensities close to that of cerebrospinal fluid and do not enhance. They may result in mass effect on adjacent structures, but their presentation would be more insidious than pituitary apoplexy. (D) Aneurysms can have unusual signal intensities due to thrombosis and also can present with acute headache if they rupture. The lesion in this case arises within the pituitary gland as can be seen by small claws of enhancing tissue around the hemorrhage.

135.

D The lesion is entirely radiation sensitive and should be treated primarily by radiation.

The imaging and pathological characteristics of this mass in a young adult are most consistent with a germinoma. A normal pituitary gland is present on the sagittal images; therefore, this is not a pituitary adenoma. Germinomas usually demonstrate avid homogeneous enhancement as well as restricted diffusion on MRI apparent diffusion coefficient maps and hyperdensity on CT due to their high cellularity. Although pineal region germinomas are significantly more frequent in males (male-to-female ratio of 10:1), the gender distribution of suprasellar lesions is relatively even. Pure germinomas are exquisitely sensitive to radiation, with long-term progression-free survival rates greater than 90% for localized lesions; therefore, this constitutes the mainstay of therapy, and gross total resection is not usually recommended for pure germinomas. The role of surgery in such cases generally is limited to tissue biopsy and decompression in cases of acute visual symptoms (in suprasellar lesions) or obstructive hydrocephalus (in pineal lesions). Although most germinomas do respond to chemotherapy, chemotherapy alone is associated with high rates of relapse.

136.

B Hemiparesis

The axial FLAIR image shows increased signal in the visualized portions of the right internal carotid artery within the carotid canal due to thrombosis, which may result in left hemiparesis if there is resultant anterior circulation ischemia. (A) Vision loss may be seen as a consequence of posterior circulation infarcts involving the visual cortex. (C) Gait ataxia may result from occlusion of the cerebellar arteries. (D) Lateral medullary syndrome (also known as Wallenberg syndrome) usually results from posterior inferior cerebellar artery territory infarcts. (E) Locked-in syndrome may be secondary to infarcts of the lower pons in the proximal basilar artery territory.

137.

D High FiO_2 concentration

High FiO_2 concentrations have been shown to result in sulcal FLAIR nonsuppression and is a commonly encountered phenomenon in patients undergoing general anesthesia. Keeping FiO_2 concentrations below 50% decreases the incidence of this finding. Causes of FLAIR nonsuppression include leptomeningeal disease (infectious or carcinomatous meningitis), subarachnoid hemorrhage, prior gadolinium administration in patients with renal insufficiency, and susceptibility artifacts commonly from metallic dental orthodontia and ventriculoperitoneal shunt reservoirs. (A) Leptomeningeal tumor spread would be highly unlikely in an asymptomatic and otherwise healthy child. (B, C) Meningitis and subarachnoid hemorrhage are unlikely, given the patient's clinical background.

138.

B Well-circumscribed margins

Hydatid cysts usually have well-circumscribed margins with a thin wall that is hypointense on T1 and T2 images. They are spherical and typically occur in the middle cerebral artery distribution.

Their signal tends to follow that of cerebrospinal fluid. (A) Perilesional edema is absent in hydatid cysts unless there is superimposed infection or rupture. (C, D) Hydatid cysts do not show restricted diffusion or enhancement unless there is superimposed infection. (E) There is usually no calcification in hydatid cysts.

139.

B Eosinophilic granuloma

Eosinophilic granuloma is the localized form of Langerhans cell histiocytosis characterized by infiltration with myeloid dendritic cells. In the spine, it most commonly affects the vertebral body and can result in a vertebra plana with variable degrees of epidural or paravertebral tissue. T2 signal tends to be normal or near normal. (A) Metastases from neuroblastoma usually are more heterogeneous and ill defined. They also may present with a soft tissue component projecting outside of the vertebra. (C) Telangiectatic osteosarcomas of the spine are rare. They are heterogeneous and frequently hemorrhagic with fluid–fluid levels. (D) Diskitis-osteomyelitis is an infectious process that, in children, probably begins in the disk (which still is vascularized). It would result in increased T2 signal within the disk and variable degrees of end-plate destruction (not present in this case). (E) A fracture would not have such a homogeneous appearance with smooth margins unless it is chronic. It also would not explain the solid-appearing tissue bulging into the prevertebral region.

140.

C Inferior petrosal sinus

Shown in the image accompanying the question is the inferior petrosal sinus, which generally transmits blood from the cavernous sinus to the jugular vein or, less commonly, to the suboccipital venous plexus via the hypoglossal canal; however, there is marked anatomic variation. (A) The sphenoparietal sinus receives tributaries from the middle cerebral, middle meningeal, and anterior diploic veins, and drains into the cavernous sinus. It courses along the ridge of the lesser wing of the sphenoid bone. (B) The superior petrosal sinus runs along the superior aspect of the petrous bone and drains blood from the cavernous sinus into the transverse sinus. (D) The inferior anastomotic vein (of Labbé) drains the temporal convexity and opercular region transmitting blood from the middle cerebral vein to the transverse or sigmoid sinus. (E) The marginal sinus extends along the rim of the foramen magnum.

141.

B They arise from anomalous differentiation of the meninx primitiva.

Intracranial lipomas are congenital lesions and not true neoplasms. They arise from anomalous differentiation of the meninx primitiva. (A) The tubulonodular variant and not the curvilinear type of intracranial lipoma is associated with callosal dysgenesis. (C) Short-tau inversion recovery (STIR) sequences nonselectively suppress fat and other tissues that have a short T1 values; therefore, a lipoma would demonstrate suppressed signal. (D) Calcification is common in pericallosal and interhemispheric lipomas, particularly in association with callosal dysgenesis. (E) Approximately 85% of intracranial lipomas arise at the midline. They are less commonly seen in the quadrigeminal plate, cerebellopontine angle, suprasellar, and sylvian cisterns.

142.

D Grade 4

The coronal ultrasound image accompanying the question shows intraventricular hemorrhage involving the entire right lateral ventricle and left temporal horn. There is extensive parenchymal abnormality surrounding the right lateral ventricle due to venous ischemia. Findings are consistent with grade 4 intraventricular hemorrhage. Note ventricular dilatation. (A) Grade 1 intraventricular hemorrhage is confined to the germinal matrices, which are located in the caudothalamic grooves. (B) Grade 2 intraventricular hemorrhage is defined by intraventricular hemorrhage extension with normal-sized ventricles. (C) Grade 3 intraventricular hemorrhage is defined by intraventricular hemorrhage extension accompanied by ventricular distention. (E) There is no grade 5 intraventricular hemorrhage.

143.

C Neuroglial cyst

The axial T2 image accompanying the question shows a well-circumscribed, cystic-appearing parenchymal lesion in the right cerebellum with an imperceptible wall. There is no contrast enhancement. Findings are most consistent with a neuroglial cyst. These are benign, epithelial-lined lesions of different sizes that can be found virtually anywhere in the neuraxis. There typically is no surrounding edema. (A) Arachnoid cysts are extra-axial. This is an intra-axial lesion, as it is nearly completely surrounded by parenchyma. (B) Even though they can occur in isolation, giant perivascular spaces usually have some structure to them and often show a clustered or branching pattern. It would be very unusual for one to present as a single, well-circumscribed cyst. Giant perivascular spaces can have areas of FLAIR hyperintensity due to gliosis around them. (D) Cysticercal cysts usually are smaller than the pictured cyst. A scolex, wall enhancement, calcification, or surrounding edema may be seen depending on the Escobar stage of the parasite. The racemose form can develop within the subarachnoid space or ventricles and appears like a cluster of cysts.

144.

D Atrophy of the ipsilateral mammillary body

The image accompanying the question shows atrophy and loss of the internal architecture of the right hippocampus with increased signal. Additionally, there is atrophy of the ipsilateral mammillary body compared with the left, as can be seen in severe and long-standing cases of mesial temporal sclerosis. (A) MR spectroscopy may show decreased N-acetylaspartate and mildly increased myoinositol in mesial temporal sclerosis. (B) FDG-PET may by useful by showing decreased metabolism/uptake in the hippocampus in patients with mesial temporal sclerosis even in the absence of structural abnormalities on MRI. (C) Atrophy of the ipsilateral fornix can be seen in severe and long-standing cases of mesial temporal sclerosis.

145.

A Requires a pial-arachnoid defect

The images accompanying the question show an intracerebral pneumatocele. The coronal CT reformat *(left)* shows a fracture through the right frontal sinus and air tracking intracranially with the formation of a parenchymal air cyst, which can be characterized best on the axial T2 image *(right)*.

There also is a cerebrospinal fluid level present within the cyst. An intracerebral pneumatocele requires a defect in the pia-arachnoid membrane in close proximity to a craniodural defect. Air may accumulate due a ball valve effect or possibly due to increased cerebrospinal fluid leakage, leading to slightly negative intracranial pressures. (B) About 75 to 90% of intracerebral pneumatoceles are secondary to trauma as in this case. Pneumatoceles are present in up to 25% of all cases of pneumocephalus. (C) Pneumatoceles are not true cysts, and therefore are not lined by epithelium. (D) Arachnoid cysts are lined by arachnoid cells formed by the splitting of arachnoid membranes.

146.

C Enhancement of the paraspinal musculature

Enhancement of the paraspinal musculature is an indirect sign of avulsion injury due to denervation. Enhancement of intradural nerve roots indicates functional avulsion even in the presence of a normal-appearing nerve. (A) These lesions are fluid-filled pseudomeningoceles and would not show contrast enhancement unless they were infected. (B) Fatty lesions would show suppression of signal on STIR images. (D) Restricted diffusion may be seen in many disease processes. In the spinal cord, it can be secondary to infection or cord ischemia. The pseudomeningoceles in this case would not show restricted diffusion.

147.

C Trigeminal nerve

Shown in the image accompanying the question is the trigeminal nerve, which arises from the lateral aspects of the pons. It has a characteristic shape, with fibers that appear to spread out before piercing the dura and entering the Meckel cave. (A) The oculomotor nerves are relatively thick and can be identified exiting the brainstem at the level of the pontomesencephalic junction. They course between the posterior cerebral and superior cerebellar arteries on coronal images. (B) The trochlear nerve generally is not seen on CISS or FIESTA images due to its small caliber, unless thinner slices are acquired (0.4 mm). (D) The abducens nerves are thin and can be seen exiting the brainstem at the level of the pontomedullary junction. (E) The glossopharyngeal nerve is part of the cranial nerve IX–X–XI complex. It exits the upper medulla and leaves the skull through the pars nervosa of the jugular foramen.

148.

C Carotid artery dissection

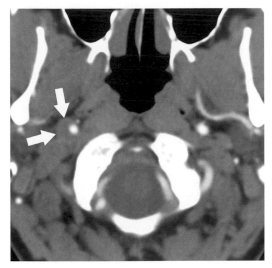

The axial CT angiogram image shown here demonstrates a crescentic, eccentric soft tissue density along the lateral aspect of the right internal carotid artery *(arrows)* consistent with a dissection. These dissections can be traumatic, as in this case, or associated with collagen vascular disease or iatrogenic causes. They may result in ischemic or embolic strokes and can be associated with pseudoaneurysm formation, Horner syndrome, or retinal ischemia. (A) There is no visible vertebral dissection. (B) Pseudoaneurysms sometimes may complicate a carotid artery dissection and may occur within hours, months, or years after the initial injury. In a pseudoaneurysm, the intima, media, and adventitia of the arterial wall are absent. (D) The visualized vertebral arteries are normal in this case. (E) The node of Rouvière is the most superior of the lateral retropharyngeal nodes. In children, it most commonly is enlarged secondary to infection, but it raises suspicion about malignancy of the upper aerodigestive tract in older patients.

149.

C Enostosis

The density of the lesion and radiating spicules that blend with the surrounding trabeculae are classic findings for an enostosis, commonly known as a bone island. These are incidental benign lesions that occur in cancellous bone. (A) Blastic metastases can be secondary to a variety of tumors. Bone islands sometimes can be mistaken for metastases when their characteristic imaging findings are not present. (B) Osteoid osteomas usually present as a lucent nidus surrounded by sclerotic bone and may have a dense, calcified center. They more commonly occur in long bones and in the spine where they preferentially involve the posterior elements. (D) Osteoblastomas are benign lesions that may be locally aggressive. They are histologically similar to osteoid osteomas but are much larger. They are predominantly lytic (unlike enostoses, which are dense), but may have matrix mineralization that can be seen on CT.

150.

C Eosinophilic granuloma

Eosinophilic granulomas, plasmacytoma/multiple myeloma, and most metastases are examples of lytic lesions with sharply circumscribed margins and no surrounding sclerosis. (A) Chondroblastomas are benign, slow-growing lesions that commonly present with a sclerotic margin. (B) Calvarial epidermoids typically present as lucent lesions with a sclerotic rim due to their slow growth. (D) Osteoid osteomas consist of a radiolucent nidus surrounded by sclerotic bone.

151.

B Hyperglycemia

Nonketotic hyperglycemia can be associated with hemiballismus. The most consistent imaging finding is the presence of hyperintensity unilaterally involving the lentiform nucleus and caudate nucleus head, which may be accompanied by T2 hypointensity and restricted diffusion. The reason for these signal changes is not entirely certain. (A) Carbon monoxide intoxication is not associated with unilateral basal ganglia lesions. Increased T2/FLAIR signal abnormalities and restricted diffusion may be present in the globi pallidi and cerebral white matter, including the corpus callosum following this type of injury. (C) The characteristic imaging finding in methanol intoxication is bilateral hemorrhagic putaminal necrosis and variable degrees of cerebral edema. (D) Liver disease can lead to T1 hyperintense basal ganglia, but the findings usually are bilateral.

152.

A Anoxic-ischemic brain injury

The "white" (or dense) cerebellum sign is secondary to a relatively increased density of the cerebellum, thalami, and brainstem due to extensive hypoattenuation of the supratentorial brain. It represents anoxic-ischemic brain injury and portends a grim prognosis. (B) Cerebellitis would result in hypoattenuation of the edematous areas, which may be focal or diffuse. (C) Cerebellar neoplasms may show increased or decreased density, depending on their histologies. Medulloblastomas, for instance, tend to be hyperdense due to their high cellularity. (D) Rhombencephalosynapsis consists of absence of the vermis with fusion of the dentate nuclei, cerebellar hemispheres, and superior peduncles.

153.

B Persistent trigeminal artery

A primitive trigeminal artery is the most common of the persistent fetal carotid-vertebrobasilar anastomoses. It arises at the junction of the cavernous and petrous segments of the internal carotid artery and courses along the trigeminal nerve or over the dorsum sellae. It may be associated with hypoplasia of the basilar artery, and a possible increased incidence of intracranial aneurysms and vascular malformations has also been described. (A) A persistent hypoglossal artery is second in frequency after a persistent trigeminal artery (although still much less common). It originates from the distal cervical internal carotid artery and courses through an enlarged hypoglossal canal to terminate in the basilar artery. (C) The primitive otic artery is the earliest fetal artery to disappear in embryonic life and represents the least common of the persistent fetal carotid-vertebrobasilar anastomoses. It arises from the internal carotid artery within the carotid canal and courses through the internal acoustic meatus to join the basilar artery. (D) The primitive stapedial artery is not part of the embryonic carotid-vertebrobasilar anastomoses. A persistent vessel may arise from the carotico-tympanic or inferior tympanic arteries at the level of the carotid canal and course along the cochlear promontory or through or parallel to the facial nerve canal. (E) A persistent pro-atlantal artery arises from the internal (type 1) or external (type 2) carotid artery and communicates with a vertebral artery. It rarely may arise from the common carotid artery.

154.

B Percheron artery infarct

In the MRI scans shown accompanying the question, there is restricted diffusion with very high signal in a particular arterial territory involving the paramedian thalami bilaterally as well as the rostral midbrain, consistent with Percheron artery territory infarcts. Although there is some variability, the paramedian arteries arise from the posterior cerebral arteries and supply this particular thalamic territory (in some patients they also may supply the anterior polar regions). The artery of Percheron is an anatomic variant, whereby a single artery supplies both paramedian thalamic territories. There is variable blood supply to the rostral midbrain, which may or may not be involved. (A) Bithalamic gliomas are rare and would not be restricted to the territory of the paramedian thalamic arteries or explain involvement of the rostral midbrain. (C) Deep venous thrombosis can result in diffuse swelling of the deep gray nuclei, but would not lead to the particular arterial territorial pattern of this case. (D) Top of the basilar syndrome occurs when a thrombus lodges at the distal basilar artery occluding both posterior cerebral arteries. This can result in occlusion of the paramedian thalamic arteries but likely will result in infarction of other posterior cerebral artery territories, which do not appear involved in this case.

155.

D Aquaporin-4 IgG seropositivity

Antibodies against the aquaporin-4 (AQP4) channels are highly specific for neuromyelitis optica (NMO). Lesions in NMO characteristically are found in areas of high AQP4 channel expression, such as around the ventricles, cerebral aqueduct, and dorsal midbrain. White matter lesions with "cloud-like" enhancement and "pencil-thin" ependymal enhancement also have been described and are thought to be relatively characteristic. NMO typically results in longitudinally extensive spinal cord signal abnormalities that may show enhancement. Optic neuritis typically is more severe in NMO than in multiple sclerosis. (A) Dawson fingers are demyelinating lesions seen in multiple sclerosis that are oriented radially from the lateral ventricles. Multiple sclerosis usually causes small lesions in short segments of the cord and does not result in longitudinally extensive signal abnormalities. The other features depicted on the MRI of the brain are not consistent with multiple sclerosis. (B) Hilar adenopathy can be seen in sarcoidosis. Neurosarcoid can present as leptomeningeal or parenchymal disease with formation of noncaseating granulomas. (C) Enhancement of ventral cauda equina roots characteristically is seen in Guillain-Barré syndrome, which does not involve the spinal cord or brain. (E) Decreased levels of B12 can result in subacute combined degeneration, which affects the posterior and sometimes lateral columns of the cord. There may be associated contrast enhancement.

156.

C Fibromuscular dysplasia

Both fibromuscular dysplasia and central nervous system vasculitis can be described as a "string of pearls" on angiogram. (A, E) Both severe carotid artery stenosis and dissection can be described as displaying a "string sign." (B) Dural arteriovenous fistulae are described as having "retrograde cortical venous drainage," implying the need for intervention. (D) Arteriovenous malformations characteristically display early draining veins.

157.

B Type 2a fractures present with minimal displacement and severe angulation.

Type 2a fractures (modification proposed by Levine and Edwards) present with severe angulation (more than 11 degrees) but minimal or no significant translation or displacement and are most commonly due to flexion-distraction injuries. Type 2 (not type 2a) fractures are associated with significant displacement (more than 3 mm) and angulation (more than 11 degrees) with translation of the anterior fragment and disruption of the C2-C3 intervertebral disk space. These are secondary to hyperextension, axial loading, and rebound flexion-compression. (A) There is no type 4 fracture in the modified Effendi grading system. (C) Type 1 fractures are hairline fractures of the ring of the axis, with no significant translation and no angulation between C2 and C3. They are the result of hyperextension and axial loading. (D) Type 3 fractures present with severe angulation and displacement of the anterior fragment with unilateral or bilateral facet dislocation, and they result from a flexion-compression injury. There is fracture of the posterior elements.

158.

A 3-mm funnel-shaped segment at the posterior communicating artery origin

An infundibulum classically is less than 3 mm at its widest portion, triangular in shape, with a vessel arising from its apex, and almost always is located at the origin of the posterior communicating artery. They are not uncommon to find, and although they can grow into an aneurysm, an infundibulum in itself is not classically associated with rupture. (B, E) A diameter greater than 3 mm would be too large for an infundibulum. By definition, there also should be a normal vessel arising from its apex. (C) A spherical dilation of the basilar artery tip is the definition of a basilar tip aneurysm and not an infundibulum. (D) Infundibula arise at the origin of a vessel and not adjacent to it (as can occur with a saccular aneurysm). Additionally, size greater than 3 mm would be too large for an infundibulum.

159.

D The apex is the most common location.

The apex (tip) is the most common location of basilar artery aneurysms, and lesions at this site represent 50 to 80% of all posterior fossa aneurysms. Aneurysms of the basilar trunk are rare. Other locations for basilar artery aneurysms include the junctions of the posterior cerebral, anterior inferior cerebellar, and superior cerebellar arteries. (A) Endovascular therapy the is mainstay for treating basilar tip aneurysms and largely has replaced traditional microsurgical techniques, which necessitate significant brain retraction and temporary arterial occlusion that may result in significant morbidity or mortality. (B) Posterior circulation aneurysms have the highest rate of rupture of all intracranial aneurysms. Basilar and internal carotid artery aneurysms also may be more likely to grow compared with aneurysms developing at other sites. (C) The epicenter of subarachnoid hemorrhage may suggest the site of the aneurysm. Anterior communicating artery aneurysms bleed primarily into the interhemispheric fissure, and those from the middle cerebral artery hemorrhage bleed into the sylvian fissure. Basilar tip aneurysms characteristically bleed into the basilar cisterns, posterior third ventricle, and fourth ventricle. That being said, hemorrhage frequently is widespread without a discernible pattern.

160.

D Meningioma

The pathological description provided in the question is that of a meningioma. Meningiomas represent the most common primary intracranial tumors in adults and most frequently are parafalcine or seen along the sphenoid wings. About 10% occur in the parasellar region. Meningiomas can arise primarily within the cavernous sinus or involve it secondarily. The patient's presentation depends on the neurovascular structures involved. Patients commonly present with oculomotor, visual, or trigeminal symptoms. (A) Hemangiopericytomas are rare intracranial lesions. Microscopically, one can find uniform spindle cells with intratumoral staghorn vessels. On imaging, they commonly present as a large and aggressive dural-based mass. (B) Secondary lymphomas are more common than primary lymphomas in the central nervous system. The great majority of primary central nervous system lymphomas are of the B-cell type and occur in the parenchyma. Most secondary lymphomas affect the leptomeninges but also may occur in the brain. Dural lymphomas are rare. (C) Schwannomas arise from Schwann cells and are seen in adults. Microscopic exam shows spindle cells with ill-defined cytoplasm and dense chromatin sometimes associated with Verocay bodies. Intracranial schwannomas most commonly are related to the vestibular nerve followed by the trigeminal and facial nerves. In the parasellar region, trigeminal schwannomas predominate.

161.

A Embryonic endoderm

This is the characteristic location of a colloid cyst, which derives from embryonic endoderm and nearly always is situated in the anterosuperior aspect of the third ventricle. These lesions may be associated with obstruction of the foramina of Monro, which can be acute and lead to rapid herniation and death. They often are hyperdense on CT, and their MRI signal characteristics vary depending on the degree of proteinaceous contents; those with lower T2 signal tend to be more viscous. The cyst is bright on both the noncontrast T1-weighted and FLAIR images shown in this case. (B, D) Colloid cysts derive from embryonic endoderm. (C) Tornwaldt cysts, among other lesions, are derived from the notochord. (E) Arachnoid cap cells give rise to meningiomas.

162.

B Calcification is common

The location and homogeneously bright T1 signal intensity of the mass displayed along with signal suppression on the fat-saturated T2 image are most consistent with a pericallosal lipoma (tubulonodular type). Note that the image to the left is without intravenous contrast (there is no mucosal enhancement in the nasopharynx or pituitary gland). Calcification is common, particularly when there is callosal dysgenesis, which is associated more frequently with tubulonodular lipomas. Curvilinear lipomas have a low incidence of associated anomalies. Note arachnoid cysts posterior to the corpus callosum and in the posterior fossa compressing the cerebellum. The callosal splenium is short. (A) Meningiomas arise from arachnoid cap cells. Lipomas develop from anomalous differentiation of the meninx primitiva. (C) Dermoids contain dermal appendages. Although they characteristically show areas of fat signal intensity, they are more heterogeneous than lipomas and commonly show dark areas of T2 hypointensity and fluid–fat levels. Dermoids have a predilection for the midline, whereas lipomas tend to occur along infoldings of the subarachnoid space. (D) Meningiomas demonstrate an alanine peak on MR spectroscopy at short TE values.

163.

C Acute infarct

There is hypoattenuation involving the left insula and lateral basal ganglia in a patient with an acute middle cerebral artery infarct. Note two hyperdense dots in the left sylvian fissure (the "MCA dot" sign), consistent with thrombosed M2 branches. (A) There is no defined fluid collection to suggest an abscess. (B) An infiltrative neoplasm potentially can mimic an infarct particularly on CT. (D) Contusions in a patient with trauma usually are peripheral and cortical but may vary in size and involve the subcortical white matter. They do not follow a vascular distribution and would not explain the hyperdense vessels. (E) Old infarcts usually show lower attenuation and well-circumscribed margins, with variable degrees of volume loss and wallerian degeneration.

164.

C Osmotic demyelination

The axial FLAIR image accompanying the question shows a triangular hyperintensity in the mid-posterior pons that demonstrates peripheral enhancement on the coronal postcontrast image. This is a characteristic location and presentation for osmotic demyelination, which commonly is seen in alcoholics after rapid correction of hyponatremia, as well as in advanced liver disease, various causes of malnutrition, and burns. Fifty percent of patients show abnormalities in the pons, and the rest of the lesions are extrapontine, occurring in the basal ganglia, thalami, brainstem, and corpus callosum. Lesions usually do not enhance, although ring enhancement of pontine lesions has been observed in the acute phase, as in this case. (A) An infiltrative glioma would have some degree of mass effect. The discrete central location and triangular configuration of the lesion in this case is more consistent with osmotic demyelination. (B) Infarction usually does not cross the midline except for some infarcts from perforator vessels. The triangular shape and central location of the lesion in this case are much more likely to be related to osmotic demyelination. (D) Edema associated with brainstem encephalitis likely would show mass effect and would be either asymmetric or diffuse.

165.
C Shows increased uptake on bone scintigraphy

These findings are most consistent with an osteoid osteoma with a lucent nidus, a calcified center, and surrounding sclerosis. These lesions typically show increased uptake on bone scintigraphy, on which they may appear as a "double density" with marked central uptake and a surrounding rim of relatively lower uptake. (A) Osteoid osteomas usually occur in adolescents and young adults, and more commonly present in the second decade of life. There is growing evidence that osteoid osteomas resolve over time. (B) Osteoid osteomas commonly occur in the long bones. In the spine, they usually involve the posterior elements and are most frequently seen in the lumbar followed by cervical spine. (D) With osteoid osteomas, pain typically is worse at night, relieved with aspirin (osteoid osteomas produce prostaglandins), and is not related to activity.

166.
B There is an increased risk of dural tears.

Depressed skull fractures are associated with an increased risk of dural tears. (A) Most pediatric skull fractures can be managed expectantly if they are depressed less than 1 cm, they are closed, there is no associated intracranial hemorrhage, and the patient is neurologically intact. (C) There is no evidence that surgical elevation decreases the incidence of posttraumatic seizures, as any potential cortical damage occurs at the time of injury.

(D) Depressed skull fractures have an increased risk of cortical laceration. (E) Linear fractures are the most common type of skull fractures, followed by depressed and basilar fractures.

167.
C It derives from arachnoid cap cells.

Meningiomas can result in thickening and enhancement along the optic nerve sheath in a parallel configuration resembling a tram track. They derive from arachnoid cap cells. (A) A retinoblastoma is a highly malignant small round blue cell tumor. It does not produce the so-called tram track sign. Retinoblastomas commonly show low intensity on T2-weighted sequences and profound restricted diffusion due to their high cellularity. (B) Optic pathway gliomas can either be sporadic or associated with neurofibromatosis type 1. Those that are syndromic more commonly involve the optic nerves than the optic chiasm or postchiasmatic tracts. MRI shows expansion of the optic nerve due to tumor infiltration with variable degrees of contrast enhancement. (D) Thyroid orbitopathy is related to leukocytic infiltration with deposition of mucopolysaccharides. It can affect any extraocular muscle with preferential involvement of the inferior, medial, and superior extraocular muscles.

168.
D Neurenteric cyst

This is a complex, cystic lesion with a component projecting into and expanding the spinal canal and a second component projecting into the posterior mediastinum. The inferior aspect of the lesion is partially intramedullary. Note also congenital vertebral anomalies with incomplete segmentation and a small size of multiple adjacent thoracic vertebrae. This constellation of findings is most consistent with a neurenteric cyst. These lesions result from incomplete resorption of the neurenteric canal, and when they occur in the spine, they are most commonly thoracic. (A) Epidermoid tumors in the spine may be developmental or acquired, and occur most commonly in the lumbar region. They rarely may be associated with spinal malformations such as hemivertebrae. (B) A traumatic pseudomeningocele would not result in congenital vertebral anomalies, and its contents would follow cerebrospinal fluid signal on all sequences. (C) An arachnoid cyst is not associated with vertebral anomalies, although it could result in osseous remodeling due to slow growth.

169.

B Melanin

Melanin has a high affinity for many metals including iron, manganese, copper, and zinc, and their paramagnetic effects result in T1 shortening; therefore, melanin is bright on T1-weighted sequences. (A) Myelin is bright on T1-weighted images due to the decreased motion of water molecules associated with macromolecules such as myelin. T1 images are helpful in the evaluation of myelination in infants. (C) High vascular flow results in a flow void and therefore looks dark on T1-weighted sequences. (D) Deoxyhemoglobin is seen in acute hemorrhage. There is no significant effect on T1 signal as the three-dimensional configuration of deoxyhemoglobin does not allow access of water molecules to the paramagnetic iron atoms, which prevents the dipole–dipole interactions that would result in T1 shortening.

170.

D Compression of the contralateral cerebral peduncle against the cerebellar tentorium

The Kernohan notch phenomenon (also known as a "false localizing sign" and the Kernohan-Woltman notch) is a result of supratentorial mass effect with extensive shift of midline structures, resulting in compression of the contralateral cerebral peduncle against the cerebellar tentorium. This manifests clinically as hemiplegia or hemiparesis ipsilateral to the primary lesion. (A) Contralateral hydrocephalus secondary to obstruction of the foramen of Monro can be seen as a complication of supratentorial mass effect. (B) The Kernohan notch phenomenon refers to compression of the contralateral (not ipsilateral) cerebral peduncle against the cerebellar tentorium. (C) Compression of the anterior cerebral artery against the falx cerebri can occur with subfalcine herniation, as the cingulate sulcus is displaced beyond the midline.

171.

A Acute demyelination

These lesions demonstrate the typical appearance of acute tumefactive demyelination: concentric rings of different intensities on the FLAIR image, a periventricular configuration along perimedullary veins (somewhat perpendicular to the lateral ventricles), and, most importantly, an incomplete ring of enhancement on the postcontrast T1 images. (B) Metastases are a cause of multifocal enhancing lesions, but the presence of incomplete ring enhancement would be unusually rare, as would be the perimedullary configuration of the lesions (metastases favor the gray matter–white matter junction and vascular border zones). In addition, metastases likely would incite a significant amount of surrounding edema for the size of these lesions. (C) Multifocal glioblastoma likely would have a more heterogeneous and infiltrative appearance rather than the discrete lesions in the distribution described above. (D) Multifocal abscesses would not present with an incomplete ring of enhancement, and the perimedullary/periventricular distribution seen in this case would be unusual for abscesses. Abscesses also demonstrate central restricted diffusion, whereas tumefactive demyelination may demonstrate restricted diffusion peripherally. (E) Vasculitides can result in multifocal white matter lesions and infarcts. Mural enhancement sometimes can be demonstrated on high-resolution vessel wall imaging. An incomplete ring enhancement is not seen.

172.

C Wackenheim line

The Wackenheim (basilar) line is drawn along the clivus and extends inferiorly to the cervical spinal canal. It should be tangential to the dorsal surface of the tip of the odontoid process. Transection of this line by the odontoid process indicates basilar invagination.

173.

A McRae line

The McRae line is drawn from the basion to the opisthion and marks the level of the foramen magnum. The odontoid process normally is located inferior to this line, and its extension above it indicates basilar invagination. (B) The Chamberlain line extends from the posterior pole of the hard palate to the opisthion. Extension of the odontoid process greater than 3 mm beyond this line indicates basilar invagination. (D) The McGregor line is a modification of Chamberlain line developed for cases where the opisthion could not be identified in radiographs. The McGregor line extends from the posterior pole of the hard palate to the most inferior aspect of the occipital curvature. Greater than 4.5 mm extension of the odontoid process beyond this line indicates basilar invagination.

174.

D Hematoma

The noncontrast CT image accompanying the question shows a large and heterogeneous retroperitoneal mass on the left side, with areas that are hyperdense relative to the adjacent psoas muscle, consistent with a retroperitoneal hematoma. This is an infrequent but important complication with a reported incidence between 0.5% and 5% that can be seen following difficult arterial or venous groin access, particularly in patients who are anticoagulated. (A) An urinoma would not be expected after femoral puncture. It also would appear more homogeneous and demonstrate lower density on CT unless it was infected. (B) The image shows a retroperitoneal process that is displacing the bowel loops anteriorly. (C) The image shows fluid that is not within the peritoneal cavity. The location of this hematoma is retroperitoneal, which can be suspected following difficult groin access and also by noticing mild enlargement of the left psoas muscle and stranding of the surrounding retroperitoneal fat.

175.

E Limited by dural reflections

This is an acute subdural hematoma with hyperdense blood, resulting in a shift of midline structures. These lesions occur between the inner layer of the dura and arachnoid membranes, and therefore are limited by dural reflections including the falx cerebri and tentorium cerebelli. (A) Epidural, not subdural, hematomas occur between the outer layer of the dura and the calvaria and are thus limited by tight dural attachments at the sutures. (B) Supratentorial subdural hematomas cannot cross the midline, as they are limited by the dural reflections that form the falx cerebri. (C) Subdural hematomas are most commonly due to the tearing of bridging veins due to a shearing injury. For this reason, they are more common in older brains where these veins may be stretched due to cerebral atrophy. (D) Subdural hematomas occur between the dura and arachnoid membranes.

176.

D Preferential involvement of the cortex is a distinctive feature.

Preferential involvement of the cortex is one of the distinctive features of oligodendroglial tumors. (A) Oligodendrogliomas occur most commonly in the frontal lobes, followed by the temporal and parietal lobes. Occipital involvement is relatively rare. (B) Calcification is a common feature of oligodendrogliomas and is found in 70 to 90% of cases. Cystic degeneration and hemorrhage may be seen occasionally. (C) In contrast to astrocytic brain tumors, perfusion-weighted imaging has had limited value in differentiating subgroups of oligodendrogliomas with significant overlap between low- and high-grade histologies. Low-grade oligodendrogliomas can present with increased perfusion. (E) Oligodendrogliomas with *1p/19q* co-deletions respond more favorably to both radiation and chemotherapy, and this is the most important factor associated with improved survival.

177.

A Pial collateral circulation

Patients with moyamoya-type vascularity may develop pial collaterals due to chronic occlusion. MRI shows nonsuppression of FLAIR signal in sulci and perivascular spaces, which may be accompanied by contrast enhancement. (B) Leptomeningeal carcinomatosis can show FLAIR nonsuppression but is not associated with an "ivy" sign and would not be an expected complication, given the patient's clinical history. (C) Meningitis can result in leptomeningeal enhancement and FLAIR nonsuppression. (D) Cerebral microhemorrhages are a complication of sickle cell disease and may be related to embolism of marrow fat or local thrombosis with subsequent hemorrhage. (E) Ischemia is one of the known complications of sickle cell disease. The cause is multifactorial and includes hypercoagulability, endothelial injury, and development of moyamoya type vessels.

178.

D Enhancement of the cyst wall

Enhancement of the cyst wall may be present in pilocytic astrocytomas, whereas the wall of a hemangioblastoma should not enhance. Two thirds of hemangioblastomas are cystic with an enhancing mural nodule, and one third is solid. (A) Hemangioblastomas are highly vascular lesions with relative cerebral blood volumes that are significantly higher than pilocytic astrocytomas. (B) Hemangioblastomas often have small vascular flow voids due to hypervascularity. (C) An enhancing nodule abutting the pia is characteristic of a hemangioblastoma.

179.

C Intrinsic T1 hyperintensity

Angiocentric gliomas are relatively indolent and slow-growing cortical masses that initially were included in the WHO classification of central nervous system tumors in 2007. Intrinsic T1 hyperintensity is suggestive of the diagnosis, but such a feature is present inconsistently. They usually do not enhance. (A) Pleomorphic xanthoastrocytomas occur most commonly in the temporal lobes and typically have an enhancing solid component abutting the meningeal surface. (B) A usually nonenhancing cortical/subcortical mass with a bubbly appearance on T2 and FLAIR images is most consistent with a dysembryoplastic neuroepithelial tumor. (D) A triangular morphology sometimes has been described in dysembryoplastic neuroepithelial tumors.

180.

A *ATP7B*

The findings described in the question are compatible with Wilson disease (hepatolenticular degeneration). The clinical exam describes the Kayser-Fleischer rings that are present in 98% of patients with neurologic manifestations. The imaging findings show the typical distribution of signal abnormalities in the basal ganglia and midbrain, with sparing of the red nuclei and substantia nigra. Wilson disease results from mutations in the *ATP7B* gene that leads to a ceruloplasmin deficiency and copper accumulation in the liver, brain, and corneas. (B) Cerebral autosomal dominant arteriopathy with subcortical infarcts and leukoencephalopathy (CADASIL) has been linked to mutations in the *NOTCH3* gene. (C) Mutations in the *SMARCB1* gene can lead to Coffin-Siris syndrome and to an increased risk of developing rhabdoid tumors such as ATRT. (D) Most syndromic cases of trigonocephaly are related to mutations in the *FGFR* genes. (E) Cowden disease (multiple hamartoma syndrome) has been linked to loss of *PTEN* gene function.

181.

A Pantothenate kinase–associated neurodegeneration

Pantothenate kinase–associated neurodegeneration is a rare disorder caused by mutations in the *PKAN2* gene that result in abnormal iron accumulation in the brain, particularly in the globi pallidi and substantia nigra. Patients present in the first or second decades of life with symptoms including progressive dystonia, dementia, choreoathetosis, and rigidity. The "eye of the tiger" sign classically is described on T2-weighted images, with central hyperintensity representing demyelination and gliosis surrounded by dark areas of iron deposition. (B) The characteristic imaging finding of Huntington disease is atrophy of the heads of the caudate nuclei, resulting in ballooning of the frontal horns of the lateral ventricles. The putamina also can show volume loss, and there may be increased T2/FLAIR signal in the basal ganglia. (C) Wilson disease shows increased signal in the basal ganglia, particularly in the lateral putamina, and brainstem, typically with sparing of the red nuclei and substantia nigra, leading to the "face of the giant panda" sign. (D) Carbon monoxide intoxication may show increased signal in the globi pallidi and white matter.

182.

A Aneurysm

Areas of profound T2 hypointensity in a well-circumscribed skull base region mass should raise concern about an aneurysm. The presence of pulsation artifact propagating along the phase-encoding direction makes this lesion an aneurysm until proven otherwise. Other sources of phase-encoding motion artifact are swallowing, breathing, peristalsis, and patient movement during the scan. (B) Meningiomas are relatively hypointense on T2-weighted images and can have irregular areas of marked hypointensity due to calcification or occasionally hemorrhage. They do not result in a phase-encoding artifact. (C, D) Chordomas and chondrosarcomas characteristically are bright on T2 images. They are not associated with pulsation artifacts.

183.

B Coronal

Premature fusion of the coronal sutures can result in the so-called harlequin-eye deformity, which may be unilateral or bilateral. Approximately 10% of craniosynostoses are syndromic and may be related to mutations involving the *FGFR* and *TWIST-1* genes, among others. Syndromic associations include Crouzon, Apert, and Pfeiffer syndromes. (A) Fusion of the sagittal suture leads to scaphocephaly. (C) Lambdoid synostosis is rare and results in flattening of the posterior head ipsilaterally. (D) Metopic craniosynostosis gives an abnormal triangular shape to the forehead (trigonocephaly), sometimes with the development of a frontal osseous ridge.

184.

A Cranioplasty

"Sunken skin flap" or "trephine" syndrome refers to an uncommon late postoperative complication following decompressive craniectomy in which there is marked concavity of the skin flap and paradoxical cerebral herniation. The pathophysiology is presumed to be related to exposure of the intracranial contents to atmospheric pressure and a negative pressure gradient that may be exacerbated by cerebrospinal fluid hypovolemia. Neurologic deterioration in this context is a surgical emergency, and the goal of treatment is to restore intracranial pressure, which generally can be achieved by cranioplasty. Other measures include placing the patient in the Trendelenburg position, tilting the head toward the craniectomy site, an epidural blood patch, or clamping the ventricular shunt tubing. (B) There are no collections to evacuate in this patient. (C) Contralateral craniectomy would not help restore the intracranial pressure. (D) Lumbar spinal fluid drain would be contraindicated in a patient with a herniation syndrome. Lumbar epidural blood patches may be useful in the management of sunken flap syndrome.

185.
D Central location

Ependymomas tend to have a central location, although such distinction usually is difficult to make and is not possible with large tumors. Ependymomas more commonly present with cysts, calcifications, and hemorrhage. (A) Patients with neurofibromatosis type 2 have an increased incidence of ependymomas, which occur most frequently in the brainstem and spinal cord. (B) Ill-defined margins more commonly are present in spinal cord astrocytomas. Ependymomas usually are well defined. (C) Heterogeneous enhancement can be seen in both astrocytomas and ependymomas and is not a helpful discriminating feature.

186.
C Subluxation of C2 on C3

The findings describe a hangman fracture, which most commonly is secondary to hyperextension, compression, and distraction. Subluxation of C2 on C3 indicates an unstable fracture. (A, B) Hangman fractures with more than 3 mm between fragments and more than 15 degrees of angulation are considered unstable. (D) In patients with a Jefferson fracture, a combined offset of the lateral C1 masses relative to C2 greater than 6 mm suggests disruption of the transverse ligament and an unstable fracture.

187.
B Pedicle subtraction osteotomy

This patient has sagittal imbalance due to loss of the expected lumbar lordosis, with acute kyphotic angulation centered at L1 above the level of the fusion. A pedicle subtraction osteotomy at L1 potentially could restore lordosis by means of a wedge-shaped vertebral resection and shortening of the posterior column. (A) Although other modalities such as MRI are more sensitive, there is no radiographic evidence of diskitis/osteomyelitis that would manifest as erosive changes centered at the disk space with variable degrees of end-plate and vertebral destruction. (C) There is no visible peri-hardware lucency to suggest loosening on this

exam. (D) Anterior interbody fusion would not restore lumbar lordosis.

188.
E Sporadic presentation

Sturge-Weber syndrome presents sporadically without a definite hereditary pattern identified to date. (A) Sturge-Weber syndrome is a disorder of neural crest cell migration and differentiation. It is characterized by an inadequate control of capillary formation, with the development of leptomeningeal angiomatosis and choroidal angiomas and the recruitment of deep medullary and choroidal veins. Cortical calcifications and cerebral volume loss ipsilateral to the port-wine stain are seen in advanced cases, possibly related to chronic ischemia. Arteriovenous malformations are not seen. (B) The port-wine stain of Sturge-Weber syndrome occurs along the distribution of cranial nerve V. The ophthalmic branch almost always is involved, followed by the maxillary division in frequency. Involvement of the mandibular division almost never occurs in isolation. (C) Glioneuronal hamartomas are known as cortical tubers and are seen in tuberous sclerosis. (D) Progressive hemifacial atrophy (also known as Parry-Romberg syndrome) is characterized by a slow and progressive unilateral atrophy of the skin, bones, and soft tissues of the face. It sometimes is accompanied by volume loss and abnormal signal in the ipsilateral and sometimes contralateral brain.

189.
A Increased relative cerebral blood volume

The necrotic mass shown with heterogeneous enhancement in an adult patient most likely represents a glioblastoma, which may arise de novo or from degeneration of a lower grade glioma. Glioblastomas show increased relative cerebral blood volume and blood flow on MR and CT perfusion studies and increased permeability values on advanced MR imaging. Approximately 10% are multicentric. They may hemorrhage and rarely calcify. (B) Because glioblastomas are highly cellular tumors, their solid components tend to show restricted diffusion and decreased (not elevated) apparent diffusion coefficient values. (C, D) On MR spectroscopy, glioblastomas and other high-grade gliomas show decreased N-acetylaspartate levels (reflecting neuronal loss) and elevated choline levels due to increased cellular turnover. Glioblastomas may show elevated lipid and lactate levels secondary to necrosis. (E) Elevated alanine levels are a characteristic feature of meningiomas on MR spectroscopy.

190.

D Hemangiopericytoma

This constellation of imaging findings and histopathology are consistent with a hemangiopericytoma. Hemangiopericytomas are locally aggressive tumors with a high incidence of recurrence. They occur more commonly in the supratentorial compartment and usually are large at presentation. Distinguishing them from meningiomas by imaging may be difficult, but hemangiopericytoma can be suggested in the setting of an aggressive, highly vascular, heterogeneous, dural-based mass in a relatively younger patient. Hemangiopericytomas also can metastasize (particularly the anaplastic subtype). On MR spectroscopy, they do not show an alanine peak, which is typical of meningiomas. (A) Hemangioblastomas can occur sporadically. They are vascular tumors with avid enhancement and frequently show prominent flow voids. They very rarely occur in the supratentorial compartment, usually are intra-axial or intraventricular, and may grow along the pial surface (rather than the dural surface). (B) Meningiomas can show variable degrees of vascularity and may be difficult to distinguish from hemangiopericytomas by imaging. Meningiomas more commonly are homogeneous and are more likely to result in hyperostosis rather than frank bone erosion, although they also may be invasive and primarily osseous. They tend to occur in patients older than 50 years of age. (C) Dural lymphoma is rare and usually shows avid but homogeneous enhancement on MRI.

191.

A Sporadic gliomas are more frequently chiasmatic or postchiasmatic.

Syndromic optic pathway gliomas (associated with neurofibromatosis type 1) more frequently involve the optic nerves, whereas sporadic ones more commonly are chiasmatic or postchiasmatic. (B) Optic pathway gliomas are the most common central nervous system neoplasms in neurofibromatosis type 1. (C) Calcification is rare in optic pathway gliomas. Cysts may be present and appear to be more common in sporadic tumors. (D) Hemorrhage is exceedingly rare in optic pathway gliomas. (E) Contrast enhancement in optic pathway gliomas is variable and does not correlate with tumor grade.

192.

C Ratio of the largest width of the frontal horns divided by the maximum internal diameter of the skull

The Evans ratio is defined as the largest width of the frontal horns divided by the maximum internal diameter of the calvaria, with a value ≥ 0.3 being used to document ventriculomegaly as per the current normal pressure hydrocephalus guidelines; however, recent studies have shown significant variability related to the plane of measurement and angulation. (A) The frontal horn ratio is defined as the largest width of the frontal horns divided by the internal diameter of the skull at the same level. (B) Dilatation of the temporal horns more than 2 mm and a frontal horn ratio more than 0.5 have been described as suggestive of hydrocephalus. Other signs that suggest hydrocephalus include ballooning of the frontal horns or third ventricle, transependymal flow, and bowing of the corpus callosum on sagittal images. (D) Occipital-frontal circumference is followed for every growing child, and abnormalities such as rapid growth, crossing growth curves, growth more than two standard deviations above or below the average, or a head circumference out of proportion to length/weight should prompt a workup for underlying conditions (e.g., hydrocephalus).

193.

C Eosinophilic granuloma

Eosinophilic granulomas, plasmacytomas, and multiple myeloma are examples of lytic processes without surrounding sclerosis. (A) Hemangiomas have sclerotic margins in 30% of cases and often have a characteristic "honeycomb" or "star-bust" pattern of trabeculation on skull radiographs. (B) Epidermoids are slow-growing lucent lesions with sclerotic borders. (D) Osteoid osteomas consist of a radiolucent and sometimes calcified nidus with surrounding zones of dense sclerosis.

194.

A Osteomyelitis of the skull with subperiosteal abscess

Pott's puffy tumor is characterized by a subperiosteal abscess and osteomyelitis, usually as a complication of frontal sinusitis. Less common causes include mastoiditis, trauma, craniotomy, and intranasal substance abuse (e.g., cocaine and methamphetamines). It has a higher incidence in adolescents but can occur at any age. Pott's puffy tumor may be complicated by cortical vein or dural sinus thrombosis, epidural abscess, subdural abscess, cerebritis, or brain abscess. (B) Tuberculosis of the spine or tuberculous spondylitis sometimes is referred to as Pott disease. The infection originates in the end plates with subsequent subligamentous spread.

There is a higher incidence of extensive paraspinal abscess formation, and the intervertebral disks more often are spared compared with bacterial infections. In addition, Pott disease has a predilection for the vertebral body with sparing of the posterior elements. (C) True (also known as idiopathic) moyamoya disease has the appearance of a "puff of smoke" on angiography due to extensive collateralization in the setting of bilateral carotid artery stenosis. Moyamoya syndrome (secondary moyamoya) is a nonspecific radiographic finding with a similar pattern of collateralization associated with conditions such as neurofibromatosis type 1, Down syndrome, sickle cell disease, and connective tissue disorders, and may be seen after radiation for treatment of sellar or suprasellar tumors. (D) Dermoid cysts originate from epithelial inclusion cysts and may develop in the skull at sites of suture closure. They contain dermal appendages (as opposed to epidermoid cysts) and are lined by keratinized squamous epithelium.

195.

D Lateral putamina and tectum

Wilson disease results from a ceruloplasmin deficiency leading to copper accumulation in brain, liver, and corneas. On MRI, T2/FLAIR signal hyperintensity typically affects the midbrain and basal ganglia, particularly the tectum and lateral putamina. The red nuclei and substantia nigra typically are preserved, resulting in the "face of the giant panda" sign on axial imaging. Diffusion restriction may be seen in the acute stage. (A) T2/FLAIR signal hyperintensity in the medial thalami, periaqueductal gray, tectum, and mammillary bodies should prompt the diagnosis of Wernicke encephalopathy. (B) The red nuclei and substantia nigra usually are spared in Wilson disease. (C) The external capsules and temporal poles characteristically are involved in cerebral autosomal dominant arteriopathy with subcortical infarcts and leukoencephalopathy (CADASIL). (E) Carbon monoxide poisoning classically shows signal abnormalities in the globi pallidi, but the subcortical white matter, hippocampi, and cerebral cortex also may be affected.

196.

A Thickening and enhancement of the cauda equina

Thickening and enhancement of the cauda equina would support the presence of an adjacent inflammatory process or infection. Myelopathy with edema of the distal cord and conus medullaris and pial enhancement may be seen depending on the severity of the infection. (B) Markedly increased diffusion-weighted imaging signal within a mass could be related to restricted diffusion from an abscess, but also can be seen in epidermoids and dermoids due to what is probably a combination of restricted diffusion and T2 shine-through effects. An infected dermoid or epidermoid is accompanied by inflammatory changes such as edema and enhancement of the surrounding tissues. (C) It is important to differentiate whether increased signal on the postcontrast T1 sequences is due to true enhancement or related to intrinsic T1 hyperintensity; therefore, both pre- and postcontrast sequences should be evaluated side by side. Hemorrhage, fatty masses, and certain tumors such as melanomas can show increased T1 signal on the precontrast images. (D) Signal dropout on gradient echo sequences can be seen with prior hemorrhage.

197.

B West Nile virus infection

Neuroimaging findings in West Nile virus infection are varied and, in the spine, include nonspecific intramedullary signal abnormalities with variable enhancement. Infection can result in progressive ascending paralysis and preferential ventral nerve root enhancement mimicking Guillain-Barré syndrome. (A) Leptomeningeal carcinomatosis is distributed more unevenly and is commonly nodular. Patients may present with "sugar coating" of the spinal cord. (C) Dural arteriovenous fistulas often can be identified by the presence of vascular flow voids surrounding an edematous spinal cord (best seen on T2 sequences). (D) Sarcoidosis can result in leptomeningeal or parenchymal disease with formation of noncaseating granulomas. It does not preferentially involve the ventral nerve roots.

17 Pathology/Histology

1.

B The basal membrane thickens, and the internal elastic lamina fragments.

In cerebral amyloid angiopathy, amyloid deposits form in the walls of vessels, making them friable and prone to hemorrhage. Congo red staining reveals the amyloid deposits.

2.

B Multiple sclerosis

Multiple sclerosis is a demyelinating disease (thus causing white matter pathology). Histologically, demyelination is seen along with a paucity of oligodendrocytes. Newly demyelinated axons are irregularly dilated and nonuniform. There is an infiltration of lymphocytes in active lesions. (A) In Creutzfeldt-Jakob disease, there are spongiform changes of the gray matter, with a loss of neurons and gliosis. Amyloid-like plaques also can be seen. (C) In subacute cerebral infarctions, macrophages predominate (after the neutrophils of acute infarctions), and neural cytoplasm is eosinophilic with pyknotic nuclei. Numerous reactive astrocytes are seen around zones of rarefaction (reduced cellular density). (D) In neurosarcoidosis, there are noncaseating granulomas with numerous surrounding lymphocytes. The absence of granulomas in this specimen argues against sarcoidosis.

3.

A Alterations in chromosome 17, S-100, and nestin

S-100 is a sensitive marker for malignant peripheral nerve sheath tumors (MPNSTs), but it is not seen in all cases, as it is positive in only 50 to 90% of MPNSTs. Higher grade tumors tend to have an even lower incidence of S-100 positivity. CD56 also is sensitive but not specific for MPNSTs. Recent studies highlight that nestin expression is one of the most sensitive and specific markers for these tumors. The tumors also are associated with chromosome 17 mutations, as about 50% of them occur in individuals with neurofibromatosis type 1. (B) Chromosome 22 abnormalities are seen in neurofibromatosis type 2. GFAP (glial fibrillary acidic protein) is a marker found in the intermediate filaments of some glial cells (primarily astrocytes). CD10 often is used as a marker for various types of lymphomas. (C) Chromosome 6 abnormalities can be associated with Parkinson disease or Dandy-

Walker malformation. Vimentin is a marker for sarcoma. MIB-1 is a proliferation marker. (D) Chromosome 4 abnormalities are associated with Huntington and Parkinson disease among other condition. AFP (α-fetoprotein) can be a useful marker for diagnosing germ cell tumors, especially yolk sac tumors. CD20 is a B-cell marker. (E) Trisomy of chromosome 18 results in Edwards syndrome. HCG is a marker for choriocarcinomas and germ cell tumors. Desmin is a marker for muscle intermediate filaments.

4.

C Meningioma

Meningiomas are marked by vimentin, epithelial membrane antigen (EMA), and sometimes progesterone receptor immunoreactivity. They typically are dural based and may contain psammoma bodies. (A) Dural arteriovenous fistulas (dural arteriovenous malformations) are as described below for answer B, except that they have dural vessels as the feeding and draining vessels. They have no distinct nidus. (B) Arteriovenous malformations appear histologically as vascular channels of various wall thicknesses, in which arteries connect to veins without an intermediate capillary. Early draining veins are demonstrated on angiograms. There is a gross nidus on imaging. (D) Like all glial tumors, high-grade gliomas stain for glial fibrillary acidic protein. High-grade gliomas also can display gross elements of cysts, degeneration, mitotic figures, and necrosis. (E) Hemangioblastomas stain richly for reticulin, are positive for vimentin, and negative for EMA. They do not have calcifications, mitotic figures, or necrosis. Microscopically, they are seen as capillaries with hyperplastic endothelial elements with stromal cells and vacuoles. They do not stain with EMA.

5.

B Adamantinomatous; wet

Adamantinomatous craniopharyngiomas typically occur in children, in contrast to papillary craniopharyngiomas, which occur more frequently in adults. The former contains "wet" keratin (keratinocytes in a loose stellate reticular zone), whereas the latter contains "dry" keratin. Both cause surrounding gliosis and have Rosenthal fibers present.

6.

C AIDS dementia complex

AIDS dementia complex is seen in 50% of AIDS patients and is characterized by the triad of cognitive dysfunction, behavioral changes, and motor deficits. (A) Toxoplasmosis is seen in 10% of AIDS cases at autopsy and is the most common cause of focal neurologic symptoms in AIDS patients. Treatment is with pyrimethamine and sulfadiazine. (B) Primary central nervous system lymphoma (B-cell origin) is seen in 5% of AIDS cases at autopsy. The Epstein-Barr virus frequently is detected in the affected cells. (D) Encephalitis is characterized by microglial nodules in white matter and subcortical gray matter, with focal demyelination and neuronal loss. Multinucleated giant cells may be seen and are unique to HIV infection. (E) Vacuolar myelopathy (diagnosed during pathological tissue examination) may be symptomatic or asymptomatic, and is detected in 50% of AIDS cases at autopsy. Myelopathy may involve the posterior and lateral columns of the lower thoracic cord and is detected clinically in less than 50% of AIDS patients.

7.

A Amiodarone

Amiodarone is associated with myelinopathy, which also may be seen with other agents such as hexachlorophene, perhexiline, and toluene. The other agents listed as options more typically cause a neuropathy.

8.

A Subgaleal hematoma

Subgaleal hematomas are associated with linear, nondisplaced skull fractures in children. They can cross sutures as they separate the galea from the periosteum. They may present as fluctuant masses. (B) Subperiosteal hematomas (also known as cephalohematomas) are seen in newborns and are associated with parturition. Bleeding elevates the periosteum, but the extent is limited by the sutures. Subperiosteal hematomas usually are firm and can calcify. (C) Subdural hematomas are not in the scalp. (D) Temporalis contusions are intramuscular and are not in the loose connective tissue of the scalp.

9.

B Secondary glioblastoma

A high-grade glial neoplasm with neovascularization and necrosis is diagnostic for glioblastoma. The younger age of this patient and the presence of a *TP53* mutation argue for a secondary glioblastoma through malignant degeneration. In con-

trast, primary glioblastomas are associated with *EGFR* amplification in older patients. (C) Rhabdoid meningiomas are grade III meningiomas that often behave aggressively and are not glial tumors. (D) Medulloblastomas have small, densely packed, undifferentiated cells and often are referred to as blue cell tumors given their hypercellularity and scant cytoplasm. They are WHO grade IV tumors. (E) Chordomas are low-grade tumors distinguished by the pathological finding of physaliphorous cells.

10.

B Neurofibromatosis type 1

Neurofibromatosis type 1 is associated with optic gliomas (usually pilocytic in nature) in which histology can demonstrate Rosenthal fibers. These fibers also are seen in Alexander disease and in areas of gliosis. (A) Von Hippel–Lindau disease is associated with hemangioblastomas, which are the most common primary tumors of the posterior fossa. Hemangioblastomas do occur in the retinae. (C) Neurofibromatosis type 2 is associated with bilateral vestibular schwannomas and the MISME syndrome (multiple inherited schwannomas, meningiomas, and ependymomas). Patients can have retinal hamartomas. (D) Tuberous sclerosis is associated with subependymal giant cell astrocytomas and cortical tubers. Retinal tumors (hamartomas) can occur. (E) Sturge-Weber syndrome is associated with cortical atrophy and calcifications, an ipsilateral port-wine facial nevus, meningeal venous proliferation, and contralateral seizures. Patients can have retinal angiomas.

11.

D Prolactin

The pituitary adenoma is characterized by a monomorphic proliferation of cells. The most common secreting adenoma is prolactinoma, followed by growth hormone adenoma.

12.

C Hirano body

Hirano bodies are eosinophilic cytoplasmic inclusions within neurons. They are composed of actin, and have a paracrystalline appearance with electron microscopy. (A) Amyloid usually does not accumulate in the cytoplasm of neurons. (B) Evidence of granulovacuolar degeneration (small dark dots inside a vacuole in the cytoplasm of neurons) also is seen in this field. (D) Lewy bodies typically are seen in Parkinson disease. (E) Neurofibrillary tangles are elongated, filamentous, cytoplasmic inclusions in neurons in Alzheimer disease.

13.
A Amyotrophic lateral sclerosis

Amyotrophic lateral sclerosis is marked by a loss of neurons in the anterior horn cell region as seen in the image accompanying the question. Patients often have symptoms of both upper and lower motor neuron disease. (C, D) The spinal muscular atrophies (types I and 2) may show a pathology similar to that of amyotrophic lateral sclerosis but present earlier in life (childhood or infancy). (E) Degeneration of the posterior columns is the hallmark of tabes dorsalis associated with syphilis.

14.
C Grade 3

Germinal matrix hemorrhages are a complication of prematurity. Grade 3 germinal matrix hemorrhages show rupture of the blood from the germinal matrix into the ventricles with ventricular expansion. (A) Grade 1 germinal matrix hemorrhages are limited to the germinal matrix. (B) Grade 2 germinal matrix hemorrhages show rupture of the blood from the germinal matrix into the ventricles without ventricular expansion. (D) Grade 4 germinal matrix hemorrhages show intraventricular hemorrhage and hemorrhage into hemispheric parenchyma (periventricular venous infarct). Parenchymal involvement is worse than ventricular involvement because the latter can be treated with cerebrospinal fluid diversion. (E) Grade 5 germinal matrix hemorrhages do not exist in this schema.

15.
B Amyotrophic lateral sclerosis

Bunina bodies are a feature of amyotrophic lateral sclerosis and are seen in areas of neuronal loss in the anterior horn cell region of the spinal cord. (A) Hirano bodies are eosinophilic cytoplasmic inclusions within neurons seen in patients with Alzheimer disease. (C–E) Prominent neuronal inclusions typically are not seen in Huntington chorea, Machado-Joseph disease, or olivopontocerebellar atrophy of Menzel.

16.
C Contusion

A contusion is defined as a bruise when referring to skin and soft issue. In the brain, a contusion translates into an infarct secondary to trauma. (A) An abrasion represents a scrape of the skin (i.e., a surface injury). (B) An avulsion is a large tear of the tissue creating a tissue flap. (D) A laceration is the result of blunt force injury causing a tear in the skin and underlying soft tissues.

17.
C Melan-A and HMB-45 positivity

Melanomas stain with antibodies to S-100 protein, melan-A (MART 1), and HMB-45 and do not stain with the other antibodies listed as options.

18.
E Notochord remnants

The tumor shown in the image accompanying the question represents a chordoma. It contains epithelioid cells with a vacuolated cytoplasm arranged against a chondromyxoid-like stroma. These tumors arise from notochordal remnants, especially in the clival or the sacrococcygeal regions.

19.
C Normal pineal gland

The tissue sample shown in the image accompanying the question demonstrates a vaguely lobular arrangement of cells against a fibrillary-type background, consistent with normal pineal gland tissue. Calcifications commonly are seen in the gland. Occasionally, gliotic cysts, sometimes with Rosenthal fibers, also are present.

20.
A CD1a

CD1a is the best and most specific stain to highlight Langerhans histiocytes. By electron microscopy, these cells contain Birbeck granules (likened to tennis rackets). (D, E) CD68 and HAM56 are macrophage markers that are not specific for Langerhans cells.

21.
B Lysosomes

The cytoplasmic granularity of the tumor shown in the image accompanying the question is due to an increased number of large lysosomes.

22.
A *NF2*

The tumor shown in the image accompanying the question represents a schwannoma. Tumor cells typically are elongated with pointed nuclear ends. The pleomorphism displayed represents what is sometimes referred to as "ancient change," which does not impact prognosis. Schwannomas are associated with neurofibromatosis type 2 and may show alterations in the *NF2* gene. (B) *TP53* gene mutations are seen in Li-Fraumeni syndrome. (C) *PTEN* gene mutations are observed in a variety of cancers including secondary glioblastomas. (D) *SOD1* gene mutations occur in apoptosis and amyotrophic lateral sclerosis. (E) *TSC2* gene mutations are seen in tuberous sclerosis.

23.

D Breast

(A–E) Each of these tumors generally is described as being highly resistant to radiation therapy, with the exception of breast cancer, which is moderately sensitive. Highly sensitive tumors include small and germ cell tumors, lymphoma, leukemia, and multiple myeloma.

24.

B Chromosome 9q and 16p

Tuberous sclerosis is an autosomal dominant disease characterized by seizures, mental retardation, and sebaceous adenomas; 10 to 15% of patients present with subependymal giant cell astrocytomas, which occur at the foramen of Monro and can cause hydrocephalus. Pathology of the subependymal giant cell astrocytomas shows large cells with abundant cytoplasm and prominent nucleoli. Vascular proliferation and necrosis can be seen without being suggestive of a more malignant tumor. (A) Chromosome 17p is associated with *TP53* gene mutations. Li-Fraumeni syndrome is characterized by *TP53* mutations and is associated with a 25 times increased risk for developing malignant tumors by age 50. (C) Chromosome 1p and 19q deletions can be seen in oligodendrogliomas, and these mutations often predict a better response to chemotherapy with a longer tumor-free survival. (D) Chromosomes 3 and 7 are associated with the development of cavernomas. (E) Chromosome 15 is associated with Angelman and Prader-Willi syndromes, characterized by seizures and mental retardation but not tumors.

25.

C Dermoid cyst

The cyst lining is characterized by squamous epithelium and shows evidence of skin adnexal structures in the cyst wall that may include structures such as sebaceous glands, apocrine glands, hair, or eccrine glands. These findings are consistent with a dermoid cyst.

26.

B Chondrosarcoma

The tumor shown in the image accompanying the question is marked by a malignant spindled cell component next to an atypical cartilaginous component, consistent with a chondrosarcoma.

27.

C Most pontine tumors have high-grade histology.

The axial T2 and contrast-enhanced T1-weighted images demonstrate a nonenhancing, infiltrative, expansile lesion involving the pons, most compatible with a diffuse infiltrative pontine glioma. These lesions are more common in children than in adults. Histologically, they may originate from astrocytes, oligodendrocytes, or ependymal cells, but the great majority (95%) are astrocytic. Most brainstem gliomas arise in the pons, and most pontine tumors have a high-grade histology, being either anaplastic astrocytomas or glioblastomas. In contrast, tumors arising in the tectum and cervicomedullary junction as well as those that are cystic or exophytic usually are low grade. Enhancement is variable. Prognosis usually is poor, even for presumed low-grade histologies. (A) Diffuse intrinsic pontine gliomas are aggressive lesions, but they rarely metastasize to distant sites. Instead, they tend to infiltrate along anatomic fiber tracts and can extend cranially to involve the midbrain and thalami. (B) Hydrocephalus is a late complication of diffuse intrinsic pontine gliomas, and is more commonly seen in tectal lesions. (D) Calcifications are unusual in diffuse intrinsic pontine gliomas.

28.

E Osteosarcoma

The malignant tumor shown in the image accompanying the question is marked by bone formation (the dark purple material). Osteosarcoma is the best diagnosis for this tumor. These lesions rarely may represent a primary tumor arising in the meninges or skull or distant metastatic disease. (A) Chondrosarcomas contain atypical cartilage within the tumor. (B) Glial fibrillary acidic protein (GFAP) negativity rules out a gliosarcoma. (C) Hemangiopericytomas often are malignant meningeal tumors that lack bone formation. (D) Metaplastic meningiomas are benign tumors marked by meningothelial cells intermixed with benign mesenchymal tissue such as bone or cartilage.

29.

C 12 hours

The earliest changes indicating ischemic damage are apparent in neuronal cells at 12 to 24 hours after the precipitating event. The cells shrink in size, acquire cytoplasmic hypereosinophilia, and show nuclei shrinkage (the "red and dead" look).

30.

B Filum terminale

The tumor shown in the image accompanying the question represents a paraganglioma, which generally is marked by cells arranged in loose nests (zellballen). The nests of cells are delimited by spindled, S-100–positive staining sustentacular cells. The tumor cells in the nests stain with neural markers such as chromogranin and neuron-specific enolase. In the central nervous system, paragangliomas most commonly arise in the spinal cord region.

31.

E CD138

The lesion shown in the image accompanying the question is composed of plasma cells and represents a plasma cell dyscrasia. CD138 is an antibody that targets plasma cells. These lesions typically demonstrate evidence of monoclonality with either kappa or lambda immunostaining.

32.

A Cerebellopontine angle

This simple squamous epithelial-lined cyst represents an epidermoid cyst. It lacks the adnexal structures that mark a dermoid cyst. Epidermoid cysts most commonly arise in the cerebellopontine angle region.

33.

A Epidural space

Over 90% of epidural hemorrhages are associated with a skull fracture and are associated with a torn middle meningeal artery. Less commonly, epidural hemorrhages result from a dural sinus tear or a tear in the middle meningeal vein.

34.

A 2 hours

Usually within 2 hours of diffuse axonal injury, axonal swelling can be visualized with β-amyloid precursor protein immunostaining.

35.

A Dermatomyositis

The biopsy shown in the image accompanying the question demonstrates predominantly perivascular-based chronic inflammation and atrophy around the perimeter of the muscle fascicles (perifascicular atrophy). Perifascicular atrophy in the setting of an inflammatory myopathy is highly suggestive of dermatomyositis.

36.

B Dystrophin

The clinical history is suggestive of Duchenne muscular dystrophy. The biopsy is marked by a prominent variation in muscle fiber size with increased endomysial fibrosis. One would anticipate an absence of membrane staining with dystrophin antibody in this case.

37.

A Arachnoid cyst

The cyst shown is lined by a thin layer of meningothelial cells or arachnoid cap cells, consistent with an arachnoid cyst.

38.

E No available therapies

The pathological findings shown in the image accompanying the question are consistent with inclusion body myositis. The biopsy shows inflammation, a variation in muscle fiber size, and rimmed vacuoles (vacuoles with basophilic granularity). Currently, there is no known effective treatment for inclusion body myositis.

39.

E Ryanodine receptor gene mutation

The findings in the biopsy illustrate a core myopathy, one of the congenital myopathies marked by a focal decrease in oxidative activity as manifested by the staining pattern. The condition generally is inherited as an autosomal dominant condition and is associated with mutations in the ryanodine receptor gene. There is an association of this condition with malignant hyperthermia.

40.

A Acid maltase deficiency

Glycogen-filled vacuoles suggest a glycogen storage disease. Acid maltase deficiency is the only one of the glycogenoses that is lysosomal associated and stains with acid phosphatase (a lysosomal associated enzyme).

41.

C Kappa light chain protein

Most of the amyloid encountered in the brain is β-amyloid. Less commonly, other proteins may arrange themselves in a β-pleated sheet configuration to form amyloid. Kappa light chain protein is unlikely to deposit in the brain. (A) Cystatin C is a serum indicator of kidney function and may be involved in Alzheimer amyloid. (B) Gelsolin is a regulator of actin filament assembly/disassembly and is associated with β-amyloid formation in the brain. (D) Prion protein causes spongiform encephalopathy.

42.

D *HTT* gene

The trinucleotide repeat in the HTT gene that encodes the huntingtin protein is associated with Huntington disease. The normal CAG repeat length is up to 35 repeats, whereas in Huntington disease, there are 36 or more repeats. (A, B) Ataxin-2 and CACNA1A gene repeats are associated with forms of hereditary spinocerebellar ataxia. (C) Chorein gene alterations are associated with a rare condition known as neuroacanthocytosis. (E) The myotonin gene is implicated in myotonic dystrophy.

43.

A Alzheimer disease

The globular, extracellular structures highlighted with the silver stain represent senile plaques and are associated most classically with Alzheimer disease. Current pathological diagnostic criteria rely on plaque and neurofibrillary tangle counts as well as an assessment of the distribution of amyloid deposition. Plaques are composed variably of neuritic processes (highlighted with the silver stain), amyloid, and associated microglial cells.

44.

D Tau

The dark-staining, elongated structures located within the cytoplasm of neurons represent neurofibrillary tangles. They can be highlighted with tau immunostaining. (A) α-synuclein is a good stain to highlight Lewy bodies. (B, E) Congo red and thioflavin S stains highlight amyloid.

45.

D Lymphoma

Lymphomas often are B cell in origin and are identified by white blood cells with angiocentric growth patterns forming perivascular cuffs by tumor cells. (A) Germinomas show large, epithelioid cells with abundant PAS-positive cytoplasm. The cells have irregular nuclei that may have prominent nests of lymphocytes with occasional granulomatous inflammation. (B) Ependymomas classically have dark, small nuclei with perivascular and true rosettes. (C) Chordomas characteristically

are described by physaliphorous cells and represent a remnant of the nucleus pulposus. (E) Hemangioblastomas have numerous capillary channels lined by a single layer of endothelium surrounded by reticulin.

46.

D Froin syndrome

Froin syndrome is stagnation of the cerebrospinal fluid (CSF) from an inflammatory or neoplastic lesion, causing increased exudation from the tumor itself and activation of coagulation factors. (A) A positive Queckenstedt test is a failure of jugular vein compression to increase CSF pressure, which it will normally do in the absence of a block of the venous outflow. (B) Coup de poignard of Michon is sudden excruciating back pain with subarachnoid hemorrhage in patients with a spinal vascular malformation. (C) A positive Froment sign (during an evaluation of the ulnar nerve) occurs when a patient is unable to grasp a sheet of paper between his thumb and extended index finger and will instead pinch the paper, as the action of the weak adductor pollicis (ulnar innervated) is substituted for the action of the strong flexor pollicis longus (anterior interosseous innervated). (E) Foix-Alajouanine is an acute/subacute neurologic deterioration without hemorrhage in patients with a spinal vascular malformation.

47.

D Seizure

The epithelial-lined cyst shown in the image accompanying the question represents a colloid cyst. Seizures are not an expected presenting symptom. (A, B, E) Headaches, incontinence, and even sudden death can occur with the development of hydrocephalus secondary to colloid cysts, especially if a "ball-valving" phenomenon occurs.

48.

A β-amyloid

β-amyloid is the best and most specific stain for the type of amyloid that accumulates in patients with Alzheimer disease. (B) Luxol fast blue is a myelin stain. (C) Mucicarmine stains mucin such as in an adenocarcinoma. (D) Prussian blue is an iron stain. (E) Trichrome highlights connective tissue and collagen.

49.

B Cavernous malformation

Cavernous malformations appear on MRI with hemosiderin and a "popcorn-like" appearance, with irregular thick- and thin-walled sinusoidal vascular channels without intervening neural parenchyma, large feeding arteries, or draining veins. (A) Microscopically, capillary telangiectasias have slightly enlarged capillaries with low flow and intervening neural tissue. (C) Venous malformations (venous angiomas, also known as developmental venous anomalies) are abnormal veins draining normal brain. They often present as a starburst pattern (caput medusa on angiogram) and are associated with cavernomas. (D) Arteriovenous malformations appear as tangles of abnormal vessels of various diameters separated by gliotic tissue without an intervening capillary bed. There may be evidence of prior hemorrhage. (E) Dural arteriovenous fistulas are true arteriovenous shunts within the leaflets of the dura matter and usually are found adjacent to dural sinuses.

50.

D Sporadically with no obvious genetic transmission

Sturge-Weber disease has no known genetic transmission and is characterized by a facial nevus in the ophthalmic division of the trigeminal nerve, along with leptomeningeal venous angiomas and intracortical tram-track calcifications.

51.

A *SNCA*

The neuron displayed with the eosinophilic cytoplasmic inclusion also has brown melanin pigment in its cytoplasm, with these components representing a Lewy body. α-synuclein (encoded by the *SCNA* gene) is the best stain for highlighting Lewy bodies. The most common gene to be affected in familial cases of Parkinson disease is the *SCNA* gene. Less commonly, alterations in the various *PARK* genes have been described in the disease.

52.

A L-iduronidase

The described patient has Hurler syndrome. (B) Iduronate sulfatase deficiency (Hunter syndrome) causes symptoms similar to those seen in Hurler syndrome, except that Hunter syndrome is milder, without mental retardation, with minimal corneal involvement, slower progressing, and with a life span into adulthood. (C) Galactose 6-sulfatase and β-galactosidase deficiencies (Morquio syndrome) are inherited in an autosomal recessive manner and are characterized by severe skeletal abnormalities, ligamentous laxity, dwarfism, myelopathy, and a lack of mental retardation. (D) Sulfatase B deficiency (Maroteaux-Lamy) presents with carpal tunnel syndrome, valvular heart disease, and without mental retardation. (E) β-glucuronidase deficiency is inherited in an autosomal recessive manner and is characterized by moderate mental retardation, corneal clouding, hydrocephalus, hepatosplenomegaly, and various bony changes.

53.

A Low posterior hairline, brevicollis, and decreased neck motion

Klippel-Feil syndrome is a congenital fusion of two or more cervical vertebrae due to the failure of normal segmentation of cervical somites that is characterized by a low posterior hairline, shortened neck, and limitations in neck motion. The condition also can be associated with scoliosis, torticollis, pterygium colli (neck webbing), and Sprengel deformity (inability to raise the scapula). (B) Sebaceous adenomas, mental retardation, and seizures represent a triad associated with tuberous sclerosis. (C) Anorectal malformation, anterior sacral defects, and presacral masses are seen in the Currarino triad, which typically presents with constipation secondary to the anorectal malformation. (D) Dementia, urinary incontinence, and gait instability are seen in conjunction with normal pressure hydrocephalus.

54.

D Amyotrophic lateral sclerosis

Axonal spheroids are seen in amyotrophic lateral sclerosis, diffuse axonal injury, and Hallervorden-Spatz disease.

55.

C Myxopapillary ependymoma

The findings are most consistent with a myxopapillary ependymoma (WHO grade I). (A, D, E) These tumor types often are in the differential diagnosis due to location rather than histomorphology. (B) Metastatic adenocarcinomas also can be mucin positive but would be unusual in such a young patient and are generally glial fibrillary acidic protein negative.

56.

A Basal ganglia

PANK2 gene mutations are associated with neuronal degeneration with brain iron accumulation (formerly known as Hallervorden-Spatz disease). The increased iron accumulation preferentially deposits in the basal ganglia region and is accompanied by neuronal loss and gliosis.

57.

C CA1 and CA4

In hippocampal sclerosis, the most severely involved areas are the CA1 and CA4 regions; however, neuronal loss may be present in any of the hippocampal regions.

58.

B Dysautonomia

Dysautonomia is a feature present in multisystem atrophy in both the parkinsonian and cerebellar predominant types. The cerebellar type usually presents with gait and limb ataxia, dysarthria, and oculomotor disturbances. It is marked by atrophy of and loss of neurons in the cerebellum, middle cerebellar peduncles, and pons. Ubiquitin and tau immunoreactive glial cytoplasmic inclusions may be seen.

59.

D *SOD1*

Ten percent of patients with amyotrophic lateral sclerosis have an autosomal dominant pattern of familial disease. Twenty percent of familial cases are due to a mutation in the gene encoding the Cu/Zn superoxide dismutase 1 protein on chromosome 21. Less commonly, familial cases have been associated with mutations in the *TARDBP* gene on chromosome 1.

60.

A Cytomegalovirus infection

The occasional large cells marked by prominent intranuclear inclusions are suggestive of a viral infection (e.g., cytomegalovirus). A few of the large cells also have small, brightly eosinophilic cytoplasmic inclusions as well, which sometimes can be encountered with cytomegalovirus infection.

61.

C Radiation effects

The thickened or sclerosed appearance of the blood vessels in this case is typical of the vascular changes observed following radiation therapy. Sometimes these changes are accompanied by chronic inflammatory cells and necrosis of the adjacent tissue with infiltration by macrophages.

62.

B Fourth ventricle

The low-grade tumor shown in the image accompanying the question is marked by loose aggregates of tumor cell nuclei with intervening hypocellular zones. Microcysts frequently are present in this tumor. These pathological findings are consistent with a subependymoma (WHO grade I). Although they can arise in the spinal cord, the fourth ventricle is a more common site.

63.

C Tuberous sclerosis

As its name suggests, large astrocytic cells compose this intraventricular subependymal giant cell astrocytoma. This tumor sometimes is associated with tuberous sclerosis along with subependymal hamartomas and cortical tubers.

64.

A ATRX protein staining

Oligodendrogliomas generally show retention of ATRX protein staining (in contrast to a subset of diffuse astrocytomas).

65.

D Deletion on chromosome 1p

Prognosis for anaplastic oligodendrogliomas is best predicted by looking for large deletions on chromosomes 1p and 19q. The deletions are thought by many to be part of the definition of these tumors. Although high mitotic count and cell proliferation indices and necrosis are associated with higher grade oligodendrogliomas, the chromosome deletions are more predictive of chemoresponsiveness and outcome.

66.

B IDH-1

IDH-1 antibody does not stain reactive or inflammatory lesions including gliosis. A subset of diffuse or fibrillary astrocytomas and most oligodendrogliomas stain with IDH-1 antibody. (A, E) GFAP and S-100 antibodies stain astrocytes in both processes. (C) More cells stain with Ki-67, a cell proliferation marker in astrocytomas versus gliosis; however, there is significant overlap in the ranges of observed labeling indices with Ki-67 in both processes, so it has little value unless the labeling index is moderately high. (D) Only widespread positivity with p53 antibody would be useful in indicating a tumor, as low levels of staining may be seen in both processes and is nonspecific.

67.

D B12

A deficiency in vitamin B12 (cobalamin) can result in degeneration of the posterior columns of the spinal cord, referred to as subacute combined degeneration. The lateral columns of the upper thoracic and lower cervical spinal cord also may be involved. (A) Vitamin B1 (thiamine) deficiency can lead to Wernicke encephalopathy, Korsakoff psychosis, or Beriberi. (B) Vitamin B2 (riboflavin) deficiency can cause stomatitis and a red, scaly rash. (C) Vitamin B6 (pyridoxine) deficiency is associated with isoniazid and hydralazine use, and causes lower limb paresthesias, pain, and weakness. (E) Vitamin C deficiency results in scurvy, with early symptoms of malaise, lethargy, and painful gums.

68.

A *BRAF*

This astrocytic tumor is marked by the presence of clustered eosinophilic material known as eosinophilic granular bodies. This finding is suggestive of a pilocytic astrocytoma, which sometimes is associated with *BRAF* gene alterations. (B–D) Alterations in these genes generally are not encountered in pilocytic astrocytomas and are more common in diffuse or fibrillary astrocytomas.

69.

A Associated with focal cortical dysplasia

The image accompanying the question presents a WHO grade I dysembryoplastic neuroepithelial tumor. These tumors are associated with chronic epilepsy and most frequently arise in the temporal lobe. Ki-67 indices are typically low, often less than 5%. The tumor has a blistered appearance grossly. It often is associated with adjacent cortical architectural disorganization (focal cortical dysplasia).

70.

A Ependymoma

True rosettes (tumor cells arranged around a central lumen) are characteristic of an ependymoma. (C, E) Rosettes and perivascular pseudorosettes are not typical features of myxopapillary ependymomas and subependymomas. (D) Retinoblastomas of the eye contain similar true rosettes (Flexner-Wintersteiner rosettes).

71.

A *Streptococcus* species

Streptococcus species are the most common pathogens found in brain abscesses across all ages and typically stem from adjacent sinus or ear infections. (B, E) *Staphylococcus* species and enteric bacilli are common pathogens in brain abscesses due to trauma. (C, D) *Bacteroides* and *Proteus* species are common pathogens in brain abscesses in neonates, along with *Citrobacter* species and gram-negative bacilli.

72.

D Adjacent sinus or ear infections

Adjacent sinus or ear infections account for about 40% of brain abscesses due to the ability of pathogens to spread along valveless venous channels that are the cranial sinuses. (E) Hematogenous spread from distant infections accounts for about 30% of brain abscesses. Hematogenous spread of pathogens tends to produce abscesses in the middle cerebral artery territory and often causes multiple abscesses.

73.

C Grade III

An astrocytoma with necrosis, vascular proliferation, and moderate pleomorphism is WHO grade IV.

74.

D P53 protein mutation

The p53 tumor suppressor protein is encoded by the *TP53* gene on chromosome 17, and mutations result in Li-Fraumeni syndrome. Individuals with Li-Fraumeni syndrome are at risk for developing a variety of tumors throughout their bodies, including primitive neuroectodermal tumors and astrocytomas in the brain, breast cancer, and soft tissue and bone sarcomas. (A) Turcot syndrome has been linked to gene mutations in the *MLH1, MSH2, MSH6,* and *PMS2* genes and predisposes individuals to medulloblastomas and glioblastomas. (B) Merlin protein is a tumor suppressor protein encoded by the neurofibromin 2 gene on chromosome 22. Mutations in merlin are seen in individuals with neurofibromatosis type 2, which is associated with bilateral acoustic neuromas, meningiomas, astrocytomas, and ependymomas. (C) The neurofibromin 1 protein is mutated in individuals with neurofibromatosis type 1. This chromosome 17 abnormality predisposes possessors to optic gliomas, astrocytomas, and neurofibromas. (E) The von Hippel–Lindau tumor suppressor gene mutation (chromosome 3) is seen in von Hippel–Lindau disease and results in an increased risk for developing hemangioblastomas and endolymphatic sac tumors.

75.

E Synaptophysin

Central neurocytomas most commonly arise in the lateral ventricles and demonstrate diffuse, strong immunoreactivity with synaptophysin antibodies, consistent with their neural lineage. (A) CD34 is a vascular marker. (B) Epithelial membrane antigen stains carcinomas and meningiomas. (C, D) Glial fibrillary acidic protein and S-100 protein stain astrocytic tumors, among others.

76.

E WHO grade III anaplastic astrocytoma

Ki-67 is a cell proliferation marker that stains a nuclear protein that is produced during the proliferative phases of the cell cycle. Staining results typically are reported as a percentage of positive staining tumor cells in the area of the tumor with the most staining (labeling index). The rate of cell proliferation is more than what would be expected in a WHO grade I or II neoplasm and is most consistent with a higher grade neoplasm.

77.

B WHO grade II

This tumor represents a pleomorphic xanthoastrocytoma. It is one of the few astrocytic tumors that has a rich connective tissue matrix that can be highlighted with a reticulin stain. Despite the cellularity and marked atypia of the tumor cells in this neoplasm, the majority of these tumors are considered to be WHO grade II neoplasms. Rare WHO grade III pleomorphic xanthoastrocytomas are marked by increased mitotic activity or necrosis.

78.

E Sturge-Weber syndrome

The photomicrograph shown in the image accompanying the question demonstrates some surface cortex on the right and a proliferation of blood vessels in the meninges (angiomatosis). The history and pathological image are suggestive of Sturge-Weber syndrome. (A) There are no tumor cells between the blood vessels, as one would encounter in an angiomatous meningioma.

79.

D Nasal glioma

The presence of ectopic neural/brain tissue in the nasal area is referred to as a nasal glioma, even though it is not really a glioma in the traditional sense. The usual differential diagnosis with the described lesion is encephalocele if the lesion is connected to the brain itself. Angiofibromas,

meningiomas, and pituitary adenomas occasionally can arise as masses in the nasal cavity but look very different histologically.

80.

D Atypical teratoid/rhabdoid tumor

Atypical teratoid/rhabdoid tumors are associated with *INI1* and chromosome 22 abnormalities and stain positively for vimentin, epithelial membrane antigen, and glial fibrillary acidic protein, among others. (A) Chromosomal deletions in chromosome 17p and not 22 are seen with medulloblastomas and other primitive neuroectodermal tumors. (B) The most common chromosomal changes in ependymomas are amplification of chromosome 1q and loss of chromosomes 6q, 17p, and 22q, with chromosome 1q amplification being most likely to lead to intracranial tumor recurrence. (C) Astrocytomas can be associated with a variety of syndromes and their associated chromosomal changes, including neurofibromatosis types 1 and 2, tuberous sclerosis, retinoblastoma, Li-Fraumeni, and Turcot syndromes. (E) Chromosome 22 abnormalities can be seen with schwannomas, but *INI1* mutations are not seen.

81.

E Thiamine deficiency

The changes described are associated with thiamine deficiency and Wernicke-Korsakoff syndrome. The brownish discoloration of the mammillary bodies is due to small hemorrhages.

82.

D Syringobulbia

A glial-lined cavitation in the brainstem area is referred to as syringobulbia. In the spinal cord, a comparable lesion is called syringomyelia. (A) Diplomyelia refers to duplication of spinal cord segments. (B) Hydromyelia is a dilation of the central spinal canal. (C) Iniencephaly refers to failure of closure of the posterior vertebral arches of the rostral cervical vertebrae and usually is associated with abnormalities of the brainstem.

83.

B Hemorrhagic infarct

The acute angle branching hyphae shown in the image accompanying the question are consistent with *Aspergillus*. *Aspergillus* tends to be angioinvasive, and consequently presents most commonly with hemorrhagic infarcts. Less commonly, one can encounter an abscess or meningitis with *Aspergillus*.

84.
D Open neural tube defect

Elevated amniotic fluid levels of α-fetoprotein and acetylcholinesterase are associated with open neural tube defects (i.e., defects in which there is a lack of skin covering exposed meninges or central neuroglial tissue). The risk of such defects can be reduced with adequate maternal folate consumption.

85.
C Germinoma

The pineal region is a common location for germinomas. In addition to Parinaud (dorsal midbrain) syndrome, precocious puberty and other endocrine manifestations commonly are associated with this malignant neoplasm. Histologically, the classic findings with germinomas are aggregates of nonneoplastic lymphocytes (small dark blue cells) and large tumor cells with abundant cytoplasm, large nuclei, and prominent nucleoli.

86.
B Hemangioblastoma

A WHO grade I tumor, hemangioblastoma is commonly seen in the cerebellum as a brightly enhancing mass associated with a cystic component. Histologically, these tumors are rich in capillaries (hence their name despite their histogenesis remaining unknown), with intervening large "epithelioid" cells with foamy cytoplasm and hyperchromatic nuclei called stromal cells.

87.
C Prematurity

Germinal matrix hemorrhage is associated strongly with prematurity and results from the increased susceptibility of these patients to hypoxia/ischemia. Germinal matrix hemorrhage can extend into the ventricles, leading to intraventricular hemorrhage, which is associated with serious sequelae.

88.
D Glioblastoma, WHO grade IV

The microphotograph accompanying the question shows a hypercellular neoplasm with characteristic pale areas of necrosis surrounded by viable tumor cells. This type of necrosis is called pseudopalisading necrosis and is characteristic of glioblastomas (WHO grade IV) and other high-grade lesions.

89.
B Schwannoma

Antoni A (compact spindled areas) and Antoni B (loosely organized and less cellular areas of muci-

nous stroma and fibrillary collagen) areas are typical of schwannomas. (A) Neurofibromas often stain with neurofilament and have axons coursing through them. (C) Malignant peripheral nerve sheath tumors often involve multiple fascicles and are characterized by uniform spindle cells with hyperchromatic nuclei arranged in fascicles. Necrosis and a high mitotic index are seen.

90.
A Alzheimer disease

Pathological findings in Alzheimer disease include deposition of extracellular β-amyloid in neuritic plaques and intracellular neurofibrillary tangles composed of hyperphosphorylated tau and ubiquitin proteins. (B) Pick disease (frontotemporal dementia) is characterized by tauopathy (a neuronal/glial inclusion of tau). (C) Creutzfeldt-Jakob disease is associated with abnormal prion PrPsc, and has the classic findings of 14-3-3 protein in the cerebrospinal fluid and periodic sharp waves and spikes on electroencephalography. (D) Dementia with Lewy bodies has eosinophilic intracytoplasmic neuronal inclusions (Lewy bodies) that contain α-synuclein and tau proteins. (E) Huntington disease is due to a CAG trinucleotide repeat on chromosome 4 and is not associated with intra- or extracellular inclusion bodies.

91.
A Putamen

The basal ganglia are the most common site of hypertensive hemorrhage. Of the basal ganglia, the putamen is the most common location for hypertension-related hemorrhage. This is followed by the thalamus, the pons, and the dentate nuclei of the cerebellum. Lobar hemorrhages can occur with hypertension in the subcortical white matter, but they more often are associated with amyloidosis in the elderly.

92.
B Chromosomes 1p and 19q co-deletion

The histopathological features in this case are of an oligodendroglioma. Tumor cells have round, uniform nuclei with an artifactual perinuclear halo. Branching, delicate blood vessels are present within the tumor. Most oligodendrogliomas show a co-deletion of the short arm of chromosome 1 (1p) and long arm of chromosome 19 (19q). The presence of this co-deletion is associated with a better response to chemotherapy and longer survival.

93.

B Angiocentric glioma

Angiocentric gliomas are rare, low-grade lesions most commonly seen in the temporal lobe in young patients with chronic epilepsy. The tumor, as shown in the image accompanying the question, is marked by perivascular pseudorosette-like structures. Ependymomas also may have similar rosette structures but are predominantly intraventricular in location.

94.

D Neuroblastoma

Homer-Wright rosettes lack a central canal or capillary and are seen classically in neuroblastomas, medulloblastomas, primitive neuroectodermal tumors (PNETs), and retinoblastomas. Their lumens contain dense neuropil. Flexner-Wintersteiner rosettes are seen classically in retinoblastomas but also occur in pineoblastomas. They have no fiber-rich neuropil in their centers and resemble photoreceptor rods/cones ultrastructurally. (A) Ependymal rosettes form central lumens, whereas pseudorosettes form zones of fibrillary processes around blood vessels. Pseudorosettes are seen much more commonly in ependymomas and are more sensitive for a diagnosis of ependymoma than true rosettes. (C) Pineocytomatous/neurocytic rosettes are seen in pineocytomas/central neurocytomas and are similar to Homer-Wright rosettes but are larger and more regular.

95.

E Papillary and rhabdoid

Meningothelial, transitional, and fibrous are the most common meningioma subtypes. Clear cell, chordoid, and atypical meningiomas are WHO grade II. Atypical meningiomas are characterized by increased mitotic activity (four or more mitotic figures per high power microscopic field), brain invasion, or a tumor with three or more other worrisome features (e.g., patternless/sheet-like growth patterns, hypercellularity, small cell change, necrosis, and prominent nucleation). Anaplastic meningiomas are grade III, characterized by obvious malignant features resembling carcinoma/melanoma or high-grade sarcoma or mitotic activity in excess of 19 mitotic figures per 10 high power fields. Papillary and rhabdoid tumors also are considered WHO grade III.

96.

C Pilocytic astrocytoma

The most common histological type of optic pathway/hypothalamic glioma in the pediatric pop-

ulation is pilocytic astrocytoma, which comprises the majority of prechiasmatic tumors. Other common tumor types are low-grade fibrillary astrocytoma, ganglioglioma, and, rarely, malignant glioma.

97.

C Cytomegalovirus infection

Neurons infected by cytomegalovirus show large intranuclear eosinophilic inclusions known as Cowdry A (or just Cowdry) bodies. Smaller cytoplasmic inclusions also can be present in infected cells.

98.

E Oligodendroglioma

Oligodendrogliomas have a "chicken wire" vasculature with a delicate network of branching capillaries, whereas the "fried egg" appearance is an artifactual perinuclear clear space following delayed formalin fixation (thus not seen in frozen sections). (A) Germinomas have sheets of large cells with round nuclei, distinct cell borders, and often are infiltrated with lymphocytes. (B) Ependymomas often show rosettes or perivascular pseudorosettes. (C) Pleomorphic xanthoastrocytomas are described by their large cells with abundant intracytoplasmic vacuoles due to lipid accumulation.

99.

A *Streptococcus* species

Sixty percent of cerebral abscesses are polymicrobial. *Streptococcus* species are the most frequent organisms found, with 33 to 50% of abscesses being anaerobic or microaerophilic. *Streptococcus milleri* can be seen in frontoethmoidal sinusitis. (B) *Escherichia coli* abscesses are seen in neonates and following brain surgery. (C) *Bacteroides* is a common abscess former from otitis media/mastoiditis. (D) *Actinomyces* abscesses can be seen with odontogenic sources. (E) *Staphylococcus epidermidis* abscesses can be seen after neurosurgical procedures.

100.

E Pilocytic astrocytoma

The microphotograph shows the classic "biphasic" pattern of a pilocytic astrocytoma. Compacted eosinophilic areas *(center)* contrast with loose, microcystic zones *(sides)*. Rosenthal fibers (not shown) also are frequently seen.

101.

A Glioblastoma

Glioblastoma (high-grade astrocytoma) is the most common primary tumor of the central nervous system. The most common tumor of the central nervous system is metastasis.

102.

D Metastatic carcinoma

TTF-1 (thyroid transcription factor-1) was a marker initially designed to target thyroid cancer. The marker also stains a significant percentage of adenocarcinomas arising in the lung.

103.

C Mitotic activity

Anaplastic astrocytomas typically are more cellular than low-grade astrocytomas and have more readily observable mitotic figures. (A) Calcifications are present in about 15% of fibrillary astrocytomas and are not associated with tumor grade. (B) All diffuse or fibrillary astrocytomas have an infiltrative border. (D, E) Necrosis and vascular proliferation are features found in glioblastoma.

104.

B Low-grade diffuse astrocytoma

The tumor shown in the image accompanying the question is marked by mild increased cellularity and scattered atypical appearing tumor cells (large pleomorphic and hyperchromatic [i.e., darker staining nuclei]). These findings morphologically are most consistent with a low-grade diffuse astrocytoma, many of which are p53 mutated neoplasms. (A) Anaplastic astrocytomas would be more cellular than this tumor. (C) Oligodendroglioma nuclei are more rounded and, overall, are monomorphic in appearance. (D, E) Features that are characteristic of pilocytic astrocytomas and pleomorphic xanthoastrocytomas (granular bodies, Rosenthal fibers, lipidized astrocytes) are absent in this pathology slide.

105.

E Small cell

The vast majority of small cell glioblastomas show epidermal growth factor receptor (EGFR) alterations as compared with other glioblastoma variants. This sometimes can be useful in distinguishing this variant from anaplastic oligodendrogliomas that can look remarkably similar to glioblastomas at times.

106.

B Gemistocytic astrocytoma

Gemistocytic astrocytomas are marked by a proliferation of large cells with eccentrically placed nuclei and abundant eosinophilic cytoplasm (so-called gemistocytes). In the background is a second population of atypical cells with scant cytoplasm more typical of malignant astrocytes. (A) Epithelioid glioblastomas typically resemble carcinoma or

melanoma. (C) Giant cell glioblastomas often contain scattered, multinucleated, giant cells. (D) The cellular density is much greater in gemistocytic astrocytomas compared with gliosis. (E) Subependymal giant cell astrocytomas are intraventricular masses.

107.

D Pilocytic astrocytoma

This low-grade tumor is marked by spindled cells arranged against a fibrillary background with intermixed brightly eosinophilic, elongated structures (Rosenthal fibers). These features are typical of pilocytic astrocytomas. The optic nerve is a common site for these tumors, which most commonly arise in the first two decades of life.

108.

D Prior surgery

The histopathology shown in the image accompanying the question consists of disorganized peripheral nerve tissue intermixed with collagen tissue. These features are consistent with a traumatic neuroma. Traumatic neuromas may be a complication of prior surgery.

109.

E Prion disease

The section of gray matter shows spongiform change and the presence of starburst-like structures, which represent prion plaques. These plaques particularly are salient in the variant form of Creutzfeldt-Jakob disease. (A–D) All of these processes would have some sort of inflammatory component associated with them.

110.

E *Nocardia asteroides*

The thin, filamentous organisms highlighted with the Gomori methenamine silver stain are consistent with *Nocardia asteroides*. The hyphae of *Aspergillus fumigatus* also are elongated, but are thicker, acute angle branching, and septated. The septations often are difficult to see on this stain.

111.

E Toxoplasmosis

The large, rounded cysts containing small organisms inside of them represent the cysts of toxoplasmosis. The cysts are associated with a collection of microglial cells (a microglial nodule). Although more commonly seen in the setting of an abscess in immunocompromised patients, *Toxoplasma* occasionally may manifest as encephalitis.

112.

E Respiratory tract

The large, rounded organisms shown (some of which have an internal round structure) represent *Blastomyces*. Their internal structure is a protoplasmic body. These organisms also may show evidence of budding (like *Cryptococcus*). *Blastomyces* typically gains access to the body through the respiratory system and sometimes the skin.

113.

D Metastatic melanoma

The vignette in the question describes a patient presenting with intracerebral hemorrhage with intraoperative findings that are concerning for melanosis of the dura. The pathological specimen is hematoxylin-and-eosin stained and demonstrates epithelioid cells with melanin inclusions. The most likely diagnosis is intraparenchymal hemorrhage secondary to metastatic melanoma. (A) The diffuse presence of the infiltrating melanin-containing cells indicates abnormal tissues. (B) Although there are red blood cells observed within a vessel, the specimen is abnormal due to the melanin-containing cells. (C) Although hemorrhage is common with metastatic renal cell carcinoma, the mention of dural discoloration and the microscopic specimen are more consistent with melanoma. (E) Melanocytoma would have a similar pathological specimen, but the patient's presentation and frequency of metastatic melanoma make it the more likely diagnosis.

114.

A Abscess

The section demonstrates a collection of neutrophils most consistent with an acute abscess. The purple structures represent colonies of bacterial organisms within the abscess.

115.

D *Mucor*

The thick fungal hyphae highlighted on a PAS stain represent *Mucor*. The hyphae are nonseptate with an irregular, wide angle (approaching 90 degrees) branching pattern. (A–C, E) These organisms have different morphologies, being generally thinner and, in some cases, with septations to the hyphal structures.

116.

C Smith-Lemli-Opitz syndrome

Smith-Lemli-Opitz syndrome is associated with multiple congenital abnormalities due to an error in cholesterol synthesis. It may be associated with some cases of holoprosencephaly. (A) Cyclopia (not diprosopus [craniofacial duplication]) is a physical exam finding in holoprosencephaly that typically indicates the alobar form, which is the most severe. (B) Caudal regression syndrome but not holoprosencephaly is associated with maternal diabetes. (D) Trisomy of chromosome 5 is known as cri-du-chat (Lejeune) syndrome, and results in a characteristic cry in affected individuals. Trisomy of chromosomes 13 and 18 may be associated with holoprosencephaly. (E) Holoprosencephaly is not associated with Turner syndrome (partial or complete absence of an X chromosome in a female).

117.

E Organizing subdural hemorrhage

The section shown in the image accompanying the question demonstrates a focal hemorrhage associated with a proliferation of small blood vessels and fibroblasts with intermixed chronic inflammatory cells. The findings are consistent with an organizing subdural hematoma. Subdural hemorrhages typically are associated with tears in the cortical bridging veins and less commonly with tears in cortical arteries.

118.

D Schwannoma

The palisaded structure shown in the image accompanying the question represents a Verocay body associated with schwannomas.

119.

B Neurofibroma

The tumor shown in the image accompanying the question is marked by moderate hypercellularity and nuclear atypia with readily identifiable mitotic activity. This lesion represents a malignant peripheral nerve sheath tumor arising from a neurofibroma.

120.

E Viral infection

The peripheral nerve is marked by small foci of acute and chronic inflammation. An occasional larger size cell also is evident, and is marked by a large, intranuclear inclusion. These inclusions are typical for Cowdry A type viral inclusions (they fill up most of the nucleus and displace internal nuclear structures). The etiology of the neuritis in this example is *Cytomegalovirus*.

121.

E *Cryptococcus*

The rounded organisms, which at times appear to be paired (budding), represent *Cryptococcus*. They are about the size of one or two red blood cells in diameter, and because of their capsule (fairly unique to *Cryptococcus* in the yeast/fungus world), they stain with mucicarmine.

122.

A Cowden disease

The lesion displayed in the image accompanying the question is marked by a proliferation of large neuronal or ganglionic cells. There is no evidence of a glioma component in the background to indicate a ganglioglioma. The lesion is best classified as a dysplastic cerebellar gangliocytoma (Lhermitte-Duclos disease), which is associated with Cowden disease resulting from a mutation in the *PTEN* gene.

123.

B Ganglioglioma

Gangliogliomas are the most common tumor encountered in the setting of pharmacoresistent epilepsy. (A, C–E) These tumors also can be encountered in this setting but are less commonly seen.

124.

A Choroid plexus epithelium

The tissue sample on the biopsy shown in the image accompanying the question represents normal choroid plexus tissue, which is marked by a single layer of epithelioid cells lining fibrovascular cores. The cells are devoid of any appreciable cytologic atypia. (B) The cells lining the papilla are not piled up as they would be in a choroid plexus papilloma.

125.

D Transthyretin

The lesion displayed in the image accompanying the question represents a choroid plexus papilloma. It is marked by a proliferation of bland-looking choroid plexus epithelial cells (hyperplasia). Although these tumors may stain variably with the other antibodies listed, transthyretin is the most distinctive and readily allows this lesion's differentiation from other tumors in the differential diagnosis.

126.

A Caudate nucleus

The biopsy shown in the image accompanying the question demonstrates gray matter with bun-

dles of white matter. These bundles are referred to as pencil bundles or fibers of Wilson. The architecture demonstrated is present in only two locations in the brain—the caudate and putamen nuclei.

127.

A Chordoid meningioma

The lesion shown in the image accompanying the question represents a chordoid meningioma and is characterized by cords of epithelioid cells arranged against a chondromyxoid-like stroma. The tumor cells lack the bubble-like cytoplasmic changes (physaliferous cells) seen in chordomas. The importance of this variant of meningioma lies in its increased likelihood to recur in a shorter interval of time, hence its WHO grade II designation.

128.

B Brain invasion

The tumor shown in the image accompanying the question is marked by islands of meningothelial cells surrounded by brain parenchyma, consistent with brain invasion. Brain invasion warrants a diagnosis of WHO grade II. (A) Angiomatous meningiomas are grade I lesions. (C, D) Hypercellularity and necrosis may be seen in grade II tumors but alone are not enough to warrant a grade II designation. (E) Papillary tumors are WHO grade III lesions.

129.

C Embolization effect

The changes within the blood vessel in this meningioma represent changes related to embolization of the tumor with polyvinyl alcohol. Embolization results in irregularly shaped spaces surrounded by blood and fibrin. Embolization may cause infarct in the tumor. Necrosis in this setting should not be used in assessing tumor grade.

130.

D Progesterone receptors and EMA

The fibrous meningioma shown in the image accompanying the question, marked by spindled cells, is most likely to stain with antibodies to epithelial membrane antigen (EMA) and progesterone receptors. Solitary fibrous tumors stain with CD34 and STAT6 and do not stain with the hormonal receptors and EMA.

131.

D Hemangiopericytoma (solitary fibrous tumor)

The tumor represented in the image accompanying the question is marked by prominent cellularity and staghorn-shaped blood vessels. The findings are most consistent with a hemangiopericytoma pattern, which now is designated as a tumor on the spectrum of the solitary fibrous tumor.

132.

C Inhibin

The tumor shown in the image accompanying the question is composed of rounded stromal cells with a prominent intervening vasculature. The tumor morphologically resembles a hemangioblastoma. Given the association of this tumor with von Hippel–Lindau syndrome, ruling out metastatic renal cell carcinomas (clear cell type) is important, as these two tumors can resemble each other. Inhibin stains hemangioblastomas but not renal cell carcinomas. (A, B, D, E) These antibodies are more likely to stain renal cell carcinomas.

133.

C Intravascular lymphoma

CD20 is a B-cell lymphoid marker. The CD20-positive tumor cells shown in the image accompanying the question all are contained within the blood vessels. These findings are most consistent with an intravascular lymphoma (angiotropic large cell lymphoma).

134.

C HIV infection

The lesion shown in the image accompanying the question here represents a diffuse large B-cell lymphoma or primary CNS lymphoma. This tumor is associated with patients who are immunosuppressed and have EBV infection. HIV-infected patients are at increased risk of developing this tumor.

135.

B Medulloblastoma

The tumor is marked by a proliferation of small cells with scant cytoplasm. The synaptophysin immunoreactivity in this tumor supports a diagnosis of medulloblastoma. Because there is no evidence of tumor elsewhere, a metastasis from a neuroblastoma, which might look similar and also stain with synaptophysin, is not likely.

136.

A Germinoma

The tumor is marked by a proliferation of large cells with abundant cytoplasm and large nucleoli. Intermixed benign-appearing lymphocytes also are present. The morphology is consistent with germinoma, the most common tumor of the pineal gland.

137.

D Pineocytoma

The tumor is marked by a sheet of monomorphic-appearing cells. Occasional pseudorosette structures in which the tumor cells are arranged around pink fibrillary material (a pineocytomatous rosette) are present. These rosette structures are characteristic of a pineocytoma and are not seen in the pineal parenchymal tumor of intermediate differentiation.

138.

D Neurofibromatosis type 2

Multiple meningiomas are associated with neurofibromatosis type 2 (merlin protein mutation on chromosome 22); some patients may develop multiple tumors including bilateral acoustic neuromas (vestibular schwannomas). (A) Gorlin syndrome also is known as basal cell nevus syndrome (among other names) and is characterized by multiple basal cell carcinomas. Patients with this syndrome are very susceptible to ultraviolet light and also can be prone to developing medulloblastomas but not multiple meningiomas. (B) Li-Fraumeni syndrome results from an autosomal dominant mutation of the *TP53* tumor suppressor gene, which entails a propensity to develop multiple types of tumors including sarcomas, breast cancer, leukemia, and adrenal carcinoma. Central nervous system involvement usually includes astrocytomas or primitive neuroectodermal tumors. (C) Neurofibromatosis type 1 results in central nervous system tumors including optic gliomas, astrocytomas, and neurofibromas but not meningiomas. (E) Turcot syndrome is a rare disorder characterized by colorectal neoplasms together with neuroepithelial tumors of the central nervous system. Typical tumors seen in this condition include glioblastomas (Turcot type 1) and medulloblastomas (Turcot type 2).

139.

B Liponeurocytoma

The tumor is marked by a proliferation of rounded cells with scant cytoplasm and a salt-and-pepper nuclear chromatin pattern similar to the cells seen in a central neurocytoma. The scattered vacuolar structures seen in the tumor represent fat cells. These are features of a liponeurocytoma.

140.

D Rosette-forming glioneuronal tumor of the fourth ventricle

The clinical presentation, location, and appearance of the tumor described best fits with the rare, low-grade, rosette-forming glioneuronal tumor of the fourth ventricle.

141.

A Associated with gelastic epilepsy

Hypothalamic hamartomas are rare lesions that typically are small in size and consist of a disordered arrangement of neuronal cells. Gelastic seizures are a common presentation. (C) There is no strong gender predilection for hypothalamic hamartomas. (D) Rare cases of hypothalamic hamartomas arise in the setting of Pallister-Hall syndrome.

142.

B INI-1 loss

The tumor shown in the image accompanying the question is marked by cells with eccentric nuclei and cytoplasmic inclusion-like structures. This rhabdoid morphology is characteristic of atypical teratoid/rhabdoid tumors, which are marked by INI-1 protein loss.

143.

A Chordoid glioma

This tumor is marked by clusters and cords of epithelioid-appearing cells embedded in a mucin-rich stroma. Bright red Russell bodies and chronic inflammatory cells may be present. The location of this tumor and its appearance are most consistent with a chordoid glioma (WHO grade II).

144.

E Zellweger syndrome

Zellweger syndrome is a peroxisomal biogenesis disorder characterized by dysmorphic features, calcific stippling of the patella, liver disease, neuronal migration abnormalities resulting in cortical architectural abnormalities (perisylvian pachygyria with surrounding polymicrogyria), accumulation of lipid material in neurons, glial cells and macrophages, and abnormalities of the white matter with deficient myelin. It has an autosomal recessive pattern of inheritance. (A) Behçet syndrome is a vasculitis disorder with relapsing ocular lesions and recurrent oral and genital ulcers. Headaches occur in over 50% of diagnosed individuals, with other central nervous system manifestations such as pseudotumor cerebri, cerebellar ataxia, paraplegia, seizures, and dural sinus thrombosis. (B) Apert syndrome is a form of syndromic craniosynostosis of the bilateral coronal sutures and is associated with syndactyly. (C) Dejerine-Roussy syndrome is a rare lacunar stroke syndrome characterized by thalamic pain. (D) Gerstmann syndrome is associated with a dominant parietal lobe lesion characterized by agraphia without alexia, left-right confusion, digit agnosia, and acalculia.

145.

A Cardiac myxoma

Cardiac myxomas are associated with psammomatous melanotic schwannomas in the setting of Carney syndrome.

146.

B CHMP2B protein mutation

Frontotemporal lobar atrophy with ubiquinated inclusions represents a form of frontotemporal dementia associated with charged multivesicular body protein 2B mutations (CHMP2B). Patients present with behavior and personality changes and progressive aphasia with progression to an akinetic rigid syndrome and dystonia.

147.

D Pick disease

The argyrophilic or silver-positive staining neuronal cytoplasmic inclusions are referred to as Pick bodies and are seen in a subset of patients with Pick disease. In areas of neuronal loss and gliosis, one also can encounter large, ballooned neurons known as Pick cells. (A) Argyrophilic grain disease is a neurodegenerative disease that may be seen concomitantly with Pick disease. The ballooned neurons indicate Pick disease in this case. (B) Corticobasilar degeneration produces high-density, astrocytic plaques in the frontal lobe. (C) Multisystem atrophy is defined by parkinsonism plus idiopathic orthostatic hypotension and another sign of autonomic nervous system dysfunction. (E) Progressive supranuclear palsy is described as the triad of supranuclear ophthalmoplegia (typically involving vertical gaze), pseudobulbar palsy, and axial dystonia.

148.

D Degeneration of anterior horn cells and corticospinal tracts

The presentation of upper and lower motor neuron findings in the absence of cognitive deficits is concerning for amyotrophic lateral sclerosis (ALS). Although most cases are sporadic, up to 10% of ALS cases may be familial. The report of the brother's progression from presentation to death in 5 years also supports the diagnosis of ALS and its typical timeline of decline. (A) Degeneration of the pars compacta of the substantia nigra is typical of Parkinson disease. (B) Widespread Lewy bodies throughout different areas of the brain are typical of Lewy body dementia. Lewy bodies also may be seen in Parkinson disease but not in ALS. (C) Atrophy of the caudate nuclei can be seen in Huntington disease.

149.

D Trypanosomiasis

Given the patient's country of origin and the appearance of the organisms, Trypanosomiasis infection (Chagas disease) needs to be considered. The organisms typically fill up the cytoplasm of glial cells and are not encysted like *Toxoplasma* organisms.

150.

C Friedreich ataxia

Friedreich ataxia is an autosomal recessive condition resulting from a mutation in the *FXN* gene on chromosome 9 that encodes for the protein frataxin. The mutation results in an expansion of the GAA nucleotide triplet (70 or more repeats constitute the disease). (A) Charcot-Marie-Tooth disease types 1 and 2 make up the most common inherited peripheral nerve disorder and most commonly cause demyelination of peripheral nerves. The disease most commonly is inherited in an autosomal dominant fashion, but X-linked forms of inheritance also exist. (B) Dentatorubral-pallidoluysian atrophy is a very rare, autosomal dominant disease most similar to Huntington disease and is caused by a CAG trinucleotide repeat. (D) Spinocerebellar atrophy type 1 is caused by a CAG repeat on chromosome 6p. (E) Spinocerebellar atrophy type 2 is caused by a CAG repeat on chromosome 12q.

151.

D Motor vehicle accident

Hinge fractures, a type of basilar skull fracture in which there is a gaping fracture across the base of the skull, often transverse the petrous ridge. They most commonly are encountered in the setting of a motor vehicle accident.

152.

C Ragged red fibers

Ragged red fibers are marked by increased subsarcolemmal or peripheral red staining on the trichrome stain corresponding to an accumulation of mitochondria often in the setting of a mitochondrial disorder. A similar finding can be seen with succinate dehydrogenase staining in a subset of cases where they are called ragged blue fibers. (A) Nemaline rods are visualized best with a Gomori trichrome stain and appear as dark-blue structures mostly in the muscle fiber cytoplasm. They are seen in some congenital myopathies. (B) Nuclear chains represent centralized nuclei and may be seen in myotonic dystrophy. (D) Rimmed vacuoles are autophagic in nature and are seen in several neuromuscular diseases, including inclusion body myositis. (E) Ring fibers are peripheral myofilaments that encircle myofibers of the same bundle. They may be a marker of myotonic dystrophy.

153.

E Mucopolysaccharidoses

GAG accumulation results from impaired lysosomal degradation of mucopolysaccharides and characterizes the mucopolysaccharidoses.

154.

C Optic nerves and chiasm

Devic disease (also known as neuromyelitis optica) preferentially involves the optic nerves and chiasm and cervical spinal cord.

155.

B Gaucher disease

Gaucher disease is the most common of the lysosomal storage diseases, with a prevalence of 1.16 to 1.75 per 100,000. There is an increased risk of developing the disease in people of Ashkenazi Jewish descent. (A) Fabry disease is caused by a deficiency in α-galactosidase A and is inherited in an X-linked fashion. (C) Globoid cell leukodystrophy (also known as Krabbe disease) is caused by a mutation in the *GALC* gene and is inherited in an autosomal recessive fashion. (D) Neuronal ceroid lipofuscinosis refers to a family of neurodegenerative conditions that result in the accumulation of lipofuscin in the body's tissues and is less common than Gaucher disease. (E) Pompe disease is caused by a deficiency in α-glucosidase.

156.

A Sphingomyelinase; sphingomyelin

Sphingomyelinase is the deficient enzyme in Niemann-Pick disease that causes a buildup of sphingomyelin. (B) Sphingomyelinase is the enzyme deficiency in Niemann-Pick disease, but glucocerebroside is the metabolite that accumulates in Gaucher disease. (C) Hexosaminidase A and GM2 ganglioside are the deficient enzyme and accumulating metabolite, respectively, in Tay-Sachs disease. (D) Hexosaminidase A is the enzyme deficient in Tay-Sachs disease, whereas glucocerebroside is the metabolite that builds up in Gaucher disease. (E) Glucocerebrosidase and glucocerebroside are the enzyme deficiency and accumulating metabolite, respectively, in Gaucher disease.

157.

B Neuronal ceroid lipofuscinosis

The neuronal ceroid lipofuscinoses are a group of autosomal recessive disorders characterized by neurologic deterioration and by the accumulation of lipofuscin-like products. Ultrastructurally, these accumulations may manifest as granular osmiophilic deposits, curvilinear bodies, or fingerprint bodies. (A) Fucosidosis is an autosomal recessive disease due to a deficiency of the enzyme α-L-fucosidase, which is involved in the metabolism of complex sugars and not lipofuscin. (C) Schindler disease is an autosomal recessive lysosomal storage disease caused by a deficiency of α-N-acetyl-galactosaminidase, which leads to a buildup of glycosphingolipids. (D) Sialidosis is a lysosomal storage disease caused by a deficiency of α-N-acetyl neuraminidase, which leads to the accumulation of mucopolysaccharides and mucolipids. (E) Wolman disease is due to a deficiency of lysosomal acid lipase, which leads to an accumulation of fats in various body tissues.

158.

E Wilson disease

The changes of Alzheimer type 2 astrocytes are associated with hepatic encephalopathy, as first described in Wilson disease.

159.

B Homocystinuria

The features described are characteristic of homocystinuria resulting from a gene abnormality encoding for cystathionine β-synthase. (A) Urea cycle disorders is a broad category of diseases that result in abnormal urea metabolism and the buildup of ammonia in the body. Individuals may present at any age, depending on the severity of the enzyme deficiency. (C) Maple syrup urine disease is an autosomal recessive disorder of amino acid metabolism. It is named for the sweet smell of urine in infancy or during acute exacerbations of the disease. (D) Menkes disease results from mutations of the *ATP7A* gene and is inherited in an X-linked recessive manner. The disease results in an abnormal distribution of copper in the body, leading to a deficiency in some tissues and deposition in others. Infants typically display coarse, brittle hair, hypotonia, sagging facial features, seizures, and developmental delays. (E) Phenylketonuria results in an error in the metabolism of phenylalanine due to a deficiency of phenylalanine hydroxylase. Affected individuals must follow a phenylalanine-restricted diet. Untreated, it can lead to intellectual disability and seizures, among other problems.

160.

A Fabry disease

(B) Tay-Sachs disease is due to a deficiency of hexosaminidase A. (C) Gaucher disease is due to a deficiency of glucocerebrosidase. (D) Krabbe disease is due to a mutation in the *GALC* gene. (E) Pompe disease is due to a deficiency of the α-glucosidase enzyme.

161.

B Dandy-Walker malformation

(A) Chiari type 2 malformations typically are associated with myelomeningoceles and are characterized by a small posterior fossa with herniation of the brainstem and cerebellum through the foramen magnum. Other findings include tectal "beaking," a large third ventricle and massa intermedia, colpocephaly, hydrocephalus, and aqueductal stenosis. (C) Joubert syndrome is characterized by an underdeveloped vermis and abnormal brainstem. The most common findings are ataxia, hyperpnea, hypotonia, and sleep apnea. (D) Lhermitte-Duclos disease is characterized by a hypertrophied cerebellar granular cell layer and increased myelin in the molecular layer with thick folia. The lesion is considered a hamartoma and may demonstrate calcifications and associated hydrocephalus. The condition may be associated with Cowden syndrome. (E) Rhombencephalosynapsis is characterized by partial vermian agenesis and fusion of the cerebellar hemispheres. It typically is associated with other syndromes such as VACTERL.

162.

C Periventricular leukomalacia

The changes described are characteristic of periventricular leukomalacia, which represents a pattern of injury involving the deep white matter. The incidence is increased in premature infants.

163.

E Zellweger syndrome

The description is of Zellweger (also known as cerebrohepatorenal) syndrome, the worst disease on a spectrum of peroxin protein disorders. (A) Menkes disease is transmitted by maternal mitochondria, and affected patients suffer from encephalopathy, stroke-like episodes, cortical blindness, seizures, and mental retardation, and have characteristic sparse/coarse hair and sagging facial features. (B) Leigh disease is also known as subacute necrotic encephalomyelopathy. Inheritance is autosomal recessive. The disease manifests in bilateral, symmetric spongiform degeneration and necrosis of the thalami, basal ganglia, brainstem, and spinal cord with peripheral nerve demyelination. (C) Lowe (also known as oculocerebrorenal) syndrome is an X-linked recessive disease causing bilateral cataracts, nystagmus, large eyes, and psychomotor retardation. Death typically occurs by renal failure. (D) Lesch-Nyhan disease is caused by a deficiency of hypoxanthine-guanine phosphoribosyltransferase. Uric acid accumulates, and patients exhibit self-mutilation behaviors and choreoathetosis. Inheritance is X-linked recessive.

164.

A Lissencephaly

Miller-Dieker syndrome is associated with lissencephaly or agyria. Affected individuals have characteristic facial features (bitemporal hollowing, short nose, broad nasal bridge, upturned nares, long thin upper lip, small chin, and low-set and posteriorly rotated ears). The syndrome is associated with a defect in the gene encoding for platelet activating factor (PAF) on chromosome 17p13.3.

165.

C Rhabdomyolysis

The biopsy shows numerous necrosis muscle fibers being phagocytosed by macrophages. Widespread myonecrosis is consistent with rhabdomyolysis.

166.

A Abnormal dystrophin, fatty/fibrous infiltration, and no necrosis

The patient's gender, age, progressive symptoms, and pseudohypertrophy of his calves indicate Becker muscular dystrophy. Although Becker and Duchenne muscular dystrophy both result from dystrophin abnormalities (partially functional dystrophin in the former and nonfunctional dystrophin in the latter), the Becker form does not demonstrate necrosis whereas the Duchenne form does. (B) The absence of dystrophin and muscle fiber necrosis with regeneration is characteristic of Duchenne muscular dystrophy. (C) Chronic inflammatory cells without fiber necrosis or regeneration within the muscle are characteristic of facioscapulohumeral dystrophy. This is an autosomal dominant condition, with pathology located on chromosome 4 that involves the face, shoulders, and upper arms. The forearms are spared, resulting in a "Popeye" appearance. (D) Basophilic bodies with dark centers are typical of Lafora bodies and are due to the accumulation of polyglucosans. These bodies are seen in Lafora disease, which is a systemic and fatal autosomal recessive muscular dystrophy.

167.

E Medium range

A medium-range gunshot wound occurs when the muzzle is a few inches to a few feet from the skin. A gunshot at this range results in stippling caused by tiny pieces of burned, burning, or unburned gunpowder impacting the skin and injuring it. (A, B) Close range and contact wounds typically leave behind an imprint of the muzzle, soot, and possibly lacerations from escaping gases. (C) Distance wounds lack stippling and typically are the caliber of the projectile used. (D) Exit wounds generally are larger than entrance wounds and contain little to no soot. There also may be a beveling effect on the bone.

168.

D Sarcoidosis

The section shown in the image accompanying the question demonstrates necrotizing granulomatous inflammation. No larger organisms, such as a parasite or fungus, are discernible. The most likely etiology is tuberculosis.

18 Ophthalmology

1.

D At the junction of the left optic nerve and chiasm

A lesion at the junction of the left optic nerve and chiasm could affect the Wilbrand knee, which is a group of fibers supplying vision to the superior temporal field in the contralateral eye. In this case, the patient would have a central scotoma in the left eye due to the optic nerve involvement and a right superior temporal visual defect in the right eye. (A) A lesion in the left inferior optic radiations would produce a relatively congruous right superior quadrantanopsia. (B) A lesion in the right occipital pole would produce a left central homonymous hemifield deficit. (C) A lesion in the orbital portion of the left optic nerve would produce a central scotoma in the left eye. (E) A lesion in the optic chiasm would produce variable visual field deficits, and classically is described as producing a central bitemporal hemianopsia if only the decussating nasal-macular fibers are affected.

2.

E Ability to turn head

In oculomotor apraxia, patients have difficulty with saccade initiation in addition to a blunted or absent vestibulo-ocular reflex. Patients must turn (and typically thrust) their heads to track objects and often overshoot the target. (A) The optokinetic reflex involves smooth pursuits of the eyes followed by saccadic movement. When an object moves by, the eyes track the object until it has left the visual field and then return to the initial position through a saccade. Think about being able to fixate on telephone poles while driving by them rapidly. (B) The ability to converge on an object has no role in assisting this patient. (C) In oculomotor apraxia, patients have a blunted or absent vestibulo-ocular reflex, which is the reflex enabling the eyes to maintain fixation on an object as the head makes slight turns and movements. (D) The tonic labyrinthine reflex is a primitive reflex that disappears by 6 months of age. It involves full-body extension except for flexion of the upper extremities when the head is extended in the supine position. It would not assist this patient.

3.

D Sympathetic chain distal to the superior cervical ganglion but proximal to the off-take of the vasomotor fibers

A lesion of the sympathetic chain distal to the superior cervical ganglion proximal to the off-take of the vasomotor fibers results in a third-order Horner syndrome with anhydrosis of only the brow. The vasomotor fibers to the rest of the face emerge from the sympathetic chain proximal to the superior cervical ganglion at the level of the carotid bifurcation. Amphetamines would not cause pupillary dilation, as amphetamines cause a release of norepinephrine only in an intact neuron. (A, B) Lesions proximal to the synapse of central sympathetic fibers in the upper thoracic spinal cord result in a first-order Horner syndrome with miosis, ptosis, and anhydrosis of the ipsilateral face, arm, and trunk. Amphetamines would cause pupillary dilation, as the third-order neuron is intact. (C) A lesion of the proximal sympathetic chain results in a second-order Horner syndrome and in anhydrosis of the face as the vasomotor fibers decussate at the carotid bifurcation and follow the external carotid artery. The fibers innervating the arm and truck already have emerged from the sympathetic chain. Amphetamines would cause pupillary dilation, as the third-order neuron is intact. (E) A lesion of the sympathetic chain distal to the superior cervical ganglion distal to the off-take of the vasomotor fibers results in a third-order Horner syndrome without anhydrosis. Amphetamines would not cause pupillary dilation, as amphetamines cause a release of norepinephrine only in an intact neuron.

4.

C Ipsilateral paramedian pontine reticular formation and the ipsilateral medial longitudinal fasciculus

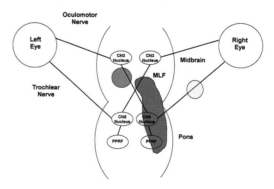

As demonstrated in this diagram by the orange lesion and with reference to the right eye, a lesion here would cause a right internuclear ophthalmoplegia with a horizontal gaze palsy. The patient would not be able to abduct his right eye, and it would not move medially when the left eye is abducted. (A) With reference to the left eye, this condition would be represented in the diagram by the purple lesion of the medial longitudinal fasciculus (MLF) combined with the yellow lesion of the right abducens nerve. By naming convention, this would be a left ipsilateral internuclear ophthalmoplegia with an abduction palsy in the right eye. The patient would have no issue gazing to the left with both eyes. (B) As seen in the diagram, bilateral pontine paramedian reticular formation (PPRF) lesions are equivalent to bilateral abducens nucleus lesions and would prevent eye abduction bilaterally. (D) This would have the same result seen in A. (E) As seen in the diagram (if the purple lesion were represented bilaterally), a lesion of the bilateral MLF will separate the abducens and oculomotor nuclei, causing a bilateral internuclear ophthalmoplegia.

5.

B Painless, slowly progressive monocular vision loss

The typical diagnostic triad of optic nerve sheath meningiomas (ONSMs) is painless, slowly progressive vision loss with optic atrophy and optociliary shunt vessels. (A) ONSMs arise from the proliferation of meningoepithelial cells lining the intraorbital or intracanalicular optic nerve. They arise from the arachnoid and not the dural layer. (C) Optic atrophy is seen. (D) ONSMs account for one third of optic nerve tumors and are the second most common cause after benign optic nerve gliomas. They usually affect women in their 40s or 50s.

6.

C Horner syndrome

In nuclear-fascicular syndrome with injury to the trochlear nucleus and fasciculus (the two almost always are injured together due to the short course of the midbrain trochlear fascicles), there may be injury to the descending sympathetic pathways through the dorsolateral tegmentum. This could manifest in a Horner syndrome contralateral to the observed trochlear nerve deficit. (A) The pupil would be miotic and not mydriatic with a Horner syndrome. (B) Although the extent of the

infarction may extend into the pons and affect the abducens nucleus, it will affect other anatomy first. (D) Although the oculomotor nucleus is located in the midbrain, it is more likely that the patient would suffer other deficits prior to oculomotor involvement.

7.

D Between the third and fourth neurons

The light-near dissociation disorder described is Adie syndrome, as the other two primary causes were ruled out. Adie syndrome results from a viral or bacterial infection of the ciliary ganglion. This is the synapse of the third and fourth neurons in the pupillary reflex pathway. (B) The first neurons in the pupillary reflex pathway originate in the retinal ganglion cells in the eye and project to the pretectal nucleus through the optic nerve. (C) The second neurons in the pupillary reflex pathway originate in the pretectal nucleus and synapse in the Edinger-Westphal nucleus of the rostral midbrain. The third neurons then emerge and run along the oculomotor nerves. (E) The fourth neurons in the pupillary reflex pathway run from the ciliary ganglion through the short ciliary nerves to innervate the iris sphincter muscle.

8.

B A right olfactory groove meningioma

The patient has signs and symptoms consistent with Foster-Kennedy syndrome. The syndrome is defined as optic atrophy and a central scotoma (loss of vision in the middle of the visual field) in the ipsilateral eye, disk edema in the contralateral eye, and ipsilateral anosmia. These symptoms typically are caused by an olfactory groove lesion.

9.

A Hunt-Hess score

More severe aneurysmal subarachnoid hemorrhage as identified by a greater Hunt-Hess score is the major predictor of the incidence of Terson syndrome. The syndrome is defined as intraocular hemorrhage associated with intracranial hemorrhage and elevated intracranial pressure and occurs in 10 to 50% of cases of aneurysmal subarachnoid hemorrhage. Visual acuity may or may not be affected. (D) There is no definite association with the occurrence of Terson syndrome and the location of a ruptured aneurysm.

10.

A Myasthenia gravis

The relaxation of the orbicularis oculi after prolonged contraction fits well with the symptom manifestation of myasthenia gravis, in which muscles fatigue with sustained use. Symptoms tend to be worse with drowsiness and can be improved after a short period of ice application to the muscle. (B) Hemifacial spasm would manifest in a tonic or clonic contraction of the orbicularis oculi. It can be treated with botulinum toxin injections. (C) The orbicularis oculi demonstrates good strength at the start of the examination and thus is not paretic. (D) Disinsertion of the levator palpebrae would cause a ptosis. (E) Botulinum toxin injection into the orbicularis oculi would cause a sustained paresis.

11.

B Ophthalmoplegic migraine

Ophthalmoplegic migraines are characterized by recurrent migraine headache attacks with subsequent periorbital pain and diplopia often lasting for days to months once the initial headaches have resolved. The diplopia is due to cranial neuropathies most commonly involving the oculomotor nerve. Ophthalmoplegic migraines are seen mainly in children but can occur in adults. (A) The patient is quite young to have multiple sclerosis, and severe headache episodes are not typical of the condition. A negative MRI of the brain makes multiple sclerosis less likely. (C) Although there are juvenile forms of myasthenia gravis and patients with myasthenia gravis can have episodic weakness of extraocular muscles, the disease is not associated with severe headaches. (D) Patients with classic migraines can have photophobia and nausea recurring in the described pattern, but the ophthalmoplegia best fits with a diagnosis of an ophthalmoplegic migraine. (E) Orbital cellulitis would not have the recurrent nature seen with this patient.

12.

C They present with optic atrophy and disk edema with an afferent pupillary defect.

Often occurring unilaterally except in syndromic cases, optic nerve gliomas present with optic atrophy, disk edema, proptosis, and a relative afferent pupillary defect. (A) Optic nerve gliomas typically are of the pilocytic astrocytoma variety, which means WHO grade I. (B) Most optic nerve gliomas (70%) occur in the first rather than the third decade; 90% present by the end of the second decade. (D) Observation or chemotherapy is the first-line treatment for optic nerve gliomas. Surgery is reserved for aggressive tumors invading the chiasm with significant vision loss in that surgery itself often compromises vision. (E) Optic nerve gliomas are associated with neurofibromatosis type 1 and can be seen bilaterally.

13.

B Superior arcuates of the retina

In the eye, deficits tend to respect the horizontal midline, whereas lesions beyond the eye tend to respect the vertical midline. This visual field result is indicative of a retinal lesion involving the superior arcuates.

14.

B Tolosa-Hunt syndrome

Tolosa-Hunt syndrome is characterized by painful ophthalmoplegia secondary to cavernous sinus granulomatous inflammation. Patients with the syndrome can have recurrent attacks occurring over intervals of months to years with spontaneous remission between attacks. Steroids can help to abate symptoms more rapidly. Although this is a diagnosis of exclusion, the finding of isolated elevation in cerebrospinal fluid lymphocytes can help. (A) Ramsay Hunt syndrome is due to a reactivation of the *Varicella zoster* virus in the geniculate ganglion, causing ear pain, facial weakness, and possibly a vesicular rash on the skin of the ear. (C) Sarcoidosis is characterized by multisystem granulomatous disease typically arising in young to middle-aged women of Northern European or African descent. It can present with ophthalmoplegia with spontaneous remission and recurrence, but usually is associated with disease elsewhere in the body and can be followed by elevated serum angiotensin-converting enzyme levels. (D) Multiple sclerosis is characterized by the presence of demyelinating lesions in the central nervous system. Although patients can have remission and relapse of symptoms including ophthalmoplegia, ophthalmoplegia is not painful. (E) In tuberculosis meningitis, granulomatous disease would be expected beyond just the cavernous sinus, and the whole body MRI likely would have found primary pulmonary disease. The cerebrospinal fluid in tuberculosis meningitis reveals an elevated lymphocyte and protein count, with a decrease in glucose.

15.

C Infectious neuroretinitis

Infectious neuroretinitis in an inflammation of the optic nerve due to an infectious source that causes unilateral loss of visual acuity and disk edema. Although not always present, macular exudates confirm the diagnosis in an otherwise healthy patient and are most common with *Bartonella henselae*. (A) Pseudotumor cerebri can present with disk edema, but the edema appears bilaterally and not necessarily symmetrically. It is extremely rare to present unilaterally. The condition is associated with young, overweight females and can be characterized by headaches and decreased visual acuity, but these are common and incidental findings in this patient. Macular exudates also are not characteristic of the disease. (B) An optic nerve glioma or any tumor causing mass effect on the optic nerve can decrease visual fields and acuity as part of a compressive optic neuropathy. In addition, due to axoplasmic stasis, unilateral disk edema can occur, but optic nerve gliomas are overall rare. (D) Glaucoma would be rare in a young female and typically causes a loss of the peripheral vision after the disease is advanced. It may occur unilaterally, but the disease is not associated with disk edema. (E) Nonarteritic anterior ischemic optic neuropathy is a disease characterized by an acute ischemic event in the optic nerve, and it typically presents in individuals 50 years of age and older who have cardiovascular risk factors and small, crowded disks. Unilateral disk edema can be seen in the acute phase of the disease. This patient is much too young for this condition.

16.
E Refractive error

The most common cause of unilateral diplopia is a refractive error, as is well observed with severe astigmatism in one eye (multiple focal points of the light rays). (A–D) These conditions are associated with bilateral diplopia (double vision when both eyes are open) due to misalignment of the eyes.

17.
E Poor prognosis with little recovery of vision

Perioperative idiopathic optic neuropathy is associated with prolonged prone positioning, induced hypotension, and anemia but typically is idiopathic. It occurs in 0.2% of spinal procedures, and the risk may be reduced by keeping the head elevated above the heart and by aggressive fluid replacement.

18.
A Start high-dose steroids

High-dose steroids should be given immediately as soon as arteritic anterior ischemic optic neurop-

athy (A-AION) (i.e., giant cell temporal arteritis) is suspected, as the biopsy results take at least 2 weeks to be affected by steroid administration. Steroids should not be delayed pending a biopsy. (B) Plasmapheresis plays no mainstream role in the first-line treatment of A-AION. (C) Fluorescein angiography is a useful ancillary test, as no test for A-AION is 100% specific. Steroids should be administered before any ancillary testing, however. (D) A 2- to 3-cm biopsy of the superficial temporal artery with pathology analysis is very useful to diagnose a case of A-AION, but it should not be the first step in intervention. (E) Observation may result in symptom progression and loss of vision.

19.
B < 50 Gy total and < 2 Gy fractionated

(E) Under 8 Gy of radiation is a safe maximal dose of radiation during radiosurgery.

20.
D There is a 50% risk of developing MS across all patients with optic neuritis.

(A) There is a 25% chance of developing multiple sclerosis (MS) in the 15 years following optic neuritis when there is an MRI without plaques at the time of the optic neuritis. (B) More than one demyelinating plaque on MRI at the time of optic neuritis yields a 72% chance of developing MS in the next 15 years. (C) Male gender, more severe optic disk swelling, and hemorrhage in the optic disk all are factors that lower the risk of developing MS following optic neuritis.

21.
C Dural venous sinus thrombosis

Dural venous sinus thrombosis can cause an elevation in intracranial pressure and can be the underlying etiology of pseudotumor cerebri in some individuals. In addition, congenital transverse sinus abnormalities have been linked to pseudotumor cerebri. These conditions should be investigated with CT or MR venography. (A, B) An empty sella sign is the appearance of the "flattened" pituitary gland by elevated intracranial pressure in pseudotumor cerebri. Along with flattening of the globes, it is a sign rather than an etiology of elevated intracranial pressure. (D) Although there have been rare case reports linking thyroid supplementation medications to pseudotumor cerebri, thyroid disease is not known to be associated with pseudotumor cerebri. (E) An excessive consumption of vitamin A can lead to pseudotumor cerebri.

22.

A Methylmalonic acid and homocysteine levels

The described patient may have pernicious anemia (B12 deficiency) following bariatric surgery or nutritional deficiency due to dietary changes. B12 deficiency is a leading cause of bilateral acute optic neuropathy. (B) Hereditary optic neuropathies (e.g., Leber hereditary optic neuropathy) often but not always are mitochondrial in origin and tend to present in younger individuals. These conditions are possible in this patient but are quite rare overall. (C) MRI of the orbits may reveal lesions such as optic nerve gliomas and meningiomas, but these typically are benign and grow slowly. Optic neuropathies caused by these lesions would not be acute in occurrence. (D) Methanol as an unintended by-product of homemade alcohol is neurotoxic and can cause an acute bilateral optic neuropathy typically 10 to 30 hours after ingestion.

23.

D Vaso-occlusive disease

(A–E) Although all answer choices are explanations for a third nerve palsy, vaso-occlusive disease is the leading cause of spontaneous oculomotor nerve palsy. Vaso-occlusive disease can include giant cell arteritis and nerve ischemia and has the risk factors of hypertension, heart disease, and diabetes.

24.

D Chest imaging

As the patient presents with a second-order Horner syndrome (amphetamine dilating the pupils rules out a third-order Horner syndrome), concern arises about a chest/lung lesion (Pancoast tumor), causing compression and injury to the sympathetic chain proximal to the superior cervical ganglion. As the vasomotor fibers to the face follow the common and then the external carotid arteries, there would be facial anhidrosis. Apraclonidine is an α_2-adrenergic agonist and a weak α_1-adrenergic agonist, but because in Horner syndrome the denervated pupillary dilator muscle up-regulates its α_1 receptors, the miotic, affected pupil dilates more than the normal pupil, resulting in a reversed anisocoria. (B) Orbital imaging is not necessary as part of the patient's workup. (C) Imaging of the medulla would be useful when trying to diagnose lateral medullary (Wallenberg) syndrome caused by infarction in the distribution of the posterior inferior cerebellar artery. This could cause a first-order Horner syndrome, but anhidrosis would be expected to be seen in the arm and trunk in addition to the face. (E) CT angiography of the neck would assist when looking for carotid artery dissections, and the patient's history and exam is consistent with a second-order Horner syndrome; however, the vasomotor fibers that would need to be disrupted to cause anhidrosis to the face travel with the external carotid. Common carotid artery dissection could result in the picture described. Internal carotid artery imaging would not be helpful.

25.

D Check the blood pressure.

Undiagnosed hypertensive retinopathy can be suggested by headaches and decreased visual acuity. On funduscopic exam, there can be disk edema in severe cases, arteriovenous nicking, and hard exudates in a ring around the retina (the first and latter of these are seen in the image). (A) Diabetic retinopathy is associated with macular edema, flame hemorrhages (secondary to vascular proliferation), and cotton wool spots (axoplasmic material within the nerve fiber layer). These are not seen in this image. (B) Mass effect from a tumor may be the etiology of disk edema but not macular exudates. (C) Glaucoma can present with an increased cup-to-disk ratio on funduscopic exam, but typically is not associated with retinal hard exudates.

26.

C Duane syndrome

Duane syndrome is congenital strabismus of various forms, with the most common involving unilateral abduction limitation with or without esotropia. Patients often assume a squint or head turn to maintain binocular fixation. More common in females and mostly unilateral and sporadic, the syndrome is thought to be due to a maldevelopment of the abducens nucleus and nerve along with a lack of innervations of the lateral rectus. (A) In Duane syndrome, the abducens nucleus and nerve are hypoplastic or missing, and thus the condition is not due to a palsy of an otherwise developmentally normal neural pathway. (B) Although an intracranial mass cannot be ruled out, the long-standing, stable symptoms would argue against mass effect on the abducens nerve. (D) Multiple sclerosis is rare in this age group, and typically would not have isolated and stable symptoms. (E) Trauma is a possibility that could explain a left abducens nerve palsy, but Duane syndrome is much more likely.

27.

A More symmetrical visual field deficits tend to localize lesions closer to the occipital lobes.

28.

D Thyroid

Thyroid disease (especially Graves disease) is the most common cause of bilateral exophthalmos in an otherwise healthy patient. Graves disease is an autoimmune attack on the thyroid gland causing hyperthyroidism. (A) Thymus pathology may be present with such conditions as myasthenia gravis, but this would present with a ptosis and not an exophthalmos. (B) Brain tumors with bilateral orbital invasion or severely raised intracranial pressure can cause bilateral exophthalmos, but this is a rare condition. (C) Eye pathology likely would be unilateral, as would such conditions as orbital cellulitis. (E) Acute leukemia can present with bilateral exophthalmos, but this is not the most common scenario.

29.

B Upgaze with "doll's eyes" test

Although all upgaze eventually can be lost with Parinaud syndrome, reflex upgaze with the "doll's eyes" test typically is the most preserved upgaze, as Parinaud represents a supranuclear process. The vertical response portion of the vestibulo-ocular reflex is due to an intact medial longitudinal fasciculus circuitry. (A) Voluntary upgaze classically is lost with Parinaud syndrome. (D) Lying supine should increase the intracranial pressure and should induce symptoms of Parinaud syndrome.

30.

B Disk edema and enlargement of the blind spot

This visual field is the result of a patient with a left sphenoid wing meningioma with optic canal invasion. Such a lesion could produce axoplasmic stasis, causing disk edema and enlargement of the blind spot. The central vision is deteriorated along with the lateral and inferior visual fields. This indicates that the tumor may be compressing on all aspects of the nerve except for its inferolateral aspect. (A) Quadrantanopsia would present with a 90-degree wedge-shaped deficit. (C) Ptosis typically occludes the superolateral portion of the visual periphery (represented in the upper left portion of this visual field). (D) There is no spiraling seen, which would be indicative of an unreliable exam. There are lesions that could conceivably produce this visual field.

31.

D Trauma

The patient has a bilateral trochlear nerve palsy, and trauma should be the primary suspicion until proven otherwise.

32.

B Superiorly

The mnemonic is CUWD: "cold, up; warm, down". Bilateral stimulation results in a vertical fast phase of nystagmus. The fast phase is opposite the direction of the slow eye movements, which are elicited by movement of endolymph with respect to the ampulla. Cold water moves the endolymph in the superior semicircular canals, giving the sensation that the head is being raised. The eyes compensate with slow movements downward and fast movements upward. For reference, the mnemonic for unilateral cold caloric testing is COWS ("cold, opposite; warm, same"), where the fast phase of nystagmus is expected to be in the direction away from the cold water injection.

33.

C Optic neuritis

Optic neuritis variably affects the visual fields but typically does not produce a wedge or hemispheric visual field cut. Patients simply may present with a global loss of visual or color acuity in the affected eye. (A) A pituitary tumor classically produces a bitemporal hemianopsia or at least visual deficits that respect the vertical midline. (B) Methyl alcohol poisoning creates a central scotoma, as it damages the interior portions of the optic nerve first. (D) A left middle cerebral artery territory infarction could produce as much as a right homonymous hemianopsia or quadrantanopsia. The vertical midline would be respected.

34.

E 14 years old

Strabismic amblyopia becomes refractory to therapy as patients leave their critical periods for the development of their visual pathways. With strabismus in childhood, the brain essentially learns to use only one eye and neglects the other in order to avoid diplopia. Although early intervention is better, some improvement in vision can be attained in children up to 14 years of age.

35.

A Laterally

The patient described has a cavernous sinus thrombosis due to the spread of a skin infection intranasally and into the intracranial space. Given its location not against the lateral wall of the cavernous sinus, the abducens nerve is the most likely cranial nerve to be affected by this condition. (B–D) These functions all are controlled by the oculomotor nerve. (E) The trochlear nerve innervates the superior oblique, which has the action of bringing the eye downward when looking medially.

19 Critical Care

1.

E Mercury

Dimercaprol can increase mercury concentrations in the blood and brain in cases of methylmercury poisoning. DMSA does not increase blood or brain mercury concentrations. (A) Lead chelation historically has been accomplished with EDTA or dimercaprol but now is accomplished with DMSA. (B) Arsenic chelation can be accomplished with dimercaprol, DMPS, or DMSA and less effectively with penicillamine. (C) Cadmium chelation can be accomplished with dimercaprol. (D) Chromium chelation can be accomplished with dimercaprol.

2.

B Phenytoin

Side effects of phenytoin include lupus-like syndromes, Stevens-Johnson variant syndrome, hepatic granulomas, megaloblastic anemia, hirsutism, and gingival hypertrophy. In chronic use, there may be cerebellar degeneration. (A) Side effects of levetiracetam include psychiatric disturbances, somnolence, gait instability, anxiety, gastrointestinal disturbances, and skin pigmentation changes. (C) Side effects of primidone include drowsiness, ataxia, nystagmus, visual disturbances, nausea, and, rarely, Dupuytren contractures. (D) Side effects of valproic acid include dyspepsia and weight gain and, less commonly, peripheral edema and acne. Hair loss, tremors, and severe liver dysfunction also are possible side effects. (E) Side effects of lamotrigine include somnolence, dizziness, diplopia, and, rarely, severe rashes/Steven-Johnson syndrome in a subacute fashion.

3.

C Febrile nonhemolytic

Febrile nonhemolytic transfusion reactions occur in about 1% of transfusions. They are characterized by fevers and rigors occurring within 6 hours of transfusion and are due to antibodies against donor white blood cells and cytokines released from cells in blood products. Febrile nonhemolytic transfusion reactions are treated with acetaminophen. (A) Acute hemolytic transfusion reactions occur in 1/250,000 transfusions and are characterized by fever, hypotension, flank pain, and renal failure within 24 hours of transfusion. These reactions are secondary to ABO incompatibility. (B) Delayed

hemolytic transfusion reactions occur 5 to 7 days after a transfusion and are due to undetected alloantibodies against minor antigens. They occur in 1/10,000 transfusions. (D) Allergic transfusion reactions manifest as urticaria and rarely anaphylaxis (patients with an IgA deficiency are most prone to anaphylaxis). Bronchospasm and laryngeal edema also may occur. Allergic transfusion reactions occur in 1% of blood transfusions. (E) Transfusion-related acute lung injury (TRALI) complicates 1/5,000 blood transfusions. TRALI is characterized by noncardiogenic pulmonary edema due to donor antibodies binding recipient white blood cells, which then aggregate in the pulmonary vasculature.

4.

D Vitamin B6

All patients taking isoniazid should be co-treated with vitamin B6 (pyridoxine). Isoniazid induces a state of functional pyridoxine deficiency by directly inactivating pyridoxine species and by inhibiting pyridoxine phosphokinase.

5.

A Decreased right atrial pressure, decreased pulmonary capillary wedge pressure, decreased cardiac output, and increased systemic vascular resistance

The pattern described is reflective of decreased blood volume and thus hypovolemic shock. (B) This pattern is reflective of poor pumping capacity and thus cardiogenic shock. (C) This pattern is reflective of distributive shock, such as neurogenic or septic shock. (D) This pattern is reflective of acute shock in the setting of right ventricular failure or a massive pulmonary embolism. (E) This pattern is reflective of shock secondary to restrictive cardiac disease, such as cardiac tamponade.

6.

A Desmopressin

Von Willebrand disease (vWD) is the most common congenital bleeding disorder and is characterized by a low level of von Willebrand factor (vWF) and subsequently a low level of factor VIII. Patients with vWD have bleeding patterns characteristic of a platelet deficiency. Treatment options include factor VIII concentrate or desmopressin administration, with the latter increasing levels of endogenous vWF by triggering its release from endothelial cells. (B) Von Willebrand factor concentrates should be given in conjunction with factor VIII, but would be helpful only at the time of surgery. (C) Factor VII is not deficient in the setting of vWD. (D) Intravenous crystalloids are not helpful in this situation. (E) Factor IX is not deficient in the setting of vWD.

7.

B $PaCO_2$ of 65 mm Hg with a 20 mm Hg rise over the patient's baseline after 12 minutes of testing with no spontaneous respirations

Hospital protocols may vary slightly, but almost all are based on the Harvard Brain Death Criteria. Although apnea testing is not part of these criteria, the test is relatively standardized. Apnea testing includes 15 minutes of preoxygenation with 100% FiO_2, maintenance of normal blood pressure, preservation of oxygenation saturation greater than 80% with passive oxygen, and the absence of conditions that would prevent the patient from breathing at higher levels of $PaCO_2$ (e.g., severe COPD, congestive heart failure).

8.

C Opening pressure 30, 1,500 WBC with more than 80% PMN, protein 400, glucose 10

This profile represents bacterial meningitis characterized by an elevated opening pressure, low glucose, high protein, white blood cell count over 200 with a polymorphonuclear leukocyte dominance, and a turbid appearance.

9.

D Opening pressure 21, 110 WBC with more than 50% lymphocytes, protein 80, glucose 50

This profile represents viral meningitis characterized by a slightly elevated opening pressure, normal glucose, normal protein, white blood cell count under 200 with a mononuclear dominance, and a clear appearance. (A) This profile represents a normal cerebrospinal fluid sample. (B) This profile represents tubercular meningitis characterized by a high opening pressure, low glucose, high protein, low white blood cell count, and a cobweb appearance.

10.

A Its lack of analgesia

Although it is a poor analgesic, propofol has excellent properties including an ability to lower

intracranial pressure, induce rapid anesthesia, and provide hypnotic and euphoric effects. Propofol does lower seizure thresholds and can mask the clinical signs of a patient being in status epilepticus.

11.

A Stop the anesthetic agent.

The diagnosis in this case is malignant hyperthermia, and the first step in the management is to discontinue volatile anesthetic agents and succinylcholine. The patient should then be hyperventilated to 100% FiO_2 in order to flush volatile anesthetics from her system and lower the end tidal PCO_2. Intravenous dantrolene then should be given until the patient has a decrease in the end tidal PCO_2. Calcium chloride, glucose, and insulin can be given for hyperkalemia resulting from malignant hyperthermia.

12.

C Nitrous oxide

Nitrous oxide is a unique inhalational agent in that it greatly increases cerebral blood flow with only a small increase in cerebral metabolism. Most other agents lower cerebral metabolism. Nitrous oxide also can be associated with a risk of air embolism and pneumocephalus due to its high solubility.

13.

A They suppress EEG activity.

All halogenated agents suppress EEG activity, which may be neuroprotective; however, the EEG effects must be considered when performing intraoperative neuromonitoring. Some anesthetics, such as enflurane, counterintuitively lower the seizure threshold despite EEG suppression. (B–D) All halogenated anesthetics tend to increase cerebral blood flow while reducing cerebral metabolism. This results in increases in intracranial pressure to some extent. (E) At high, and even normal, therapeutic doses, halogenated anesthetics can show signs of hepatotoxicity in some patients.

14.

B No analgesic effect

Propofol is a sedative hypnotic that reduces cerebral metabolism and intracranial pressure without any analgesic effects.

15.

D Nitroglycerin and nitroprusside raise intracranial pressure.

Nitroglycerin and nitroprusside raise intracranial pressure through their vasodilatory effects. (A) Nitroglycerin and nitroprusside have no significant effect on the seizure threshold. (B) Nitroglycerin and nitroprusside can cause neurologic symptoms as patients develop thiocyanate and cyanide toxicity with elevated doses or prolonged use. (C) Nitroglycerin and nitroprusside both have a vasodilatory effect, with the former having more of an effect on the venous system and the latter having a greater effect on the arterial system. (E) Nitroglycerin and nitroprusside have variable effects on cerebral perfusion pressure depending on the degree of intracranial pressure increase and decrease in mean arterial pressure.

16.

B Colloids (e.g., dextran, hetastarch)

Colloids as a whole (but especially certain ones like dextran and hetastarch) have been shown to worsen coagulopathies.

17.

A Obtaining a muscle biopsy for in vitro testing

The gold standard to test for the risk of developing malignant hyperthermia is contracture testing. It relies on the in vitro measurement of the muscle contracture response of a biopsied muscle to graded concentrations of caffeine, halothane, and other calcium-releasing agents. (B) More recently, two genes predisposing individuals to developing malignant hyperthermia have been identified, the most common of which is the *RYR1* gene mutation (accounting for 70% of malignant hypothermia cases).

18.

B Phenylephrine

In spinal shock, there is sympathetic dysfunction with an intact parasympathetic system. Bradycardia is a manifestation; therefore, an agent with positive inotropic effects is required. Phenylephrine (unlike the other choices) is non-inotropic and thus should be avoided.

19.

D In primary adrenal insufficiency, both glucocorticoids and mineralocorticoids need to be replaced.

Primary adrenal insufficiency (adrenal gland failure) requires the replacement of both glucocorticoids and mineralocorticoids, whereas min-

eralocorticoid secretion tends to be preserved with secondary adrenal insufficiency. It is important to select a steroid with the appropriate properties.

20.

A Hypertension and hypokalemia

Hypertension and hypokalemia may occur when cortisone is used in the setting of secondary adrenal insufficiency even when the steroid is dosed appropriately to provide glucocorticoid support. This is due to the mineralocorticoid effects of cortisone in addition to the adrenal glands' endogenous production of mineralocorticoids.

21.

A Thiopental

Thiopental is a short-acting barbiturate general anesthetic that decreases intracranial pressure in a fashion superior to pentobarbital. In addition, thiopental decreases cerebral blood flow and cerebral metabolic rate/oxygen consumption. Recently, propofol and etomidate have been used increasingly, as they have similar neuroprotective effects and a shorter duration of action.

22.

C Thrombotic thrombocytopenic purpura

Thrombotic thrombocytopenic purpura (TTP) is characterized by severe thrombocytopenia, microangiopathic hemolytic anemia, fluctuating neurologic status, renal failure, and fever. (A) Idiopathic thrombocytopenic purpura is a diagnosis of exclusion; it occurs in patients with normal red blood cells. (B) Disseminated intravascular coagulation (DIC) has a presentation similar to that of TTP, with an elevation in the INR and partial thromboplastin time. Although in TTP the problem mainly is thrombocytopenia, in DIC there is a consumptive coagulopathy that manifests with decreased platelets and increased fibrin split products and d-dimers. DIC typically occurs following trauma or in the presence of sepsis. (D) Neurologic changes are rare in hemolytic uremic syndrome.

23.

D The patient is volume depleted.

In both cerebral salt wasting (CSW) and syndrome of inappropriate antidiuretic hormone secretion (SIADH), the serum sodium concentration may be low due to salt loss (CSW) or hemodilution (SIADH). A patient with either condition may have accompanying cerebral edema due to the reduction in serum sodium concentration. Low urine output can occur because of high levels of antidiuretic hormone (SIADH) or volume depletion (CSW). Although volume status is low in CSW, it is normal to increased in SIADH.

24.

B Central pontine myelinolysis

Central pontine myelinolysis (CPM) is the likely cause of a sudden quadriplegia with pseudobulbar palsies. Confusion and other mental status changes can occur. CPM has an acute onset when a hyponatremia is corrected rapidly (usually a correction of the serum sodium of more than 25 mEq/L within 48 hours). This patient's acute alcohol use in the setting of chronic alcoholism would tend to cause hyponatremia in addition to a nutritional deficiency. With sudden nutritional supplementation in the form of regular meals and the likely sodium correction he received, the patient would be prone to developing CPM. (A) Beriberi is a syndrome due to thiamine deficiency. It can either be "dry," characterized by wasting, peripheral neuropathies, and confusion, or "wet," characterized by heart failure and peripheral edema. Although the patient may be deficient in thiamine due to his chronic alcoholism, this is a chronic condition unlikely to present acutely. (C) Pseudohyponatremia is a decreased serum sodium lab value in the setting of hyperglycemia. The clinical picture does not support a diagnosis of hyperglycemia in this patient. (D) Cerebral edema is possible in the setting of cerebral contusions and the likely hyponatremia, as explained above, but the patient was preparing for discharge home and was neurologically intact. Sudden cerebral edema is not expected with this clinical picture. (E) A missed cervical spinal cord contusion would not have a sudden onset, nor would it cause the confusion or pseudobulbar palsies described.

25.

C Hyperventilation to achieve a $PaCO_2$ of 30 to 35 mm Hg is appropriate to use as a temporizing measure for patients with signs of progressive neurologic deterioration when ICP monitoring is not yet established.

Hyperventilation to achieve a $PaCO_2$ of less than 30 mm Hg should not be used, because it will reduce cerebral blood flow and exacerbate cerebral ischemia without a further reduction in intracranial pressure. (B) Level 2 guidelines indicate that prophylactic hyperventilation is not recommended.

26.

D 10 mg/kg intravenous bolus over 30 minutes followed by a 1 mg/kg/h infusion

10 mg/kg intravenous bolus over 30 minutes followed by a 1 mg/kg/h infusion is the regimen for the treatment of intracranial hypertension using a pentobarbital coma. The dosing is modified to sustain the coma and is followed by serum pentobarbital levels. (A) 20 mg/kg intravenous bolus followed by 100 mg every 8 hours represents a phenytoin loading/maintenance dose for seizure prophylaxis. (B) 100 mg intravenously every 4 hours is a pentobarbital dosing regimen for increased intracranial pressure when used as a sedating agent (not to induce a pentobarbital coma). (C) 20 to 75 µg/kg/min intravenous continuous drip is a standard dosing range for propofol sedation.

27.

A Clozapine

Agranulocytosis is a characteristic side effect of clozapine and occurs in 1 to 2% of patients; therefore, patients on clozapine need to be monitored with regular complete blood counts. Other side effects of clozapine include extrapyramidal symptoms and tardive dyskinesia, with a rarer side effect being sialorrhea (drooling). (B) Thioridazine can lead to pigmentary retinopathy and atropine-like effects. (C) Chlorpromazine can lead to abnormal skin pigmentation and "gray man" syndrome. (E) Quetiapine can lead to an increase in suicide attempts in major depression.

28.

A Equivalent level = Observed level/(0.1(Albumin level) + 0.1)

The key to deriving the conversion equation is knowing that 90% of phenytoin is protein bound, and in the setting of hypoalbuminemia, the equivalent phenytoin level will be higher that the observed phenytoin level. The equation in answer A is the only one that would yield an equivalent level greater than the observed level.

29.

C Nitrous oxide

The use of nitrous oxide has been linked to the development of tension pneumocephalus following surgery in the supine position. Nitrous oxide is known to increase cerebral blood flow and can diffuse into air-filled spaces and expand gaseous volume. On CT, a "Mount Fuji" sign (compression of the bilateral frontal lobes with separation of the frontal poles by air) is a characteristic feature of postoperative tension pneumocephalus.

30.

A Noncollapsible vein and negative pressure in the vein

Injury to a noncollapsible vein (diploic vein or dural sinus) and negative pressure inside the vein are essential factors in the pathogenesis of air emboli. Negative pressure created by elevating the head above the level of the heart is necessary to entrain air into the venous circulation. A collapsible venous structure would collapse under negative pressure, which is why injury to a noncollapsible structure is another essential factor in the pathogenesis of air emboli. The presence of a patent foramen ovale or a pulmonary arteriovenous fistula can lead to paradoxical air emboli with the production of ischemic strokes.

31.

C *Streptococcus pneumoniae*

Most posttraumatic meningitis in the setting of nonpenetrating and nondepressed skull injuries are pneumococcal in nature, and therefore empiric treatment should be targeted against these bacteria. Of note, the standard use of prophylactic antibiotics in such patients is debatable, and antibiotics should be used on a case-by-case basis.

32.

A Calcium gluconate

The first step in the management of symptomatic hyperkalemia is to administer calcium gluconate for its cardioprotective effect. Only then should potassium levels be lowered with medications including insulin and glucose, Kayexalate, and β-agonists.

33.

C Flumazenil

The reversal agent for benzodiazepines is flumazenil. It works as a competitive inhibitor competing with benzodiazepines for the binding site on GABA-A receptors.

34.

F Naloxone

The reversal agent for morphine is naloxone. Naloxone is a mu-receptor competitive antagonist with a high affinity for the mu-opioid receptors in the central nervous system.

35.

B Physostigmine

The antidote for anticholinergics is physostigmine. It is a reversible cholinesterase inhibitor.

36.

E Phentolamine

The antidote for dopamine overdose is phentolamine. It works through α_1-blockade. (A) Atropine is a competitive antagonist of muscarinic acetylcholine receptors. (D) Glucagon is a pancreatic peptide hormone that has an effect opposite that of insulin. Glucagon raises the blood glucose concentration. (G) Protamine is used to reverse the effects of heparin. (H) Dimercaprol is a chelating agent used to treat heavy metal poisoning.

37.

B Nonselective β-adrenergic agonism

Isoproterenol is a β_1- and β_2-adrenoreceptor agonist and a trace amine associated receptor 1 (TAAR1) agonist. It has a positive inotropic and chronotropic effect. It also leads to arrhythmias and vasodilation that is more accentuated in skeletal muscles compared with cerebral vessels. Isoproterenol should not be administered for a patient with myocardial ischemia.

38.

A Breaths are patient- or time-triggered with a constant tidal volume for each breath.

Assist control ventilation is patient-triggered. If a patient fails to breathe, the ventilator machine will take over at a specified rate. Each breath taken has a preset tidal volume. (B) Synchronized intermittent mandatory ventilation is similar to assist control ventilation except that patient-initiated breaths are not supported. (C) Pressure support ventilation can be a stand-alone ventilation mode or combined with synchronized intermittent mandatory ventilation. The concept is to deliver additional pressure for patient-initiated breaths. (D) This answer represents continuous positive airway pressure (CPAP) ventilation where the patient must breathe independently of the ventilator.

39.

B Metabolic acidosis

A low pH indicates acidosis, whereas a low bicarbonate level and a relatively normal PCO_2 is indicative of a metabolic origin.

40.

A Respiratory alkalosis

A high pH indicates alkalosis, whereas a low PCO_2 and normal bicarbonate level is indicative of a respiratory origin. (C) A high pH indicates alkalosis, whereas a combined low PCO_2 and high bicarbonate level is indicative of a combined respiratory and metabolic origin. (D) A low pH indicates acidosis, whereas a high PCO_2 is indicative of a respiratory origin. There is partial metabolic compensation as indicated by the rise of the bicarbonate level above normal. Compensatory mechanisms never fully reverse the primary acid/base abnormality.

Normal target labs values are as follows:

pH: 7.40
PCO_2: 40 mm Hg
HCO_3^-: 24 mEq/L

41.

B Age greater than 40 years, systolic blood pressure less than 90 mm Hg, and posturing on motor exam

In a patient with a normal head CT following a concussion, if two or more risk factors are present, there is a 60% risk of developing intracranial hypertension. This risk decreases to 4% if one or no risk factor is present.

42.

A 1 mm Hg = 1.36 cm H_2O

An intracranial pressure of 15 mm Hg is approximately 20 cm H_2O (exact is 20.4 cm H_2O).

43.

C Normothermia

To this day, there is no definitive evidence in favor of hypothermia (whether it is induced or permissive) in a patient with a traumatic brain injury. There have been at least four meta-analyses that concluded that there is no evidence suggesting that hypothermic patients have better outcomes than normothermic patients. (D, E) Hyperthermia should be avoiding in patients with a traumatic brain injury.

44.

C Etomidate

Etomidate is used for induction and can produce adrenal insufficiency. (A) Propofol's exact mechanism of action is unknown. It is a good agent for total intravenous anesthesia and can be used for burst suppression. (B) Dexmedetomidine is an α_2-agonist that can be used for sedation. (D) Ketamine is an NMDA antagonist that produces a dissociative anesthesia and increases intracranial pressure.

45.

A Bilateral absence of the N20 waveform

The N20 waveform reflects activity in the thalamocortical radiations and sensory cortex. Bilat-

eral absence of the N20 waveform at least 3 days after CPR, therefore, is a predictor of a poor neurologic outcome. (B) The N9 waveform reflects peripheral nerve activity and usually is expected to be present. It does not indicate the state of the central nervous system. (C) The N13 waveform reflects activity in the dorsal horns of the spinal cord and would be expected to remain present in the described patient.

46.

C Breaths are patient-triggered, and inspiratory pressure is added to patient-initiated breaths.

Pressure support ventilation can be a stand-alone ventilation mode or combined with synchronized intermittent mandatory ventilation. The concept is to deliver additional pressure for patient-initiated breaths. (A) Assist control ventilation is patient-triggered. If a patient fails to breathe, the ventilator machine takes over at a specified rate. Each breath taken has a preset tidal volume. (B) Synchronized intermittent mandatory ventilation is similar to assist control ventilation except that patient-initiated breaths are not supported. (D) This represents continuous positive airway pressure (CPAP) ventilation where the patient must breathe independently of the ventilator.

47.

D Toxoplasmosis

Toxoplasmosis is one of the most common neurologic complications of AIDS. Patients present with fever, headaches, seizures, and possibly focal neurologic deficits. Multiple ring-enhancing lesions are seen in 70% of patients with toxoplasmosis. Distinguishing toxoplasmosis from lymphoma can be difficult, and a trial of antitoxoplasmosis medications may be used for 2 weeks to confirm the diagnosis.

48.

F JC virus

JC virus leads to progressive multifocal leukoencephalopathy (PML). This fatal disease has no effective treatment. Symptoms develop over several weeks and include clumsiness, progressive weakness, and vision, speech, and personality changes. Characteristic imaging findings include multifocal hypointense T1 and hyperintense T2 lesions.

49.

E West Nile virus

West Nile virus causes poliomyelitis and meningitis, with poliomyelitis being the most common manifestation. Patients typically have fever, myalgias, and encephalopathy along with asymmetric weakness that quickly can progress to quadriplegia. Cerebrospinal fluid studies show pleocytosis and elevated protein. (A) *Tenia solium* is a tapeworm found in pigs that causes neurocysticercosis. Symptoms include seizures, decreased vision, papilledema, and parkinsonism. Although the pork supply in the United States is free of the organism, pork in Central and South America may be colonized. (B) *Herpes simplex* causes temporal encephalitis and temporal epileptiform discharge on electroencephalogram. (C) Central nervous system *Cryptococcus* infection can manifest with multiple focal mass lesions called cryptococcomas. The opening pressure during a lumbar puncture is high, cryptococcal antigen titer is positive, and cerebrospinal fluid India ink staining is positive with this condition, which is common in patients with HIV. Treatment is with amphotericin B and flucytosine.

50.

C Needle thoracotomy

This patient developed a right-side tension pneumothorax most likely secondary to the rupture of a lung bulla precipitated by mechanical ventilation. Because he is unstable, emergent needle decompression of the right lung should be performed at the bedside to decompress the intrapleural space and enable adequate venous return. (A) A chest tube will be needed in this patient with a tension pneumothorax, but needle decompression should be done first. (B) The diagnosis in this case is obvious. Obtaining a chest radiograph will only delay a lifesaving treatment. (D) Ultrasounds are readily available in most intensive care units. They can be used to diagnose pneumothorax effectively; however, in this patient, an ultrasound will only delay a lifesaving treatment. (E) Decreasing the respiratory rate and tidal volume help to prevent tension pneumothoraces in predisposed patients.

51.

C Fat embolism

Fat emboli occur 1 to 3 days following long bone or pelvic fractures. Patients develop tachypnea, tachycardia, hypotension, mental status changes, thrombocytopenia, and petechiae. The petechial rash is pathognomonic for a fat embolism. (A) Although subdural hematoma expansion cannot be ruled out,

it is unlikely to occur in a patient stable for 2 days. (B) A pulmonary embolism is a possibility; however, a long bone fracture with a petechial rash in a young patient favors a diagnosis of fat embolism. (D) Myocardial contusions usually manifest with arrhythmias. (E) Pulmonary contusions are most likely to appear on a chest radiograph.

52.

B Aseptic meningitis

Penicillins and cephalosporins have been linked to aseptic meningitis, with the exact pathophysiology being unknown. Other medications linked to aseptic meningitis are trimethoprim-sulfamethoxazole, ciprofloxacin, metronidazole, and isoniazid.

53.

A Benign intracranial hypertension

Amphotericin B can lead to benign intracranial hypertension.

54.

C Cerebellar ataxia

Ethambutol is known for causing optic neuritis; however, another side effect of this antituberculous drug is cerebellar ataxia. Patients need routine ophthalmologic exams while on the medication. (D) Vancomycin can cause cochlear and vestibular dysfunction. (E) Side effects of temozolomide include nausea, vomiting, constipation, diarrhea, blurred vision, sleep problems, unusual or unpleasant tastes, and headaches. Patients also may have temporary hair loss.

55.

A In a patient with central DI, DDAVP will cause a 50% increase in urine osmolality, whereas it will cause an increase of 5% in a normal individual.

Patients with central diabetes insipidus (DI) have an impaired production of antidiuretic hormone, and therefore have a significant response to the injection of DDAVP. Patients with nephrogenic DI do not show a response to DDVAP injection.

56.

B Neuroblastoma

Opsoclonus-myoclonus is composed of involuntary arrhythmias and chaotic multidirectional saccades with myoclonic jerks of the limbs and trunk as well as cerebellar ataxia, tremors, and encephalopathy. In children, 50% of cases are secondary to a neuroblastoma, whereas in adults the condition can be secondary to small cell lung, ovarian, or breast cancer.

57.

A Hodgkin lymphoma

Paraneoplastic cerebellar degeneration is characterized by a loss of Purkinje cells. Symptoms include gait unsteadiness that evolves into ataxia, diplopia, and dysarthria. This condition most commonly is seen in patients with lung, ovarian, or breast cancer, and Hodgkin lymphoma.

58.

D Thymoma

Limbic encephalitis presents with mood and sleep disturbances, seizures, hallucinations, and short-term memory loss. Electroencephalography shows foci of epileptic activity in the temporal lobes, and MRI demonstrates hyperintense T2 and FLAIR sequence signals in the mesial temporal lobes. Most commonly, the condition involves tumors including small cell lung cancer, germ cell tumors, thymomas, and teratomas. Of these tumors, thymomas are associated with myasthenia gravis.

59.

C Small cell lung cancer

Lambert-Eaton myasthenia syndrome involves the muscles of the trunk, shoulder and pelvic girdles, and lower extremities. It is most commonly associated with small cell lung cancer and is due to antibodies against the presynaptic calcium channels at neuromuscular junctions. (E) Carcinoid tumors can secrete hormones such as serotonin, resulting in carcinoid syndrome (characterized by flushing, wheezing, diarrhea, abdominal cramping, and peripheral edema).

60.

C 28 mm Hg

Decreasing PCO_2 leads to cerebral vasoconstriction, and with decreased cerebral blood volume, intracranial pressure can be reduced significantly. When PCO_2 decreases below 28 mm Hg, the cerebral blood volume can decrease to a level at which ischemia occurs. A recommended typical long-term goal for hyperventilated patients is a PCO_2 of 35 mm Hg. A PCO_2 of 28 to 32 mm Hg can be tolerated for 4 to 8 hours in the acute setting.

61.

A Asystole or pulselessness will occur within 1 hour of withdrawal of care.

When proceeding with attempted donation after cardiac death, the expectation is that the potential donor will progress rapidly to cardiac arrest. This criterion is intended to minimize warm ischemia time. The convention is that warm ischemia time of up to 1 hour can be tolerated. If cardiac arrest does not occur within 1 hour after withdrawal of care, organ donation is cancelled. (B) Patients who undergo donation after cardiac death do not meet brain death criteria and are declared deceased by cardiac criteria before proceeding with donation. (C) The transplant surgeons usually are excluded from the donation after the cardiac death procedure until arrest is declared. (D) The heart cannot be donated after asystole.

62.

C 800 mL

The estimated blood volume in infants and children is approximately 8% of total body weight or 80 mL of blood per kilogram of body weight.

63.

C Carbamazepine

Although all of the options are used as first-line therapies for trigeminal neuralgia, carbamazepine alone provides complete or tolerable relief in almost 70% of patients. Its common side effect is mild leukopenia with a lesser frequency of rash and even Stevens-Johnson syndrome in rare cases.

64.

A Alcoholic hallucinosis

Patients experiencing alcohol withdrawal can start developing minor symptoms within 6 hours of their last drink. These symptoms include tremulousness, anxiety, sweating, and palpitations. This initial stage of alcohol withdrawal is followed by alcoholic hallucinosis, which occurs between 24 and 48 hours following the last drink. Symptoms include visual, auditory, or tactile hallucinations without autonomic changes. (E) The last stage of alcohol withdrawal is delirium tremens, with symptoms including hallucinations, disorientation, tachycardia, hypertension, low-grade fever, agitation, and diaphoresis. Delirium tremens occurs 3 to 10 days following the last drink.

65.

A 70 mm Hg + 2(Age in years)

The lower limit of a normal systolic blood pressure (fifth percentile) for a given age may be estimated by this formula:

$$\text{Systolic blood pressure} = 70 \text{ mm Hg} + 2(\text{Age in years})$$

66.

C Left atrial pressure

Pulmonary capillary wedge pressure (PCWP) is obtained by wedging a pulmonary catheter with an inflated balloon into a small pulmonary arterial branch. Because the pulmonary circulation has a very high compliance and minimal resistance, the PCWP is an indirect measure of the left atrial pressure. It can be used to determine the causes of pulmonary edema in critically ill patients.

67.

E No ammonia level is predictive of cerebral herniation.

Although an ammonia level above 200 µmol/L most often is associated with cerebral edema and herniation, there is no established relationship between ammonia level and herniation. Elevated intracranial pressures (ICP) can be seen at a much lower ammonia level, and therefore ICP monitoring is recommended in a patient with an altered level of consciousness and an elevated ammonia level, as dependence on the ammonia level alone is not predictive of herniation risk.

68.

C Distal renal tubule

Antidiuretic hormone (ADH) acts primarily in the distal renal tubule, where it increases its permeability to water, resulting in the reabsorption of water into the blood, producing concentrated urine and decreased plasma osmolarity.

69.

C NMDA receptor antagonist

Ketamine produces a dissociative anesthesia by antagonizing the NMDA receptor, and this mechanism can account for ketamine's hallucinogenic properties in adults.

70.

B 0.9% normal saline

The official guidelines for blood transfusions recommend administering normal saline while transfusing blood products. The rationale is that a hypotonic solution would lead to hemolysis. (A) Lactated Ringer's solution is slightly hypotonic as compared with normal blood, and its calcium content can bind the sodium citrate in the transfusing blood, making it more prone to clot.

71.

E Thiamine 100 mg intravenously

Often, medication administration can be performed simultaneously or in quick succession. In the event of hypoglycemia or severe nutrition deficiencies (as seen in alcoholics), rapid administration of thiamine prior to glucose (glucose administration may precipitate Wernicke encephalopathy if given prior to thiamine) is a fast and effective therapy to abort seizures in these disorders. The first antiepileptic drug (AED) given thereafter is lorazepam 0.1 mg/kg intravenously at a rate less than 2 mg/min. (B) Phenytoin 20 mg/kg intravenous load is a second-line AED.

72.

B Thiamine

Chronic thiamine (B1) deficiency causes beriberi with polyneuropathy, whereas an acute deficiency (Wernicke encephalopathy seen in alcoholics) leads to ophthalmoplegia (most commonly nystagmus and abducens palsies), ataxia, and confusion, with prominent deficiencies of immediate recall and recent memories. After treatment, ocular abnormalities usually resolve first followed by ataxia and confusion. (A) Cyanocobalamin (B12) deficiency causes subacute combined degeneration of the spinal cord, leading to peripheral neuropathy, gait ataxia, and spastic paraparesis. The most common cause is pernicious anemia, which results in a gastrointestinal absorption issue. (C) Pyridoxine (B6) deficiency leads to polyneuropathy and seizures, and can be related to the drug isoniazid. (D) Folate deficiency can lead to neural tube defects (myelomeningoceles). (E) Niacin (B3) deficiency leads to pellagra and the "3 D's" (diarrhea, dementia, and dermatitis).

73.

E Medulla

Ataxic breathing is a completely irregular pattern with regard to rate and depth of respiration and is seen in preterminal medullary lesions. (A) Cheyne-Stokes breathing often indicates diencephalon or bilateral cerebral hemisphere dysfunction due to processes such as elevated intracranial pressures or metabolic abnormalities. The pattern is characterized by gradual crescendos in respiratory amplitude that trail off and are followed by expiratory pauses. (B) Hyperventilation can be due to pontine dysfunction, but also may suggest a psychiatric origin if no other localizing sign is found. (C) Cluster breathing characterized by periods of rapid irregular breaths separated by apneic spells may be found with superior medullary or inferior pontine lesions. (D) Apneustic breathing is a pause at full inspiration seen with pontine lesions.

74.

A Pheochromocytoma

Von Hippel–Lindau disease is an autosomal dominant disease, the locus of which is on chromosome 3. Characteristics of the disease include cerebellar and spinal cord hemangioblastomas, retinal angiomas, pheochromocytomas, and renal cell carcinoma. In this patient, the most likely etiology of his symptoms is pheochromocytoma.

75.

A Dehydration

A fractional excretion of sodium (FENa) is defined by this equation:

$$FENa = 100 \times ((\text{Urinary sodium}) \times (\text{Plasma creatinine}))/((\text{Plasma sodium}) \times (\text{Urinary creatinine}))$$

A FENa of less than 1% indicates a prerenal disease process such as dehydration. A FENa greater than 2% is suggestive of acute tubular necrosis or other kidney damage.

76.

B Transesophageal echocardiogram

A transesophageal echocardiogram is the most sensitive way to detect a venous air embolism through the visualization of air bubbles. (A) A right atrial central venous pressure catheter is the best way to treat an air embolism once detected. It enables the aspiration of the embolism with the patient in the left lateral decubitus position. (C) Precordial Doppler monitoring is an alternative monitoring method for venous air embolism. It is easier to use than transesophageal echocardiography, but it is slightly less sensitive. A machinery sound will be heard when air emboli occur. (D) An arterial line has no role in the management of venous air emboli. (E) A sudden decrease in end-tidal PCO_2 may be the earliest clue to the occurrence of an air embolism, but is not as sensitive as transesophageal echocardiography for monitoring.

77.

D Emergent vascular consultation and abdominal CT angiogram

In this patient with a pulmonary embolus, abdominal pain with a negative abdominal exam is most suggestive of vascular occlusion and possible mesenteric ischemia. Emergent vascular evaluation is required.

78.

A RSBI = Breath frequency/Tidal volume

The rapid shallow breathing index (RSBI) is defined as the ratio of the respiratory frequency to tidal volume. This ratio is designed to identify people who cannot tolerate independent breathing and tend to breathe rapidly and shallowly, resulting in a high RSBI.

79.

B Pressure generated by a patient during forced inspiration

The negative inspiratory force (NIF) is the force/pressure generated by a patient above the minimal subambient pressure. It is dependent on patient cooperation and effort as well as on the practitioner to assist. A NIF less than –25 may be predictive of successful extubation.

80.

A Acute lowering of the systolic blood pressure to 140 mm Hg is safe and can be effective in improving functional outcome.

It was long thought that acute blood pressure lowering in the presence of intracranial hemorrhage was associated with poor outcomes; however, recent studies demonstrate that acute lowering of blood pressure is associated with improved functional outcomes.

81.

E Thiamine

Emergent thiamine administration is indicated in the setting of Wernicke encephalopathy and alcohol withdrawal in order to prevent progression of the disease. (A) Wernicke encephalopathy is a potentially fatal complication of thiamine deficiency. This deficiency is exacerbated if a large dose of glucose is given, as it leads to a rapid depletion of brain thiamine and the development of the encephalopathy. On pathological examination, patients with Wernicke encephalopathy have hemorrhagic necrosis in the periventricular gray matter and extensively damaged mammillary bodies. (B) Magnesium is not indicated for the management of Wernicke encephalopathy. (C) There is no role for beta-blockers in the management of alcohol withdrawal. (D) Although nicotine patches may be helpful in a nicotine-dependent patient to control agitation, they are not indicated in the acute setting.

82.

A Polymyositis more often is associated with malignancy and T-cell infiltration more than B-cell infiltration.

Both polymyositis and dermatomyositis are diseases more prevalent among women.

83.

B Withdraw fluid through myelogram needle.

Serious reactions might occur secondary to inadvertent injections of ionic contrast agents intrathecally. Seizures, intracerebral hemorrhages, cerebral edema, arachnoiditis, myoclonus, and respiratory compromise are possible side effects of the injection, and there is a significant mortality rate. Recommended management of inadvertent intrathecal injection of ionic contrast agents includes starting with immediate removal of cerebrospinal fluid if the error is recognized while there still is access to the intrathecal space. The head of the bed also should be elevated to keep the contrast as caudal as possible. Attention then should be given to securing an airway followed by antihistamine administration. Blood pressure control, intravenous hydration, steroids, and antiepileptic drugs follow.

84.

D Does not affect the risk of vasospasm but decreases the mortality rate

Administration of nimodipine has been proven to decrease mortality rates in patients with aneurysmal subarachnoid hemorrhage. Although it initially was thought to decrease the risk of vasospasm, most studies have shown no direct effect of nimodipine on decreasing the risk of developing vasospasm in aneurysmal subarachnoid hemorrhage patients.

85.

E Washing the transfused cells

Febrile reactions are due to antibodies against donor white blood cells and cytokines released from cells in the transfused blood product. Leukocyte depletion techniques can reduce the potential for a transfusion reaction. Leukocyte depletion techniques include creating frozen deglycerolized red cells, using leukocyte depletion red blood cell filters, and cell washing. (A) Warming transfused blood products is recommended during rapid, massive trauma transfusions to avoid hypothermia. (B) Transfusing whole blood carries an increased risk of febrile reactions because whole blood has more donor leukocytes than most other blood prod-

ucts. (C) Clerical error is the most common cause of ABO incompatible transfusion reactions (not febrile reactions). (D) Although premedication with acetaminophen can be helpful during transfusions, it does not reduce the risk of febrile, nonhemolytic transfusion reactions.

86.

A Anaphylactic transfusion reaction

Selective IgA deficiency syndrome is the most common human immunodeficiency, with most individuals being asymptomatic but having a higher propensity for respiratory and gastrointestinal infections. These patients have anti-IgA antibodies that can lead to anaphylactic reactions when they are transfused with regular packed red blood cells (RBCs). When a patient has an established diagnosis of an IgA deficiency, he should be transfused with washed RBCs. If a reaction occurs, frozen-thawed deglycerolized RBCs can be given. Other alternatives include autologous RBCs or RBCs from IgA deficient donors.

87.

A Avoiding contrasted MRI studies

The symptoms described in this case are those of nephrogenic systemic fibrosis. It is a rare but serious complication of gadolinium contrast use in patients with renal dysfunction/failure. It can develop days to years after contrast use and is characterized by fibrosis of the skin and internal organs. Currently, gadolinium use is absolutely contraindicated in patients with a glomerular filtration rate (GFR) less than 30 mL/min and relatively contraindicated in patients with a GFR between 30 and 60 mL/min. (B) Stopping metformin prior to receiving CT contrast agents would help decrease renal injury following contrast injection but is not the cause of this patient's symptoms. (C) For patients on dialysis, the use of contrast agents should be followed by dialysis. (D) Blood glucose management would have little effect on the patient's condition. (E) Antihistamine use prior to contrast-enhanced studies can be prescribed for patients with allergic reactions to contrast agents.

88.

A Tachycardia

(A–E) All of these signs are common with pulmonary embolism, but tachycardia is the most sensitive clinical sign. Other signs and symptoms of pulmonary embolism include dyspnea, pleuritic chest pain, cough, hemoptysis, cyanosis, and hemodynamic collapse. (B) Hypotension can be seen with pulmonary embolism secondary to decreased filling of the left atrium; however, it is a late sign and exclusive for severe emboli. (C) Tachypnea occurs with pulmonary embolism and is secondary to oxygen desaturation and difficulty perfusing peripheral tissues. (D) Oxygen desaturation occurs with pulmonary embolism and is secondary to blood shunting in the lungs. (E) Low-grade fever is most likely to occur when a pulmonary embolism is associated with pulmonary hemorrhage or infarction. Fever is secondary to the degradation of blood products.

1.

C Positive predictive value

The positive predictive value indicates how often a patient has a disease given a positive test result. (A) The sensitivity indicates how often a test will be positive if a person has a disease. (B) The specificity indicates how often a test will be negative if a person does not have a disease. (D) The negative predictive value indicates how often a patient does not have a disease given a negative test result.

2.

A Selection and placebo effect biases

The goal of randomization is to minimize selection bias, which occurs when subjects are included in a study in a nonrandom fashion. The goal of single blinding is to minimize the placebo effect, which occurs when a treatment improves a patient's condition simply because he has the expectation that the treatment will help. (B) Observer bias (interviewer bias) occurs when a researcher intentionally or unintentionally pays more attention or provides more weight to one type of response or treatment. (C) Design bias occurs when the case and control groups are not matched properly. (D) Definition bias describes a lack of clarity of the concepts used in and goals of the study.

3.

E Unprofessional behavior during medical school

Multiple recent studies have demonstrated a very strong association between medical school unprofessional behavior and subsequent disciplinary actions during the career of a physician. (A–D) These factors are much weaker predictors of future disciplinary actions.

4.

A Sort, Assess, Lifesaving interventions, and Treatment/Transport

The SALT algorithm prioritizes the concept of triage. Patients should be triaged first, and then resources should be allocated and lifesaving procedures performed accordingly.

5.

A Immediate, delayed, minimal, expectant

In a mass casualty scenario, the Centers for Disease Control and Prevention recommends triaging casualties into four categories. The lives of Category 1 patients with a red triage tag and "immediate" or "T1 priority" designation are in immediate danger and require immediate treatment. The lives of Category 2 patients with a yellow triage tag and "delayed" or "T2 priority" designation are not in immediate danger and will require urgent but not immediate medical care. Category 3 patients with a green triage tag and "minimal" or "T3 priority" designation have minor injuries but eventually will require treatment. Category 4 patients with a black triage tag and "expectant" or "no priority" designation are either dead or have very severe injuries precluding survival with the limited available resources.

6.

B Identifying the characteristics of successful performance

The positive deviance theory focuses on identifying the attributes of successful performance and replicating these attributes in similar scenarios.

7.

A Inform the family of the mistake, complete the procedure at the correct level, and inform the risk management team.

Informing the patient and family of anything that has gone wrong during a surgery is proper patient care and even may help to decrease liability. Most experts also agree that acknowledging the mistake will lead to a better trust relationship between the physician and the patient and family. Although the next most appropriate course of action in this situation is debated, after full disclosure and if the patient's family agrees, completing the surgery is an option that should be considered to relieve symptoms and eliminate the need for further surgeries. It always is a good idea to contact the risk management team in such situations for advice on how to proceed following surgery.

8.

D It is not unreasonable to perform the procedure, but there are limited data to endorse it.

This table summarizes the levels and classes of evidence.

Applying Classification of Recommendations and Level of Evidence

Size of Treatment Effect

	Class I	Class IIa	Class IIb	Class III
	Benefit >>> Risk *No additional studies needed*	**Benefit >> Risk** *Additional studies with focused objectives needed*	**Benefit ≥ Risk** *Additional studies with broad objectives needed. Additional registry data would be helpful*	**Risk ≥ Benefit** *No additional studies needed*
	Procedure/Treatment SHOULD be performed/administered	**IT IS REASONABLE to perform procedure/administer treatment**	**IT IS NOT UNREASONABLE to perform procedure/administer treatment**	**Procedure/Treatment should NOT be performed/administered SINCE IT IS NOT HELPFUL AND MAY BE HARMFUL**
Level A *Multiple (3–5) population risk strata evaluated* *General consistency of direction and magnitude of effect*	• Recommendation that procedure or treatment is useful/effective • Sufficient evidence from multiple randomized trials or meta-analyses	• Recommendation in favor of treatment or procedure being useful/effective • Some conflicting evidence from multiple randomized trials or meta-analyses	• Recommendation's usefulness/efficacy less well established • Greater conflicting evidence from multiple randomized trials or meta-analyses	• Recommendation that procedure or treatment not useful/effective and may be harmful • Sufficient evidence from multiple randomized trials or meta-analyses
Level B *Limited (2–3) population risk strata evaluated*	• Recommendation that procedure or treatment is useful/effective • Limited evidence from single randomized trial or non-randomized studies	• Recommendaiton in favor of treatment or procedure being useful/effective • Some conflicting evidence from single randomized trial or non-randomized studies	• Recommendation's usefulness/efficacy less well established • Greater conflicting evidence from single randomized trial or non-randomized studies	• Recommendation that procedure or treatment not useful/effective and may be harmful • Limited evidence from single randomized gtrial or non-randomized studies
Level C *Very limited (1–2) population risk strata evaluated*	• Recommendation that procedure or treatment is useful/effective • Only expert opinion, case studies, or standard-of-care	• Recommendation in favor of treatment or procedure being useful/effective • Only diverging expert opinion, case studies, or standard-of-care	• Recommendation's usefulness/efficacy less well established • Only diverging expert opinion, case studies, or standard-of-care	• Recommendation that procedure or treatment not useful/effective and may be harmful • Only expert opinion, case studies, or standard-of-care

Estimate of Certainty (Precision) of Treatment Effect

9.

A Stark law

The Stark law (also known as the physician self-referral law) prohibits physicians from referring patients to institutes in which they or a close family member have financial interests. (B) The federal anti-kickback statue prevents physicians from receiving compensation in exchange for using specific instruments or prescribing specific drugs. (C) Antitrust law regulates the conduct and organization of businesses to promote fair competition for the benefit of consumers. (D) The false claim act is a federal law that imposes liabilities on people and companies that defraud governmental programs.

10.

A Proceed with the donation.

The recently revised Uniform Anatomical Gift Act states, "In the absence of an expressed, contrary indication by the donor, a person other than the donor is barred from making, amending, or revoking an anatomical gift of a donor's body or a part if the donor made an anatomical gift" [194.240.1]. In this situation, proceeding with the donation is the most appropriate course of action; however, it always is prudent to attempt to reconcile the wishes of the donor with those of the family. (E) Obtaining a court order to proceed with the donation is not necessary in this situation, but discussing the situation with the ethics committee might be a good option.

11.

A Incidence: 1/3,200,000; prevalence: 1/50,000

The incidence of a disease is defined as the annual number of new cases (in this example, 100) out of the total population (320 million). The prevalence of a disease is defined as the total number of cases at a certain point in time (6,400) out of the total population (320 million). These ratios often are simplified to have a numerator of 1 or a denominator of 100,000.

12.

B Randomized, single-blinded, prospective clinical study

This study is an example of a randomized, single-blinded, prospective clinical study. In the HEAT (Hydrogel Endovascular Aneurysms Treatment) trial, patients were randomly allocated to one of two groups, making the study randomized. The study was prospective, as patients were allocated to the groups prior to their procedures and were fol-lowed after their procedures. Because the patients did not know which type of coil they were receiving, and because the physicians did know, the study was single-blinded. Of note, in the actual trial, a blinded imaging core lab evaluated all imaging to minimize reporting bias.

13.

C Interpersonal skills and communication

Interpersonal skills and communication skills refer to a resident's ability to communicate effectively among colleagues in his and other specialties. It also refers to the ability of a resident to share his research and demonstrate leadership skills. (A) Patient care describes the ability to provide compassionate and effective health care. (B) Medical knowledge describes the ability to acquire and apply current medical knowledge and use advanced search engines to stay current on medical knowledge and data. (D) Practice-based learning and improvement describes the ability to appraise information critically on a daily basis and to analyze it in a way that improves patient care. (E) Systems-based practice describes multidisciplinary approaches to patient care and the ability to optimize care by involving multiple teams in patient management.

14.

B Federal anti-kickback statute

The federal anti-kickback statue prevents physicians from receiving compensations for using or prescribing specific instruments or drugs. (A) The Stark law (also known as the physician self-referral law) prohibits physicians from referring patients to institutes in which they or a close family member have financial interests. (C) Antitrust law regulates the conduct of organizations and businesses to promote fair competition for the benefit of consumers. (D) The false claim act is a federal law that imposes liabilities on people and companies who defraud governmental programs.

15.

A Reliable

Reliability is an evaluation of random error. Reliability is maximal when a test gives similar results on repeat measurements (has high precision). (B, C) Validity and accuracy are defined as the ability of a test to measure a given outcome. Accuracy is determined by comparing data from a test to a predefined gold standard. (D, E) Sensitivity and specificity are obtained by comparing test results to a gold standard.

16.

D The sample size in the second study is small.

The lack of statistical significance in the second study (the 95% confidence interval includes the value of 1) is secondary to the study being underpowered with a small sample size. We know from the first study that there is an association between smoking and atherosclerosis; therefore, increasing the sample size in the second study should lead to the same result. (A) The first study is statistically significant, as the 95% confidence interval does not include the null value of 1. (B) Bias cannot be assessed from the information. (C) Accuracy cannot be assessed from the information. (E) The sample size in the first study is adequate, as the study has reached statistical significance with a 95% confidence interval that does not include the value of 1.

17.

A ANOVA

The analysis of variance (ANOVA) test is used to compare two or more independent, quantitative, continuous, normal variables. An example of its use would be when answering the question "Are neurosurgery board exam scores different between residents who have read one, two, or three Thieme review books?" (B) The Student (unpaired) *t*-test is used to analyze one continuous, normal variable in two groups. It could be used when answering the question "Is there a difference in the resting heart rates of diabetics compared with nondiabetics?" (C) The paired *t*-test is used to analyze one continuous, normal variable in two groups. It often is used when data are being evaluated pre- and post-treatment. It could be used when answering the question "How do the heart rates of diabetics differ before and after using an antihypertensive?" (D) The chi-square test compares one independent variable in two independent groups of the categorical type. For example, it would be used to answer the question "Is the distribution of gender and drinking behavior due to chance, or is there a statistical significant difference?" (E) The Fisher exact test compares one independent variable in two independent groups of the categorical type; it works well for small sample sizes. It provides an exact *p* value instead of estimating a *p* value (the latter needed as groups move toward infinity); therefore, it is more accurate than the chi-square test.

18.

A Equipoise

Equipoise provides the ethical basis for medical research. It means that there is genuine uncertainty within the expert medical community about whether the treatment will be beneficial. Patients with large posterior fossa hemorrhages most likely will die if they are not surgically treated; therefore, it is unethical to randomize such patients to the two groups and withhold the known therapy. (B) Autonomy refers to the capacity to think, decide, and act based on one's own free initiative. The patients with the hemorrhages most likely will be unable to make decisions regarding their care, but this is true regardless of their enrollment in the study. (C) Nonmaleficence is the principle of do no harm. (D) Justice is to account for limited resources by justly allocating resources. (E) Disclosure refers to making patients aware of the risks of surgery and nonoperative care. This would have to be done prior to enrollment in any such trial.

19.

C Practice-based learning and improvement

Practice-based learning and improvement describes the ability to appraise information critically on a daily basis and to analyze it in a way that improves patient care. (A) Patient care describes the ability to provide compassionate and effective health care. (B) Medical knowledge describes the ability to acquire and apply current medical knowledge and use advanced search engines to stay current on medical knowledge and data. (D) Systems-based practice describes multidisciplinary approaches to patient care and the ability to optimize care by involving multiple teams in patient management. (E) Professionalism describes the ability to demonstrate the principles of ethical behavior.

20.

D 4%

Posttest probability is the probability that a patient has or does not have the disease after obtaining test results. In this case, the question is asking for the negative predictive value (NPV). The NPV depends on the prevalence of the disease in a tested population and can be calculated using the formulas given below. The NPV expresses the probability of the patient not having the disease following a negative test. In this situation, the probability of the patient not developing Alzheimer disease is 96%, giving him a 4% chance of developing the disease.

$$NPV = \text{Number of true negatives}/(\text{Number of true negatives} + \text{Number of false negatives})$$

$$NPV = (\text{Specificity})(1 - \text{Prevalence})/[(1 - \text{Sensitivity})(\text{Prevalence}) + (\text{Specificity})(1 - \text{Prevalence})]$$

21.

C Lead-time bias

For screening tests, a lead-time bias occurs when there is an incorrect assumption that a screening test prolongs apparent survival. This happens when a screening test leads to early detection of a disease, resulting in patients living longer after diagnosis but not actually altering the clinical course of the disease. (A) An observer bias (also known as the observer expectancy effect) is seen in non-blinded studies. This bias is a form of reactivity in which researches tend to influence consciously or unconsciously the participants in studies. (B) A measurement bias refers to errors in evaluating obtained data. (D) A confounding bias occurs when an extraneous variable correlates with dependent and independent variables. A classic example of confounding bias occurred in a study correlating the number of ashtrays in a home with the risk of lung cancer. Although there was a real mathematical correlation between both variables, there was no causality. The number of ashtrays was a reflection on smoking habits, and smoking was the confounding variable that led to a higher number of ashtrays and to an increased risk of developing lung cancer. (E) A sampling bias is a flaw in study design such that a specific group of patients is overly included or excluded from the studied sample.

22.

B Class 2A

Class 2A indicates that the benefits outweigh the risk but that additional studies with focused objectives are needed to classify further the benefit/risk ratio. It is reasonable to perform the procedure. (A) Class 1 indicates that the benefits outweigh the risks. The procedure should be performed. (C) Class 2B indicates that the benefits are equal to or outweigh the risks, and that additional studies with broad objectives or additional registry data are needed to classify further the benefit/risk ratio. The procedure may be considered. (D) Class 3 indicates there is no benefit or harm; therefore, the procedure should not be performed. (E) There is no class 4 benefit.

23.

D Proceed with transfusion after documenting the indication in the chart.

In emergent situations, physicians always should act in the best interest of minors even when their parents object. It is important to document the situation properly, however. (A) Withholding the transfusion is considered illegal in this situation, as it jeopardizes the patient's survival. (B) Although it always is preferable to obtain the family's consent prior to transfusion in an emergency situation (if there is time), from a legal prospective parents cannot place their minor children at the risk of death regardless of their religious beliefs. (C) The hospital legal counsel can be informed after performing any emergent and lifesaving interventions for the patient. Contacting them in an emergent situation would take too much time. (E) It is unethical to wait for a court order prior to proceeding with a lifesaving intervention.

24.

B 225

In a box plot, 50% of the data (when placed in order of increasing value) falls within the box area. The bar in the box indicates the mean, and with a normal distribution of data it is found in the center of the box. The upper limit of the first quartile is denoted by the inferior edge of the box, whereas the lower limit of the fourth quartile is denoted by the superior edge of the box.

25.

B The greatest non-outlier

The whiskers in a box plot denote the largest/smallest non-outlier data points. (A) Outlier data points are indicated by points beyond the whiskers. (C) The lower limit of the fourth quartile occurs at the superior edge of the box. (D) Box plots do not indicate the deciles of data. (E) Box plots do not illustrate confidence intervals.

26.

A 14, 14, 14.4

When all data points are ordered from low to high, the median is the data point separating the lower half of the data sample from the higher half. If there is an even number of data points, then the median is the average of the two middle data points. The mode is the data point that occurs most frequently in the data set. The mean (average) is obtained by adding all of the data points and dividing the sum by the number of data points.

27.

A HR = OBS/INTER

The hazard ratio (HR) is the chance of a harmful event occurring in the treatment arm (the interventional therapy group, INTER) divided by the chance of a harmful event occurring in the control arm (the observation group, OBS). An HR of 1 means that patients in both groups have a similar rate of complications. An HR > 1 means that patients in the treatment arm are more likely to have harmful events (hazards), whereas an HR < 1 means that patients in the treatment arm are less likely to have harmful events.

28.
E The interval of 0.14–0.54 represents the values of the HRs for which the difference between the real population HR and the calculated HR is not statistically significant.

The confidence interval represents values for the population parameter (in this case the HR) for which the difference between the parameter (real HR) and the observed estimate (calculated HR) is not statistically significant at a predefined level of significance. (A–D) These answer choices represent common misinterpretations of confidence intervals. Specifically, a confidence interval of 95% does not mean that the chance of the result being within this interval is 95%. A confidence interval of 95% also does not mean that the certainty of the study is 95%.

29.
B The neurosurgeon should document the need for surgery in the chart and then proceed with surgery.

Surgical emergencies are one of the few circumstances where the limits of patient autonomy are acknowledged freely, and surgeons are empowered by laws and ethics to work in the best interest of the patient without obtaining consent in the illustrated scenario. (A) Withholding treatment is unethical and against the principles of beneficence. In the absence of a documented will and family, the surgeon should proceed with what he believes is in the best interest of the patient. (C) There is no obligation to obtain the opinions of other physicians prior to proceeding with surgery. (D) It would be unethical to withhold surgery from this patient while awaiting a court order. (E) It would be unethical to withhold surgery from this patient while awaiting a decision from the ethics committee.

30.
A Will decrease
The positive predictive value represents the test's ability to identify patients with the disease cor-

rectly. It is equal to the ratio of the true positives to the sum of the true positives and false positives combined. Moving the cutoff point from point A to B will increase the number of true positives in addition to the number of false positives. (B) An increase in the positive predictive value will result in fewer false positives.

31.
A Selection bias
Selection bias is common in most prospective trials. If a large number of initially enrolled patients are lost to follow-up, it is always possible that the lost people are different and would have showed result patterns different from those of the people who remain enrolled. This bias can misinterpret associations between interventions and outcomes. (B) Recall bias occurs mostly in studies based on questionnaires, in which affected individuals tend to recall exposure to factors more that those who are unaffected. This bias type is unlikely in prospective studies. (C) Confounding bias occurs when an extraneous variable correlates with the dependent and independent variables. This may lead to the conclusion that two factors correlate without actually having a causal relationship. (D) Observer bias also is known as the observer expectancy effect and is seen in non-blinded studies. This bias is a form of reactivity in which researchers tend to consciously or unconsciously influence the participants in studies. (E) Ascertainment or sampling bias is a flaw in study design such that a specific group of patients is overly included or excluded from the studied sample.

32.
A Linear with a positive correlation coefficient
The relationship in the graph accompanying the question is linear, as the points can be approximated by a straight line. In addition, the correlation coefficient is positive, as there is a direct relationship between the two measurements (i.e., both variables increase together). A negative correlation coefficient would be seen as an inverse relationship (i.e., when one variable increases, the other decreases). (D, E) A direct logarithmic relationship would be seen on a non-logarithmic axis scale as a line increasing indefinitely but at an ever-deceasing rate.

33.

D Cross-sectional

A cross-sectional study looks at exposures and outcomes simultaneously at a specific point in time. There is no "following" of patients in this study type. (A, B) Cohort studies are designed by selecting patients with a particular exposure status and following them prospectively or retrospectively. (C) A case-control study is designed by selecting patients with and without a particular disease and then determining their previous exposure statuses. (E) Randomized clinical trials compare two or more treatments or interventions and follow patients prospectively to observe outcomes due to the manipulated variables.

34.

A Change in how a task is performed

A process change is defined by the International Health Institute as a change in the way a task is performed. Process changes are essential to helping improve the overall health system performance. (B, D) A change in the way the team perceives a task and a change in the work culture/environment are defined as culture changes. These changes are necessary to institute a process change. (C) Changes in outcome are likely to result from a process change.

35.

A Medical knowledge

Medical knowledge describes the ability to acquire and apply current medical knowledge and use advanced search engines to stay current on medical knowledge and data. (B) Professionalism describes the ability to demonstrate the principles of ethical behavior. (C) Systems-based practice describes multidisciplinary approaches to patient care and the ability to optimize care by involving multiple teams in patient management. (D) Practice-based learning and improvement describes the ability to appraise information critically on a daily basis and to analyze it in a way that improves patient care. (E) Interpersonal skills and communication skills refer to a resident's ability to communicate effectively among colleagues in his and other specialties. It also refers to the ability of a resident to share his research and demonstrate leadership skills.

III Practice Exam

21 Practice Exam Questions

Section 1: 60 Minutes, 75 Questions

1.

What structure is deep to the arrow in this view from the endoscope during a resection of a pituitary macroadenoma using a transnasal transsphenoidal approach?

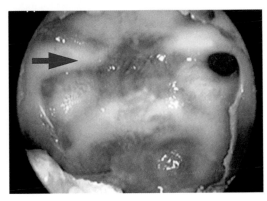

A. Pituitary gland
B. Pituitary stalk
C. Internal carotid artery
D. Optic nerve
E. Sella turcica floor

2.

A 42-year-old, otherwise healthy woman presented to clinic with a several-month history of increasing headaches that worsened over the past few days. On physical exam, she had papilledema but otherwise no focal neurologic deficits. Representative scans from an MRI of the brain are shown in these images. What is the most likely diagnosis?

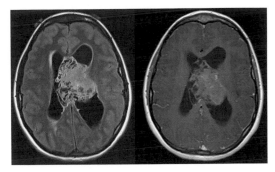

A. Central neurocytoma
B. Meningioma
C. Metastasis
D. Choroid plexus papilloma
E. Subependymal giant cell astrocytoma

3.

What is thought to be the source of the intrinsic T1 hyperintensity normally seen in the posterior pituitary gland on MRI?

A. Neurosecretory vesicles–neurophysin complex
B. High calcium content within pituicytes
C. High concentration of iron
D. Manganese

4.

A patient with severe, large-amplitude hemiballismus in his right upper extremity most likely has a lesion involving what basal ganglia structure?

A. Ipsilateral putamen
B. Contralateral putamen
C. Ipsilateral subthalamic nucleus
D. Contralateral subthalamic nucleus

5.

What target for deep brain stimulation is thought to provide the best control of essential tremors?

A. Globus pallidus pars externa
B. Subthalamic nucleus
C. Head of the caudate nucleus
D. Ventral intermediate nucleus of the thalamus
E. Globus pallidus pars interna

6.

The meningeal lesion shown in this image most likely would be demonstrated with a stain directed against what marker?

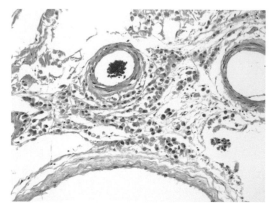

A. CD3
B. CD20
C. Cytokeratin AE1/AE3
D. GFAP
E. S-100 protein

7.

What structure is indicated by the arrow in this image from an endoscopic third ventriculostomy?

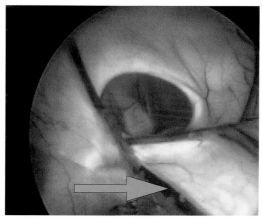

A. Septal vein
B. Internal cerebral vein
C. Caudate vein
D. Thalamostriate vein
E. Choroid vein

8.

The lesion shown in these images demonstrated avid uptake on a ^{111}In-DTPA-pentetreotide scan. What is a characteristic of this lesion?

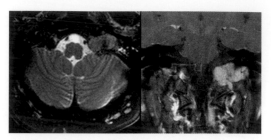

A. The majority of these lesions are multicentric.
B. It arises at the Obersteiner-Redlich zone.
C. Sporadic lesions are more common in males.
D. The majority of these lesions are malignant.
E. It may be associated with *SDHx* gene mutations.

9.

What low-grade brain tumor has been shown to be responsive to chemotherapy?

A. Meningioma
B. Epidermoid
C. Choroid plexus papilloma
D. Vestibular schwannoma
E. Ependymoma

10.

A neurosurgical attending physician consults a cardiologist after a patient had an intraoperative myocardial infarction. The anesthesiologist during the procedure was able to draw and send a panel of cardiac enzymes to the lab. This best represents which ACGME Core Competency?

A. Medical knowledge
B. Professionalism
C. Systems-based practice
D. Practice-based learning and improvement
E. Interpersonal skills and communication

11.

A patient presents with a T4 vertebra burst fracture. He has sensation to light touch in the upper and lower extremities in addition to sensation in the S4 and S5 dermatomes. Upper extremity motor function is normal, but the patient has no motor function in the lower extremities. What is the patient's ASIA classification?

A. A
B. B
C. C
D. D
E. E

12.

What are the steps, in order, in a rapid sequence intubation?

A. Induction agent, paralytic agent, intubation
B. Bag valve mask preventilation, induction agent, paralysis, intubation
C. Paralysis, bag valve mask preventilation, intubation
D. Paralysis, induction agent, intubation
E. Bag valve mask preventilation, paralysis, intubation

13.

Fibers from the flocculonodular lobe of the cerebellum synapse on the vestibular nuclei after first synapsing on what nuclei?

A. Dentate nuclei
B. Emboliform nuclei
C. Globose nuclei
D. Fastigial nuclei
E. No additional nuclei

14.

What limits facilitated diffusion across a neuronal membrane?

A. Numerous receptor binding sites for the diffusing molecule
B. Lipophilic membranes
C. Large concentration gradients
D. Amount of ATP available
E. Number of transmembrane channels specific for the diffusing molecule

15.

The intracranial hemorrhage score is used as a(n):

A. Indicator for surgery
B. Predictor of morbidity
C. Predictor of mortality
D. Indicator for the need for intracranial pressure monitoring

16.

A 60-year-old woman is being examined by her primary care physician when he notices fine twitching movements beneath the surface of her tongue with "wasting" on one side. What cranial nerve is most likely to be involved in the patient's condition?

A. V
B. VII
C. IX
D. X
E. XII

17.

A 17-year-old boy presents with increasing thoracic kyphosis. MRI shows multilevel Schmorl nodes and more than 5 degrees of anterior wedging in more than three adjacent vertebrae. What is the patient's diagnosis?

A. Scheuermann disease
B. Osteopoikilosis
C. Baastrup disease
D. Alkaptonuria
E. Osteopetrosis

18.

What organ would respond to systemic cocaine administration but not to systemic atropine administration?

A. Heart
B. Salivary glands
C. Pancreas
D. Sweat glands
E. Pupils

19.

A 20-year-old man with a history of bipolar disease presents with an acute onset of right-sided hemiparesis and expressive aphasia. According to the CT shown in this image, and assuming the most likely diagnosis, what is the risk of re-hemorrhage?

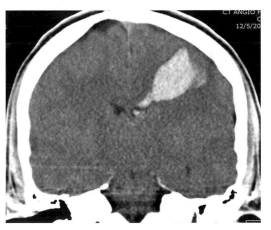

A. 4% in the first 24 hours after hemorrhage
B. 20% in the first 2 weeks after hemorrhage
C. 50% in the first 6 months after hemorrhage
D. 4 to 6% per year
E. Less than 1% over a lifetime

20.
In what spinal disease is sacroiliac joint involvement not seen?

A. Diffuse idiopathic skeletal hypertrophy
B. Ankylosing spondylitis
C. Both diffuse idiopathic skeletal hypertrophy and ankylosing spondylitis
D. Rheumatoid arthritis
E. Gout

21.
What is the definitive host for the most common opportunistic infection in an individual with HIV/AIDS?

A. Bird
B. Cat
C. Mosquito
D. Rodent
E. Sheep

22.
A deep brain stimulator lead was placed medial to the subthalamic nucleus. What side effects could be expected?

A. Increased akinesia with reduced rigidity
B. Reduced tremor with persisting akinesia
C. Tetanic muscular contraction and dysarthria
D. Double vision, ocular deviation, and postural imbalance
E. Perspiration, mydriasis, and dysesthesias

23.
A 32-year-old man underwent an MRI of the brain that demonstrated a nonenhancing intracranial lesion. An MRI sequence based on measuring the random brownian motion of water molecules at the cellular level showed this lesion to be markedly bright; therefore, the lesion likely is a(n):

A. Epidermoid
B. Lymphoma
C. Meningioma
D. Craniopharyngioma
E. Arachnoid cyst

24.
Back pain, low-grade fever, and destruction of the vertebral bodies with disk preservation are most associated with what condition?

A. Tuberculosis
B. *Staphylococcus aureus* diskitis
C. Fungal infection
D. Hemangioma
E. Osteoid osteoma

25.
A 32-year-old man suffered a severe neurologic injury in a motor vehicle collision. The patient progresses to presumed brain death. During the brain death exam, the patient is intubated, his PaO_2 is 89, systolic blood pressure is 105 mm Hg, diastolic blood pressure is 75 mm Hg, and core body temperature is 35.2°C. What prevents completing the brain death examination in this patient?

A. Core body temperature < 35.5° C
B. PaO_2 < 90
C. Systolic blood pressure < 110 mm Hg
D. The fact that the patient is intubated
E. Diastolic blood pressure < 80 mm Hg

26.
A woman presents to the emergency department with dizziness, nystagmus, and a feeling of falling toward the left. An MRI of the brain was performed, and a representative scan is shown in this image. What vessel likely is involved in this patient's condition?

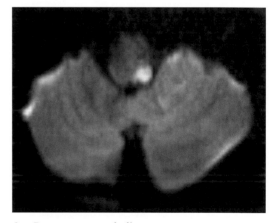

A. Pontomesencephalic artery
B. Anterior inferior cerebellar artery
C. Superior cerebellar artery
D. Posterior inferior cerebellar artery

27.
The primary neurotransmitter of Purkinje cells in the cerebellum is:

A. Glutamate
B. Glycine
C. GABA
D. Acetylcholine
E. Substance P

28.
The most common immediate postoperative endocrine abnormality encountered in children following craniopharyngioma resection surgery is:

A. Diabetes insipidus
B. Diabetes mellitus
C. Hypothyroidism
D. Growth hormone deficiency
E. Acromegaly

29.
How do steroids affect bony density?

A. Inhibit osteoclast function
B. Inhibit bone reabsorption
C. Increase urine calcium excretion
D. Prevent urine calcium excretion
E. Induce gastrointestinal calcium absorption

30.
A 25-year-old woman is discovered to have a cluster of paraspinal neurofibromas involving multiple nerves and a family history of similar lesions throughout multiple family members. What other lesion or condition may be found on physical exam?

A. Bilateral acoustic neuromas
B. Iris hamartomas
C. An increased risk of meningiomas
D. Pigmented spots encircling the iris
E. Multiple schwannomas

31.
How would nerve action potential as measured by peripheral nerve conduction testing be affected by a herniated disk with nerve root compression?

A. Unaffected
B. Slowed conduction velocity
C. Decreased amplitude
D. Increased velocity

32.
A 20-year-old man presenting with hearing loss and vertigo underwent an MRI examination, shown in this image. What is an additional expected associated feature of the entity shown?

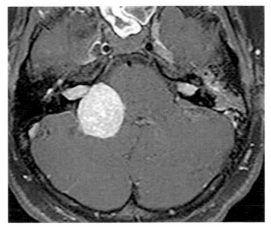

A. Ependymomas
B. Sphenoid wing dysplasia
C. Calcified subependymal nodules
D. Leptomeningeal angiomatosis
E. Endolymphatic sac tumors

33.
What antibiotic can be used to treat a patient with chronic syndrome of inappropriate antidiuretic hormone secretion (SIADH)?

A. Vancomycin
B. Cefazolin
C. Doxycycline
D. Demeclocycline
E. Erythromycin

34.
This histological image represents what disease process?

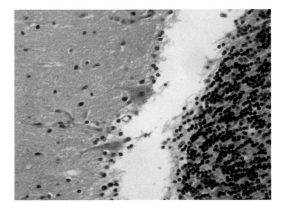

A. Alzheimer disease
B. Parkinson disease
C. Lafora disease
D. Creutzfeldt-Jakob disease
E. Rabies

35.
A sharply circumscribed, lucent lesion with beveled edges is demonstrated on a skull radiograph of a child. What is the likely diagnosis?

A. Langerhans cell histiocytosis
B. Hemangioma
C. Intraosseous meningioma
D. Metastasis

36.
What types of fibers are targeted for destruction during a percutaneous trigeminal rhizotomy for trigeminal neuralgia?

A. A-alpha and beta fibers
B. A-alpha and A-delta fibers
C. A-delta and C fibers
D. A-delta and beta fibers
E. C and beta fibers

37.
The afferents from the mammillothalamic tract project from the mammillary bodies to what thalamic nuclei?

A. Centromedian nuclei
B. Anterior nuclei
C. Ventral lateral nuclei
D. Lateral posterior nuclei
E. Medial dorsal nuclei

38.
A woman presents to a neurologist with complaints of being unable to walk down a flight of stairs due to an ability to "see the stairs clearly." The neurologist notes that the patient is tilting her head to the left when in primary gaze. What type of ophthalmoplegia does the patient have?

A. Left trochlear nerve palsy
B. Left oculomotor nerve palsy
C. Right trochlear nerve palsy
D. Right oculomotor nerve palsy
E. Internuclear ophthalmoplegia

39.
A basion–axial interval greater than 12 mm on a lateral cervical spine radiograph is indicative of what process?

A. Anterior atlanto-occipital dislocation
B. Atlantoaxial instability
C. Longitudinal dislocation
D. A normal finding
E. Transverse ligament injury

40.
A patient with amyotrophic lateral sclerosis may present with what symptoms?

A. Tongue fasciculations, atrophy of the hands, and lower extremity hyporeflexia
B. Forehead-sparing facial weakness, spasticity of the hands, and lower extremity hyperreflexia
C. Progressive weakness (proximal more than distal), areflexia, and bilateral facial weakness
D. Weakness (upper more than lower extremity), decreased sensation with dysesthesias, and urinary retention
E. Tongue fasciculations, atrophy of the hands, and lower extremity hyperreflexia

41.
What is the incidence of symptomatic hydrocephalus in patients with a Dandy-Walker malformation?

A. 20%
B. 50%
C. 70%
D. 90%
E. 100%

42.
What is the standard radiation regimen for stereotactic radiosurgery for trigeminal neuralgia?

A. 20 Gy in four doses directed at the center of the lesion
B. 20 Gy in four doses directed to extend beyond the periphery of the lesion
C. 80 Gy in a single dose directed at the center of the lesion
D. 80 Gy in a single dose directed to extend beyond the periphery of the lesion
E. 100 Gy in a single dose directed at the center of the lesion

43.
A 65-year-old divorced man is brought to the hospital following a severe head injury. The patient's ex-wife had legal power of attorney prior to the divorce and states that the patient would not want to be intubated or receive any further medical care. In most states, what is the best course of action?

A. Follow the ex-wife's orders, and do not provide any further medical care.
B. Consult the hospital's ethics committee.
C. Obtain a court order to proceed with necessary treatments.
D. Attempt to contact the patient's children to discuss plans of care.
E. Proceed with the necessary treatments regardless of the ex-wife's wishes.

44.

An axial noncontrast CT of the head is shown in this image. What does the arrow point to?

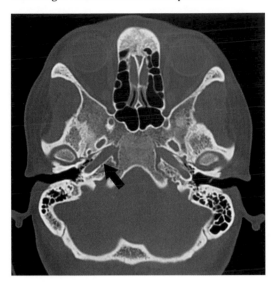

A.   Petroclival fissure
B.   Pars nervosa of jugular foramen
C.   Carotid canal
D.   Foramen rotundum
E.   Foramen ovale

45.

A 28-year-old man weighing 60 kg remains intubated following a craniotomy. His serum sodium is 153 mEq/L. What is his approximate free water deficit?

A.   0.8 L
B.   3.2 L
C.   4.0 L
D.   6.2 L

46.

The vertebral CT findings shown in this image are compatible with what process?

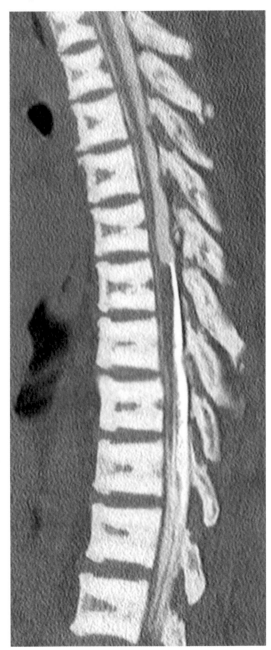

A.   Ochronosis
B.   Paget disease
C.   Blastic metastases
D.   Osteopetrosis

47.

A non–terminally ill patient has medically intractable pain in the lower extremities bilaterally due to cancer. What is the best procedure to perform for pain relief in this patient?

A. Bilateral cervical cordotomies
B. Punctate midline myelotomy
C. Commissural myelotomy
D. Spinal cord stimulation
E. Dorsal root entry zone (DREZ) lesioning

48.

How do the characteristics of optic nerve gliomas in children differ from those in adults?

A. Optic nerve gliomas have more of an association with neurofibromatosis type 1 in adults.
B. Optic nerve gliomas tend to be low grade in children and high grade in adults.
C. Rosenthal fibers are absent in presentations of optic nerve gliomas in children.
D. There is a stronger association with optic nerve gliomas and neurofibromatosis type 2 in adults than in children.

49.

A 3-year-old boy is diagnosed with a posterior fossa tumor and undergoes tumor resection. This image depicts the pathology of the lesion. What associated syndrome might he also have?

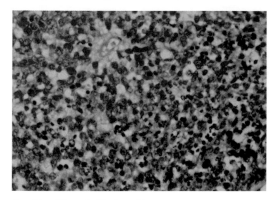

A. Von Hippel–Lindau disease
B. Gorlin syndrome
C. Tuberous sclerosis
D. Lynch syndrome

50.

What muscle typically is innervated by the radial nerve itself and not by one of its terminal branches?

A. Extensor carpi radialis longus
B. Extensor carpi radialis brevis
C. Extensor carpi ulnaris
D. Supinator
E. Abductor pollicis longus

51.

At what day of human embryogenesis does the primitive streak first appear?

A. Day 8
B. Day 12
C. Day 15
D. Day 20
E. Day 26

52.

A 45-year-old man patient with history of hypertension and diabetes presents with progressive myelopathy. A contrast enhanced MRI study was performed, shown in these images. What is the likely diagnosis?

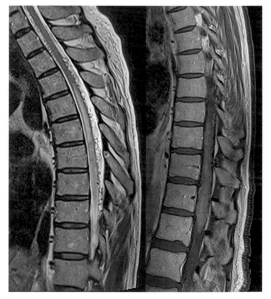

A. Acute spinal cord ischemia
B. Arteriovenous fistula
C. Infiltrating neoplasm
D. Demyelinating process
E. Infectious myelitis

53.

What is the effect of antiepileptic drugs (AEDs) on seizures following a traumatic brain injury?

A. AEDs decrease the rate of acute and delayed-onset seizures.
B. AEDs decrease the rate of acute but not of delayed-onset seizures.
C. AEDs decrease the rate of delayed-onset but not of acute seizures.
D. AEDs do not decrease the rate of acute or delayed-onset seizures.
E. AEDs have an indeterminate effect on post-traumatic seizures.

54.

A 78-year-old woman presents to the emergency room complaining of weakness and long-standing headaches. She reports that the weakness began in the right upper extremity and then proceeded to involve the right lower extremity followed by the left lower extremity and, most recently, the left upper extremity. Based on these clinical findings, what is the most likely pathological cause of the patient's symptoms?

A. Interhemispheric mass
B. Brainstem infarct
C. Cervical spine epidural hematoma
D. Foramen magnum tumor
E. Third ventricle tumor

55.

What triangle of the skull base is delineated by the greater superficial petrosal nerve and the mandibular division of the trigeminal nerve?

A. Oculomotor
B. Parkinson (infratrochlear)
C. Glasscock
D. Kawase
E. Inferolateral

56.

With relation to intracranial hypertension, to what does the Cushing triad refer?

A. Hypertension, tachycardia, and respiratory irregularity
B. Hypotension, tachycardia, and respiratory irregularity
C. Hypertension, bradycardia, and respiratory irregularity
D. Hypotension, tachycardia, and respiratory irregularity

57.

The most important predictor of outcome in children with pediatric ependymomas is:

A. Gross total resection
B. Radiosurgery
C. Dose of conformal radiation
D. Chemotherapy
E. Steroids

58.

A 5-month-old boy underwent an MRI of the brain, shown in these images. What may be a related finding?

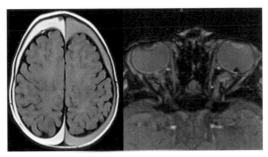

A. Abdominal mass
B. Opisthotonos
C. Fever
D. Cutaneous bruising

59.

A Parkinson patient is having a deep brain stimulating electrode placed in the globus pallidus, and the lead is passed too far inferiorly. What symptom(s) may arise when the system is activated?

A. Perspiration and mydriasis
B. Muscle contractions
C. Dysarthria
D. Visual flashes

60.

If additional sodium channels were opened on a neuron at its maximal point of depolarization during an action potential, what would happen to sodium ion flux and membrane potential?

A. Sodium flux and membrane potential would not change as they are maximized at this point in the action potential.
B. Sodium ions would enter the neuron, and membrane potential would become more positive.
C. Sodium ions would leave the neuron, and membrane potential would become more positive.
D. Sodium ions would enter the neuron, and membrane potential would become less positive.
E. Sodium ions would leave the neuron, and membrane potential would become less positive.

61.

A 60-year-old man presents with a fairly sudden onset of severe vertigo and left-side hearing loss. What is the most likely diagnosis?

A. Labyrinthitis
B. Vestibular neuronitis
C. Benign positional vertigo
D. Meniere disease
E. Stroke

62.

This image shows cerebral vessels stained with Congo red. What is the underlying disease process represented in the image?

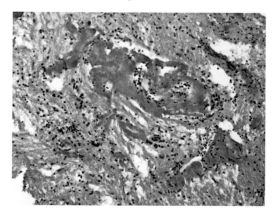

A. Moyamoya disease
B. Cavernous hemangioma
C. Cerebral angiopathy
D. Mucormycosis
E. Radiation necrosis

63.

The sural nerve is formed from the combination of two nerves arising from what larger branches?

A. Deep and superficial peroneal nerves
B. Tibial and common peroneal nerves
C. Tibial and femoral nerves
D. Common peroneal and femoral nerves
E. Superficial peroneal and tibial nerves

64.

MRI scans of the brain of a newborn are shown in these images. What is the patient's likely diagnosis?

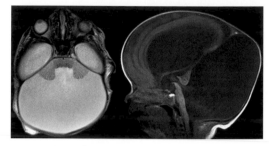

A. Arachnoid cyst
B. Blake pouch cyst
C. Dandy-Walker malformation
D. Mega cisterna magna

65.

A patient presents with exophthalmos and an orbital bruit. What is the likely finding on CT of the brain and orbits?

A. Orbital mass
B. Engorgement of the extraocular muscles
C. Enlarged ophthalmic artery
D. Unruptured cavernous sinus aneurysm
E. Flattening of the posterior aspect of the globe

66.

The cerebral venous angle occurs at what junction?

A. Internal cerebral vein and basal vein of Rosenthal
B. Septal and thalamostriate veins
C. Vein of Galen and inferior sagittal sinus
D. Caudate and thalamostriate veins
E. Torcular

Use the following answers for questions 67 and 68:

A. Respiratory alkalosis
B. Metabolic acidosis
C. Combined respiratory and metabolic alkalosis
D. Partially compensated respiratory acidosis

67.
What pathology is represented by the following arterial blood gas values?

pH: 7.15
PCO_2: 79 mm Hg
HCO_3^-: 29 mEq/L

68.
What pathology is represented by the following arterial blood gas values?

pH: 7.70
PCO_2: 29 mm Hg
HCO_3^-: 40 mEq/L

69.
A 14-year-old boy presents to his pediatrician with short stature, delayed puberty, and anosmia. He otherwise is developmentally normal without focal neurologic deficits. What is a characteristic of his likely condition?

A. The disease is more common in women.
B. The disease typically is inherited in an autosomal dominant fashion.
C. This disease typically is inherited in an X-linked fashion.
D. MRI of the brain is expected to show no abnormalities.

70.
Crouzon syndrome is mostly associated with premature closure of what skull suture(s) during infancy?

A. Bicoronal sutures
B. Sagittal suture
C. Lambdoid suture
D. Metopic suture
E. Unilateral coronal suture

71.
What characteristic is most likely to be associated with intracranial aneurysms?

A. Whole brain radiation exposure
B. Type 2 Ehlers-Danlos syndrome
C. Illicit drug use
D. Bacterial endocarditis
E. Male gender

72.
A 24-year-old man presents with progressive back pain. Imaging demonstrates an osteolytic lesion in the posterior elements of the middle thoracic spine with a fluid–fluid level. What is the most likely pathology?

A. Spinal metastatic lesion
B. Aneurysmal bone cyst
C. Osteoid osteoma
D. Osteoblastoma
E. Eosinophilic granuloma

73.
The reticulin rich mass shown in this image presented in the right frontal lobe of a 4-year-old boy. The tumor stains with glial fibrillary acidic protein and contains focal areas of synaptophysin positive staining neuronal cells. What is the most likely diagnosis for this tumor?

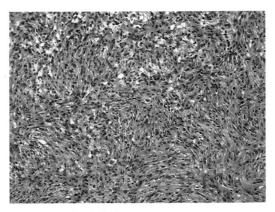

A. Desmoplastic infantile astrocytoma
B. Desmoplastic infantile ganglioglioma
C. Extraventricular neurocytoma
D. Gangliocytoma
E. Pleomorphic xanthoastrocytoma

74.
A 56-year-old man comes to clinic at the behest of his wife because of an increasing number of falls at home. During the interview, the physician notices that the patient has a masklike expression. The patient's wife also states that he has been choking during meals and holding reading materials straight in front of his face. Vertical gaze paresis, axial rigidity, and dysarthria are noted on exam. What is the most likely diagnosis?

A. Parkinson disease
B. Corticobasal degeneration
C. Progressive supranuclear palsy
D. Multiple system atrophy

75.
A 49-year-old woman presents to the emergency room with the "worst headache of my life" and a third nerve palsy with ptosis and a dilated pupil. She is noted to have subarachnoid hemorrhage on a head CT. What is her Hunt and Hess grade?

A. 1
B. 2
C. 3
D. 4
E. 5

End of Section 1. Take a 10-minute break.

Section 2: 60 Minutes, 75 Questions

1.
Assuming that this image is the only finding on a noncontrast cervical spine CT, this patient may have what pathology?

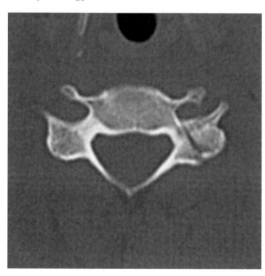

A. Intra-abdominal injuries
B. Spinal cord transection
C. Anterior circulation infarcts
D. Cerebellar infarcts

2.
What is the risk of stroke per year in patients with atrial fibrillation and a CHADS$_2$ score of 2, and what is the relative risk reduction for stroke in prescribing warfarin for patients with a CHADS$_2$ score of 2 or greater?

A. 1 to 3%; 74% reduction
B. 3 to 5%; 64% reduction
C. 5 to 6%; 54% reduction
D. 6 to 8%; 44% reduction
E. 8 to 10%; 84% reduction

3.
Mutations in the MCPHi or cyclin-dependent kinase 5 regulatory associated protein 2 are associated with what clinical condition?

A. Autosomal dominant macrocephaly
B. Autosomal dominant microcephaly
C. Autosomal recessive macrocephaly
D. Autosomal recessive microcephaly
E. X-linked microcephaly

4.
The tumor shown in these images was found to have rosettes and perivascular pseudorosettes on microscopic examination, and stained positive for glial fibrillary acidic protein. What is a characteristic of the lesion?

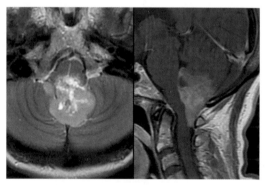

A. It commonly arises from the roof of the fourth ventricle.
B. It is associated with neurofibromatosis type 1.
C. It may be complicated by polycythemia.
D. Calcification and hemorrhage are common.

5.
Cheyne-Stokes respirations are characterized by increasing followed by decreasing tidal volumes separated by periods of apnea. They are seen in heart failure, with rapid blood sugar changes, and in stroke. Where do Cheyne-Stokes respirations originate?

A. Carotid bodies, pons, and cerebral hemispheres
B. Diencephalon, medulla, and dorsal pons
C. Basal ganglia, pons, and cerebral hemispheres
D. Diencephalon, pons, and carotid bodies
E. Diencephalon, basal ganglia, and cerebral hemispheres

6.
A patient is doing well and recovering after a lumbar diskectomy. She requests pain medications and has a first-time seizure shortly after administration of a pain medication known to cause histamine release. Tachycardia is noted. What part of her medical care may account for the postoperative developments?

A. Cerebral hypotension due to a cerebrospinal fluid leak
B. Vasovagal response to pain
C. Administration of meperidine
D. Acute recurrent disc
E. Chemical meningitis related to surgery

7.
What is a characteristic of the lesion found in the MRI scan shown in this image?

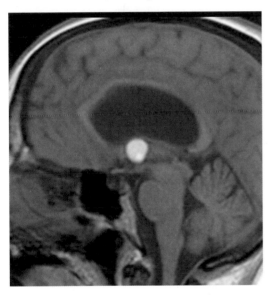

A. It is derived from embryonic mesoderm.
B. It most commonly presents with cranial neuropathies.
C. It is associated with elevated levels of alanine on MR spectroscopy.
D. It may present with acute brain herniation and death.
E. Calcification and regions of nodular enhancement are common.

8.
What triangle of the skull base is formed by the interclinoidal dural fold, posterior petroclival ligament, and anterior petroclival ligament?

A. Oculomotor
B. Parkinson (infratrochlear)
C. Glasscock
D. Kawase
E. Inferolateral

9.
The most common suprasellar contrast-enhancing solid and cystic mass during childhood as seen on the MRI shown in this image is:

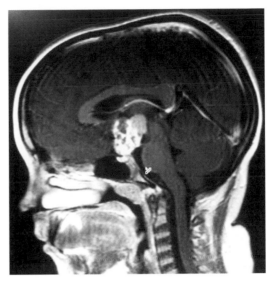

A. Suprasellar astrocytoma
B. Suprasellar teratoma
C. Craniopharyngioma
D. Suprasellar ependymoma
E. Optic pathway glioma

10.
A 14-year-old girl with a long-standing history of epilepsy presents to clinic with progressive headaches. Medical history is otherwise unremarkable. An MRI examination of the brain was performed. Shown in these images, from left to right, are axial FLAIR, T1-weighted, and contrast-enhanced T1-weighted scans of the brain. This lesion likely represents:

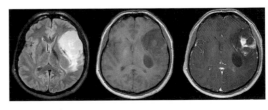

A. Lymphoma
B. Pleomorphic xanthoastrocytoma
C. Meningioma
D. Dysembryoplastic neuroepithelial tumor
E. Pilocytic astrocytoma

11.
When explaining the risks and benefits of undergoing surgery to a patient, a vascular neurosurgeon cites the ARUBA trial, which is a multicenter, international, randomized clinical trial. What level of evidence is the physician providing?

A.   Level 1
B.   Level 2
C.   Level 3
D.   Level 4
E.   Level 5

12.
What is the diagnosis of a patient with the Goldman visual field testing result shown in this image?

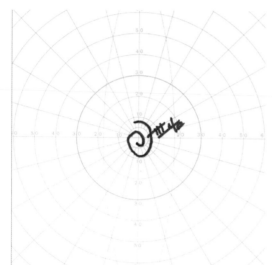

A.   Malingering/inability to participate in the exam
B.   Severe glaucoma
C.   Optic nerve atrophy
D.   Chiasmatic lesion
E.   Afferent papillary defect

13.
What T-score defines osteoporosis?

A.   +1 to 2.5
B.   −1 to +1
C.   −1 to −2.5
D.   Less than −2.5
E.   T-score definition is age dependent

14.
A patient with bluish pigmentation of the auricles and sclerae presents for evaluation. Levels of homogentisic acid in his urine are elevated. What finding is likely to be seen on a CT of the patient's spine?

A.   Wedging of adjacent vertebrae
B.   Multifocal Schmorl nodes
C.   Extensive intervertebral disk calcification
D.   H-shaped vertebrae

15.
What is the best deep brain stimulation target for Parkinson disease–related gait and postural instability, falls, and freezing?

A.   Subthalamic nucleus
B.   Ventralis intermedius nucleus of the thalamus
C.   Pedunculopontine nucleus
D.   Globus pallidus internus

16.
The histological appearance of the hippocampus shown in this image suggests:

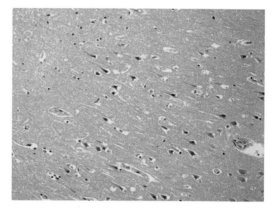

A.   Tumor
B.   Mesial temporal lobe sclerosis
C.   Hypoxia/anoxia
D.   Trauma/cerebral contusion

17.
A 58-year-old man presents with delusions and hallucinations. His wife reports that he has been complaining recently of headaches, irritability, and sleep disturbance, and that he has had a progressive memory decline over the past month. Brain MRI shows high T2 signal without enhancement, mostly in the left mesial temporal lobe. Chest radiograph shows a centrally located pulmonary mass. Cerebrospinal fluid examination shows elevated lymphocytes, elevated protein, normal glucose, elevated IgG index, and oligoclonal bands. Herpes virus PCR is negative. What is the most likely diagnosis?

A. Herpes simplex encephalitis
B. Limbic encephalitis
C. Pontine stroke
D. Paraneoplastic cerebellar degeneration
E. Multiple sclerosis

18.
A preterm infant undergoes a cranial ultrasound. Coronal and sagittal images are presented here. What is the likely diagnosis?

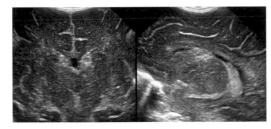

A. Acute infarction
B. Germinal matrix hemorrhage
C. Hypoxic-ischemic injury
D. Periventricular leukomalacia

19.
Which structure runs through the cavernous sinus but does not pass through the superior orbital fissure?

A. Optic nerve
B. Oculomotor nerve
C. Ophthalmic division of the trigeminal nerve
D. Maxillary division of the trigeminal nerve
E. Abducens nerve

20.
What type of receptor is found on sweat glands along postganglionic sympathetic fibers?

A. Muscarinic
B. Adrenergic
C. AMPA
D. NMDA
E. Nicotinic

21.
Sagittal balance is measure from what two positions?

A. C1 to L5
B. Opisthion to L5
C. T1 to sacrum
D. C7 to sacrum
E. C7 to L5

22.
A patient has unilateral twitching of her left eye when looking downward and nasally. She denies pain and discomfort but describes her vision in that eye as "shaky." The rest of her ophthalmological workup is unremarkable. What is the likely diagnosis?

A. Hemifacial spasm
B. Duane syndrome
C. Myasthenia gravis
D. Superior oblique myokymia

23.
What letter in this image represents the portion of the primary motor cortex most devoted to control of the hand intrinsic muscles?

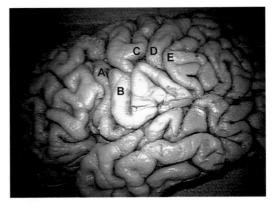

A. A
B. B
C. C
D. D
E. E

24.

An established patient with multiple sclerosis presents to clinic. He has a known lesion in his medial longitudinal fasciculus affecting his right eye. What is found on examination of his extraocular movements?

A. Conjugate gaze to the right, plegia of right eye adduction, and left eye nystagmus with left gaze

B. Conjugate gaze to the left, plegia of right eye abduction, and left eye nystagmus with left gaze

C. Conjugate gaze with left and right gaze and nystagmus of the right eye when looking to the left

D. Normal extraocular movements

25.

A 33-year-old, otherwise healthy man underwent an MRI, shown in these images. Histological analysis of his lesion revealed a large amount of mucin with formation of rosettes and pseudorosettes. "Collagen balls" were evident on periodic acid-Schiff staining. This lesion is consistent with a:

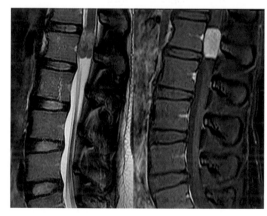

A. Schwannoma

B. Metastasis

C. Myxopapillary ependymoma

D. Neurofibroma

E. Paraganglioma

26.

A 53-year-old woman is status post–resection of a 2.5-cm vestibular schwannoma. Preoperatively, her House-Brackmann facial function was grade 1. Postoperatively, the patient had obvious weakness with facial asymmetry. There was no movement

of her forehead with incomplete eye closure and asymmetry of her mouth with maximum effort. What is her House-Brackmann grade?

A. Grade 2

B. Grade 3

C. Grade 4

D. Grade 5

E. Grade 6

27.

The lesion shown in this image most commonly is associated with what underlying disease?

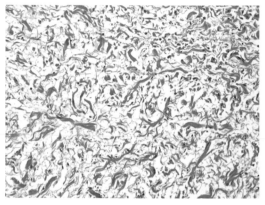

A. Multiple endocrine neoplasia (MEN) type 1

B. MEN type 2a

C. Neurofibromatosis type 1

D. Neurofibromatosis type 2

E. Tuberous sclerosis

28.

What parameter change in a neuron favors a signal temporal summation rather than a spatial summation?

A. A smaller membrane resistance

B. A larger internal resistance

C. A lower membrane capacitance

D. A larger intracellular space

29.

What is the best route for vitamin K administration in the setting of life-threatening hemorrhage in a patient on warfarin?

A. Oral

B. Intravenous bolus

C. Subcutaneous

D. Intravenous slow continuous infusion

E. Intra-arterial

30.
As a screening tool for a disease, a physician orders a diagnostic test with a sensitivity of 80% and specificity of 90%. The result returns as positive for the disease, which happens to have a 25% prevalence in the general population. What is the chance that the patient actually has the disease?

A. 100%
B. 90%
C. 89%
D. 73%
E. 57%

31.
What is a characteristic of the tumor shown in this image?

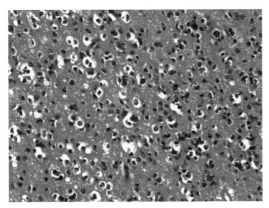

A. Calcifications are infrequent.
B. Necrosis warrants a WHO grade IV designation.
C. Pericellular clearing is an artifact of delayed formalin fixation.
D. It represents a WHO grade I tumor.
E. It is generally circumscribed and amenable to gross total resection.

32.
A 68-year-old man with a history of diabetes, hypertension, and multiple prior transient ischemic attacks presents to the emergency department with left-sided hemiplegia and a facial droop. Conventional angiography is performed after MRI of the brain. A digital subtraction image of the patient's right carotid artery bifurcation is shown in this image. What is the angiographic finding?

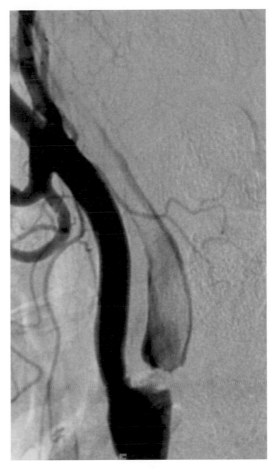

A. Internal carotid artery dissection
B. Complete occlusion of the internal carotid artery
C. Fibromuscular dysplasia
D. Formation of a pseudoaneurysm with flow artifact
E. Critical carotid artery stenosis with intraluminal thrombus

33.
A 32-year-old man presents to the hospital with seizures. Imaging reveals a 4-cm arteriovenous malformation (AVM) in the right frontal basal ganglia. The venous drainage is to the internal cerebral veins. What is the Spetzler-Martin grade of this AVM?

A. 1
B. 2
C. 3
D. 4
E. 5

34.
What nerve(s) provide(s) parasympathetic innervation to the kidneys?

A. Vagus nerve
B. Lumbar splanchnic nerves
C. Thoracic splanchnic nerves
D. Inferior mesenteric plexus nerves
E. Superior mesenteric plexus nerves

35.
A 9-month-old, nonvaccinated girl is brought to the emergency room for generalized seizures. She has a stiff neck, is poorly responsive, and has a temperature of 39.1°C. Her parents report that she had one episode of diarrhea earlier in the day. Cerebrospinal fluid Gram stain is negative. What pathogen most likely is the origin of these symptoms?

A. *Cryptococcus*
B. *Haemophilus influenzae*
C. *Neisseria meningitidis*
D. *Streptococcus pneumoniae*
E. Herpes simplex virus

36.
Representative scans of a brain MRI examination in a child are shown in these images. What likely is related directly to the neuroimaging findings?

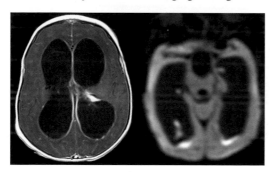

A. Nonaccidental trauma
B. Congenital aqueductal stenosis
C. Sepsis
D. Medulloblastoma

37.
What is the most important factor to determine the stability and need for surgical fixation of a Jefferson fracture?

A. Disruption of the transverse ligament
B. Disruption of the alar ligament
C. Posterior arch fracture
D. Lateral mass fractures
E. Disruption of tectorial membrane

38.
What triangle of the skull base is formed by the lateral border of cranial nerve IV, medial border of the ophthalmic division of the trigeminal nerve, and dura between the dural entry points of both cranial nerves IV and the ophthalmic division of V?

A. Oculomotor
B. Parkinson (infratrochlear)
C. Glasscock
D. Kawase
E. Inferolateral

39.
A 9-year-old boy presents to the emergency department with progressive throat and neck pain after tonsillectomy. The emergency room physician consults neurosurgery for evaluation for Grisel syndrome. What radiographic finding supports this diagnosis?

A. Power ratio greater than 1
B. Overhang of the C1 lateral masses on C2 is at least 7 mm
C. Rotatory subluxation with inflammation of the C1/C2 facet capsule
D. "Kissing" spinous processes
E. Significant anterior cervical "flowing" osteophytes

40.
Two axial noncontrast CT scans of the head are shown in these images. What is the patient's likely clinical presentation?

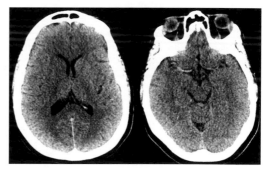

A. Rapid-onset dementia
B. Acute left-sided hemiplegia
C. Fever and nuchal rigidity
D. Progressive encephalopathy

41.

What is the most common location of choroid plexus papillomas in children?

A. Lateral ventricles
B. Third ventricle
C. Fourth ventricle
D. Foramen of Monro
E. Cerebral aqueduct

Use the following answers for questions 42 to 45:

A. Hyperkalemia
B. Hypokalemia
C. Hypercalcemia
D. Hypomagnesemia
E. Hypophosphatemia

42.

What is the likely electrolyte abnormality in a patient presenting with ileus, weakness, U waves, and a prolonged QT interval?

43.

What is the likely electrolyte abnormality in a patient presenting with polyuria, dehydration, mental status changes, abdominal pain, anorexia, nausea, vomiting, and fatigue?

44.

What is the likely electrolyte abnormality in a patient presenting with weakness, muscle cramps, tremors, nystagmus, and tetany?

45.

What is the likely electrolyte abnormality in a patient presenting with weakness, nausea, peaked T waves, and an increased PR interval?

46.

Axial and sagittal postcontrast T1 scans of the brain of a child are shown in these images. What is the likely diagnosis?

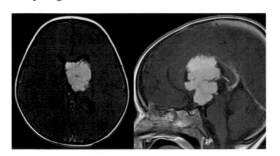

A. Choroid plexus papilloma
B. Meningioma
C. Ependymoma
D. Subependymoma
E. Central neurocytoma

47.

What feature of a burst fracture may imply instability and the need for surgery?

A. Loss of height of 25%
B. Angulation of 5 degrees
C. Residual canal diameter 80% of normal
D. Pain that improves with bracing
E. Injury to the posterior ligamentous complex

48.

A patient presents with a nystagmus described as the eyes moving up and down discordantly with intorsion of the rising eye and extorsion of the falling eye. What visual field abnormality might be seen on exam?

A. Loss of peripheral vision (tunnel vision)
B. Bitemporal hemianopsia
C. Central scotoma
D. Binasal hemianopsia
E. Unilateral inferior hemianopsia

49.

On MRI, a cerebral hematoma is noted to be hyperintense on T1 and hypointense on T2-weighted sequences. These signal characteristics are related to what blood component?

A. Oxyhemoglobin
B. Deoxyhemoglobin
C. Intracellular methemoglobin
D. Extracellular methemoglobin
E. Hemosiderin

50.

How does hypertension affect the risk of developing a hemorrhagic stroke?

A. Hypertension does not increase the risk.
B. Hypertension increases the relative risk by 3.9 to 5.4%.
C. Acute hypertension secondary to sympathomimetics or preeclampsia is not thought to elevate the risk.
D. Hypertension increases the risk of developing a supratentorial but not an infratentorial intracranial hemorrhage.

51.
Compared to primary glioblastomas, secondary glioblastomas tend to express what histopathological characteristics?

A. *EGFR* gene amplification
B. *PTEN* gene mutations
C. *TP53* gene mutations
D. Allelic gain of chromosomes 10q and 19q
E. Increased GFAP staining

52.
You perform surgery on a patient with a far lateral herniated disk at L4/L5. You use a lateral approach, and the pars interarticularis is identified. The L4 nerve root can be found anterior to what structure?

A. L4 pedicle
B. L5 pedicle
C. Intertransverse ligament
D. Disk space
E. Multifidus muscle

53.
What muscle is innervated by the superior laryngeal nerve?

A. Transverse arytenoid
B. Posterior cricoarytenoid
C. Stylopharyngeus
D. Cricothyroid
E. Geniohyoid

54.
What hydrolyzes cAMP?

A. Adenyl cyclase
B. Phosphodiesterase
C. Protein kinase A
D. CREB
E. Phospholipase C

55.
The "empty delta" sign on a contrast-enhanced head CT implies what pathology?

A. Arterial thrombosis
B. Dural sinus thrombosis
C. Expansion of a parenchymal hematoma
D. Impending herniation

56.
What aspect of newer "atypical" antipsychotics is thought to be responsible for the lower rate of extrapyramidal side effects when compared with older "typical" antipsychotics?

A. More antihistaminergic and anticholinergic activity
B. Less antihistaminergic and anticholinergic activity
C. More antidopaminergic activity
D. Less antidopaminergic activity
E. Serotonin receptor agonism

57.
According to the Gardener and Robertson modified hearing classification, serviceable hearing has at least what percentage of speech discrimination?

A. 15%
B. 30%
C. 50%
D. 70%
E. 90%

58.
The cerebellum projects to what thalamic nucleus (nuclei)?

A. Anterior nuclei group
B. Ventral lateral nucleus
C. Ventral posterior lateral nucleus
D. Ventral posterior medial nucleus
E. Medial geniculate body

59.
What type of nystagmus can be associated with Parinaud syndrome?

A. Downbeat nystagmus
B. Seesaw nystagmus
C. Nystagmus retractorius
D. Abducting nystagmus

60.
A 70-year-old man presents to the emergency room with neck pain after a fall. The patient is reported to be neurologically intact. CT scan shows imaging consistent with ankylosing spondylitis. Imaging suggests a Chance fracture through the C5/C6 disk space extending through the posterior elements. Upon the neurosurgeon's arrival, the patient is found to be quadriparetic. What is the most likely cause of the patient's sudden quadriparesis?

A. Poor initial neurologic exam by the emergency room physician
B. Epidural hematoma alone
C. Unstable fracture exacerbated by external stabilization alone
D. Unstable fracture exacerbated by external stabilization with potential epidural hematoma
E. Over medication/sedation

61.

A 65-year-old man undergoes an MRI of the brain. The enhancing lesion shown in these images demonstrates diffuse low apparent diffusion coefficient values. What is the patient's likely diagnosis?

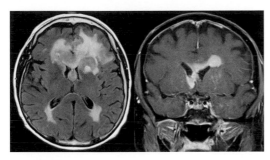

A. Glioblastoma
B. Lymphoma
C. Tumefactive demyelination
D. Infection

62.

For infants with positional plagiocephaly, what is a characteristic finding on examination?

A. Contralateral frontal bossing
B. Ridging over the ipsilateral lambdoid suture
C. Anterior displacement of the ipsilateral ear
D. Posterior displacement of the ipsilateral ear
E. Presence of torticollis

63.

Sympathetic activity of what organ/action most likely would be affected by atropine administration?

A. Heart rate
B. Pupillary constriction
C. Peristalsis inhibition
D. Sweating
E. Ejaculation

64.

A young adult with a history of headaches and seizures underwent a brain MRI and was found to have the lesion shown in these images. What characteristic predicts a high surgical risk on the Spetzler-Martin grading system?

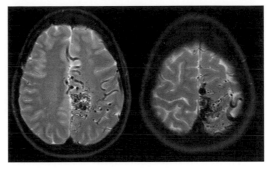

A. Superficial venous drainage
B. Involvement of eloquent brain
C. Retrograde cortical venous drainage
D. Venous ectasia

65.

What inborn error of metabolism is inherited in an X-linked recessive fashion?

A. Farber disease
B. Fragile X syndrome
C. Rett syndrome
D. Hurler syndrome
E. Fabry disease

66.

By quantity, the predominant type of neuron in the human brain is found in what cerebral or cerebellar layer?

A. Molecular layer
B. External pyramidal layer
C. Purkinje layer
D. Internal pyramidal layer
E. Granular layer

67.

Two large hospitals are the only tertiary care centers in a city. The hospitals are planning a merger. This merger is a violation of what law?

A. Antitrust law
B. Stark law
C. Federal anti-kickback statue
D. Emergency Medical Treatment and Active Labor Act (EMTALA)

68.

What feature can distinguish a foot drop caused by L5 nerve root pathology from a foot drop caused by a common peroneal nerve (CPN) palsy?

A. An L5 nerve root palsy will include weakness of anterior tibialis, which is spared with a CPN palsy.

B. There is weak internal rotation of the hip with a CPN palsy, which is spared with an L5 nerve root palsy.

C. There is weakness of foot inversion with an L5 nerve root palsy, which is spared with a CPN palsy.

D. There is weakness in plantarflexion with a CPN palsy, which is spared with an L5 nerve root palsy.

69.

The American Spinal Injury Association (ASIA) motor scoring system is an international classification for spinal cord injury. A patient presents with a suspected cervical spine injury and the following strength exam: deltoids 5/5 bilaterally; biceps 5/5 bilaterally; wrist extensors 5/5 bilaterally; triceps 5/5 on the right and 3/5 on the left; and 0/5 in the grip, hand intrinsics, and bilateral lower extremities. What is the patient's ASIA motor scale score?

A. 23
B. 28
C. 37
D. 73
E. 87

70.

The most successful commonly used treatment for recurrent strokes in a child younger than 10 years of age with moyamoya disease is:

A. Direct revascularization using a superficial temporal artery to middle cerebral artery bypass

B. Indirect revascularization using an encephaloduroarteriosynangiosis procedure

C. Conservative observation

D. Medical therapy (daily aspirin administration)

E. Endovascular treatment

71.

The best diagnosis for the enhancing mass shown in this image, presenting in the left parietal lobe in a 70-year-old man, is:

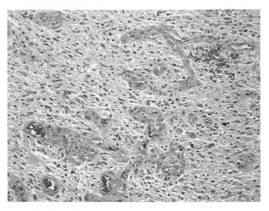

A. Anaplastic astrocytoma
B. Anaplastic oligodendroglioma
C. Glioblastoma
D. Lymphoma
E. Medulloblastoma

72.

According to the Sunderland classification for peripheral nerve injuries, a nerve with a disrupted endoneurium with an intact epineurium and perineurium has what degree of injury?

A. First degree
B. Second degree
C. Third degree
D. Fourth degree
E. Fifth degree

73.

What characteristic is consistent with malignant transformation of a plexiform neurofibroma?

A. FDG uptake
B. Heterogeneous enhancement
C. "Target" sign
D. Slow growth

74.

A patient presents with nausea, vomiting, nystagmus, dysphagia, decreased facial sensation on the left side, decreased pain and temperature sensation on the right side, and a Horner syndrome on the left. Where is his lesion?

A. Right anterior medulla
B. Left lateral medulla
C. Right lateral medulla
D. Left ventrocaudal pons

75.

Though not clinically reliable, what exam finding can be used to differ between the "classic" presentation of an epidural hematoma and the presentation of a subdural hematoma?

A. Degree of nausea
B. Irritability
C. Presence of a lucid interval
D. Progressive neurological deficits

End of Section 2. Take a 10-minute break.

Section 3: 60 Minutes, 75 Questions

1.

What is the historic procedure used for the treatment of Parkinson disease with the unintended and frequent consequence of hemiparesis?

A. Ligation of recurrent artery of Heubner
B. Ligation of the superior hypophyseal artery
C. Surgical resection of the contralateral supplementary motor association area
D. Ligation of the anterior choroidal artery

2.

What finding on MRI is suggestive of a brachial plexus avulsion injury?

A. Lateral meningoceles
B. Nerve root enhancement
C. Presence of fluid within the root sleeve
D. Spinal cord hematoma

3.

What are the electroencephalographic changes seen in herpetic encephalitis?

A. Alpha activity over occipital areas
B. Beta activity over temporal areas
C. Alpha activity over frontal areas
D. 3-Hz spike-and-wave discharges
E. Periodic sharp wave complexes

4.

An MRI of the brain was obtained in an 8-year-old boy during a workup for macrocephaly. Axial T2 and FLAIR scans are shown in these images. What is the boy's likely diagnosis?

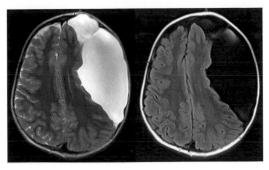

A. Porencephalic cyst
B. Arachnoid cyst
C. Neurenteric cyst
D. Schizencephaly

5.

Postmortem brain examination of a 66-year-old man with cognitive impairment found the changes shown in this image in the hippocampal neurons. This finding is the result of the abnormal accumulation of what substance?

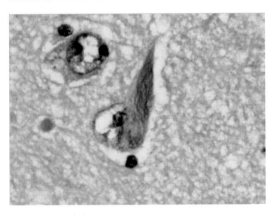

A. α-synuclein
B. Amyloid precursor protein
C. β-amyloid
D. Hyperphosphorylated tau protein
E. Prion protein

6.

The superior limit of the thalamic surface in the third ventricle is marked by what structure(s)?

A. Habenula
B. Corpus callosum
C. Internal medullary lamina
D. Thalamic fasciculus
E. Striae medullaris thalami

7.

A 21-year-old man presents to the emergency room with a radial fracture and wrist drop. What finding supports the diagnosis of injury to the radial nerve and not the posterior cord?

A. Lack of weakness in the deltoid and latissimus dorsi
B. Lack of weakness in the serratus anterior
C. Lack of weakness in the rhomboids
D. Lack of sensation loss in the medial forearm
E. Weakness of the brachioradialis

8.

A patient was found to have a T2 hypointense odontoid/periodontoid lesion on MRI. A postcontrast T1-weighted scan is shown in this image. What is a characteristic of the demonstrated lesion?

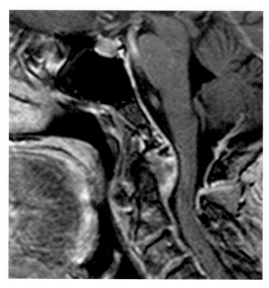

A. Requires surgical removal
B. Arises from notochordal elements
C. Associated with atlantoaxial subluxation
D. Arises from arachnoid cap cells

9.

A 12-year-old boy presents rather acutely with signs of a central nervous system infection. A brain biopsy specimen is shown in this image. The etiology of the infection is:

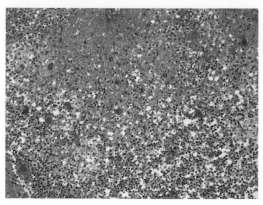

A. Amoebiasis
B. *Aspergillus*
C. *Cryptococcus*
D. *Mucormycosis*
E. *Toxoplasma*

Use the following answers for questions 10 to 12:

A. *Tenia solium*
B. *Herpes simplex*
C. *Cryptococcus*
D. Toxoplasmosis
E. West Nile virus
F. JC virus

10.

A 40-year-old man with 2 days of fever and seizures has an electroencephalogram demonstrating left temporal periodic lateralized epileptiform discharges and slowing. What is the most likely diagnosis?

11.

A 35-year-old patient with HIV has a headache, stiff neck, and altered metal status. MRI shows enhancing lesions with little mass effect, and a lumbar puncture demonstrates organisms with India ink stain. What is the patient's most likely diagnosis?

12.

A 27-year-old man from Mexico presents with generalized tonic-clonic seizures. Diffuse parenchymal lesions are seen on CT scan, and the patient has focal weakness, papilledema, decreased vision, and parkinsonian symptoms. What is the most likely diagnosis?

13.

The photomicrograph shown in this image demonstrates the microscopic appearance of a posterior fossa mass in a 6-year-old patient. What is the most likely diagnosis?

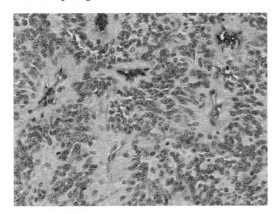

A. Astroblastoma
B. Ependymoma
C. Hemangioblastoma
D. Medulloblastoma
E. Neuroblastoma

14.

When considering a surgical approach to the L4/L5 level, what complication is seen with an anterior lumbar interbody fusion (ALIF) that generally is avoided with an extreme lateral interbody fusion (XLIF)?

A. Vascular injury
B. Neurologic injury
C. High-volume blood loss
D. Sexual dysfunction
E. Interbody subsidence

15.

A 56-year-old man underwent an uneventful craniotomy for the resection of a meningioma. On the second postoperative day, he started complaining of increasing headaches and subsequently became unresponsive. An emergent CT of the head is shown in this image. What therapy should be administered or performed next?

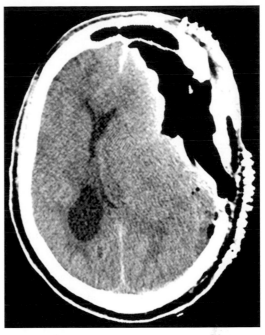

A. Lumbar puncture
B. Hypertonic saline
C. Surgical decompression
D. Mannitol

16.

Where in the action potential does the peak potassium conductance occur?

A. Before the peak of sodium conductance
B. During the peak of sodium conductance
C. After the peak of sodium conductance but before hyperpolarization
D. At maximal hyperpolarization
E. Following maximal hyperpolarization

17.

A 44-year-old man presents to clinic with new double vision and uncoordinated walking. You notice that he has trouble smiling due to weakness on both sides of his face. No other weakness is noted on physical exam. He states that he just recovered from the flu. What is the most likely diagnosis?

A. Multiple sclerosis
B. Cerebellar stroke
C. Miller Fisher syndrome
D. Ethanol intoxication
E. Myasthenia gravis

18.
What is the term for stimulation of the median or tibial nerve with averaging of the electroencephalographic waveforms to null out activity that is not time locked to the stimulus?

A. Motor evoked potential
B. Brainstem auditory evoked response
C. Somatosensory evoked potential
D. Electroencephalogram
E. Electromyography

19.
A 12-year-old child with shunted hydrocephalus since birth presents with severe abdominal pain and vomiting. Ultrasound is concerning for a large pseudocyst around the peritoneal catheter tip. The next step in this patient's management should involve:

A. Antibiotics alone
B. Complete shunt removal and placement of a ventricular drain
C. Peritoneal tap
D. Shunt externalization
E. Observation

20.
The histological section shown in this image represents what type of neural tissue?

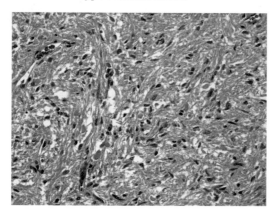

A. Corpus callosum
B. Cranial nerve
C. Dural fibrosis
D. Neurohypophysis
E. Schwannoma

21.
Which Modic type change is hyperintense on T1 and iso- to hyperintense on T2 MRI?

A. Type 1
B. Type 2
C. Type 3
D. Type 4

22.
What is the function of the nucleus ambiguus?

A. Provides special visceral efferent fibers to the stylopharyngeus and the laryngeal, pharyngeal, and palatine musculature
B. Provides special visceral afferent fibers from the posterior one third of the tongue
C. Provides general visceral efferent fibers to the otic ganglion and eventually the parotid gland
D. Provides general visceral efferent fibers to the greater petrosal nerve and eventually the pterygopalatine ganglion
E. Provides special visceral efferent fibers to stylohyoid, stapedius, and posterior belly of the digastric

23.
A study was conducted to evaluate two types of deep brain stimulation electrodes. The results showed that electrode 1 consistently lasted 0.5 months longer than electrode 2, with a p value of < 0.001. The authors concluded that electrode 1 should be used consistently instead of electrode 2. What is the error committed by the researchers?

A. The results are not actually statistically significant.
B. The results are not clinically significant.
C. The confidence interval is not reported.
D. Other confounding variables are not reported.
E. The authors might have conflicts of interest.

24.
What happens to the H-band during muscle contraction?

A. Disappears
B. Stays the same
C. Lengthens
D. Shortens
E. Has a variable change

25.

What abnormality is seen on the axial T1-weighted MRI of the lumbar spine shown in this image?

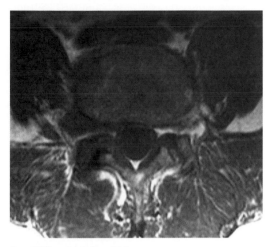

A. Diffuse bulging disk
B. Paracentral protrusion
C. Central extrusion
D. Foraminal/extraforaminal extrusion
E. Asymmetrically bulging disk

26.

The most likely organism responsible for the changes seen in the pathological specimen shown in this image, from a 72-year-old, otherwise healthy man, is:

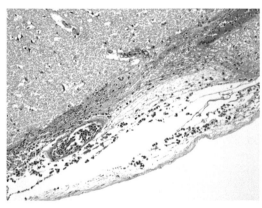

A. *Escherichia coli*
B. *Haemophilus influenzae*
C. *Listeria monocytogenes*
D. *Neisseria meningitidis*
E. *Streptococcus pneumoniae*

27.

After suffering a skull base fracture in a motor vehicle collision, a patient presents with persistent rhinorrhea. The most specific finding to determine if this fluid is cerebrospinal fluid is:

A. Presence of β_2-transferrin
B. Presence of glucose
C. Positive ring sign
D. Positive reservoir sign
E. Salty taste reported by the patient

Use the following answers for questions 28 and 29:

A. Weakness of dorsiflexion and ankle inversion
B. Weakness of plantarflexion and ankle eversion
C. Weakness of dorsiflexion and ankle eversion
D. Weakness of plantarflexion and ankle inversion

28.

What deficit is expected with a tibial nerve injury?

29.

What deficit is expected with an S1 nerve injury?

30.

What is a characteristic of the lesion depicted on the CT scans shown in these images?

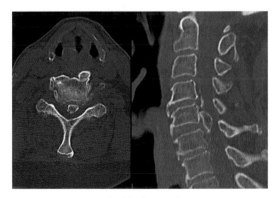

A. Most common in black people
B. More common in women
C. Arises from arachnoid cap cells
D. Associated with ankylosing spondylitis

31.

A patient presents with unilateral decreased visual acuity over 2 days. She complains of severe eye pain. What is the most likely cause of the symptoms?

A. Atherosclerosis
B. Arteritis
C. Demyelination
D. Retinal artery embolism
E. Increased intracranial pressure

32.
Where is the cleft in the spinal canal that is associated with diastematomyelia most commonly located?

A. Cervical region
B. Thoracic region
C. Lumbar region
D. Sacral region
E. Foramen magnum

33.
A study is conducted to assess the risk of lumbar disk herniation among patients with desk jobs. What type of bias will occur if patients change their behaviors (e.g., start exercising more frequently) because they are aware they are being studied?

A. Sample distortion bias
B. Information bias
C. Hawthorne effect
D. Observer bias
E. Lead time bias

34.
What is the Evans ratio?

A. Largest width of the frontal horns divided by the internal diameter of the skull from the inner table to the inner table at this level
B. Largest width of the frontal horns divided by the largest width of the third ventricle
C. Largest width of the frontal horns divided by the maximal biparietal diameter of the skull from the inner table to the inner table
D. Occipital-frontal circumference divided by age (in months) of the child

35.
During a retrosigmoid craniotomy, an artery is seen looping into the internal carotid artery. This is most likely a branch of what artery?

A. Vertebral artery
B. Posterior inferior cerebellar artery
C. Anterior inferior cerebellar artery
D. Superior cerebellar artery
E. Basilar artery

36.
When sodium flux into a neuron increases and all other ion fluxes remain the same, what happens to the excitatory postsynaptic potential (EPSP) and inhibitory postsynaptic potential (IPSP)?

A. EPSP decreases and IPSP increases
B. EPSP increases and IPSP decreases
C. EPSP and IPSP both increase
D. EPSP and IPSP both decrease
E. EPSP and IPSP both remain the same

37.
A 34-year-old woman presents to the emergency room with altered mental status and a suspected seizure. A 4.5-cm peripherally enhancing mass near the lateral ventricle is demonstrated on MRI that shows diffusion restriction and significant vasogenic edema with 7 mm of midline shift. The WBC is 30,000, and the C-reactive protein is elevated. What is the appropriate next step?

A. Lumbar puncture
B. Ventriculostomy
C. Urgent craniotomy and resection of lesion
D. CT of chest/abdomen/pelvis
E. Medical treatment

38.
What characterizes an upper motor neuron lesion?

A. Hypotonicity, muscle fasciculations, hyporeflexia, and a negative Babinski response
B. Hypertonicity, muscle fasciculations, hyperreflexia, and a positive Babinski response
C. Hypotonicity, absence of muscle fasciculations, hyporeflexia, and a positive Babinski response
D. Hypertonicity, muscle fasciculations, hyporeflexia, and a negative Babinski response
E. Hypertonicity, no muscle fasciculations, hyperreflexia, and a positive Babinski response

39.
What paralytic has the shortest time to onset and duration?

A. Succinylcholine
B. Rocuronium
C. Atracurium
D. Pancuronium
E. Vecuronium

40.

What is the etiology of the lesion shown in this image from an MRI study?

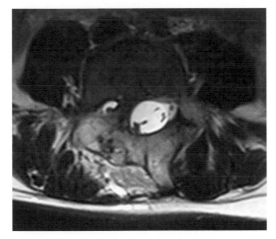

A. Persistence of the accessory neurenteric canal
B. Failure of closure of the rostral neuropore
C. In utero infarction
D. Infection
E. Partial resorption of the accessory neurenteric canal

41.

What structures form the boundaries of the lateral recess of the spine?

A. Posterior vertebral body, pedicle, and superior articular facet
B. Superior articular facet, inferior articular facet, and pars interarticularis
C. Posterior vertebral body, posterior disk space, and posterior longitudinal ligament
D. Transverse process, superior articular facet, and pedicle
E. Ligamentum flavum, superior articular facet, and pars interarticularis

42.

The sodium-glucose transporter is an example of what type of transport process?

A. Facilitated diffusion
B. Simple diffusion
C. Secondary active transport
D. Primary active transport
E. Gap junctions

43.

What feature favors a chordoma over a chondrosarcoma?

A. Lower apparent diffusion coefficient values
B. Well-circumscribed lesion margins on MRI
C. Marked T2 hyperintensity
D. Heterogeneous enhancement
E. Location at the petroclival synchondrosis

44.

A patient presents with severe back pain that is worse at night and improves when taking aspirin. CT shows an expansile, radiolucent, 2-cm sclerotic lesion in the thoracic pedicle with cord compression and a contralateral spondylolysis. The optimal treatment includes:

A. Curettage
B. Complete resection
C. X-ray therapy
D. External bracing
E. Needle biopsy

45.

A patient is asked to hold a piece of paper between his thumb and index finger. When the examiner attempts to pull the paper out of the subject's hand, he flexes the flexor pollicis longus and pinches the paper, as shown in this image. What is the patient's diagnosis?

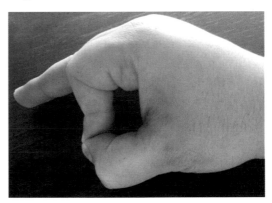

A. Ulnar nerve palsy
B. Median nerve palsy
C. Radial nerve palsy
D. Injury of the anterior interosseous branch of the median nerve
E. Injury of C5 nerve root

46.

The tumor shown in this image most commonly is associated with what cancer?

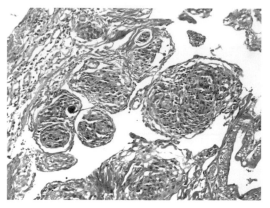

A. Breast carcinoma
B. Colon carcinoma
C. Lung adenocarcinoma
D. Lung small cell carcinoma
E. Melanoma

47.

What cervical level corresponds to the level of the thyroid cartilage?

A. C1–C2
B. C3–C4
C. C4–C5
D. C5–C6
E. C6–C7

48.

What is a delayed (more than 6 hours) finding after ischemic stroke?

A. Hyperdense artery sign
B. Decreased attenuation of the lentiform nucleus
C. Loss of the insular ribbon
D. Effacement of the cerebral sulci
E. Enhancement following contrast administration

49.

Subthalamic nucleus deep brain stimulation is a surgical treatment for Parkinson disease. Where is the subthalamic nucleus located?

A. Ventral to the thalamus, dorsal to the substantia nigra, and medial to the internal capsule
B. Ventral to the thalamus, posterior to the third ventricle, and lateral to the globus pallidus
C. Dorsal to the thalamus, ventral to the substantia nigra, and medial to the internal capsule
D. Ventral to the splenium of the corpus callosum, dorsal to the quadrigeminal plate, and medial to the thalamus
E. Ventral to the thalamus, dorsal to the lamina terminalis, and ventral to the red nucleus

50.

A 45-year-old man has been in the intensive care unit for 4 days and has had persistent hypercapnia. What is the best change that can be made to his tube feeds?

A. Minimize fats
B. Minimize carbohydrates
C. Minimize proteins
D. Add magnesium
E. Add phosphate

Use the following answers for questions 51 and 52:

A. Benign intracranial hypertension
B. Aseptic meningitis
C. Cerebellar ataxia
D. Cochlear and vestibular damage
E. Unpleasant taste

51.

What are the major potential side effects of vancomycin?

52.

What are the major potential side effects of temozolomide?

53.

A 34-year-old woman on oral contraceptive pills is being evaluated for a posttraumatic headache and blurry vision. Her head CT is shown in this image. What is the most likely diagnosis?

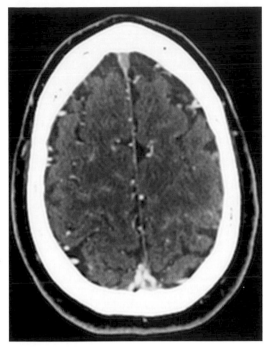

A. Cerebral venous thrombosis
B. Subdural hematoma
C. Subarachnoid hemorrhage
D. Dural arteriovenous fistula
E. Acute ischemic stroke

54.

What is the most common abnormality observed in premature infants with cerebral palsy?

A. Agyria
B. Dandy-Walker variant
C. Craniosynostosis
D. Periventricular leukomalacia
E. Septum cavum

55.

A 40-year-old man with a history of seizures underwent an MRI examination of the brain. Axial T2, noncontrast T1, and susceptibility weighted scans are shown in these images. What is a characteristic of the lesion depicted?

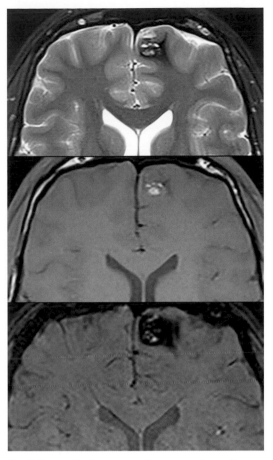

A. It is usually hypervascular on angiography.
B. Diffusion-weighted imaging is the most sensitive technique for its detection.
C. It is associated with developmental venous anomalies.
D. Normal interspersed brain parenchyma is present throughout the lesion.
E. Early venous drainage is diagnostic.

56.

What is the disease course for a patient with idiopathic intracranial hypertension (IIH) who refuses treatment?

A. IIH is self-limiting and will resolve with age regardless of weight and lifestyle changes.
B. IIH will continue to progress indefinitely without treatment.
C. IIH will stabilize at some point.
D. IIH will go into remission and relapse many times throughout a lifetime despite stable weight and lifestyle.
E. IIH prognosis is too variable to predict.

57.
A patient is found to be in a hypertensive crisis after a suicide attempt in which he drank a bottle of wine after taking several pills from the monoamine oxidase inhibitor class of medications. What substance accumulating in his plasma likely accounts for his hypertension?

A. Epinephrine
B. Tyramine
C. Monoamine oxidase
D. Tyrosine
E. Serotonin

58.
When performing deep brain stimulation of the ventral intermediate nucleus of the thalamus (VIM) to treat essential tremor, what side effect is expected if the lead is placed posterior to the VIM?

A. Involuntary muscle contractions
B. Visual deficits
C. Paresthesias
D. Facial contractions
E. Dysarthria

59.
A 10-year-old boy with a history of epilepsy, autism, and developmental delay underwent a CT and an MRI of the brain. What is a characteristic of the entity shown in these images?

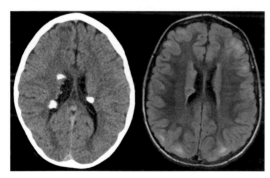

A. Eighty percent of cases are familial.
B. It usually spares the white matter.
C. It occurs as a result of mutations in tumor-suppressor genes.
D. Subependymal lesions should not enhance unless malignant transformation is present.

60.
What ligament is the cephalad extension of the anterior longitudinal ligament?

A. Apical odontoid ligament
B. Anterior atlanto-occipital membrane
C. Posterior atlanto-occipital membrane
D. Tectorial membrane

61.
The medulloblastoma shown in this image represents what subtype?

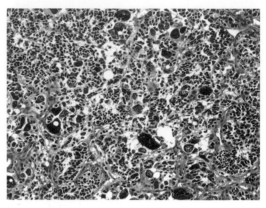

A. Anaplastic
B. Classic
C. Desmoplastic
D. Large cell
E. Excessive nodularity

62.
A 31-year-old previously healthy woman was found unconscious in her apartment. The noncontrast head CT shown in this image demonstrates:

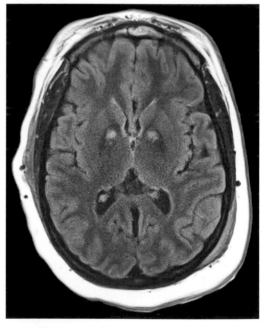

A. Carbon monoxide intoxication
B. Abnormal accumulation of copper
C. Lead poisoning
D. Methanol intoxication

63.
A neuro-oncologist is comparing the effects of drug A and drug B on his patients with glioblastomas. He falsely concludes there is a difference in clinical outcomes between the two drugs when in fact there is no difference. This is an example of what type of statistical error?

A. Type 1 and type 2 error
B. Type 1 and type 3 error
C. Type 1 error only
D. Type 2 error only
E. Type 3 error only

64.
What is the Hook effect?

A. Elevated prolactin levels secondary to pituitary stalk compression
B. A false-negative result when assessing prolactin levels for a suspected prolactinoma
C. Infertility, sexual dysfunction, and amenorrhea
D. Hyponatremia and decreased extracellular fluid volume from the renal loss of sodium
E. High output of hypotonic urine due to insufficient release of antidiuretic hormone

65.
What is the acute respiratory distress syndrome (ARDS) diagnostic triad?

A. Capillary wedge pressure less than 18 mm Hg, bilateral chest infiltrates, and PaO_2/FiO_2 ratio less than 200
B. Capillary wedge pressure less than 30 mm Hg, bilateral chest infiltrates, and PaO_2/FiO_2 ratio less than 200
C. Central venous pressure less than 8 mm Hg, bilateral chest infiltrates, and PaO_2/FiO_2 ratio less than 200
D. Central venous pressure less than 8 mm Hg, bilateral chest infiltrates, and PaO_2/FiO_2 ratio greater than 200
E. Capillary wedge pressure less than 30 mm Hg, bilateral chest infiltrates, and PaO_2/FiO_2 ratio greater than 100

66.
Following a fall on his shoulder, a patient is suspected of having a brachial plexus injury. On exam, his arm hangs by his side and is adducted and medially rotated while his forearm is extended and pronated. Where is the site of this patient's injury?

A. Upper trunk of the brachial plexus
B. Middle trunk of the brachial plexus
C. Lower trunk of the brachial plexus
D. Avulsion of the C5 nerve root
E. Avulsion of the C6 nerve root

67.
A 40-year-old woman is brought to medical attention with rapidly progressive dementia, ataxia, and myoclonus. Her electroencephalogram shows periodic high-voltage sharp waves. MRI of her brain demonstrates cortical ribboning and signal hyperintensity involving the pulvinar and dorsomedial thalamic nuclei on diffusion-weighted imaging (DWI). This thalamic abnormality is thought to be characteristic of what form of the patient's likely disease?

A. Sporadic
B. Variant
C. Familial
D. Iatrogenic

68.
What do type 1 (slow oxidative) muscle fibers possess relative to type 2A (fast oxidative/glycolytic) muscle fibers?

A. Less fatigue resistance
B. Less acidic ATPase activity
C. Greater twitch force
D. Less myoglobin
E. Smaller Z-band width

69.
What are the radiographic and clinical incidences, respectively, of vasospasm after aneurysmal subarachnoid hemorrhage?

A. 50% and 50%
B. 10% and 90%
C. 30% and 70%
D. 70% and 30%
E. 100% and 50%

70.
What percentage of children with a Chiari 2 malformation become clinically symptomatic and require surgical decompression?

A. 10%
B. 30%
C. 50%
D. 80%
E. 100%

71.
What triangle of the skull base is formed by cranial nerves IV and VI and the junction of the superior petrosal sinus and a vein just lateral to the porus trigeminus?

A.   Oculomotor
B.   Parkinson (infratrochlear)
C.   Glasscock
D.   Kawase
E.   Inferolateral

72.
Curvilinear and fingerprint bodies are characteristic ultrastructural (electron microscopic) findings occurring in what disorder?

A.   Fucosidosis
B.   Neuronal ceroid lipofuscinosis
C.   Schindler disease
D.   Sialidosis
E.   Wolman disease

73.
Horner syndrome can be associated with what lesion or pathology?

A.   Thoracic outlet syndrome and Pancoast tumors
B.   Pancoast tumors and shoulder dislocation
C.   Thoracic outlet syndrome and shoulder dislocation
D.   Pancoast tumors and T5 Chance fractures
E.   Thoracic outlet syndrome and T5 Chance fractures

74.
A 39-year-old man presents with progressive back pain. MRI shows a disk space and adjacent vertebral bodies to have decreased signal on T1 sequences and increased signal on T2 sequences. In addition, the disk space and vertebral bodies enhance. What pathology is most consistent with these image findings?

A.   Metastatic tumor
B.   Recurrent disk herniation
C.   Diskitis/osteomyelitis
D.   Tuberculosis

75.
A patient with history of motor weakness, muscular wasting, and progressive bulbar palsy underwent an MRI of his brain, shown in these images. What are possible additional findings of this disease process?

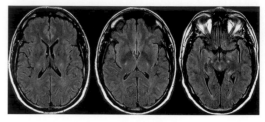

A.   Homogeneous enhancement
B.   Decreased mean diffusivity (MD) in white matter on diffuse tensor imaging
C.   Increased fractional anisotropy (FA) in white matter on diffuse tensor imaging
D.   Elevated choline and myoinositol

End of Section 3. Take a 30-minute lunch break.

Section 4: 60 Minutes, 75 Questions

1.
Noncontrast steady-state free precession (SSFP)-based sequences such as CISS or FIESTA-C are useful to evaluate what segment of the trigeminal nerve?

A.   Nuclear
B.   Parenchymal fascicular
C.   Cisternal
D.   Interdural
E.   Foraminal

2.

What is the enzyme deficiency in Niemann-Pick disease, and what metabolite accumulates?

A. Sphingomyelinase; sphingomyelin
B. Sphingomyelinase; glucocerebroside
C. Hexosaminidase A; GM2 ganglioside
D. Hexosaminidase A; glucocerebroside
E. Glucocerebrosidase; glucocerebroside

Use the following answers for questions 3 and 4:

A. Dorsal root entry zone lesioning
B. C1-C2 cordotomy
C. Spinal cord stimulation
D. Selective dorsal rhizotomy
E. Midline myelotomy

3.

What pain procedure is best for neuropathic leg pain following failed back surgery?

4.

What pain procedure is best for nerve avulsion pain?

5.

As opposed to a proximal median nerve injury, what is preserved on examination of the hand in carpal tunnel syndrome?

A. Thenar eminence muscle strength
B. Flexor pollicis brevis strength
C. Palmar sensation
D. Finger sensation
E. Opponens pollicis strength

6.

A patient with a history of intracranial hemorrhage has been in the hospital for 2 weeks. He suddenly becomes tachypneic and tachycardic, and his capillary oxygen saturation falls. The electrocardiogram is shown in this image. What is the most likely diagnosis for the patient's current condition?

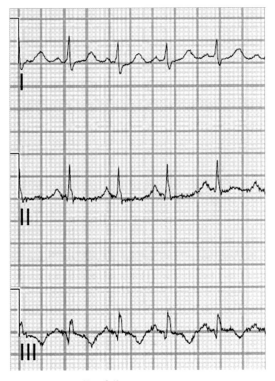

A. Acute cardiac failure
B. Myocardial infarction
C. Pulmonary embolism
D. Spontaneous pneumothorax
E. Pericarditis

7.

What class of medications should most be avoided in a patient with bradykinesia, dementia, and likely ubiquitin-positive Lewy bodies in the cortex on pathological examination?

A. Anticholinergic
B. Dopamine agonist
C. Typical antipsychotic
D. Atypical antipsychotic
E. Nonsteroidal anti-inflammatory

8.

A representative scan from a susceptibility-weighted MRI sequence of a patient's brain is shown in this image. What is correct about this patient's disease entity?

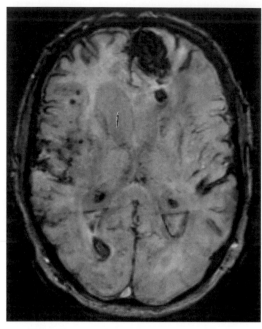

A. Related to poorly controlled hypertension
B. May be related to mutations in the *CCM* gene family
C. May be seen in young patients with sickle cell disease
D. Characterized by β-amyloid peptide deposits

9.

A study has been designed to test the association between weight lifting and the likelihood of developing lumbar back pain. The following results have been obtained:

	No Back Pain	Back Pain	Total
Weight Lifting	80	73	153
No Weight Lifting	72	75	147
Total	152	148	200

What is the best statistical test to assess the association between weight lifting and back pain?

A. Z-test
B. T-test
C. Rank-sum test
D. Chi-square
E. ANOVA

10.

What ganglion receives fibers from the anterior two thirds of the tongue?

A. Pterygopalatine
B. Gasserian
C. Otic
D. Geniculate
E. Nodosal

11.

A 2-year-old boy presents with an inability to track objects without turning his head. He is noted on exam to have a static facial expression, and no movement in the facial musculature is seen bilaterally. He also is noted by his parents to be able to push up when he is in the prone position. What is the patient's diagnosis?

A. Mobius syndrome
B. Duane syndrome
C. Kallmann syndrome
D. Poland anomaly
E. Klippel-Feil anomaly

12.

When attempting to reduce jumped/perched facets, how much weight is used?

A. Enough weight to cause distraction of the disk space more than 10 mm
B. 10 pounds per cervical vertebral level initially, with 10-pound increases until the facets are reduced, neurologic changes occur, disk space height exceeds 10 mm, or occipitocervical instability develops
C. 30 pounds for facet dislocations in the C2 through C5 region and 50 pounds for facet dislocations in the C5 through T1 region
D. 3 pounds, with 1-pound incremental increases
E. 3 pounds per cervical vertebral level, 5- to 10-pound incremental increases not to exceed 5 to 10 pounds per vertebral level

13.

Alzheimer type 2 astrocyte changes marked by astrocytes with large, clear nuclei and marginated chromatin are encountered most commonly with what pathological process?

A. Acute tubular necrosis of the kidney
B. Central pontine myelinolysis
C. Crohn disease
D. Progressive multifocal leukoencephalopathy
E. Wilson disease

14.

Babies with postinfectious and posthemorrhagic hydrocephalus can have the highest success rate of treatment with what procedure?

A. Endoscopic third ventriculostomy (ETV)
B. ETV and choroid plexus coagulation (CPC)
C. Acetazolamide therapy
D. Shunt placement
E. Septum pellucidotomy

15.

What nerve endings are nonencapsulated and are found in the alimentary tract, between epithelial cells of the skin, in the cornea, and in connective tissues?

A. Free nerve endings
B. Merkel disks
C. Hair follicle receptors
D. Meissner corpuscles
E. Pacinian corpuscles

16.

A man with HIV, who is a poorly compliant patient, presents with new-onset seizures. An MRI of the brain shows a ring-enhancing lesion with an eccentric "target" sign on contrast enhanced T1 images. This finding likely represents:

A. Cryptococcosis
B. Toxoplasmosis
C. Lymphoma
D. Cytomegalovirus

17.

The effect of succinylcholine at the neuromuscular junction is most similar to the effect of what other agent?

A. Tubocurarine
B. Decamethonium
C. Vecuronium
D. Acetylcholinesterase
E. Diazepam

18.

A patient is status post–resection of a skull base meningioma. There was a gross total resection; however, the hyperostotic bone and dura were not resected. What is the anticipated recurrence rate?

A. 9%
B. 16%
C. 29%
D. 39%
E. 54%

19.

Areflexia, proximal muscle weakness, and fascicular atrophy on a muscle biopsy in a 2-month-old boy are most likely due to:

A. Duchenne muscular dystrophy
B. Kugelberg-Welander disease
C. Myotonic dystrophy
D. Nemaline rod myopathy
E. Werdnig-Hoffmann disease

20.

What is a characteristic imaging finding of metachromatic leukodystrophy?

A. "Tigroid" pattern
B. Leading edge of enhancement
C. Symmetric basal ganglia lesions
D. T2 hyperintensity in the dorsomedial and pulvinar thalamic nuclei

21.

What extraocular muscle does not originate from the annulus of Zinn?

A. Inferior rectus
B. Inferior oblique
C. Superior oblique
D. Medial rectus
E. Superior rectus

22.

How does synchronized intermittent mandatory ventilation work?

A. Breaths are patient- or time-triggered with a constant tidal volume for each breath.
B. Breaths are patient- or time-triggered, flow limited, and volume cycled; breaths taken by patients are not assisted.
C. Breaths are patient-triggered, and inspiratory pressure is added to patient-initiated breaths.
D. Breaths are not triggered, and continuous pressure is applied to the ventilation circuit throughout the breathing cycle.

23.

A 20-year-old patient with Down syndrome undergoes flexion and extension cervical spine radiographs. The presence of atlantoaxial subluxation is determined by an atlantodental distance greater than:

A. 3 mm
B. 5 mm
C. 7 mm
D. 10 mm

24.

What cranial nerve is not tested during a brain death exam?

A. Cranial nerve II
B. Cranial nerve V
C. Cranial nerve VII
D. Cranial nerve IX
E. Cranial nerve XI

25.

What percentage of children with neurofibromatosis type 1 develops an optic pathway glioma?

A. 5%
B. 20%
C. 50%
D. 70%
E. 100%

26.

A 67-year-old man presents to your office with a complaint of progressive weakness in his hands and problems ambulating. He is hyporeflexic in the upper extremities and hyperreflexic in the lower extremities with nonsustained clonus bilaterally. He has noticeable atrophy in both hands. The sensory exam is unremarkable. The MRI is shown in these images. What is the next step in this patient's management?

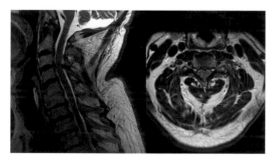

A. Lumbar puncture
B. Cervical myelogram
C. Electromyography
D. Anterior cervical diskectomy and fusion
E. Posterior cervical laminoplasty

27.

A child presents to the pediatric ophthalmologist who finds unilateral glaucoma and a cavernoma of the choroid layer. Family history fails to reveal any genetic abnormalities. What is the patient's likely diagnosis?

A. Neurofibromatosis type 1
B. Neurofibromatosis type 2
C. Tuberous sclerosis
D. Sturge-Weber
E. Von Hippel–Lindau

28.

What is the most common cause of lawsuits and sentinel events?

A. Poor medical knowledge
B. Substandard patient care
C. Poor communication skills
D. Unprofessional behavior
E. Quality of hospital food

29.

What artery is involved in the subacute infarct at the arrow on the head CT study shown in this image?

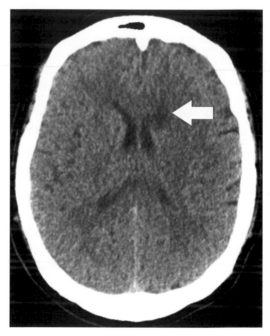

A. Recurrent artery of Heubner
B. Anterior choroidal artery
C. Posterior choroidal artery
D. Lateral lenticulostriate arteries

30.

What is the preferred drug for elevating blood pressure in the setting of vasospasm?

A. Norepinephrine
B. Dopamine
C. Dobutamine
D. Epinephrine
E. Phenylephrine

31.
Regarding radiation, what is the greatest factor determining exposure?

A. Shielding
B. Duration of exposure
C. Distance from source
D. Magnification
E. Collimation

32.
What is the enzyme deficiency in metachromatic leukodystrophy, and what metabolite accumulates?

A. Arylsulfatase A; Sulfatide
B. Sphingomyelinase; Sphingomyelin
C. Hexosaminidase A; G_{M2} Ganglioside
D. Hexosaminidase A; Glucocerebroside
E. Glucosidase; Glucocerebroside

33.
A 32-year-old man underwent a CT of the spine following a motor vehicle collision. What is a characteristic of the pathology shown in this image?

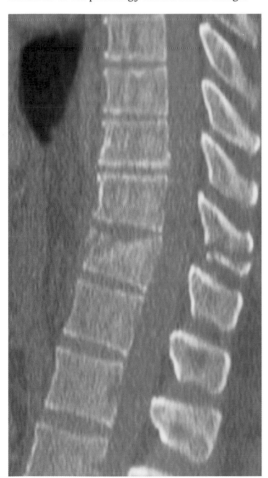

A. The underlying mechanism of injury is hyperextension.
B. It occurs most commonly in the cervical spine.
C. It is secondary to a shear injury.
D. There is a high incidence of concurrent abdominal injuries.
E. Neurologic deficits are more common than with other serious spine injuries.

34.
What is the correct calculation for the equilibrium potential across a neuronal membrane that is permeable to only one ion? The variables and constants are defined as follows:

V_{eq} is the equilibrium potential
R is the universal gas constant
T is the absolute temperature
  z is the number of moles of electrons transferred
F is the Faraday constant
[X]out is the concentration of ions outside the membrane
[X]in is the concentration of ions inside the membrane

A. $V_{eq} = (RT/zF)\ln([X]out/[X]in)$
B. $V_{eq} = (zF/RT)\ln([X]in/[X]out)$
C. $V_{eq} = (RF/zT)\ln([X]out/[X]in)$
D. $V_{eq} = (RT/zF)\ln([X]in/[X]out)$
E. $V_{eq} = (zF/RT)\ln([X]out/[X]in)$

35.
What triangle of the skull base is delineated by the posterior aspect of the mandibular division of the trigeminal nerve and greater petrosal nerve?

A. Oculomotor
B. Parkinson (infratrochlear)
C. Glasscock
D. Kawase
E. Inferolateral

36.
The most commonly involved gene in syndromic craniosynostosis is:

A. *FGFR1*
B. *FGFR2*
C. *FGFR3*
D. *TWIST1*
E. *TWIST2*

37.
A 27-year-old woman is referred to clinic due to bifrontal headaches and a progressive difficulty with breast-feeding and lactation over the past 2 months. She had been breast-feeding successfully for the previous 3 months. On exam, a visual field deficit is noted. The MRI is shown in this image. What is the patient's likely diagnosis?

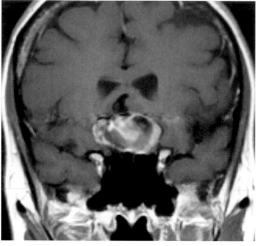

A.   Sheehan syndrome
B.   Anterior communicating artery aneurysm
C.   Prolactinoma
D.   Pituitary apoplexy
E.   Normal physiological decrease in lactation

38.
What inhalation agent is associated with tension pneumocephalus?

A.   Isoflurane
B.   Nitrous oxide
C.   Desflurane
D.   Sevoflurane

39.
What is the outcome of activating the carotid sinus reflex in a patient with a normal blood pressure and heart rate?

A.   Bradycardia and hypertension
B.   Tachycardia and hypotension
C.   Bradycardia and hypotension
D.   Tachycardia and hypertension

40.
What agent reverses angiographic vasospasm following aneurysmal subarachnoid hemorrhage?

A.   Intravenous magnesium sulfate
B.   Intravenous erythropoietin
C.   Intravenous nicardipine
D.   Oral verapamil
E.   Oral nimodipine

41.
A 40-year-old man underwent an MRI of the brain, demonstrating the lesion shown in these images. The lesion was resected and stained positive for vimentin and CD34, with histological analysis demonstrating uniform spindle cells and staghorn vessels. What is the patient's likely diagnosis?

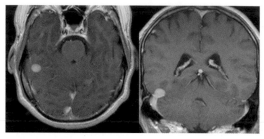

A.   Neurosarcoid
B.   Lymphoma
C.   Meningioma
D.   Hemangiopericytoma

42.
According to the North American Symptomatic Carotid Endarterectomy Trial (NASCET), a carotid endarterectomy is indicated for what type of carotid artery stenosis?

A.   Asymptomatic carotid artery stenosis greater than 60% if the patient is younger than 75 years of age
B.   Symptomatic carotid artery stenosis greater than 60%
C.   Asymptomatic carotid artery stenosis greater than 50%
D.   Symptomatic carotid artery stenosis 70 to 99%
E.   Symptomatic carotid artery stenosis less than 30%

43.
What medication is the first choice for treating partial or secondarily generalized seizures in adults?

A.   Topiramate
B.   Phenobarbital
C.   Valproic acid
D.   Carbamazepine
E.   Levetiracetam

44.

A 45-year-old woman who underwent total bilateral adrenalectomies for Cushing disease 3 years ago returns to clinic with skin hyperpigmentation. What is cause of the hyperpigmentation in this patient?

A. Melanin-stimulating hormone (MSH) over-production

B. Increased production of ACTH secondary to recurrence of Cushing disease

C. New-onset hemochromatosis

D. Postinflammatory hyperpigmentation secondary to decreased total steroids

E. Skin hypersensitivity to the sun

45.

A 24-year-old man presents with progressive back pain. Imaging demonstrated an expansile osteolytic lesion in the posterior elements of the middle thoracic spine with a fluid–fluid level. What is the patient's likely pathology?

A. Spinal metastatic lesion

B. Aneurysmal bone cyst

C. Osteoid osteoma

D. Osteoblastoma

E. Eosinophilic granuloma

46.

What ophthalmologic finding typically is used to screen for suspected nonaccidental trauma in infants?

A. Retinal detachment

B. Retinal hemorrhages

C. Cherry red spot on the retinae

D. Ophthalmoplegia

E. Ptosis

47.

A 4-week-old neonate presents with progressive macrocrania. The Brain MRI, shown in this image, suggests:

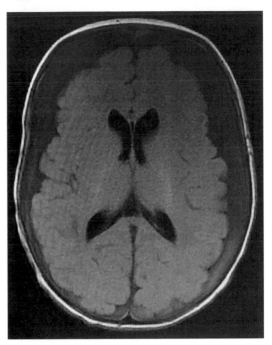

A. Benign extra-axial hygromas

B. Chronic subdural hematomas

C. Hydrocephalus

D. Epidural hematomas

E. Subdural empyemas

48.

In the electron micrograph shown in this image, what component of the sarcomere contains only myosin?

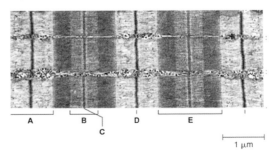

A. A

B. B

C. C

D. D

E. E

49.

At what segment of the vertebral artery shown in this image is the arrow pointing?

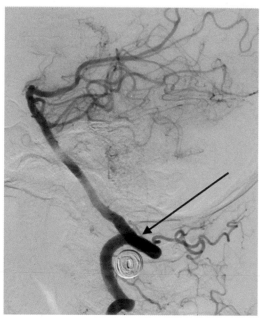

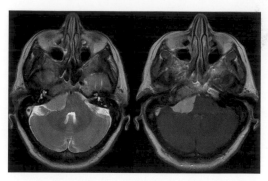

A. V1
B. V2
C. V3
D. V4
E. V5

50.

A 14-year-old boy presents due to progressive difficulty, over the past 2 years, with moving his eyes and forehead. He also is noted to have an ataxic gait and an unknown heart condition. What is the mode of inheritance of the likely disease?

A. Autosomal dominant
B. Autosomal recessive
C. Sex-linked dominant
D. Sex-linked recessive
E. Sporadic mitochondrial

51.

What is a characteristic of the intracranial lesion demonstrated in the MRI scans shown in these images?

A. Most commonly arises from the vestibulocochlear nerve
B. Derives from the inclusion of ectodermal rests during neural tube closure
C. Shows an increased frequency in patients with neurofibromatosis type 1
D. May show a lactate peak on MR spectroscopy

52.

What chemotherapy agent used for central nervous system tumors works by carbamylating amino groups and inducing DNA cross-linking?

A. Carmustine
B. Tamoxifen
C. Temozolomide
D. Cyclophosphamide
E. Cisplatin

53.

What is the blood supply for the intracranial optic nerve?

A. Branches of the middle cerebral, anterior cerebral, and anterior communicating arteries
B. Branches of the internal carotid, anterior cerebral, and anterior communicating arteries
C. Branches of the middle cerebral, posterior cerebral, and anterior communicating arteries
D. Ophthalmic artery alone
E. Branches of the internal carotid, posterior cerebral, and anterior cerebral arteries

54.

During a petrosal approach to a petroclival meningioma, the tentorium is cut where?

A. Anterior to the oculomotor nerve
B. Anterior to the trochlear nerve
C. Lateral to the petrosal sinus
D. Posterior to the trochlear nerve
E. Lateral to greater superficial petrosal nerve

55.

What is the infusion volume of one unit of packed red blood cells in children, and by how much is it expected to increase hemoglobin?

A. 10 cc/kg; 1 g/dL
B. 10 cc/kg; 2 to 3 g/dL
C. 20 cc/kg; 1 g/dL
D. 20 cc/kg; 2 to 3 g/dL
E. 40 cc/kg; 1 g/dL

56.

The lesion seen on the lumbar spine MRI shown in this image is classified as a:

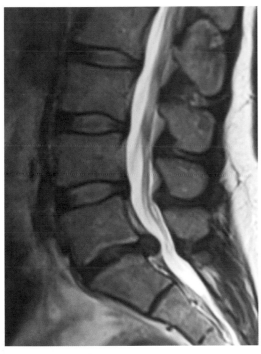

A. Disk protrusion
B. Disk extrusion
C. Disk bulge
D. Sequestered disk
E. Migrated disk

57.

What is true regarding the use of 18-fluoro-2-deoxyglucose (FDG) PET in temporal epilepsy?

A. The area of hypometabolism is smaller than the epileptogenic zone.
B. Studies usually are performed in the ictal phase.
C. There is increased ictal perfusion in the epileptogenic region.
D. There is reduced interictal metabolism in the epileptogenic region.

58.

What is the most likely cause of alexia without agraphia?

A. Left posterior cerebral artery stroke
B. Right posterior cerebral artery stroke
C. Left superior cerebellar artery stroke
D. Right superior cerebellar artery stroke
E. Occlusion of the basilar tip

59.

The results of a meta-analysis are reported using the forest plot shown in this image. What is indicated by the horizontal line length?

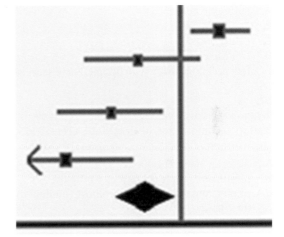

A. The 95% confidence interval range
B. The odds ratio of the study
C. The relative risk of the study
D. The range of values reported by the study
E. The weight of the study as defined by the number of patients

60.

A 40-year-old man presents with a life long history of easy fatigability with exercise and muscle cramping that is relieved with rest. Frustrated by his symptoms, he seeks evaluation. Physical examination and initial laboratory workup is unremarkable. The patient undergoes EMG and nerve conduction studies that show an isolated myopathy with contraction. The patient undergoes a muscle biopsy. Based on the suspected diagnosis, what enzyme deficiency is expected on histochemistry staining?

A. Glucose-6-phosphatase
B. Alpha-1,4 glucosidase
C. Alpha-1,6 glucosidase
D. Branching enzyme
E. Phosphorylase

61.

A patient presents with the visual fields on Goldman visual field testing shown in this image. Where is the patient's lesion?

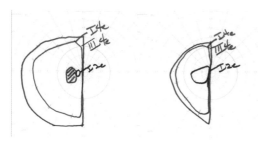

A. Left optic nerve
B. Optic chiasm
C. Left optic tract
D. Left Meyer loop
E. Left occipital cortex with occipital pole sparing

62.

What is the most effective operating room sterilization technique for dealing with Creutzfeldt-Jakob disease (CJD)?

A. Autoclaving for 1 hour at 132°C
B. Immersion in 1 N NaOH for 15 minutes
C. Immersion in sodium hypochlorite (undiluted) for 1 hour
D. Standard sterilization procedures are effective against CJD.

63.

What is a characteristic of the condition illustrated on the MRI shown in these images?

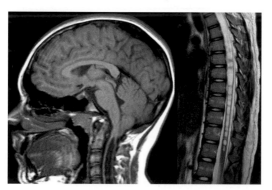

A. An open myelomeningocele is required for its development.
B. It can be associated with Klippel-Feil syndrome.
C. It is related to failure of diverticulation of the brain.
D. It is related to persistence of the embryonic Blake pouch.

64.

A 43-year-old man undergoing treatment for HIV is admitted after subarachnoid hemorrhage from a mycotic cerebral aneurysm. The patient develops a seizure on hospital day 2, with ensuing left-sided hemiplegia that lasts for 24 hours. CT of the head shows no new hemorrhage. What is the most likely diagnosis for the patient's hemiplegia?

A. Cerebral vasospasm
B. Todd paralysis
C. Extension of cerebral edema
D. Electrolyte imbalance
E. Re-hemorrhage

65.

What fibers connect the septal nuclei to the habenula?

A. Stria terminalis
B. Stria medullaris
C. Tract of Vicq d'Azyr
D. Lenticular fasciculus
E. Ansa lenticularis

66.

A woman underwent an MRI of the brain, shown in this image. What is a characteristic of the disease entity presented?

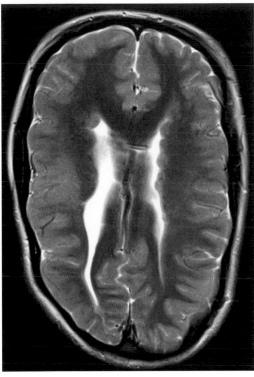

A. It is associated with glioneuronal hamartomas.
B. Enhancement is common.
C. Calcification is common.
D. It may result in ventricular obstruction.
E. It may be associated with callosal abnormalities.

67.

A patient has hypokalemic alkalosis and low serum adrenocorticotropic hormone (ACTH) levels. Where is the patient's lesion?

A. Hypothalamus
B. Pituitary gland
C. Lungs
D. Adrenal glands
E. Kidneys

68.

An 8-year-old child is found to have the lesion shown in this image. What is a characteristic of this entity?

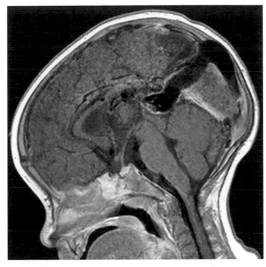

A. Develops due to a high-flow arteriovenous malformation draining into the vein of Galen
B. Characterized by progressive enlargement of the inferior sagittal sinus
C. Usually drains through a dilated inferior petrosal sinus
D. Usually presents as a dilated median prosencephalic vein draining through a persistent falcine sinus
E. Usually drains through a dilated occipital sinus

69.

A woman elects to proceed with stereotactic radiosurgery treatment for trigeminal neuralgia. You counsel her that the average time for treatment response is:

A. 2 to 3 weeks
B. 3 months
C. 6 months
D. 1 year
E. 2 to 3 years

70.

Children with Down syndrome should be screened for what spinal anomaly?

A. Chiari malformation
B. Basilar invagination
C. Odontoid fracture
D. Spinal cord tumor
E. Atlantoaxial instability

71.

A cerebral blood flow less than what rate is associated with the beginning of reversible ischemia?

A. 10 mL per 100 g of tissue/min
B. 15 mL per 100 g of tissue/min
C. 20 mL per 100 g of tissue/min
D. 45 to 60 mL per 100 g of tissue/min
E. 75 to 80 mL per 100 g of tissue/min

72.

What anatomic structure is indicated by the arrow in this image?

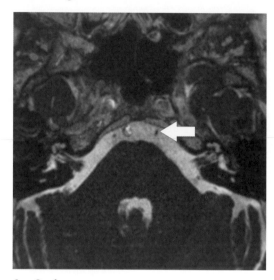

A. Oculomotor nerve
B. Trochlear nerve
C. Trigeminal nerve
D. Abducens nerve
E. Glossopharyngeal nerve

73.

The macula represents:

A. The blind spot
B. The retinal area for vision during good light
C. Closely packed cones where vision is sharpest and color discrimination is most acute
D. The optic nerve
E. Invagination of the hyaloid extending from the optic disk to the lens

74.

An alteration in what protein is responsible for Duchenne muscular dystrophy?

A. Myosin
B. Dystrophin
C. Actin
D. ATP
E. Troponin

75.

What type of visual field deficit may accompany an ophthalmic artery aneurysm?

A. Ipsilateral, monocular, inferior nasal quadrantanopsia
B. Bitemporal, superior quadrantanopsia
C. Ptosis, dilated unreactive pupils, and "down and out" eye deviation
D. Ipsilateral, monocular, inferior temporal quadrantanopsia
E. Ipsilateral, monocular, superior temporal quadrantanopsia

End of Section 4. Take a 10-minute break.

Section 5: 60 Minutes, 75 Questions

1.

Axial contrast-enhanced T1- and T2-weighted MRI scans of the brain of a 33-year-old man are shown in these images. What is the patient's likely diagnosis?

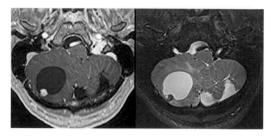

A. Ependymoma
B. Hemangioblastoma
C. Medulloblastoma
D. Juvenile pilocytic astrocytoma
E. Metastasis

2.
Single-voxel MR spectroscopy was performed at 1.5 tesla in a left frontal lobe lesion (TR/TE 1,500/135 ms). The spectral profile obtained, shown is this image, is compatible with what process?

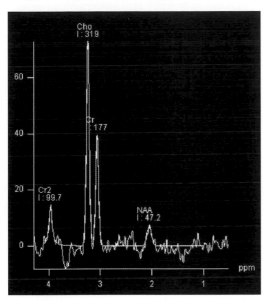

A. Radiation necrosis
B. Abscess
C. High-grade glioma
D. Infarction

3.
What is the formula for estimating a patient's lumbar lordosis (LL)?

A. LL = Pelvic tilt + 10
B. LL = Sacral slope + 5
C. LL = Pelvic tilt + 5
D. LL = Pelvic incidence + 10
E. LL = Pelvic incidence − 10

4.
Meningiomas often are immunoreactive to what antigens?

A. Epithelial membrane antigen and S-100
B. Transthyretin and S-100
C. Vimentin and CD45
D. CD45 and S-100
E. Epithelial membrane antigen and vimentin

5.
A 9-year-old boy presents with a headache, upgaze palsy, and pineal region mass. A cerebrospinal fluid analysis was performed showing elevated β-HCG levels. What tumor type is suspected?

A. Choriocarcinoma
B. Embryonal carcinoma
C. Germinoma
D. Teratoma
E. Yolk sac tumor

6.
What retinal disturbance is produced by prenatal *Cytomegalovirus* infection?

A. Chorioretinitis
B. Microaneurysms
C. Flame-shaped hemorrhages
D. Cotton wool spots
E. Cherry red spots

7.
What is the best description for the acidotic/alkalotic state for a patient with the following set of lab values?

pH: 7.44
P_aCO_2: 26 mm Hg
HCO_3^-: 20 mEq/L
P_aO_2: 53 mm Hg

A. Respiratory alkalosis with no metabolic compensation
B. Metabolic alkalosis with respiratory compensation
C. Respiratory alkalosis with metabolic compensation
D. Mixed respiratory alkalosis and metabolic acidosis
E. Combined respiratory and metabolic alkalosis

8.

The microscopic finding shown is this image corresponds to what histological element?

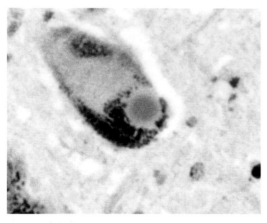

A. Cowdry body
B. Lewy body
C. Melanoma cell
D. Negri body
E. Neurofibrillary tangle

9.

Light-touch fibers from the trigeminal nerve synapse on the main (principal) trigeminal nucleus and pass through the trigeminothalamic tract to synapse on what thalamic nucleus?

A. Ventral posterior medial nucleus
B. Ventral posterior lateral nucleus
C. Ventral anterior nucleus
D. Dorsal medial nucleus
E. Ventral medial nucleus

10.

In a patient with optic neuritis, what characteristics differentiate neuromyelitis optica (NMO) from multiple sclerosis (MS)?

A. NMO-IgG antibodies are found only in NMO, not in MS.
B. There typically is a secondary progressive phase with NMO.
C. NMO but not MS has spinal lesions.
D. MS clearly is an autoimmune disease, whereas NMO is not.
E. The brain lesions in NMO are more acute in onset than those in MS.

11.

According to recommendations from the 7th American College of Chest Physicians Conference on Antithrombotic and Thrombolytic Therapy: Evidence-Based Guidelines, what are the level 1 recommendations for the prevention of venous thromboembolism in neurosurgery patients?

A. There is no level 1 evidence for the use of thromboprophylaxis in neurosurgical patients.
B. The use of intermittent pneumatic compression with or without graduated compression stockings is recommended in all patients undergoing intracranial neurosurgery.
C. The use of low-dose unfractionated heparin and postoperative low molecular weight heparin is recommended in patients undergoing intracranial neurosurgery.
D. The combination of mechanical prophylaxis (graduated compression stockings and/or intermittent pneumatic compression) is recommended in high-risk neurosurgery patients.
E. Thromboprophylaxis should be used in all neurosurgical spinal patients.

12.

What is an inheritance pattern of the condition shown on the MRI scans shown in these images?

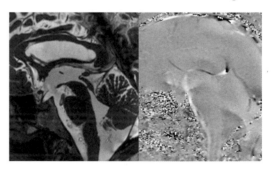

A. X-linked recessive
B. X-linked dominant
C. Autosomal dominant
D. Autosomal recessive

13.

From what developmental division of the embryonal nervous system does the facial nucleus arise?

A. Myelencephalon
B. Diencephalon
C. Telencephalon
D. Metencephalon
E. Mesencephalon

14.

A 68-year-old woman with chronic atrial fibrillation and hypertension maintained on warfarin presents for a pure sensory stroke affecting her right side. What is the most likely stroke etiology and site of injury?

A. Atrial thrombus; primary sensory cortex
B. Atrial thrombus; posteroventral nucleus of the thalamus
C. Lacunar infarct; primary sensory cortex
D. Lacunar infarct; posteroventral nucleus of the thalamus
E. Carotid thrombus; primary sensory cortex

15.

A 62-year-old man with a history of smoking and chronic exposure to wood dust presents with symptoms of nasal obstruction, facial pain, and nasal discharge. An MRI was performed, and a representative scan is shown in this image. What is the likely diagnosis?

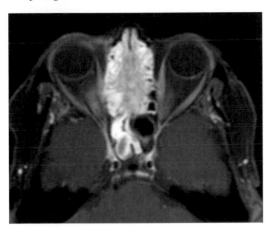

A. Mucocele
B. Sinusitis
C. Nasopharyngeal angiofibroma
D. Sinonasal carcinoma
E. Rhabdomyosarcoma

16.

Using the International League Against Epilepsy (ILAE) classification for focal cortical dysplasia, the pattern shown in this image is best categorized as what type?

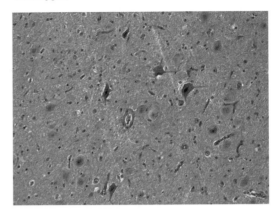

A. Type 1a
B. Type 1b
C. Type 1c
D. Type 2a
E. Type 2b

17.

What are the criteria for monitoring personnel to notify the surgeon about during somatosensory evoked potential recording intraoperatively?

A. More prominent waveforms
B. Decrease in peak amplitude more than 50% and decrease in latency more than 10%
C. Increase in peak amplitude more than 50% and decrease in latency more than 50%
D. Decrease in peak amplitude more than 50% and increase in latency more than 50%
E. Decrease in peak amplitude more than 50% and increase in latency more than 10%

18.

In patients with intracranial pressure monitors, what waveform is characterized by Traube-Hering arterial waves that have variable intracranial pressure elevations with a frequency of 4 to 8 per minute?

A. Lundberg A waves
B. Lundberg B waves
C. Lundberg C waves
D. Lundberg D waves

19.

A 38-year-old woman with a history of Hodgkin lymphoma treated with brentuximab presents with altered mental status. Axial T2- and postcontrast T1-weighted images of the brain are shown in these images. The lesions did not show restricted diffusion. What is the likely diagnosis?

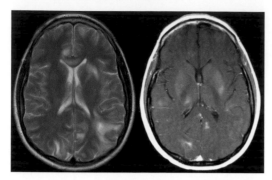

A. Immune reconstitution inflammatory syndrome
B. Acute disseminated encephalomyelitis
C. Tumefactive demyelination
D. Central nervous system lymphoma

Use the following information to answer questions 20 to 22:

A scientist has developed an innovative blood test for the early diagnosis of brain tumors in mice. When conducting his test on a group of 100 mice, he finds the following results:

	Positive Test	Negative Test
Have Disease	40	10
No Disease	20	30

20.
What is the specificity of the test?

A. 10%
B. 20%
C. 60%
D. 80%
E. 90%

21.
What is the sensitivity of the test?

A. 10%
B. 30%
C. 60%
D. 80%
E. 90%

22.
What is the positive predictive value of the test?

A. 33%
B. 67%
C. 75%
D. 80%
E. 90%

23.
A 7-year-old child has a history of recurrent pneumococcal meningitis. Brain MRI likely will demonstrate what congenital lesion?

A. Dandy-Walker malformation
B. Agenesis of the corpus callosum
C. Temporal arachnoid cyst
D. Ethmoidal encephalocele
E. Chiari malformation

24.
What is a neuroimaging characteristic of adamantinomatous craniopharyngiomas compared with the papillary subtype?

A. The adamantinomatous subtype more commonly is solid.
B. The adamantinomatous subtype occurs more commonly in older individuals.
C. The adamantinomatous subtype more commonly calcifies.
D. The adamantinomatous subtype more commonly is located at the infundibulum.
E. The adamantinomatous subtype more avidly enhances.

25.
Alzheimer type 2 astrocyte changes marked by astrocytes with large, clear nuclei and marginated chromatin are encountered most commonly with what pathological process?

A. Acute tubular necrosis of the kidney
B. Central pontine myelinolysis
C. Crohn disease
D. Progressive multifocal leukoencephalopathy
E. Wilson disease

26.
What is the precursor amino acid involved in the synthesis of melatonin?

A. Tryptophan
B. Glycine
C. Threonine
D. Proline
E. Tyrosine

27.

Nociceptive pain travels along what spinal tract?

A. Lateral spinothalamic tract
B. Anterior spinothalamic tract
C. Dorsal spinocerebellar tract
D. Dorsal columns

28.

A 45-year-old man has paralysis in cranial nerves IX through XII. What is the most likely diagnosis?

A. Medial medullary syndrome
B. Brainstem stroke
C. Glomus jugulare tumor
D. Lateral medullary syndrome
E. Lateral pontine syndrome

29.

What is the Magerl technique for placement of lateral mass screws?

A. Use a starting point 1 mm medial to the midpoint of the lateral mass and the midpoint of the mass in the craniocaudal axis, and aim 30 degrees laterally and 15 degrees cephalad.
B. Use a starting point 2 mm medial and 1 to 2 mm superior to the center of the lateral mass, and aim 20 to 25 degrees laterally and 30 degrees superiorly (parallel to facet joint).
C. Use a starting point at the midpoint of the mediolateral and craniocaudal axes of the lateral mass, and aim 0 to 10 degrees laterally and 0 degrees in the craniocaudal axis.
D. Use a starting point at the contralateral spinolaminar junction, and aim toward the junction of the transverse process and contralateral superior facet.
E. Use a starting point at the mid–facet line where the superior facet joins the transverse process, and aim 5 to 10 degrees medially and 10 to 20 degrees caudally

30.

A 53-year-old man patient with a sudden onset of headache and meningismus underwent a CT of the head that showed a small amount of subarachnoid blood limited to the prepontine and interpeduncular cisterns. Conventional angiography at admission and 2 weeks later was negative for a vascular lesion. What is a characteristic of this patient's likely entity?

A. It has a high incidence of re-hemorrhage.
B. It has a high incidence of hydrocephalus.
C. It represents an aneurysm often obscured by vasospasm.
D. A sentinel headache usually is absent.

31.

An 8-year-old girl presents with medically intractable seizures and focal atrophy of the right frontal lobe. Tissue is resected from the area of atrophy and is shown in this image. What is the most likely diagnosis?

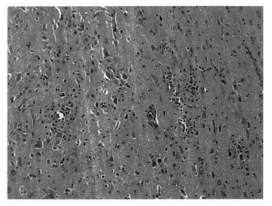

A. Focal cortical dysplasia
B. Low-grade glioma
C. Normal
D. Rasmussen encephalitis
E. Remote infarct

32.

Propofol acts primarily through:

A. Potentiation of $GABA_A$ and $GABA_B$ receptors
B. Sodium and potassium channel blockade
C. Only the endocannabinoid system
D. Glutamate inhibition and potassium channel potentiation
E. Potentiation of $GABA_A$ receptors, sodium channel blockade, and the endocannabinoid system

33.

How do baroreceptors in the aortic arch signal increasing pressure?

A. They all are tonically active and increase the frequency of action potentials.
B. They all are tonically active and increase the amplitude of action potentials.
C. They all are inactive at rest and begin firing action potentials.
D. Both the receptors at rest and the tonically active receptors begin firing action potentials.
E. Both the receptors at rest and the tonically active receptors begin firing and increase the frequency of action potentials.

34.
Schizencephaly is a condition of what broad etiology?

A. Demyelinating illness
B. Neurodegeneration
C. Improper neuronal migration
D. Neoplastic processes
E. Psychiatric disorder

35.
At what dermatomal level is the nipple located?

A. C1
B. C7
C. T2
D. T4
E. T10

36.
A patient presents with polytrauma after a motor vehicle collision, with multiple skull base and facial fractures. The patient is discharged and returns with chemosis, pulsatile proptosis, and an ocular bruit. Angiogram reveals a low-flow shunt feeding from meningeal branches of the external carotid artery. What type of carotid-cavernous fistula does this patient have?

A. Type A
B. Type B
C. Type C
D. Type D

37.
What is an expected imaging finding in a patient with intracranial hypotension?

A. Collapsed dural venous sinuses
B. Increased mamillopontine distance
C. Increased pontomesencephalic angle
D. Increased leptomeningeal enhancement
E. Engorged pituitary gland

38.
How does the syndrome of inappropriate antidiuretic hormone secretion (SIADH) affect cerebral edema?

A. SIADH decreases cerebral edema.
B. SIADH increases cerebral edema.
C. SIADH has no effect on cerebral edema.
D. SIADH decreases and then increases cerebral edema.

39.
During a neuron's absolute refractory period, what is the approximate equilibrium potential of its membrane?

A. -90 mV
B. -65 mV
C. -55 mV
D. 0 mV
E. $+30$ mV

40.
The histological section shown in this image, which is taken from a 6-month-old infant, demonstrates widespread positive staining with an antibody to herpes. This infection is thought to represent a congenital infection related to maternal transmission of the virus during pregnancy. What potential intra-amniotic infectious agent presents in a different fashion?

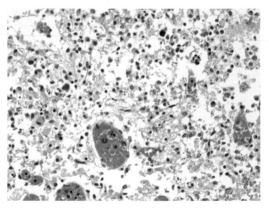

A. *Candida*
B. Cytomegalovirus
C. HIV
D. Rubella
E. Toxoplasmosis

41.

A 73-year-old woman without a pertinent medical history presents with persistent lower back pain for several weeks. A CT scan is performed, shown in this image. It demonstrates a(n):

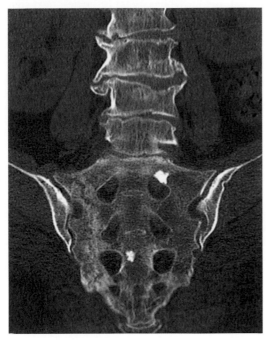

A. Blastic metastasis
B. Sacral insufficiency fracture
C. Acute traumatic fracture of the sacrum
D. Chordoma
E. Sacroiliitis

42.

The superior salivatory nucleus gives rise to axons that project along which cranial nerve?

A. Cranial nerve V
B. Cranial nerve VII
C. Cranial nerve IX
D. Cranial nerve X
E. Cranial nerve XII

43.

A 3-year-old boy is referred for evaluation due to progressive blindness, deafness, and an inability to swallow. The patient is found to have infantile Tay-Sachs disease. Absence of what functional enzyme is responsible for this patient's neurologic deficit?

A. Glucocerebrosidase
B. Alpha-galactosidase
C. Sphingomyelinase
D. Hexosaminidase A
E. Phosphofructokinase

44.

A patient underwent an endoscopic transsphenoidal resection of a pituitary adenoma. There was significant bleeding during the enlargement of the sphenoid opening. He presents 5 days later with significant epistaxis requiring transfusion. An angiogram of the internal cerebral artery is unremarkable. What is the most likely cause of the epistaxis?

A. Pseudoaneurysm of the internal carotid artery not seen during angiogram
B. Injury to the ophthalmic artery
C. Delayed oozing from the superior turbinate resection
D. Injury to the sphenopalatine artery
E. Injury to the inferior hypophyseal artery

45.

Axonal transport of materials within the neuron occurs at what overall maximal speed and in what direction?

A. Vesicles at 400 mm per day in the retrograde direction
B. Cytoskeletal proteins at 400 mm per day in the orthograde direction
C. Vesicles at 400 mm per day in the orthograde direction
D. Cytoskeletal proteins at 8 mm per day in the retrograde direction
E. Vesicles at 8 mm per day in the orthograde direction

46.

An MRI of the brain of a child shows absence of the septum pellucidum and diminutive optic nerves. What may be an additional finding with this patient's syndrome?

A. Monoventricle
B. High-riding third ventricle
C. "Viking helmet" appearance of the lateral ventricles
D. Hypoplastic or absent infundibulum

47.

What skin lesion is most likely to be present in an 8-year-old patient with epilepsy and with the findings shown in this image from a brain histological specimen?

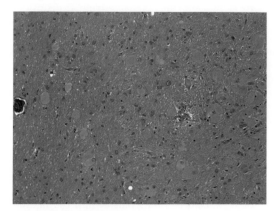

A. Adenoma sebaceum
B. Basal cell carcinoma
C. Café-au-lait spot
D. Epidermal inclusion cyst
E. Tricholemmoma

48.

What finding is demonstrated on this funduscopic image?

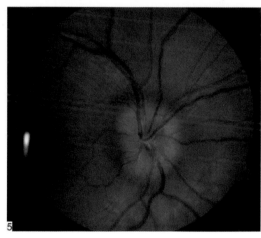

A. Drusen
B. Normal fundus
C. Pseudopapilledema
D. Papilledema
E. Neuroretinitis

49.

A 39-year-old woman undergoes general anesthesia for an elective diskectomy. As the anesthesia begins, her jaw muscles become tense, and she becomes rigid. She then develops fever, tachycardia, and tachypnea. What is the best next step in the management of this patient?

A. Apply cooling blankets.
B. Administer an intravenous fluid bolus.
C. Administer dantrolene.
D. Administer phenobarbital.
E. Administer succinylcholine.

50.

Fill in the blanks.

Wallenberg syndrome classically is defined as occlusion of the _____ but most commonly occurs from occlusion of the _____.

A. Superior cerebellar artery; posterior inferior cerebellar artery
B. Vertebral artery; superior cerebellar artery
C. Anterior inferior cerebellar artery; vertebral artery
D. Posterior inferior cerebellar artery; vertebral artery
E. Posterior inferior cerebellar artery, superior cerebellar artery

51.

The origin of the recurrent artery of Heubner occurs most commonly off of what segment of the anterior cerebral artery (ACA) circulation?

A. A1
B. At the junction of the anterior communication artery and the ACA
C. A2
D. Anterior communicating artery

52.

What is a primary central nervous system lymphoma?

A. High-grade, non-Hodgkin B-cell neoplasm
B. Hodgkin lymphoma
C. Burkitt lymphoma
D. Lymphomatous meningitis

53.

A man with clinical hypercortisolism undergoes a dexamethasone suppression test. He has no changes in his cortisol levels with low-dose dexamethasone administration; however, cortisol is suppressed with high-dose dexamethasone. What is the most likely diagnosis?

A. Cushing syndrome
B. Ectopic ACTH production
C. Cushing disease
D. Addison disease

54.

Bcl-2 plays what role in apoptosis?

A. Inhibits apoptosis
B. Promotes apoptosis
C. Can either promote or inhibit apoptosis
D. Acts as a caspase
E. Blocks p53 signaling

55.

A woman with Bell palsy is treated with prednisone and recovers slowly over the next 2 months. Despite her recovery, she notices involuntary twitching in the right corner of her mouth each time she tries to blink her right eye. What is the cause of the patient's symptoms?

A. Aberrant regeneration of the facial nerve
B. Transient ischemic attack
C. Steroid side effects
D. New injury to the facial nerve
E. Trigeminal neuralgia

56.

An atlantodental interval of 5 mm on CT imaging in an adult is indicative of:

A. Anterior atlanto-occipital dislocation
B. Atlantoaxial instability
C. Longitudinal atlanto-occipital dislocation
D. A normal finding
E. Alar ligament injury

57.

On axial sections, the claustrum separates what two structures?

A. Internal capsule and lentiform nucleus
B. Insula and lentiform nucleus
C. Insula and extreme capsule
D. Globus pallidus and putamen
E. External capsule and extreme capsule

58.

A 35-year-old pregnant woman with eclampsia, agitation, and headaches underwent an MRI examination of the brain, shown in these images. What is the likely diagnosis?

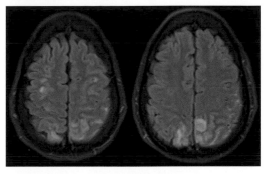

A. Posterior reversible encephalopathy
B. Superior sagittal sinus thrombosis
C. Posterior circulation infarction
D. Hypoxic ischemic encephalopathy

59.

What is the most common cause of nyctalopia?

A. Xeroderma pigmentosum
B. Retinitis pigmentosa
C. De Morsier syndrome
D. Wyburn-Mason syndrome
E. Balint syndrome

60.

What is the likely diagnosis represented in the gradient echo based and diffusion-weighted sequences shown in these images?

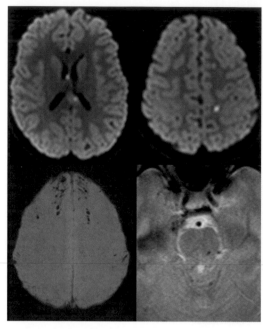

A. Chronic hypertensive encephalopathy
B. Cortical contusions
C. Fat embolism
D. Septic emboli
E. Diffuse axonal injury

61.

A 7-month-old baby underwent a posterior fossa tumor resection in the prone position. A postoperative CT, shown in this image, was performed to evaluate poor mental status. The next step in this patient's management should be:

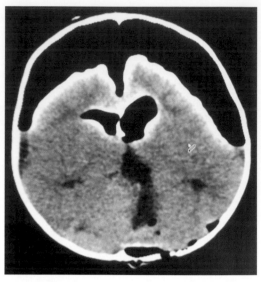

A. Conservative observation
B. Placement of an external ventricular drain
C. Percutaneous aspiration of pneumocephalus
D. Posterior fossa exploration
E. Obtaining an MRI

62.

What is the etiology of blindness unique to the transseptal approach to the sella turcica?

A. Damage to cranial nerves from a cavernous sinus hematoma
B. Orbital wall fracture
C. Devascularization of the optic chiasm
D. Injury to the ophthalmic artery
E. Injury to the optic radiations

63.

Fill in the blanks.

In addition to nausea, vomiting, and vertigo, Wallenberg (lateral medullary) syndrome includes _____ loss of pain and temperature sensation in the face, _____ loss of pain and temperature sensation in the body, _____ limb ataxia, and _____ Horner syndrome.

A. Ipsilateral; ipsilateral; contralateral; ipsilateral
B. Ipsilateral; contralateral; contralateral; ipsilateral
C. Ipsilateral; contralateral; ipsilateral; ipsilateral
D. Contralateral; ipsilateral; ipsilateral; ipsilateral
E. Contralateral; contralateral; ipsilateral; contralateral

64.

A patient has the following serum labs:

Sodium (Na): 144
Potassium (K): 3.5
Chloride (Cl): 102
CO_2: 24
Blood urea nitrogen (BUN): 14
Creatinine (Cr): 0.5
Glucose: 180

What is the calculated serum osmolarity?

A. 258.5
B. 305.5
C. 307.5
D. 305
E. 302

65.

Activation of which receptor primarily produces hallucinations and tachycardia?

A. Delta opioid receptor
B. Mu opioid receptor
C. Sigma receptor
D. Nociceptin receptor
E. Kappa opioid receptor

66.

What is the blood supply for the superior cerebellar peduncle?

A. Basilar perforators
B. Posterior inferior cerebellar artery
C. Superior cerebellar artery
D. Anterior inferior cerebellar artery
E. Posterior cerebral artery

67.

Posterior communicating artery aneurysms usually have what orientation and origin compared to the parent vessel?

A. Oriented anteriorly and arising from the anterior wall
B. Oriented posteriorly and arising from the posterior wall
C. Oriented anteriorly and arising from the posterior wall
D. Oriented posteriorly and arising from the anterior wall
E. Oriented medially and arising from the anterior wall

68.

A patient had an acute exacerbation of his epilepsy and developed hives throughout his entire body after receiving an intravenous narcotic. What agent did he likely receive?

A. Morphine
B. Meperidine
C. Fentanyl
D. Sufentanil
E. Alfentanil

69.

Presence of or abnormalities in what genes have been shown to increase susceptibility for development of the pathology shown on these CT images?

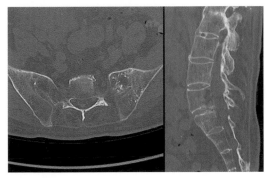

A. PTPN22
B. HLA-DRB1
C. HLA-B27
D. PHEX

70.

What is the recommended treatment for peripheral neuropathy of chronic renal failure?

A. Phenytoin
B. Renal transplantation
C. Thiamine
D. Gabapentin
E. Vitamin B12

71.

The patient with the pathology shown in this image presented at 9 months of age with psychomotor retardation, myoclonus, hypotonia, and a cherry red spot in his macula. The patient has a deficiency in hexosaminidase A. What is the most likely diagnosis?

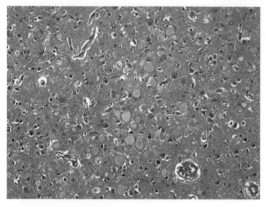

A. Fabry disease
B. Neuronal ceroid lipofuscinosis
C. Niemann-Pick disease
D. Tay-Sachs disease
E. Wolman disease

72.

What is a feature of the lesion shown in these images?

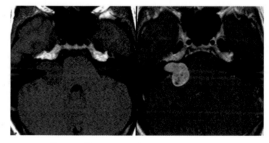

A. Confers a diagnosis of neurofibromatosis type 1 if occurring bilaterally
B. Propensity for perineural spread
C. Low incidence of cystic changes
D. Origin at the glial–Schwann cell junction
E. Origin from arachnoid cap cells

73.

Pedicle screws often fail along what portion of the screw?

A. Threads
B. Point of minimal diameter
C. Screw tip
D. Point of maximal stress
E. Screw head

74.

Subependymal giant cell astrocytomas are found in patients with what disease/syndrome?

A. Sporadic (nonsyndromic)
B. Neurofibromatosis type 2
C. Tuberous sclerosis
D. Von Hippel–Lindau disease
E. Osler-Weber-Rendu syndrome

75.

What disease process is most likely to result in the vertebral abnormalities shown in these images?

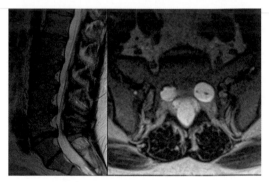

A. Multiple myeloma
B. Neurofibromatosis type 2
C. Diskitis
D. Mucopolysaccharidoses

22 Practice Exam Answers

Section 1

1.

D Optic nerve

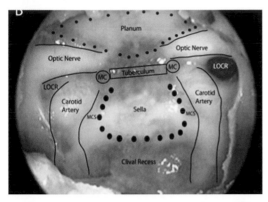

The anatomy during the transnasal transsphenoidal approach is shown in this image. MC, middle clinoid process; MCS, medial cavernous sinus; LOCR; lateral opticocarotid recess.

2.

A Central neurocytoma

The MRI scans accompanying the question show a heterogeneous intraventricular mass attached to the septum pellucidum that has solid components and areas of cystic change, with a bubbly or spongiform appearance. Of the given options, the features are most consistent with a central neurocytoma, although ependymomas can sometimes have a similar appearance. Central neurocytomas are WHO grade II neuroepithelial neoplasms that occur most commonly in patients between 20 and 40 years of age. Enhancement is variable and may be minimal, as seen in this case. Patients typically present with headaches, seizures, or symptoms of increased intracranial pressure. (B) Most intraventricular meningiomas are solid appearing and enhance avidly, although they can be heterogeneous and show cystic changes, calcifications, and even hemorrhage. (C) Intraventricular metastases are rare and usually demonstrate moderate to marked contrast enhancement. (D) Choroid plexus papillomas enhance avidly and typically show a frond-like margin with a texture that is similar to that of the normal choroid plexus. (E) Subependymal giant cell astrocytomas are seen almost exclusively in the setting of tuberous sclerosis. They almost always enhance avidly, and most commonly occur in the frontal horns in or around the foramina of Monro.

3.

A Neurosecretory vesicles–neurophysin complex

Several studies support neurosecretory granules (particularly antidiuretic hormone) as being the cause of the expected T1 shortening (hyperintensity) in the posterior pituitary gland. Specifically, antidiuretic hormone generally is accepted as the source, although oxytocin has been implicated by some sources. Neurosecretory granules form a complex with neurophysins, which are carrier proteins for transportation from the supraoptic and paraventricular nuclei of the hypothalamus. The presence of hyperintensity indicates the functional integrity of the posterior pituitary gland. It can be absent in diabetes insipidus or surgical or traumatic transection of the stalk. It also can be absent in about 10% of the population. (B) Calcification most typically is associated with signal intensity loss on T1; however, at lower concentrations of calcium, T1 shortening effects (hyperintensity) predominate, whereas at higher concentrations there usually is signal loss due to susceptibility effects. This is not the cause of the posterior pituitary bright spot. (C) Ferritin-bound iron has T1 shortening effects and can look bright; however, this is not the source of the posterior pituitary hyperintensity. Hemosiderin-bound iron does not have a significant T1 shortening effect. (D) Manganese has T1 shortening effects such as in the basal ganglia in liver disease, but this is not present in sufficient concentrations in the pituitary gland to result in significant hyperintensity.

4.

D Contralateral subthalamic nucleus

The basal ganglia are composed of the caudate nucleus, putamen, globus pallidus (GP), subthalamic nucleus (STN), and substantia nigra. These structures connect to other areas of the brain and are involved in numerous functions, including motor control. The STN is located just inferior to the thalamus and makes glutamatergic, excitatory connections to the globus pallidus and the substantia nigra. This is the only purely excitatory pathway among the intrinsic pathways of the basal ganglia. Injury to the subthalamic semilunar nucleus of Luys or its efferent or afferent connections can induce hemiballismus. The STN itself is a regulator of motor function and is involved in associative and limbic functions. It traditionally was thought that hemiballismus was only caused by injury to the STN, but new studies are showing that it can occur with damage to other areas of the brain. Hemiballismus arising from the STN is more severe than other forms of the disorder. Recent studies show that hemiballistic movements also may be associated with a decreased output from the GP. Decreased activity in the GP prevents inhibition of the motor portion of the thalamus, leading to characteristic large, irregular hemiballistic movements. Finally, the caudate nucleus helps control voluntary movement, and damage to this area may result in hemiballismus due to its involvement with voluntary movement. (A, B) The putamen projects to the premotor cortex through the globus pallidus. Damage to the putamen also can cause hemiballistic movements.

5.

D Ventral intermediate nucleus of the thalamus

Stimulation of the ventral intermediate nucleus of the thalamus offers the best control of essential tremors and "tremor dominant" Parkinson disease. (A) The globus pallidus pars externa is not a standard target for deep brain stimulation. (B, E) Stimulation of both the subthalamic nucleus and globus pallidus pars interna produces similar symptom relief with regard to the motor symptoms of parkinsonism (e.g., bradykinesia, tremor, and rigidity). Stimulation of the globus pallidus interna is effective especially at relieving symptoms of dystonia. (C) Stimulation of the head of the caudate nucleus is used for symptom relief in obsessive-compulsive disorder.

6.

C Cytokeratin AE1/AE3

The meninges shown in the image accompanying the question are marked by increased cellularity. Many of the cells appear to have eccentric nuclei and cytoplasm, with more cytoplasm present than is usually seen with lymphoid cells. The pathology is that of leptomeningeal carcinomatosis. Keratin antibody stains such as cytokeratin AE1/AE3 best highlight these cells.

7.

D Thalamostriate vein, as shown in this image.

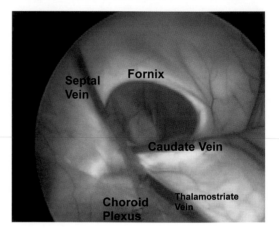

8.

E It may be associated with *SDHx* gene mutations.

The images accompanying the question show an avidly enhancing mass in the left jugular foramen that is compatible with a glomus jugulare, given its high uptake on the ^{111}In-DTPA-pentetreotide scan. These lesions are highly vascular masses that may show a "salt-and-pepper" appearance on noncontrast T1 images due to areas of hemorrhage and small vascular flow voids, respectively. About one third of paragangliomas may be part of a germline mutation particularly related to the succinate dehydrogenase gene group. Other associations include von Hippel–Lindau and multiple endocrine neoplasia type 2 syndromes. (A) Only 3% of paragangliomas are multicentric except for familial lesions, which may be multiple in 25% of patients. (B) It is believed that vestibular schwannomas arise at the glial–Schwann cell (Obersteiner-Redlich) transition zone. (C) Sporadic paragangliomas are much more common in females. Hereditary paragangliomas have a more or less equal distribution across the genders. (D) The majority of paragangliomas are benign, with malignant tumors being rare.

9.

D Vestibular schwannoma

Chemotherapy has shown some promise in treating neurofibromatosis type 2–related vestibular schwannomas with demonstrated progressive growth. (A–C) Most meningiomas, epidermoids, and choroid plexus papillomas are WHO grade I lesions and are not treated with chemotherapy. (E) Ependymomas do not respond well to chemotherapy, although there are some newer protocols that show some promise. In addition, chemotherapy may be used in children under 3 years of age in an attempt to delay radiotherapy.

10.

C Systems-based practice

Systems-based practice describes multidisciplinary approaches to patient care and the ability to optimize care by involving multiple teams in patient management. (A) Medical knowledge describes the ability to acquire and apply current medical knowledge and use advanced search engines to stay current on medical knowledge and data. (B) Professionalism describes the ability to demonstrate the principles of ethical behavior. (D) Practice-based learning and improvement describes the ability to appraise information critically on a daily basis and to analyze it in a way that improves patient care. (E) Interpersonal skills and communication skills refer to a resident's ability to communicate effectively among colleagues in his and in other specialties. It also refers to the ability of a resident to share his research and demonstrate leadership skills.

11.

B B

The American Spinal Injury Association (ASIA) impairment scale indicates the completeness of a spinal cord injury. An A classification represents a "complete" injury, whereas classifications B through D represent "incomplete" injuries. With a B classification, there is preservation of sensation in the S4 and S5 dermatomes but no motor function below the level of injury. A C classification indicates that more than half of the muscles below the level of injury have a motor grade less than 3. Classification D indicates that more than half of the muscles below the level of injury have a motor grade of at least 3. The E classification is reserved for full motor and sensory function and is used to describe patients with spinal cord injuries (i.e., it is not a way to document a normal neurologic exam in a patient without injuries).

12.

A Induction agent, paralytic agent, intubation

Rapid sequence intubation (RSI) is designed to intubate patients who are at risk of vomiting and thus aspiration. Its use does not require preventilation with a bag valve mask. RSI involves administration of an induction agent (typically etomidate) followed by a paralytic agent (succinylcholine or rocuronium). The goal is to render the patient unconscious and paralyzed within 1 minute. This then is followed by intubation.

13.

E No additional nuclei

(A–D) The dentate, emboliform, globose, and fastigial nuclei are the deep cerebellar nuclei and can be remembered by the mnemonic "*D*on't *e*at *g*reasy *f*ood."

14.

E Number of transmembrane channels specific for the diffusing molecule

Facilitated diffusion requires transmembrane channels to allow molecules to diffuse across an otherwise impermeable membrane along a concentration gradient. This process thus is limited by the number of transmembrane channels. (A) A molecule undergoing facilitated diffusion must have a binding site on its transmembrane channel. More binding sites mean that more molecules can diffuse across the membrane. (B) Cell membranes with their phospholipid bilayer are lipophilic and prevent the simple diffusion of certain molecules across the membranes. These hydrophilic molecules are the ones that require the use of transmembrane channels; thus, the actual process of facilitated diffusion avoids the membranes' limitations and is not affected by cell membrane composition. (C) Large concentration gradients assist with facilitated diffusion. (D) ATP is involved in active transport. Facilitated diffusion requires no direct energy input.

15.

C Predictor of mortality

Although other uses for the intracranial hemorrhage (ICH) score have been extrapolated, the ICH score was designed to predict mortality. An ICH score of 0 is associated with a 0% 30-day mortality, whereas patients with a score of 5 or 6 have a 100% 30-day mortality. Scores of 1, 2, 3, and 4 are associated with 30-day mortalities of 13%, 26%, 72%, and 97%, respectively.

16.

E XII

All tongue muscles except the palatoglossus are innervated by the hypoglossal nerve. Fasciculations of the tongue indicate injury to the hypoglossal nerve and denervation of the tongue. Such findings are presumed to occur secondary to acetylcholine hypersensitivity at the denervated neuromuscular junction. Atrophy also occurs when the tongue is denervated. Lesions of the hypoglossal nerve typically are secondary to amyotrophic lateral sclerosis. (A) The lingual branch of the mandibular division of the trigeminal nerve provides sensation to the anterior two thirds of the tongue through special visceral afferent fibers. (B) The chorda tympani of the facial nerve carries taste from the anterior two thirds of the tongue. (C) The glossopharyngeal never carries taste and sensation from the posterior one third of the tongue. (D) The vagus nerve innervates the palatoglossus muscle.

17.

A Scheuermann disease

Scheuermann disease is defined by the presence of anterior vertebral wedging measuring 5 degrees or greater involving at least three adjacent vertebrae. It usually presents in early adolescence. The etiology is not certain, but there may be a genetic component. (B) Osteopoikilosis is a rare, inherited sclerosing dysplasia characterized by multiple enostoses that may involve the spine. (C) Baastrup disease occurs due to chronic apposition of spinous processes in the lumbar spine, with resultant sclerosis and degenerative change. Back pain tends to improve with flexion and is exacerbated with extension of the spine. (D) Alkaptonuria (also known as ochronosis) can result in widespread calcification of the intervertebral disks. (E) Osteopetrosis is caused by deficient osteoclastic activity and leads to diffuse sclerosis of the bones. In the spine, thick sclerotic bands can be seen paralleling the end plates.

18.

D Sweat glands

Cocaine would cause an activation of the sympathetic nervous system, whereas atropine administration would block the parasympathetic nervous system. Sweat glands are unique in that they are the only organs with sympathetic but no parasympathetic innervations. Although the kidneys have parasympathetic input, they also rely mainly on the sympathetic nervous system.

19.

D 4 to 6% per year

The patient likely has an arteriovenous malformation (AVM) that has hemorrhaged. AVMs are thought to have a consistent yearly hemorrhage rate of approximately 4%, which may be slightly higher in patients who have had a previously hemorrhage, deep-seated hemorrhage, or deep-draining veins. AVMs usually do not receive emergent surgical intervention given these re-hemorrhage rates, unless there is significant mass effect reduction expected from resection of the hematoma. Note the classic appearance of the hemorrhage tapering toward the ventricle in the image. (A–C) These figures are consistent with re-hemorrhage rates following aneurysmal subarachnoid hemorrhage. (E) Cavernous hemangiomas have a less than 1% risk of re-hemorrhage over a lifetime, although documented hemorrhage and re-hemorrhage rates are very inconsistent in the literature.

20.

A Diffuse idiopathic skeletal hypertrophy

Ankylosing spondylitis starts in the sacroiliac joints and progresses rostrally, whereas diffuse idiopathic skeletal hyperostosis (DISH) spares the sacroiliac joints and primarily involves the thoracic spine. Both conditions may predispose to fractures and spinal cord injuries from minor trauma. (D, E) Rheumatoid arthritis and gout can affect the sacroiliac joints as well as numerous other joints throughout the skeleton.

21.

B Cat

Toxoplasmosis is the most common opportunistic infection found in an individual with HIV/AIDS. Its definitive host is a cat. (A) Cryptococcus is the second most common opportunistic infection found in an individual with HIV/AIDS. Its definitive host is a bird.

22.

D Double vision, ocular deviation, and postural imbalance

(A) Increased akinesia with reduced rigidity might be seen if the lead was positioned caudal to the target and hit the substantia nigra. (B) Reduced tremor with persistent akinesia might be seen with a lead placed superficially to the target in the zona incerta. (C) Tetany and dysarthria are seen with laterally placed leads in the internal capsule. (E) Perspiration, mydriasis, and dysesthesias are seen with leads placed too far posteriorly in the hypothalamus.

23.

A Epidermoid

The description of this sequence corresponds to diffusion-weighted imaging (DWI). Epidermoid tumors may be cystic appearing on T1- and T2-weighted sequences (sometimes appearing similar to cerebrospinal fluid) but are characteristically markedly bright on DWI. This latter feature can be particularly useful in differentiating epidermoid tumors from arachnoid cysts. In addition, in contrast to arachnoid cysts, epidermoids do not suppress their signal on FLAIR sequences, on which they typically show a "dirty" appearance. (B) Lymphomas show restricted diffusion of DWI due to their dense cellularity, although they usually are not as bright as epidermoid tumors. Untreated lymphomas enhance avidly and homogeneously, except in patients with HIV/AIDS, who commonly present with necrotic changes. (C) Meningiomas may show some degree of diffusion restriction on DWI, but their appearance is variable. Atypical and malignant meningiomas tend to show greater restricted diffusion with lower apparent diffusion coefficient values. These tumors enhance. (D) Marked hyperintensity on DWI is not a usual characteristic of craniopharyngiomas, which also would enhance. These tumors are heterogeneous with 90 to 95% showing calcifications. (E) Arachnoid cysts have the same signal appearance as cerebrospinal fluid on all sequences and do not show restricted diffusion.

24.

A Tuberculosis

Tuberculosis in the vertebral bodies (Pott disease) classically is associated with back pain, a low-grade fever, and destruction of the vertebral bodies with disk preservation. (B) *Staphylococcus aureus* infection (often from hematogenous spread) can result in vertebral body osteomyelitis or diskitis. The latter is seen radiographically as disk space destruction, whereas both the former and latter are characterized by more substantial signs of infection and fever relative to Pott disease. (D) Vertebral body hemangiomas often are asymptomatic, but may cause vertebral body collapse and associated pain. (E) An osteoid osteoma is a benign osteoblastic bone tumor characterized by a dull, nonradiating pain often relieved by nonsteroidal anti-inflammatory medications.

25.

B PaO$_2$ < 90

The prerequisites for determination of brain death include the absence of reversible causes of coma (e.g., hepatic, diabetic, and uremic causes); imaging supporting the clinical exam findings; lack of respiratory effort; lack of severe acid-base, electrolyte, or endocrine abnormalities; PaO$_2$ > 90 for at least 30 minutes; systolic blood pressure > 100 mm Hg for at least 30 minutes; negative drug screen; no residual paralytics; and core body temperature > 35°C.

26.

D Posterior inferior cerebellar artery

The patient's clinical symptoms are consistent with Wallenberg syndrome due to a lateral medullary infarction, which can be confirmed on the diffusion-weighted image. Infarction of the lateral medulla can occur secondary to occlusion of the posterior inferior cerebellar artery or one of its branches with or without involvement of the vertebral artery. (A) The pontomesencephalic segment belongs to the superior cerebellar artery and supplies part of the pons and mesencephalon. (B) The anterior inferior cerebellar artery supplies the anterior and inferior portions of the cerebellar hemispheres as well as the inferolateral aspect of the pons and flocculus. (C) The superior cerebellar artery supplies the superior cerebellum, superior vermis, dentate nuclei, and part of the midbrain.

27.

C GABA

GABA is released by Purkinje cells in the cerebellum as they make inhibitory projections to the deep cerebellar nuclei and supply the sole motor coordination output of the cerebellar cortex. (A) Glutamate is the most abundant excitatory neurotransmitter in the central nervous system and is the primary neurotransmitter released by cerebellar granule cells. (B) Glycine is an inhibitory neurotransmitter found most predominantly in the brainstem, retinae, and spine. In the spine, it is released by Renshaw cells. (D) Acetylcholine is found throughout the nervous system but is a prominent neurotransmitter in the autonomic nervous system and at neuromuscular junctions. (E) Substance P is a neuropeptide that acts as a neurotransmitter for transmitting pain to the central nervous system.

28.

A Diabetes insipidus

Preoperative central diabetes insipidus has been reported in 8 to 35% of patients affected by a craniopharyngioma. The condition occurs in 70 to 90% of patients after surgery.

29.

C Increase urine calcium excretion

Urine calcium excretion is increased by steroids, resulting in a lower serum calcium concentration and promotion of parathyroid hormone to induce bony reabsorption. (A) Steroids inhibit osteoblast function to slow bony modeling. (B) Steroids promote osteoclast reabsorption of the bony matrix. (E) Gastrointestinal calcium absorption is decreased by steroids.

30.

B Iris hamartomas

Iris hamartomas (Lisch nodules) are seen in neurofibromatosis (NF) type 1. This patient has NF type 1, as she has two of the diagnostic criteria, which include family history, Lisch nodules, optic gliomas, café-au-lait spots, axillary or groin freckling, multiple neurofibromas or a single plexiform neurofibroma (a cluster of neurofibromas involving multiple nerves), and skeletal abnormalities (e.g., sphenoid dysplasia). (A) Bilateral acoustic neuromas are found in NF type 2. (C) An increased risk of meningiomas and other intracranial tumors (e.g., ependymomas) is associated with NF type 2. (D) Pigmented spots encircling the iris is descriptive of Kayser–Fleischer rings seen in Wilson disease. (E) Multiple schwannomas are seen in schwannomatosis, which results from mutations on both chromosomes 17 and chromosome 22.

31.

A Unaffected

Sensory nerve action potentials (SNAPs) are unaffected with lesions proximal to the dorsal root ganglion (e.g., nerve root avulsions, herniated disks) because the cell bodies are unaffected. Postganglionic lesions reduce the SNAP amplitude and/or slow the velocity.

32.

A Ependymomas

This patient has avidly enhancing masses in his internal auditory canals bilaterally, with extension into the cerebellopontine angle cistern on the right, consistent with vestibular schwannomas. The presence of bilateral vestibular schwannomas satisfies the modified NIH criteria for NF type 2, which also may present with schwannomas and ependymomas, the latter usually in the brainstem and spinal cord. Schwannomas usually are hyperintense on T2 sequences, and larger tumors commonly have

cystic changes. (B) Sphenoid wing dysplasia is a distinctive osseous lesion of NF type 1 and constitutes a major criterion for diagnosis. (C) Calcified subependymal nodules are seen in tuberous sclerosis and show calcification in the majority of patients, except in early life. (D) Leptomeningeal angiomatosis is a capillary venous malformation seen in Sturge-Weber-Dimitri syndrome, usually accompanied by a port-wine stain along the ophthalmic and maxillary trigeminal nerve distributions. (E) Endolymphatic sac tumors are seen in 10% of patients with von Hippel–Lindau syndrome and are not a feature of neurofibromatosis.

33.

D Demeclocycline

Demeclocycline is a tetracycline that can be used to treat chronic syndrome of inappropriate antidiuretic hormone secretion, in that it is a partial antagonist of the actions of antidiuretic hormone on the distal renal tubules. It can be given orally every 6 hours.

34.

E Rabies

The image accompanying the question shows Negri bodies, which are intracytoplasmic eosinophilic collections of ribonucleoproteins seen in rabies. (A) Alzheimer disease is characterized histologically by intracellular neurofibrillary tangles (silver staining and immunoreactive for tau protein) and extracellular senile plaques (silver staining with a core of protein amyloid). Hirano bodies can be seen, and these are rod-shaped eosin inclusions. There also can be diffuse cortical vacuolization where the vacuoles appear glassy or eosinophilic. (B) Parkinson disease is characterized by intracellular Lewy bodies that derive from neurofilaments and are laminated with an eosinophilic core and a clear halo. (C) Lafora bodies are seen in Lafora disease, and these are round, basophilic polyglucosans. (D) Creutzfeldt-Jakob disease displays diffuse cortical vacuolization as sometimes seen in Alzheimer disease.

35.

A Langerhans cell histiocytosis

Langerhans cell histiocytosis is characterized by infiltration of the soft tissues with myeloid dendritic cells. In children, the skull is the most common site of involvement and represents 40% of cases. Lesions usually are well marginated and may have a beveled edge on skull radiographs or CT due to unequal involvement of the inner and outer tables. This also can lead to the appearance of a "hole within a hole" if viewed en face. (B) Calvarial hemangiomas are slow-growing lesions that can result in a characteristic sunburst-like trabecular thickening or radiating spicules. Margins usually are not sclerotic. (C) Primary intraosseous meningiomas are rare. They also can present with a radiating pattern but are not associated with a beveled edge. (D) Metastases can have various presentations from ill-defined and infiltrative to relatively well marginated. They usually are not associated with a beveled edge.

36.

C A-delta and C fibers

A-delta and C fibers are nociceptive fibers that are thought to be the cause of pain in trigeminal neuralgia, and these are the theoretical targets of lesioning procedures. In reality, it is impossible to select completely for these fibers, but creating a retrogasserian lesion tends to reduce pain while best avoiding hypesthesia. (A) A-alpha and beta fibers are sensory (fine touch) fibers that should be preserved during a percutaneous trigeminal rhizotomy.

37.

B Anterior nuclei

The anterior nuclei are part of the limbic system and project to the cingulate gyrus. (A) The centromedian nuclei are part of the intralaminar nuclei and project to the putamen and subthalamic nuclei. They receive input from multiple structures including the cerebral cortices. They are involved in attention and arousal. (C) The ventral lateral nuclei are involved in motor coordination and receive projections from the cerebellum and basal ganglia. (D) The lateral posterior nuclei are associated with the pulvinar nuclei and have similar inputs and outputs. They are part of the visual pathways. (E) The medial dorsal nuclei receive inputs from the olfactory cortices and amygdalae and project to the limbic system and prefrontal cortices.

38.

C Right trochlear nerve palsy

A right trochlear nerve palsy results in a right pupil that deviates superiorly and extorts in primary gaze as the superior oblique muscle (supplied by the nerve) has the action of moving the eye inferiorly when adducted and intorting the eye. A tilt of the head to the side contralateral of the palsy and a slight tilt downward enables the contralateral eye to align its sight with the paretic eye when looking at objects on a level plane. When looking downward, the ipsilateral eye fails to align the gaze with the contralateral eye. (A) A left trochlear nerve palsy typically results in the patient compensating with a head tilt to the right due to the loss of the intorsion action of the superior oblique. (B) A left oculomotor nerve palsy results in the left pupil being directed downward and laterally due to the unopposed action of the lateral rectus and superior oblique muscles. A patient should have no difficulty aligning her gaze when looking downward. (D) A right oculomotor nerve palsy results in the right pupil being directed downward and laterally. (E) Internuclear ophthalmoplegia results from a medial longitudinal fasciculus lesion and does not cause convergence deficits but does manifest in an adduction deficit in the ipsilateral eye when gaze is directed contralateral to the lesion. Abduction nystagmus also appears in the contralateral eye when gaze is directed contralateral to the lesion.

39.

A Anterior atlanto-occipital dislocation

The basion-axial interval (BAI) represents the distance measured between a line drawn along the dorsal aspect of the dens (posterior axial line) and the tip of the basion. Studies have demonstrated that this distance measures less than 12 mm in more than 95% of adults, and this is considered to be the upper limit of normal. A BAI greater than 12 mm is indicative of anterior atlanto-occipital dislocation where the cranium is displaced anteriorly in relation to the spine. (B) Atlantoaxial instability would present as an abnormally increased distance between the anterior surface of the dens and the posterior tubercle of C1 (the atlantodental interval). This distance normally measures 3 mm or less in adults and 5 mm or less in children. (C) Longitudinal dislocation can present with a normal BAI if there is no anterior translocation of the cranium. (D) A BAI greater than 12 mm is abnormal. (E) Atlanto-occipital dislocation results from traumatic injury to the alar and apical ligaments and tectorial membrane, which allows the cranium to move with respect to the cervical spine. Injury to the transverse ligament would result in atlantoaxial instability.

40.

E Tongue fasciculations, atrophy of the hands, and lower extremity hyperreflexia

Amyotrophic lateral sclerosis (ALS) classically is an upper and lower motor neuron disease with sparing of cognition and autonomic function. Classically, there is sparing of the eye muscles, sensation, and urinary sphincter control. ALS is due to the degeneration of the anterior horn α-motor neurons in the spinal cord and brainstem nuclei. The condition often is sporadic; however, familial forms are associated with the superoxide dismutase gene (*SOD*) mutation. (A) Tongue fasciculations, atrophy of the hands, and lower extremity hyporeflexia are lower motor neuron findings. (B) Forehead-sparing facial weakness, spasticity of the hands, and lower extremity hyperreflexia are signs of pure upper motor neuron disease. (C) Progressive weakness (proximal more than distal), areflexia, and bilateral facial weakness with little to no sensory involvement may be seen in Guillain-Barré syndrome. This condition may occur after *Campylobacter jejuni* enteritis. Cerebrospinal fluid analysis shows albuminocytologic dissociation. (D) Central cord syndrome classically results in a motor deficit worse in the upper than lower extremities, with varying degrees of sensory findings and myelopathy (usually urinary retention) that occurs with hyperextension injury or central cervical canal stenosis.

41.

D 90%

Dandy-Walker variant is a less severe posterior fossa anomaly characterized by partial agenesis of the cerebellar vermis as compared with the more severe, classic Dandy-Walker malformation, in which there is complete agenesis of the cerebellar vermis. Hydrocephalus is present and typically symptomatic in 90% of children with a Dandy-Walker malformation compared with 25% of children with a Dandy-Walker variant.

42.

C 80 Gy in a single dose directed at the center of the lesion

During stereotactic radiosurgery for trigeminal neuralgia, 70 to 80 Gy of radiation in a single dose should be directed at the center of the lesion in such a way as to keep the 80% isodose curve away from the brainstem. Pain relief usually occurs 3 months after treatment but is highly variable.

43.

A Follow the ex-wife's orders, and do not provide any further medical care.

There are two types of power of attorney: (1) immediate and (2) springing. An immediate power of attorney becomes effective as soon as it is signed, whereas a springing power of attorney becomes effective when the principal becomes incapacitated. In most states, a divorce decree does not revoke a financial or health care power of attorney in favor of the ex-spouse. Exceptions to this rule occur in Alabama, California, Colorado, Illinois, Indiana, Kansas, Minnesota, Missouri, Ohio, Pennsylvania, Texas, Washington, and Wisconsin, where divorce does revoke such a designation. In these states, or when there is not someone available with the legal right to make medical decisions for the patient, the physician should act in the best interests of the patient, providing all reasonable care that is not considered futile. (B, C) Consulting the hospital's ethics committee and obtaining a court order require a substantial amount of time and are difficult to do in emergent situations. (D) Regardless of who has the legal right to make medical decisions, if time permits it always is prudent to attempt to obtain a family consensus regarding care plans, as this tends to mitigate any potential legal implications and unrest within a family.

44.

C Carotid canal

The structure indicated by the arrow in the image accompanying the question corresponds to the carotid canal, which transmits the internal carotid artery and sympathetic plexus. (A) The petroclival fissure is seen more posteriorly, coursing somewhat parallel to the petrous carotid canal. (B) The pars nervosa is the smaller anteromedial component of the jugular foramen and is separated from the larger pars vascularis by the jugular spine. It carries cranial nerve IX and the inferior petrosal sinus. (D) The foramen rotundum courses anteriorly along the medial aspect of the middle cranial fossa and transmits the maxillary branch of cranial nerve V, artery of the foramen rotundum, and emissary veins. (E) The foramen ovale is seen in the right greater wing of the sphenoid bone. It contains the mandibular branch of cranial nerve V, accessory meningeal artery, otic ganglion, emissary veins, and sometimes the lesser petrosal nerve.

45.

B 3.2 L

The estimated water deficit is either 3.1 or 3.3 L depending on which of the following equations is used:

Free water deficit = ((Current sodium – 140)/(Current sodium)) × 0.6 × (Weight in kg)

or

Free water deficit = ((Current sodium/140) – 1) × 0.6 × (Weight in kg))

46.

D Osteopetrosis

Osteopetrosis is secondary to defective osteoclastic function, with a resultant dense appearance of the bone. In the spine, thick and dense bands of sclerosis can be seen paralleling the end plates as in this case. (A) Ochronosis may result in widespread calcification of the intervertebral disks. (B) Paget disease usually is more focal, and characteristically results in expansion of the involved bone. A "picture frame" appearance of the vertebra with a squared morphology often is seen. (C) Blastic metastases can be diffuse, particularly in patients with breast cancer. They would not be as densely homogeneous as in this case.

47.

C Commissural myelotomy

Commissural myelotomies are used for either unilateral or bilateral pain below the thoracic levels. They are not the ideal choice for visceral pain, as they work through disruption of the lateral spinothalamic tract fibers as they cross in the anterior commissure. (A) A bilateral cervical cordotomy carries a risk of an Ondine curse, with a loss of respiratory automaticity. Bilateral procedures should be staged in selected patients, with cordotomies as a whole being reserved mostly for terminally ill patients due to a variety of complications. In addition, a unilateral cordotomy often accentuates contralateral pain. (B) Punctate midline myelotomies are used best for visceral and pelvic pain and can be used in non–terminally ill patients. (D) Spinal cord stimulation is an excellent choice for bilateral lower extremity pain but has a poor response on pain secondary to cancer. It is not a good procedural choice for a patient with a short life expectancy. (E) Dorsal root entry zone (DREZ) lesioning typically helps with noncancer pain that can be isolated to specific nerve roots. It is used often following nerve root avulsions. In the patient described, there seems to be pain involving numerous nerve roots.

48.

B Optic nerve gliomas tend to be low grade in children and high grade in adults.

Optic nerve gliomas tend to be of a higher grade with advancing age of presentation. (A) Optic nerve gliomas can occur at any age but appear earlier in life, when they are associated with neurofibromatosis type 1. (C) Rosenthal fibers occur in optic nerve gliomas, especially when they are low-grade pilocytic tumors. They are more common in childhood. (D) Optic nerve gliomas typically are not a manifestation of neurofibromatosis type 2 in children or adults.

49.

B Gorlin syndrome

The image accompanying the question shows a medulloblastoma. Gorlin syndrome (autosomal dominant inheritance) occurs in approximately 1 to 2% of medulloblastomas and is characterized by the propensity to develop multiple invasive basal cell carcinomata. Other syndromes associated with medulloblastomas are Li-Fraumeni and Turcot syndromes. (A) Von Hippel–Lindau (VHL) disease results from an autosomal dominant mutation of the *VHL* gene on chromosome 3. VHL disease is associated with central nervous system hemangioblastomas; retinal hemangioblastomas; renal cell carcinomas; pheochromocytomas; cysts in the liver, pancreas, and kidneys; and epididymal cystadenomas. (C) Tuberous sclerosis can be an autosomal dominant disease but usually occurs sporadically. The associated mutation is located on chromosomes 9 and 16. Tuberous sclerosis can be characterized by the classic triad (in less than 50% of cases) of mental retardation, seizures, and adenoma sebaceum. The condition is associated with cortical tubers; subependymal giant cell astrocytomas; cardiac rhabdomyomas; renal angiomyolipomas; cysts in the lungs, liver, and spleen; pancreatic adenomas; and retinal hamartomas. (D) Lynch syndrome is a cancer syndrome primarily involving the colon, but may affect many other organ systems including the brain. It is formerly known as hereditary nonpolyposis colon cancer syndrome.

50.

A Extensor carpi radialis longus

The extensor carpi radialis longus is innervated by the radial nerve itself but may occasionally have innervations from the superficial sensory branch of the radial nerve. (B–E) These muscles are innervated by the posterior interosseous nerve, a terminal branch of the radial nerve.

51.

C Day 15

The primitive streak appears around day 15 of embryogenesis due to signaling from the notochord, and it marks the initiation of gastrulation. During this process, the bilaminar disk becomes trilaminar with the development of the endoderm, mesoderm, and ectoderm. The primitive streak defines the various axes of the embryo and continues to transform into the primitive groove. This groove further develops into the neural tube during neurulation. (A) The bilaminar disk forms during the first part of the second week of embryogenesis. (B) Around or before the start of the second week of embryogenesis, the notochord forms. (D) Primary neurulation (the creation of the neural plate to create the neural tube) begins around the start of the third week of embryogenesis. The notochord plays an integral role in this process through signaling and mechanical support. (E) In secondary neurulation, the neural tube arises from a solid cord that then cavitates, resulting in a hollow tube. This tube eventually forms the medullary and spinal cords that then connect to the cord arising from primary neurulation. This process begins around day 26 of embryogenesis.

52.

B Arteriovenous fistula

The presence of longitudinally extensive signal abnormality in the spinal cord associated with vascular flow voids (which are best seen on the T2 image) is compatible with a spinal dural arteriovenous fistula. These typically occur in older males who present with progressive myelopathy and sometimes neurogenic claudication (thought to be related to venous hypertension and vascular congestion). As in this case, ill-defined contrast enhancement may be present. (A) Acute spinal cord ischemia can result in longitudinally extensive intramedullary signal abnormalities, but usually has a hyperacute presentation and would not explain the presence of vascular flow voids. (C) Infiltrating neoplasms such as astrocytomas usually result in more focal spinal cord expansion than shown in the image accompanying the question. They may show variable degrees of contrast enhancement, which tends to be more heterogeneous. (D) Demyelination related to neuromyelitis optica can lead to longitudinally extensive signal abnormalities in the spinal cord, with a central gray matter pattern with possible patchy enhancement. This would not explain the patient's clinical presentation, as attacks in neuromyelitis optica usually occur over days with variable degrees of recovery over weeks

to months on the flow voids on the MRI scan. The lesions in multiple sclerosis are more focal and peripheral in the white matter, although they may coalesce over time in severe disease. (E) The most common etiology of infectious myelitis is viral. This would have a more rapid clinical course and would not be associated with vascular flow voids.

53.

B AEDs decrease the rate of acute but not delayed-onset seizures.

Phenytoin has been demonstrated to decrease the risk of early posttraumatic seizures by fourfold; however, it has this effect on seizures only within the first week after injury.

54.

D Foramen magnum tumor

Foramen magnum tumors (most commonly meningiomas) classically present with rotating paralysis as described in the vignette presented in the question. Other symptoms may include craniocervical pain, myelopathy, and intrinsic hand muscle atrophy (lower motor neuron findings from venous infarction). Another classic sign of cervicomedullary compression is downbeat nystagmus.

55.

C Glasscock

The Glasscock triangle (posterolateral) contains the middle meningeal artery in the floor of the triangle as it exits the foramen spinosum, the horizontal petrous internal carotid artery, and the infratemporal fossa. The triangle is useful, as it enables the surgeon to gain proximal control of the internal carotid artery for more distal vascular procedures. Approximately 10 mm of the carotid artery is accessible through this triangle. (A) The oculomotor triangle, also known as the medial or Hakuba triangle, contains the oculomotor nerve and horizontal segment of the internal carotid artery. It is the triangle by which access to most intracavernous aneurysms and tumors is gained. (B) Historically, the Parkinson triangle was accessed to treat carotid-cavernous fistulas. It also contains the abducens nerve. (D) The Kawase (posteromedial) triangle contains the petrous apex, internal carotid artery, cochlea, and vertebrobasilar junction. It can be used to perform an anterior petrosectomy so that the posterior fossa, anterior brainstem, and root of the trigeminal nerve can be visualized. (E) The porus trigeminus is the entrance to the Meckel cave and is contained within the inferolateral triangle.

56.

C Hypertension, bradycardia, and respiratory irregularity

The Cushing reflex is a physiological response to an increase in intracranial pressure. It manifests with an increase in blood pressure, decrease in heart rate, and irregular breathing. The proposed mechanism for the Cushing triad is an increase in intracranial pressure leading to decreased cerebral blood flow, and the sympathetic system causes peripheral vasoconstriction to elevate the mean arterial pressure in an attempt to restore normal cerebral blood flow. As this happens, baroreceptors in the aortic arch detect the blood pressure increase, and trigger a parasympathetic response to decrease the heart rate. Increased intracranial pressure leads to brainstem compression and irregular breathing.

57.

A Gross total resection

Approximately 85% of ependymomas present as localized disease. Gross total resection is the most important predictor of outcome. (C) Conformal field radiotherapy is recommended as an adjuvant therapy in most patients with ependymomas. (D) Early chemotherapy for ependymomas is recommended in infants to delay or avoid the need for radiotherapy, which can be very detrimental to brain development.

58.

D Cutaneous bruising

In the images accompanying the question, the MRI scan on the left shows hemispheric subdural hematomas bilaterally, with different signal intensities and therefore likely different ages. The susceptibility-weighted image on the right shows a dark focus of signal drop along the posterior aspect of the left globe compatible with retinal hemorrhage. Together, these findings are highly concerning for nonaccidental trauma. Subdural hematomas are associated significantly with nonaccidental trauma compared with unintentional trauma, and retinal hemorrhages have a specificity of approximately 94%. Cutaneous bruising may be present and should raise suspicion for trauma in a nonambulatory child. (A) An abdominal mass would not explain the findings of this case. (B) Opisthotonos is abnormal rigidity with arching of the body and may be seen in infants with meningitis. (C) Fever may be seen in infectious meningitis.

59.

D Visual flashes

If a deep brain stimulating electrode contacts the optic tract (inferomedial to the globus pallidus), a patient can experience phosphenes, which are flashes or sparkles of light in the contralateral visual field. (A) To cause perspiration and mydriasis, a lead would have to be inserted significantly medial to the globus pallidus to contact the hypothalamus. (B, C) If a deep brain stimulating electrode is passed too medially to the globus pallidus, stimulation of the internal capsule can cause contractions of the tongue, face, and throat as well as dysarthria, gagging, and visible muscle contractions.

60.

B Sodium ions would enter the neuron, and membrane potential would become more positive.

Even at maximal sodium conductance at the peak of an action potential, the neuronal membrane potential is not equal to the equilibrium potential for sodium ions. This is due to the baseline conductance of other ions including chloride and potassium. Additional open sodium channels would allow more sodium ions to enter the cell, increasing the relative concentration of sodium ions, and bringing the cell to a more positive membrane potential (closer to the sodium equilibrium potential).

61.

A Labyrinthitis

Labyrinthitis (as opposed to vestibular neuritis) involves the vestibular nerve as well as the cochlea and thus also affects hearing. (B) Vestibular neuronitis presents with acute vertigo without hearing loss, usually after an upper respiratory tract infection. (C) Benign positional vertigo is associated with nystagmus and vertigo without hearing loss that are associated with positional changes. (D) Meniere disease includes vertigo and prominent tinnitus with hearing loss that classically is fluctuating and episodic, lasting minutes to hours. (E) Stroke (Wallenberg or lateral medullary syndrome) causing vertigo, nystagmus, and hearing loss also would produce prominent nonvestibular symptoms such as loss of pain/temperature sensation in the contralateral body, Horner syndrome, and brainstem findings such as dysphagia, ataxia, diplopia, and dysarthria.

62.

C Cerebral angiopathy

In cerebral angiopathy, there is a deposition of β-amyloid protein into hyalinized cerebral vessels. Congo red stains the amyloid protein red. (A) Arteries in moyamoya disease display varying degrees of stenosis due to thrombosis, luminal collapse, and fibrous intimal thickening. (B) Cavernous hemangiomas (cavernomas) appear as dilated, thin-walled capillaries without normal intervening brain tissue. There can be surrounding hemosiderin. (D) Mucormycosis is a family of invasive fungal infections typically associated with diabetes. Histologically, thin-walled hyphae appear arranged and folded haphazardly and branching from the parent hyphae at right angles. (E) Radiation necrosis appears as areas of anuclear brain tissue with reactive astrocytes. Arteriosclerosis (vessel thickening) also can be seen.

63.

B Tibial and common peroneal nerves

The sural nerve is composed of contributions from the lateral and medial sural cutaneous nerves. The lateral sural cutaneous nerve arises as a terminal branch of the tibial nerve, whereas the medial sural cutaneous nerve is a branch of the common peroneal nerve before it bifurcates into the deep and superficial peroneal nerves.

64.

C Dandy-Walker malformation

The combination of a large posterior fossa cyst in communication with the fourth ventricle, elevation of the torcular, and vermian hypoplasia is compatible with Dandy-Walker malformation, in this case resulting in obstructive hydrocephalus. Associated findings may include corpus callosum agenesis and lipomas, neuronal migration anomalies, and cephaloceles. (A) An arachnoid cyst rarely occupies the entire posterior fossa and is not accompanied by vermian hypoplasia. (B) A Blake pouch cyst develops due to failure of regression of the embryonic Blake pouch, which then balloons posteriorly into the cisterna magna. The vermis is not hypoplastic. (D) A mega cisterna magna has an intact vermis and normal fourth ventricle, and would not result in this degree of posterior fossa expansion.

65.

B Engorgement of the extraocular muscles

This patient has a cavernous-carotid fistula characterized by exophthalmos and possibly an optic bruit when a stethoscope is placed over the ipsilat-eral closed eye. This type of arteriovenous fistula increases the venous pressure in the cavernous sinus, resulting in inhibited drainage of blood from the extraocular muscles. (A) An orbital mass can produce exophthalmos but would not produce an orbital bruit. (C) It is the ophthalmic vein and not the artery that becomes enlarged in a cavernous-carotid fistula as the venous pressure increases. (D) A cavernous sinus aneurysm produces the described symptoms only if it ruptures and results in a carotid-cavernous fistula. (E) In conditions such as elevated intracranial pressure there can be flattening of the posterior aspect of the globe. A carotid-cavernous fistula is not expected to produce global elevations in intracranial pressure.

66.

B Septal and thalamostriate veins

(A) The internal cerebral vein joins with the basal vein of Rosenthal to form the vein of Galen. (C) The vein of Galen joins the inferior sagittal sinus to form the straight sinus. (D) The caudate vein drains into the thalamostriate vein.

67.

D Partially compensated respiratory acidosis

A low pH indicates acidosis, whereas a high PCO_2 is indicative of a respiratory origin. There is partial metabolic compensation as indicated by the rise of the bicarbonate level above normal. Compensatory mechanisms never fully reverse the primary acid/base abnormality.

68.

C Combined respiratory and metabolic alkalosis

A high pH indicates alkalosis, whereas a combined low PCO_2 and high bicarbonate level is indicative of a combined respiratory and metabolic origin. (A) A high pH indicates alkalosis, whereas a low PCO_2 and normal bicarbonate level is indicative of a respiratory origin. (B) A low pH indicates acidosis, whereas a low bicarbonate level and a relatively normal PCO_2 is indicative of a metabolic origin.

Normal target labs values are as follows:

pH: 7.40
PCO_2: 40 mm Hg
HCO_3^-: 24 mEq/L

69.

C This disease typically is inherited in an X-linked fashion.

The patient has underproduction of the pituitary hormone gonadotropin, resulting in Kallmann syndrome (hypogonadotropic hypogonadism). It is an X-linked (typically) condition that is more common in men (incidence of 1:10,000) than in women (incidence of 1:50,000). Imaging would be expected to demonstrate aplasia/hypoplasia of the olfactory bulbs. Of note, there are some reported forms of Kallmann syndrome inherited in an autosomal dominant pattern.

70.

A Bicoronal sutures

Crouzon syndrome first was described in 1912. Inheritance is autosomal dominant with virtually a complete penetrance. It is due to multiple mutations in the fibroblast growth factor receptor 2 gene (*FGFR2*). Features of the skull are variable, but the skull may have associated brachycephaly, trigonocephaly, or oxycephaly. These conditions occur with premature fusions of the sagittal, metopic, or coronal sutures, with bilateral coronal sutures being the most commonly affected. In addition, the orbits are shallow, with resulting exorbitism due to anterior positioning of the greater wing of the sphenoid. The middle cranial fossa is displaced anteriorly and inferiorly, which further shortens the orbit anteroposteriorly.

71.

D Bacterial endocarditis

Conditions associated with aneurysms include autosomal dominant polycystic kidney disease, fibromuscular dysplasia, arteriovenous malformations, Ehlers-Danlos syndrome type 4, Marfan syndrome, familial intracranial aneurysm history, aortic coarctation, Osler-Weber-Rendu syndrome, and endocarditis. Intracranial aneurysms also are associated with hypertension, smoking, alcohol, trauma, obesity, and advancing age. Bacterial endocarditis can cause mycotic aneurysms mainly in the distal, smaller arteries. (A) Radiation exposure is more likely to cause meningiomas than aneurysms. (B) Ehlers-Danlos syndrome is a connective tissue disorder with six types. Each type shares features of joint laxity and soft skin. Types 1 and 2 are the classic types with hypermobile, stretchy skin. Type 3 is the most common and is marked by joint hypermobility. Type 4 is vascular and makes those affected prone to aneurysm development. Type 6 is characterized by a progressive kyphoscoliosis, thin conjunctiva, and severe muscle weakness. Types 7A and B comprise the arthrochalasia types and are characterized by very loose joints and bilateral hip dislocations. These types can be considered severe forms of the hypermobility type. Type 7C is the extremely rare dermatosparaxis type

characterized by extremely fragile and sagging skin. Note that the six subtypes are not numbered consecutively. (C) Illicit drug use indirectly can cause mycotic aneurysms in rare cases if a patient has bacterial endocarditis. (E) There is no gender predisposition for aneurysm development.

72.

B Aneurysmal bone cyst

Aneurysmal bone cysts are expansile, tumor-like, osteolytic lesions often occurring in the posterior elements of the spine. There is a high recurrence rate if they are not excised completely. (C, D) Osteoid osteomas (less than 1 cm) and osteoblastomas (1 cm and larger) characteristically respond well to aspirin. (E) Eosinophilic granulomas often present with an osteolytic defect and progressive vertebral collapse (vertebra plana) most commonly affecting the cervical spine.

73.

B Desmoplastic infantile ganglioglioma

The tumor shown in the image accompanying the question best fits with a desmoplastic infantile ganglioglioma. (A) Desmoplastic infantile astrocytomas lack the ganglion cell component highlighted with synaptophysin staining. (E) Pleomorphic xanthoastrocytomas also are reticulin rich but show more atypia and are rare in the frontal lobe.

74.

C Progressive supranuclear palsy

Progressive supranuclear palsy (PSP) causes paresis of primary vertical gaze, with preservation of the vertical doll's eyes maneuver, pseudobulbar palsy, and axial dystonia. PSP may be distinguished from Parkinson disease in that patients with PSP walk upright (not bent forward), have no tremor, and have a short-lived response to anti-Parkinson medications.

75.

B 2

Hunt and Hess grade 2 indicates a severe headache, nuchal rigidity, and cranial nerve palsies. Of note, serious systemic disease can increase the Hunt and Hess grade of the patient. (A) Grade 1 indicates an asymptomatic patient or one with only a mild headache. (C) Grade 3 indicates focal neurologic deficits, lethargy, and confusion, and should be an indicator for possible external ventricular placement. (D) Grade 4 indicates stupor, hemiparesis, and decorticate posturing. (E) Grade 5 indicates coma, decerebrate posturing, and a moribund appearance.

Section 2

1.

D Cerebellar infarcts

This patient has a minimally displaced fracture of the left lateral mass of a cervical vertebra extending to the foramen transversarium. These patients are at an increased risk of vertebral artery injury, which may be complicated by posterior circulation infarcts. This finding warrants additional evaluation with CT or MR angiography. (A) Intra-abdominal injuries are a common finding with Chance type fractures of the thoracolumbar spine, particularly in children. (B) Spinal cord transection may be present with more severe cervical spine injuries, although patients with underlying spinal canal stenosis are at an increased risk of spinal cord injury with relatively minor trauma. (C) Anterior circulation infarcts can result from carotid artery dissection or other injury.

2.

B 3 to 5%; 64% reduction

The $CHADS_2$ score is used to assess the annual risk of stroke in patients with atrial fibrillation, and it increases for patients with congestive heart failure, hypertension, diabetes, previous transient ischemic attacks (TIAs) or strokes, and an age greater than 75 years. When calculating a $CHADS_2$ score, each of these variables receives 1 point, except for previous TIAs/strokes, which receives 2 points. A $CHADS_2$ score of 2 imparts a 4% annual stroke risk, which is a three- to fivefold increase in the risk of stroke compared with non–atrial fibrillation patients. Warfarin use increases complications related to bleeding (0.4% per year risk of bleeding complications, with a 0.2% per year risk of intracranial hemorrhage), but decreases the relative risk of stroke by 64% and the absolute risk of stroke by 2.7% per year. Warfarin also performs better than antiplatelet agents with regard to stroke risk reduction.

3.

D Autosomal recessive microcephaly

Mutations in the MCPHi or cyclin-dependent kinase 5 regulatory associated protein 2 are associated with autosomal recessive microcephaly (microcephaly vera). Microcephaly refers to a head circumference more than two standard deviations below the mean for age and gender after factoring in intrauterine growth retardation and low birth weight/body length.

4.

D Calcification and hemorrhage are common.

The microscopic and staining properties of the lesion shown in the images accompanying the question as well as its imaging characteristics are compatible with an ependymoma. On the MRI, this lesion shows cystic or necrotic changes and avid enhancement, and extrudes through the foramen magnum (sagittal image) and right foramen of Luschka (axial image) in a "toothpaste" configuration. Calcification and hemorrhage are common and contribute to the heterogeneity of these lesions. Ependymomas most commonly are found in children but can occur at any age. (A) Ependymomas can occur anywhere but typically arise from the floor of the fourth ventricle. Medulloblastomas classically arise from the roof of the fourth ventricle but also can occur in the cerebellar peduncles and cerebellar hemispheres. (B) Ependymomas are associated with neurofibromatosis type 2 and not type 1. (C) Hemangioblastomas are tumors that most commonly occur in the posterior fossa and spinal cord and may be complicated by polycythemia due to their production of erythropoietin.

5.

E Diencephalon, basal ganglia, and cerebral hemispheres

The Cheyne-Stokes respiration pattern originates in telencephalic and diencephalic structures.

6.

C Administration of meperidine

Meperidine is an opioid agonist that can lower the seizure threshold. (A) Cerebral hypotension causes postural headaches rather than seizures. (B) The vasovagal response to pain causes bradycardia rather than tachycardia. (D) A recurrent disk herniation reproduces radicular symptoms rather than seizures. (E) Chemical meningitis is theoretically possible but very unlikely in this case.

7.

D It may present with acute brain herniation and death.

The displayed sagittal, noncontrast T1 sequence shows a bright lesion in the anterior aspect of the third ventricle compatible with a colloid cyst. Note a brighter spot within it (known as "fried egg" appearance) and enlargement of the lateral ventricles with thinning and bowing of the corpus callosum. Patients with a colloid cyst may present with rapid brain herniation, hydrocephalus, and death if there is acute ventricular obstruction.

(A) Colloid cysts are derived from embryonic endoderm. (B) Symptoms in colloid cysts are related to ventricular obstruction (intermittent or acute), and patients may present with headaches, nausea, and vomiting. Patients with acute obstruction, herniation, and hydrocephalus can have mental status changes and deteriorate rapidly. (C) In colloid cysts, MR spectroscopy may show a large peak that resembles N-acetylaspartate; however, normal brain metabolites are absent. Elevated levels of alanine at short TE are seen in meningiomas and not in colloid cysts. (E) Calcification and regions of nodular enhancement are features of craniopharyngiomas. Calcification in colloid cysts is rare, and they do not enhance.

8.

A Oculomotor

The oculomotor triangle, also known as the medial or Hakuba triangle, contains the oculomotor nerve and horizontal segment of the internal carotid artery. It is the triangle by which access to most intracavernous aneurysms and tumors is gained. (B) Historically, the Parkinson triangle was accessed to treat carotid-cavernous fistulas. It also contains the abducens nerve. (C) The Glasscock triangle (posterolateral) contains the middle meningeal artery in the floor of the triangle as it exits the foramen spinosum, horizontal petrous internal carotid artery, and infratemporal fossa. The triangle is useful, as it enables the surgeon to gain proximal control of the internal carotid artery for more distal vascular procedures. Approximately 10 mm of the carotid artery is accessible through this triangle. (D) The Kawase (posteromedial) triangle contains the petrous apex, internal carotid artery, cochlea, and vertebrobasilar junction. It can be used to perform an anterior petrosectomy so that the posterior fossa, anterior brainstem, and root of the trigeminal nerve can be visualized. (E) The porus trigeminus is the entrance to the Meckel cave and is contained within the inferolateral triangle.

9.

C Craniopharyngioma

Craniopharyngiomas are benign histologically, extra-axial, and slow-growing tumors that predominantly involve the sella and suprasellar space. On CT, the adamantinomatous-type tumor appears as a predominately cystic mass with a solid component in more than 90% of cases. On MRI, the tumors predominantly are cystic suprasellar masses with a solid, contrast-enhancing component as well. Characteristic calcifications commonly are seen.

10.

B Pleomorphic xanthoastrocytoma

The patient's age and history as well as the imaging characteristics of this intra-axial mass strongly favor pleomorphic xanthoastrocytoma (PXA). PXAs usually are supratentorial, occur most commonly in the temporal lobes, and have areas of mixed cystic change and enhancing nodules. They typically show extension peripherally to the dura, which may be thickened, and sometimes a dural tail is present. These tumors are seen in children and young adults who usually have a long-standing history of epilepsy with or without headaches or other focal neurologic symptoms. PXAs are slow-growing tumors categorized as WHO grade II. (A) Primary central nervous system lymphoma is very rare in children. It would show avid homogeneous enhancement in immunocompetent individuals, but tends to have areas of necrosis and hemorrhage in the immunocompromised. Primary central nervous system lymphoma favors the deep and periventricular white matter and corpus callosum as opposed to the cortical/subcortical location of the tumor in this case. Secondary lymphoma usually is leptomeningeal or dura based, although it rarely may be parenchymal. (C) The mass in the current case is intra-axial. Anteriorly it clearly abuts the white matter directly without intervening cortex. The cyst along the posterior and medial aspect of the mass also is clearly intraparenchymal. This feature rules out a meningioma, which otherwise also can show variable morphology with cystic and hemorrhagic changes and necrosis. Additionally, meningiomas are rare in children except when they are syndromic (e.g., in neurofibromatosis type 2). (D) Dysembryoplastic neuroepithelial tumors (DNETs) constitute another cause of epilepsy in young patients. These tumors are most common in the temporal lobes. They are cortically based, well circumscribed, and usually have a bubbly appearance. In contrast to PXAs, DNETs usually do not enhance, although 20% may have punctate or ring-like contrast-enhancement patterns. (E) The classic pilocytic astrocytoma presents as a cystic mass with an avidly enhancing mural nodule. They rarely occur in a supratentorial location except in adults, in whom they are most common in the cerebral hemispheres. Supratentorial pilocytic astrocytomas in children tend to favor the optic chiasm (particularly in patients with neurofibromatosis type 1) and hypothalamic region.

11.

B Level 2

Level 2 evidence consists of randomized clinical trials. (A) Level 1 evidence consists of meta-analyses of multiple level 2 studies. (C) Level 3 evidence consists of quasi-experimental studies (e.g., large observational/cohort studies). (D) Level 4 evidence consists of nonexperimental studies (e.g., small observational studies). (E) Level 5 evidence consists of case reports and narrative literature reviews. Of note, level 6 evidence consists of the opinions of respected authorities.

12.

A Malingering/inability to participate in the exam

(A–E) Although the patient may have any of these diagnoses, Goldman visual field testing in this patient is inaccurate and unreliable as evidenced by the spiraling result. This indicates that the patient is guessing at what is and is not in his visual field, as patients almost never can indicate consistently and falsely where their visual fields end.

13.

D Less than –2.5

Osteoporosis is evaluated by assessment of bone mineral density and reported as a T-score. This value represents the number of standard deviations from normal. Osteoporosis is determined by a T-score of less than –2.5 (meaning that the bone mineral density is less than normal by 2.5 standard deviations). (B) T-scores of –1 to +1 are normal, expected values. (C) A T-score of –1 to –2.5 corresponds to low bone mineral density (osteopenia) without osteoporosis. (E) The definition of osteoporosis is not age dependent, as all individuals are compared to a reference healthy 30-year-old adult of the same sex when it comes to evaluating for osteoporosis.

14.

C Extensive intervertebral disk calcification

The patient's clinical presentation and elevated homogentisic acid levels in his urine are diagnostic of alkaptonuria (ochronosis). Widespread calcification involving multiple intervertebral disks may be seen in the spine along with osteoporosis. (A, B) Wedging of at least three adjacent vertebrae associated with thoracic or thoracolumbar kyphosis is a finding seen in Scheuermann disease. (D) H-shaped vertebrae result from infarction and increased pliability of the end plates in patients with sickle cell disease.

15.

C Pedunculopontine nucleus

The pedunculopontine nucleus is a newer target of deep brain stimulation as it plays a role in the postural instability seen in Parkinson disease that is not addressed well with other stimulation targets. (A) Stimulation of the subthalamic nucleus or globus pallidus internus can relieve the Parkinson disease symptoms of tremor, bradykinesia, and rigidity. (B) Stimulation of the ventralis intermedius nucleus of the thalamus is used for tremor reduction. (D) Stimulation of the globus pallidus internus is often performed for primary dystonias.

16.

C Hypoxia/anoxia

As shown in the image accompanying the question, the CA1 region of the hippocampus is highly vulnerable to hypoxic insults and subsequent necrosis, whereas the CA3 region and dentate gyrus are more resistant. The CA2 region is the most resistant to hypoxic insults. The hippocampal regions are shown in this image.

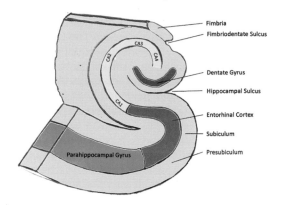

17.

B Limbic encephalitis

Limbic encephalitis (also known as autoimmune limbic encephalitis or paraneoplastic limbic encephalitis) is an autoimmune condition that arises mostly in patients with non–central nervous system tumors. It rarely is limited only to the limbic system and usually extends to other areas of the brain. Clinically, it is almost identical to herpes simplex encephalitis. The most recent system for diagnosis of herpes simplex encephalitis is the Graus and Saiz criteria, all of which need to be met to make the diagnosis: (1) subacute onset (less than 12 weeks of symptoms) of seizures, short-term memory loss, confusion, and psychiatric symptoms; (2) neuropathological or radiological evidence of involvement of the limbic system; (3) exclusion of other possible etiologies of limbic dysfunction; and (4) demonstration of a cancer within 5 years of the diagnosis of neurologic symptoms or the development of classic symptoms of limbic dysfunction in association with a well-characterized paraneoplastic antibody (e.g., antibodies to Hu, Ma2, CV2, amphiphysin, Ri). (A) Herpes simplex encephalitis is indistinguishable clinically from limbic encephalitis; however, cerebrospinal fluid PCR sensitivity has been reported to exceed 98%. In light of the concomitant diagnosis of a lung lesion, limbic encephalitis is more likely. (C) Pontine stroke is more acute in onset and would include dysfunction of the lower cranial nerves. (D) Paraneoplastic cerebellar degeneration is a paraneoplastic syndrome associated with lung, ovarian, and breast cancers as well as with Hodgkin lymphoma. It is a rare condition that occurs in less than 1% of patients with these conditions and usually affects middle-aged women. Symptoms include dysarthria; truncal, limb, and gait ataxia; nausea; vomiting; and diplopia. (E) Multiple sclerosis is not associated with psychiatric symptoms, and imaging findings are localized to white matter structures.

18.
B Germinal matrix hemorrhage
In the images accompanying the question, there are germinal matrix hemorrhages bilaterally seen as echogenic (bright) foci along the inferior aspect of the lateral ventricles on the coronal image *(left)* and focally expanding the caudothalamic groove on the sagittal image *(right)*. (A) Acute infarction presents as edema in a distinct arterial territory or in a nonarterial distribution (in the case of a venous infarction), which may be accompanied by hemorrhage. (C) Hypoxic-ischemic injury may be seen in ultrasound as increased echogenicity of the deep gray nuclei and brainstem or accentuated gray-white matter distinction peripherally due to edema. (D) Periventricular leukomalacia presents with increased echogenicity in the periventricular regions and more characteristically in the peri-atrial white matter.

19.
D Maxillary division of the trigeminal nerve
The maxillary division of the trigeminal nerve passes through the foramen rotundum.

20.
E Nicotinic
Nicotinic receptors on the target cells are an exception to the rule that adrenergic receptors are

the primary postganglionic sympathetic receptors. (A) Muscarinic receptors are the only postganglionic parasympathetic receptors.

21.
D C7 to sacrum
Global sagittal balance is a reflection of the position of the head in relationship to the pelvis and is most commonly measured on a standing, full-length lateral scoliosis radiograph by drawing a plumb line that extends from the mid–C7 vertebra to the sacrum. Such a measurement also is known as the sagittal vertical axis and should course anteriorly to the thoracic spine and intersect the L1 vertebra when neutral. A neutral sagittal vertical axis also intersects the posterosuperior corner of the S1 vertebra and, by convention, a spine with a plumb line that falls anterior or posterior to this point (the sagittal vertical axis offset) is said to be in positive or negative balance, respectively. There is no consensus on normal values. Sagittal imbalance may be compensated to a certain extent (depending on the degree of deformity) through mechanisms such as hip or knee flexion or hyperlordosis and hypokyphosis through muscular effort. Children tend to have negative imbalance compared with adults.

22.
D Superior oblique myokymia
Superior oblique myokymia is a condition with adult onset that manifests as contractions of the superior oblique that are most intense and pronounced when the eye is in the position of the action of the superior oblique (looking downward and medially). Patients describe a shaking of their vision, a feeling of a trembling eye, or tilted vision. The condition often is treated with carbamazepine. (A) Hemifacial spasm is a unilateral spasm/tonic contraction of the muscles innervated by the facial nerve. Although it can be caused by compression of the facial nerve by the anterior inferior cerebellar artery and thus corrected with microvascular decompression, patients often opt for the less invasive botulinum toxin injections into the affected muscles. (B) Duane syndrome is a congenital strabismus with three subtypes. The most common subtype involves an inability to abduct the affected eye due to maldevelopment of the abducens neural pathway. (C) Although patients with myasthenia gravis can present with variable ophthalmoplegia, the unilateral symptoms described and the isolation of the symptoms to action of the superior oblique make superior oblique myokymia more likely.

23.

C C

C represents the portion of the primary motor cortex most devoted to control of the hand. Due to the many fine motor movements required in the hand, the precentral gyrus tends to be wider in this region as supported by functional MRI studies. (A) A represents the inferior frontal gyrus. (B) B represents the precentral gyrus and primary motor cortex, but an area most likely devoted mostly to control of the facial musculature. (D) D represents the postcentral gyrus and primary somatosensory cortex. (E) E represents part of the supramarginal gyrus.

24.

A Conjugate gaze to the right, plegia of right eye adduction, and left eye nystagmus with left gaze

The median longitudinal fasciculus (MLF) is the main connection between the nuclei of cranial nerves III, IV, and VI. A lesion in the MLF causes internuclear ophthalmoplegia, and the affected eye shows impaired adduction. The contralateral eye abducts with nystagmus. This leads to horizontal diplopia when looking opposite the affected eye.

25.

C Myxopapillary ependymoma

This tumor shows the classic presentation of a myxopapillary ependymoma as an avidly enhancing intradural extramedullary mass at the level of the conus medullaris and filum terminale. Although a large mass filling the lumbosacral spinal canal (three or more vertebral segments) is highly suggestive, the imaging appearance is otherwise nonspecific, and other neoplasms such as peripheral nerve sheath tumors and paragangliomas may look similar. Myxopapillary ependymomas tend to be well circumscribed and lobulated, and sometimes show intrinsic T1 hyperintensity presumably due to the presence of mucin or hemorrhage. These tumors rarely can constitute a cause of subarachnoid hemorrhage and superficial siderosis. They are classified as WHO grade I lesions, usually are indolent, and are more common in males with a median age of 35 years at presentation. (A) Schwannomas can be solitary and may be found in this location, where they can mimic a small myxopapillary ependymoma. Both of these tumors can show cystic changes. (B) A solitary leptomeningeal metastasis of this size is a relatively rare presentation, particularly in the absence of systemic disease. Histological features in this case are consistent with a myxopapillary ependymoma. (D) Neurofibromas usually show heterogeneous enhancement. Central

hypointensity and peripheral hyperintensity on T2 images ("target sign") are suggestive of a neurofibroma, although they are not entirely specific. (E) Myxopapillary ependymomas are much more common than paragangliomas in this region; however, both may be indistinguishable by imaging. Histological features in this case are consistent with a myxopapillary ependymoma.

26.

C Grade 4

House-Brackmann grading ranges from 1 (normal) to 6 (no movement of the face). Grade 4 is moderate to severe facial weakness with obvious asymmetry. People with grade 4 function are not able to close their eyes fully. (A) Grade 2 is mild dysfunction with slight facial weakness noticeable on close inspection with normal resting tone. (B) Grade 3 is moderate, with obvious but not disfiguring asymmetry with complete eye closure with effort. (D) Grade 5 is severe with barely perceptible facial motion. (E) Grade 6 is complete facial paralysis.

27.

C Neurofibromatosis type 1

The lesion shown in the image accompanying the question represents a neurofibroma characterized by a loose arrangement of spindled cells with tapered nuclear ends and scant cytoplasm. Neurofibromas most commonly are associated with neurofibromatosis type 1. (A) Pituitary adenomas are the primary central nervous system manifestation of multiple endocrine neoplasia type 1. (D) Schwannomas are more commonly seen with neurofibromatosis type 2. (E) Subependymal giant cell astrocytomas are the hallmark of tuberous sclerosis.

28.

B A larger internal resistance

The time constant (T_c) is a measure of the amount of time required to change the voltage of the neuron (its potential). A larger time constant favors temporal summation of a signal, as a shorter time constant means that the potential will change more quickly with spatial summation. The equation is as follows:

$$T_c = \sqrt{(r_m r_i)}C_m$$

where r_m is the neuronal membrane resistance, r_i is the internal neuronal resistance, and C_m is the membrane capacitance. A larger intracellular space lowers internal resistance.

29.

D Intravenous slow continuous infusion

The usual route of administration of vitamin K is oral, which has been shown to be faster than the subcutaneous route in reversing and abnormal INR. The risk of administering vitamin K intravenously is anaphylaxis, and therefore intravenous administration should be limited strictly to patients with life-threatening bleeding. In such cases, administration is not recommended at a rate faster than 1 mg/minute.

30.

D 73%

The question is asking for the positive predictive value (PPV) of the test which can be calculated using this formula:

$$PPV = \frac{Sensitivity \times Prevalence}{Sensitivity \times Prevalence + (1 - specificity) \times (1 - Prevalence)}$$

31.

C Pericellular clearing is an artifact of delayed formalin fixation.

The tumor shown in the image accompanying the question is typical for a low-grade oligodendroglioma (WHO grade II). Calcifications are a frequent finding. Like fibrillary astrocytomas, oligodendrogliomas are infiltrative neoplasms. Oligodendrogliomas are either WHO grade II or III lesions. Tumors with necrosis are usually WHO grade III lesions.

32.

E Critical carotid artery stenosis with intraluminal thrombus

Carotid artery atherosclerosis usually is most severe within 2 cm of the bifurcation and arises opposite to the external and internal carotid artery flow divider. This lateral angiographic view shows near-complete occlusion at the level of the carotid bulb due to an atherosclerotic plaque. There is near-complete critical stenosis (> 99%) with a small amount of contrast material in the proximal internal carotid artery. There is a large, elongated filling defect within the internal carotid artery due to thrombosis. This patient also had thrombosis of the intracranial internal carotid artery, which was seen on the MRI of the brain. (A) Carotid artery dissection usually spares the carotid bulb, occurring 2 to 3 cm above this level. Dissections typically show abrupt tapering of the contrast column, resulting in a "flame-shaped" configuration in the acute phase and also may demonstrate an intimal flap with true and false lumina. (B) Although there is critical stenosis of the internal carotid artery in this case (> 99%), there is no complete occlusion, as there is still some contrast material going through the stenotic bulb and staining the proximal internal carotid artery. (C) The most common type of fibromuscular dysplasia classically presents with a beaded appearance. It can also look corrugated with small diverticula and less commonly may present with long segment stenosis (not the short segment narrowing in this case). Atypical (carotid bulb or septal type) fibromuscular dysplasia can present with a wedge-shaped defect in a nonatheromatous bulb, but this is rare. (D) Although pseudoaneurysms can thrombose due to stagnation of flow, there is no vascular dilatation or outpouching to suggest this.

33.

D 4

The described arteriovenous malformation (AVM) is grade 4. AVMs are graded on a scale of 0 to 5. AVMs less than 3 cm score 1 point, AVMs of 3 to 6 cm score 2 points, and AVMs more than 6 cm score 3 points. AVMs in eloquent areas score 1 point (0 points for non-eloquent area involvement), and 1 point is given for deep venous drainage (0 points for superficial drainage). Grading is related to surgical morbidity.

34.

A Vagus nerve

Although sympathetic input to the kidneys decreases the glomerular filtration rate through vasoconstriction, there are no definitive data to support the idea that parasympathetic activation has the reverse, vasodilatory effect. Renal activity mostly is increased through hormonal mechanisms. The parasympathetic response mainly is concerned with renal inflammatory reflexes. (B, C) The lumbar and thoracic splanchnic nerves provide sympathetic innervations to the kidneys. (D, E) The inferior and superior mesenteric plexuses provide sympathetic innervations to the various abdominal organs.

35.

B *Haemophilus influenzae*

Haemophilus influenzae is the most common cause of viral meningitis in nonvaccinated children and is uncommon among vaccinated populations. Neurologic symptoms usually are preceded by gastrointestinal symptoms such as diarrhea. (A) *Cryptococcus* is a cause of meningitis in immunosuppressed individuals. (C) *Neisseria meningitidis* is a leading cause of bacterial meningitis. (D) *Streptococcus pneumoniae* is a leading cause of viral meningitis. (E) Herpes simplex virus usually causes temporal encephalitis.

36.

C Sepsis

This child has meningitis and ventriculitis complicated by hydrocephalus. In the images accompanying the question, the postcontrast T1-weighted MRI *(left)* shows marked ventriculomegaly and enhancement of the ependymal surface, consistent with ventriculitis as well as diffuse leptomeningeal enhancement. The diffusion-weighted MRI *(right)* shows very bright material layering in the occipital horns of the lateral ventricles, which likely represents pus in this context (although blood also can show restricted diffusion). (A) Recurrent nonaccidental trauma potentially can result in ventriculomegaly related to intracranial hemorrhage. It would not explain the presence of layering debris within the occipital horns (unless there is intraventricular hemorrhage), leptomeningitis, or ventriculitis. (B) Congenital aqueductal stenosis can result in variable degrees of obstructive hydrocephalus but would not explain the other findings in this case. (D) A medulloblastoma in the posterior fossa potentially can result in obstructive hydrocephalus and leptomeningeal spread of disease. It would not explain the presence of layering material in the occipital horns unless there is associated hemorrhage or superimposed infection and ventriculitis.

37.

A Disruption of the transverse ligament

There are three types of C1 fractures: type 1, fracture of a single arch; type 2, burst fracture (Jefferson fracture); type 3, involves the lateral mass(es) of C1. The most important factor for the stability of the atlanto-occipital joint is ligamentous integrity, mostly from the integrity of the transverse ligament. Disruption of the transverse ligament can be determined by MRI or radiograph. Integrity can be determined by the rule of Spence (on an AP radiograph, the total overhang of the C1 lateral masses over C2 should be less than 7 mm, or a ligamentous disruption is likely) and by the atlantodental interval (ADI) (an ADI more than 3 mm in adults and 4 mm in children suggests ligamentous disruption).

38.

B Parkinson (infratrochlear)

Historically, the Parkinson triangle was accessed to treat carotid-cavernous fistulas. It also contains the abducens nerve. (A) The oculomotor triangle, also known as the medial or Hakuba triangle, contains the oculomotor nerve and the horizontal segment of the internal carotid artery. It is the triangle by which access to most intracavernous aneurysms and tumors is gained. (C) The Glasscock triangle (posterolateral) contains the middle meningeal artery in the floor of the triangle as it exits the foramen spinosum, the horizontal petrous internal carotid artery, and the infratemporal fossa. The triangle is useful as it enables the surgeon to gain proximal control of the internal carotid artery for more distal vascular procedures. Approximately 10 mm of the carotid artery is accessible through this triangle. (D) The Kawase (posteromedial) triangle contains the petrous apex, internal carotid artery, cochlea, and vertebrobasilar junction. It can be used to perform an anterior petrosectomy so that the posterior fossa, anterior brainstem, and root of the trigeminal nerve can be visualized. (E) The porus trigeminus is the entrance to the Meckel cave and is contained within the inferolateral triangle.

39.

C Rotatory subluxation with inflammation of the C1/C2 facet capsule

Grisel syndrome is seen in pediatric patients often after an upper respiratory tract infection or otolaryngology procedure with subsequent infection/inflammation of the C1/C2 facet joint and/or transverse atlantal ligament causing rotatory subluxation/torticollis. (A) The Power ratio (used to identify atlanto-occipital dislocation) is the ratio of the distance from the basion to opisthion (BC) divided by the distance from the opisthion to anterior arch of the atlas (OA). A ratio of 1 or less is normal, whereas a ratio of more than 1 may indicate atlanto-occipital dislocation. (B) According to the rule of Spence (a method to determine instability of the transverse ligament), an overhang of the C1 lateral masses on C2 of at least 7 mm is abnormal. (D) Baastrup syndrome is described as "kissing" spinous processes, with contact of adjacent spinous processes with enlargement/flattening/sclerosis of apposing interspinous surfaces. (E) Significant anterior cervical "flowing" osteophytes describe Forestier disease, which is characterized by dysphagia or the sensation of a lump in the throat due to compression of the esophagus between osteophytes and the larynx. This condition is part of the spectrum of diffuse idiopathic skeletal hyperostosis (DISH).

40.

B Acute left-sided hemiplegia

This is an acute, right middle cerebral artery territory infarct. On the images accompanying the question, note the loss of the gray matter–white matter distinction and the blurriness of the right basal ganglia region (*left image*) compared with the contralateral side where the caudate nucleus head and lentiform nucleus are seen well. Also shown is a hyperdense, right middle cerebral artery due to the presence of clot (*right image*). (A) Rapid-onset dementia may be seen in Creutzfeldt-Jakob disease (CJD) where the CT often is normal. The MRI in CJD may show increased cortical signal, particularly on diffusion-weighted sequences, with or without involvement of the basal ganglia and thalami. (C) The triad of fever, altered mental status, and nuchal rigidity may be seen in patients with bacterial meningitis; however, the triad is present in only 44% of bacterial meningitis patients. (D) Progressive encephalopathy is a very nonspecific presentation and is not consistent with an acute stroke.

41.

A Lateral ventricles

The majority (75%) of choroid plexus tumors arise in the lateral ventricles (usually in the atrium). The second most common (30%) location is in the fourth ventricle, which is a more common site of choroid plexus tumors in adults.

42.

B Hypokalemia

Manifestations of hypokalemia include nausea, vomiting, weakness, muscle cramps, rhabdomyolysis, polyuria, U waves on an electrocardiogram, a prolonged QT interval, and ventricular ectopy.

43.

C Hypercalcemia

Manifestations of hypercalcemia vary widely and can include polyuria, dehydration, mental status changes, nephrolithiasis, abdominal pain, anorexia, nausea, vomiting, constipation, pancreatitis, confusion, coma, and decreased deep tendon reflexes.

44.

D Hypomagnesemia

Manifestations of hypomagnesemia include weakness, muscle cramps, irritability, tremors, nystagmus, hallucinations, depression, epileptic fits, and torsade de pointes.

45.

A Hyperkalemia

Manifestations of hyperkalemia include weakness, nausea, paresthesias, palpitations, peaked T waves on an electrocardiogram, increased PR interval, increased QRS width, and loss of P waves on an electrocardiogram. (E) Manifestations of hypophosphatemia include weakness, mental status changes, white blood cell dysfunction, hemolytic anemia, rhabdomyolysis, and increased pulp chambers in teeth. It often is seen in refeeding syndrome.

46.

A Choroid plexus papilloma

The images accompanying the question show an avidly enhancing mass with frond-like margins (resembling a cauliflower), most consistent with a choroid plexus papilloma; 80% of these tumors are benign (WHO grade I), and 85% occur before age 5. The most common location is the atrium of the lateral ventricles; in adults, these tumors more frequently occur in the fourth ventricle. Twenty percent have calcifications. (B) Meningiomas are very rare in children unless they are syndromic or in patients with a prior history of radiation. (C) Ependymomas in children are much more common in the fourth ventricle. Half of supratentorial ependymomas are intraventricular, and the rest are parenchymal. Ependymomas are more heterogeneous than choroid plexus tumors and commonly show areas of calcification, cystic change, or hemorrhage. (D) Subependymomas are seen in older patients and are most common in the fourth ventricle. They characteristically do not enhance, although some may show variable degrees of enhancement. (E) Central neurocytomas most commonly occur in patients between 30 and 40 years of age. Their typical location is in a lateral ventricle abutting the septum pellucidum, but they can occur at other sites. They usually are more heterogeneous and do not enhance as avidly when compared with choroid plexus tumors.

47.

E Injury to the posterior ligamentous complex

Markers for unstable burst fractures include more than 50% loss of height, canal stenosis from retropulsion over 50%, kyphotic angulation of more than 20 degrees, increased interpedicular distance when upright, neurologic deficits, and progressive kyphosis. The Thoracolumbar Injury Classification and Severity (TLICS) score was designed to identify surgical patients. There is heavy emphasis on the integrity of the posterior ligamentous complex, as this often identifies a significant injury and is associated with excessive kyphotic angulation and/or progressive chronic kyphosis.

48.

B Bitemporal hemianopsia

The condition described is seesaw nystagmus, which can be a manifestation of a hypothalamic lesion, with a craniopharyngioma being the most common cause. Due to the association of these lesions with optic chiasmal involvement, a bitemporal hemianopsia might be present. Of note, the pathophysiology underlying seesaw nystagmus is understood poorly. (A) Loss of peripheral vision is a hallmark symptom of glaucoma. (C) A central scotoma results from such etiologies as nutritional deficiencies and methyl alcohol poisoning. (D) Binasal hemianopsia is rare in that the tracts providing vision in the nasal fields are far lateral and separated from one another. It can, however, be seen in some instances of hydrocephalus and falsely diagnosed in individuals with large, protruding noses. (E) Unilateral inferior hemianopsia is due to pathology involving the superior arcuates. Remember that pathologies in the brain create visual field deficits that tend to respect the vertical midline, whereas pathologies in the eye produce horizontal-respecting deficits.

49.

C Intracellular methemoglobin

In the early subacute stage, iron atoms are oxidized to the ferric state with resultant formation of methemoglobin, which has five unpaired electrons and is more strongly paramagnetic than deoxyhemoglobin. Because methemoglobin remains confined to the intracellular space, local susceptibility effects persist, and the hematoma appears hypointense on T2 and GRE sequences. The change in the configuration of hemoglobin enables access of water molecules to the iron atoms, and the dipole–dipole interactions result in T1 hyperintensity.

(A) Freshly extravasated erythrocytes in hyperacute hematomas contain a large proportion of oxyhemoglobin, which has no unpaired electrons and is weakly diamagnetic. Hyperacute hematomas appear isointense on T1- and hyperintense on T2-weighted sequences, sometimes with a hypointense rim on T2 and GRE sequences due to early deoxyhemoglobin formation. (B) Within several hours, acute hematomas show progressive conversion of oxyhemoglobin to deoxyhemoglobin, which proceeds centripetally. Deoxyhemoglobin has four unpaired electrons per iron atom and is strongly paramagnetic. Because deoxyhemoglobin remains restricted to the intracellular compartment, local distortions of the magnetic field lead to signal loss that appears hypointense on T2 and GRE sequences. The three-dimensional configuration of deoxyhemoglobin does not allow access of water molecules to the paramagnetic iron atoms, which prevents the dipole–dipole interactions that would increase T1 signal; therefore, both hyperacute and acute hematomas remain isointense on T1-weighted sequences. (D) In the late subacute stage, the release of methemoglobin into the extracellular compartment removes local susceptibility effects, and the hematoma now appears hyperintense on T2 while remaining hyperintense on T1-weighted images. (E) Hemosiderin in chronic hematomas appears hypointense on both T1- and T2-weighted sequences due to formation of ferritin by phagocytosing macrophages, the excess of which is accumulated as hemosiderin. Both of these substances are superparamagnetic.

50.

B Hypertension increases the relative risk by 3.9 to 5.4%.

Hypertension is a controversial cause of intracranial hemorrhage (ICH), as both ICH and hypertension are inherently more common with age. The relative risk of developing an ICH is increased by hypertension by 3.9 to 5.4%. (C) Acute surges in blood pressure not related to sympathomimetics or preeclampsia can precipitate ICH. (D) Hypertension is considered primarily a risk factor for the development of a pontine/cerebellar ICH.

51.

C *TP53* gene mutations

TP53 gene mutations are seen more commonly with malignant degradation of low-grade gliomas than with de novo glioblastomas. (A, B) *EGFR* and *PTEN* gene amplifications are seen more commonly in glioblastomas arising de novo. (D) There tends to be allelic loss of chromosomes 10q and 19q in secondary glioblastomas. (E) Both primary and secondary glioblastomas show positive staining for GFAP (glial fibrillary acidic protein).

52.

C Intertransverse ligament

The exiting nerve root (L4) travels caudal to the L4 pedicle and remains intimate with the pedicle as it exits. The nerve root is found deep to the intertransverse ligament, and care must be taken to avoid electrocautery/mechanical injury to the nerve root/dorsal root ganglion at this location. (D) The disk space is anterior and medial to the exiting nerve root.

53.

D Cricothyroid

(A, B) All intrinsic muscles of the larynx with the exception of the cricothyroid are innervated by the recurrent laryngeal nerve, which is a branch of the vagus nerve. Abduction of the vocal cords is performed solely by the actions of the posterior cricoarytenoid muscles. (C) The stylopharyngeus is innervated by cranial nerve IX. (E) The geniohyoid is innervated by the C1 nerve root via the hypoglossal nerve.

54.

B Phosphodiesterase

As a second messenger for G-protein signaling, ATP is converted to cAMP by adenyl cyclase. In the cytosol, cAMP then activates protein kinase A that then acts on CREB, which acts as a transcription factor. cAMP is converted to AMP and thus deactivated by phosphodiesterase. (E) Phospholipase C hydrolyzes and cleaves PIP_2 to IP_3 and DAG in cellular signaling. The products of this reaction then act as second messengers.

55.

B Dural sinus thrombosis

The "empty delta" sign originally was described on a contrast-enhanced head CT in thrombosis of the superior sagittal sinus. On axial images, the sign results from enhancement around the thrombus filling the superior sagittal sinus, which regularly has a triangular shape. Although there is no consensus on the pathophysiology of the surrounding enhancement, proposed mechanisms include enhancement of peridural and dural venous chan-

nels, clot organization, and partial recanalization of the thrombus. A similar appearance can be seen on MRI and in the transverse venous sinuses, where a triangular filling defect also may be seen. (A) Acute arterial thrombosis may present as a hyperdense vessel on a noncontrast CT or as a filling defect on CT, MRI, or conventional angiography. (C) The presence of a focus of enhancement within a parenchymal hematoma (the "spot" sign) is an independent predictor of expansion and poor outcome. (D) The "empty delta" sign is not related to impending herniation.

56.

A More antihistaminergic and anticholinergic activity

Old antipsychotics often are administered with antihistamine and sedating agents to counteract the expected extrapyramidal side effects. (C, D) The primary mechanism by which antipsychotics are thought to act is by dopamine receptor (D2) blockade. More D2 blockade has been associated with side effects including tardive dyskinesia and neuroleptic malignant syndrome. Increased D2 blockade does not mean increased extrapyramidal side effects, however. The side effects emerge due to a balance between the dopamine antagonizing properties of neuroleptics and their other receptor-blocking attributes. (E) The "typical" antipsychotics have more antiserotonergic properties.

57.

C 50%

58.

B Ventral lateral nucleus

The ventral lateral and ventral anterior nuclei receive information from the cerebellum and basal ganglia and project to motor cortex areas. (A) The anterior nuclei group receives afferents from the mammillary bodies and projects to the cingulate gyrus in the Papez circuit. (C) The ventral posterior lateral nucleus receives information from the spinothalamic tracts and projects to sensory cortex areas. (D) The ventral posterior medial nucleus has afferents and efferents connecting to the trigeminal sensory tracts. (E) The medial geniculate body receives signals from the inferior colliculus and projects to the auditory cortex. In contrast, the lateral geniculate body receives signals from retinal ganglion cells and projects to the primary visual cortex.

59.

C Nystagmus retractorius

Both convergence nystagmus and nystagmus retractorius are associated with Parinaud syndrome. (A) Downbeat nystagmus often is associated with Chiari 1 malformations and cervicomedullary lesions. (B) Seesaw nystagmus is associated with lesions in the diencephalon or chiasmal compression. (D) Abducting nystagmus is associated with lesions in the medial longitudinal fasciculus and occurs in internuclear ophthalmoplegia.

60.

D Unstable fracture exacerbated by external stabilization with potential epidural hematoma

Although overmedication/oversedation and poor neurologic exams may be causes of a recorded decline in the patient's condition, patients with ankylosing spondylitis are predisposed to unstable fractures after seemingly trivial trauma. This is in part due to the ossification of ligaments that create long lever arms, limiting the ability to absorb minor impacts. Patients are prone to developing epidural hematomas. An emergent MRI is indicated in this patient for this reason. In addition, fractures often are missed on radiographs, leading to improper treatment. Given the fixed deformities, strapping patients to backboards or inappropriate collars may exacerbate unstable fractures and cause damage to the neural elements.

61.

B Lymphoma

This is an avidly enhancing solid and infiltrative periventricular mass that partially involves the corpus callosum and fornix, and reportedly has low apparent diffusion coefficient values, indicating restricted diffusion. Note the surrounding edema on the images accompanying the question. The imaging findings are most compatible with lymphoma. Areas of necrosis may be seen in patients with HIV/AIDS. (A) Glioblastoma likely would show areas of necrosis. (C) Tumefactive demyelination characteristically may have an incomplete ring of enhancement. Areas of restricted diffusion sometimes are seen along the leading edge. (D) Infection could present as leptomeningeal disease, cerebritis, or infected fluid collections, which are not present in this case.

62.

C Anterior displacement of the ipsilateral ear

Positional plagiocephaly can be differentiated from lambdoid craniosynostosis (synostotic plagiocephaly) on physical examination. Lambdoidal synostosis is characterized by ipsilateral occipitoparietal flattening with the ipsilateral ear displaced posteriorly, contralateral parietal bossing, and contralateral frontal bossing.

63.

D Sweating

The sympathetic nervous system uses postganglionic norepinephrine and epinephrine receptors for end-organ activation or response. The two exceptions are that the adrenal gland and sweat glands are postganglionic and activated by acetylcholine signaling. Although sweating is a sympathetic nervous system response, the postganglionic receptors are muscarinic (bind acetylcholine), just as they are in the parasympathetic nervous system. Because atropine competitively antagonizes muscarinic receptors, sweating decreases after systemic administration of atropine. (A–C, E) These actions are only affected by atropine's blockade of the parasympathetic nervous system. Sympathetic activity remains constant with atropine administration, in that the autonomic nervous system operates by altering the relative activity of the sympathetic and parasympathetic nervous systems.

64.

B Involvement of eloquent brain

The MRI studies shown in the images accompanying the question demonstrate a large arteriovenous malformation (AVM) with extensive vascular flow voids throughout the left hemisphere. Management of AVMs is complex, and open microsurgical excision usually offers the best chance for cure in patients with a high risk of hemorrhage. The Spetzler-Martin grading system was introduced to estimate the surgical risk. It allocates points according to the size of the lesion, deep versus superficial venous drainage, and involvement of eloquent brain. Several studies have correlated higher grade lesions on the Spetzler-Martin system with worse surgical outcomes. (A) Deep-seated AVMs have an increased incidence of hemorrhage and a higher surgical risk than those with superficial venous drainage; therefore, these lesions receive a higher score on the Spetzler-Martin grading system. (C) Retrograde cortical venous drainage is associated with an increased risk of hemorrhage in dural arteriovenous fistulas. (D) Venous ectasia results in a sevenfold increase in the risk of hemorrhage in dural arteriovenous fistulas and upgrades the lesions from grade 3 to grade 4 in the Cognard classification.

65.

E Fabry disease

Fabry disease is a lysosomal storage disease resulting in full-body pain, renal dysfunction, and cardiomyopathy, among other manifestations. (A) Farber disease is an autosomal recessive lysosomal storage disease resulting from a deficiency in ceramidase. Death occurs by age 2. (B) Fragile X syndrome is the most frequent hereditary cause of mental retardation and results from an X-linked dominant inheritance of mutations in the *FMR1* gene. (C) Rett syndrome typically results from a new mutation, occurs almost exclusively in females, and is characterized by macrocephaly, developmental delays, hand-wringing difficulties, and scoliosis. (D) Hurler syndrome is an autosomal recessive mucopolysaccharidosis due to a deficiency in α_1-iduronidase and is characterized by corneal clouding, dwarfism, and mental retardation. Death occurs at ages 5 to 10 from cardiac arrest.

66.

E Granular layer

The mnemonic "miles per gallon" can be used to remember the layers of the cerebellum: *m*olecular, *P*urkinje, and *g*ranular. Granule cells (also found in the hippocampus, dorsal cochlear nucleus, olfactory bulb, and cerebral cortex) are the most prevalent type of neuron in the brain. Found in the granular layer, they communicate with the more superficial molecular layer neurons through parallel fibers. (B, D) There are six layers of the cerebral cortex, notably layer 3 (the external pyramidal layer containing the primary source of corticocortical efferents), layer 4 (the internal granular layer receiving afferents from the thalamus), layer 5 (the internal pyramidal layer containing pyramidal neurons and forming the corticospinal tracts), and layer 6 (the multiform layer, which sends efferent fibers to the thalamus).

67.

A Antitrust law

Antitrust law regulates the conduct of organizations and business to promote fair competition for the benefit of consumers. Under the antitrust laws, hospitals are perceived as business entities offering health care services. In the case discussed in the question, the merger of the two hospitals would create a monopoly of tertiary care services in the local market and can be considered a violation of antitrust law. (B) Stark law (also known as the physician self-referral law) prohibits physicians from referring patients to institutes in which they or a close family member has financial interests. (C) The federal anti-kickback statue prevents physicians from receiving compensation for prescribing or using specific drugs or instruments. (D) The Emergency Medical Treatment and Active Labor Act (EMTALA) governs hospital transfers and what patients are obligated to receive and which patients can be refused treatment. One basic premise is that patients cannot be refused emergency, stabilizing medical care, if it is within the hospital's ability, simply because of their lack of ability to pay.

68.

C There is weakness of foot inversion with an L5 nerve root palsy, which is spared with a CPN palsy.

With a common peroneal nerve (CPN) palsy, the posterior tibialis (which enables foot inversion with innervation by the posterior tibial nerve) and gluteus medius (which enables internal hip rotation with innervation by the superior gluteal nerve) are spared. L5 nerve root deficits may include weakness in ankle dorsiflexion (anterior tibialis), foot eversion (peroneus longus/brevis), and foot inversion (tibialis posterior).

69.

B 28

The ASIA motor scale awards up to five points per side to motor function at root levels C5 to T1 (biceps, wrist extensors, triceps, grip, and hand intrinsics) and L2 to S1 (iliopsoas, quadriceps, tibialis anterior, extensor hallucis longus, and gastrocnemius), for a total of 50 possible points. This exam has two motor function tests of the C5 root level (deltoid and biceps), of which only the biceps is used. Simply add up the motor grade at each level to obtain a cumulative score.

70.

B Indirect revascularization using an encephaloduroarteriosynangiosis procedure

An encephaloduroarteriosynangiosis (EDAS) procedure uses a branch of the superficial temporal artery that is laid directly on the surface of the brain without doing a direct anastomosis. Children tend to have better results with this procedure than do adults. (A) Direct revascularization using a superficial temporal artery to middle cerebral artery bypass is effective in adults. (C, D) Conservative and medical therapies result in suboptimal stroke prevention.

71.

C Glioblastoma

The vascular proliferative changes seen in the background of irregularly shaped astrocytic cells is most consistent with a glioblastoma diagnosis. Vascular proliferative changes represent a proliferation of cells that normally constitute blood vessel walls (endothelial cells, smooth muscle cells, pericytes, and fibroblasts). The significance of this finding depends on the tumor type. In a pilocytic astrocytoma, there may be vascular proliferative changes that do not have the same implication in terms of grade as they do in a fibrillary astrocytoma.

72.

C Third degree

The Seddon and Sunderland classification systems are the most commonly used classification schemes for peripheral nerve injuries. A third-degree injury is an interruption of the endoneurium. (A) A Sunderland first-degree injury (Seddon neurapraxia) is a physiological transection with the nerve and basement membrane intact. (B) A second-degree injury (Seddon axonotmesis) is an interruption of the axons and myelin with intact supporting structures. (D) A fourth-degree injury is an interruption of the endoneurium and perineurium. (E) A fifth-degree injury (Seddon neurotmesis) is a completely severed nerve. (A sixth-degree injury is a mixed lesion.)

73.

A FDG uptake

Rapid growth on serial imaging, areas of induration on clinical exam, and persistent pain are features that raise concern about malignant transformation of a plexiform neurofibroma, which can show increased FDG uptake. (B) Both benign and malignant peripheral nerve sheath tumors may show heterogeneous enhancement. (C) The "target" sign classically is seen on T2 images in neurofibromas and is related to a fibrocollagenous core. It sometimes can be seen in schwannomas and usually is not seen in malignant peripheral nerve sheath tumors. (D) Benign plexiform neurofibromas tend to grow slowly.

74.

B Left lateral medulla

Wallenberg syndrome (lateral medullary syndrome) often is attributable to vertebral artery occlusion, although classically the condition is described secondary to a posterior inferior cerebellar artery infarction. The lateral medulla essentially is the only location at which a stroke will cause an ipsilateral sensory loss in the face and a contralateral sensory loss in the body without weakness. There often are no changes in sensorium. (A) A right anterior medulla stroke (medial medullary syndrome or Dejerine syndrome) would cause deviation of the tongue to the right side, contralateral limb weakness, and loss of proprioception/vibration on the contralateral side due to occlusion of the spinal artery near its vertebral origin. (D) A stroke in the ventrocaudal pons will lead to Millard-Gubler syndrome, causing contralateral weakness, ipsilateral lateral gaze weakness, and ipsilateral whole face weakness. The deficits can be remembered by noting that there are six letters in "Gubler" and seven letters in "Millard," indicating the palsies of cranial nerves VI and VII along with the contralateral weakness.

75.

C Presence of a lucid interval

Of patients with an epidural hematoma, 10 to 27% experience the classic presentation of a brief loss of consciousness followed by a lucid interval, with further progression to obtundation, hemiparesis, and a dilated pupil. This symptom progression also can be observed with intraparenchymal and subdural hemorrhages. Eighty-five percent of epidural hematomas are due to arterial bleeding, and most often are secondary to injury to the middle meningeal artery. Skull fractures are seen in 40% of epidural hematomas, and CT scans show a lenticular shape of the hemorrhage in 84% of cases due to restrictions from the cranial sutures. Indications for surgery may include a hemorrhage volume more than 30 mL or thickness more than 15 mm, midline shift more than 5 mm, Glasgow Coma Scale score of 8 or less, and focal neurologic deficits (e.g., anisocoria).

Section 3

1.

D Ligation of the anterior choroidal artery

Surgical ligation of the anterior choroidal artery was an early procedure for Parkinson disease. It classically produces a "triple H" syndrome of hemianesthesia, hemiparesis, and a homonymous hemianopsia.

2.

B Nerve root enhancement

Enhancement of intradural nerve roots can be seen in preganglionic injuries and may indicate functional discontinuity even in the presence of a normal-appearing nerve. (A) Pseudomeningoceles (not true meningoceles) occur in more than 80% of patients with traumatic avulsion of the brachial plexus. Pseudomeningoceles may develop within the spinal canal, where they exert variable degrees of mass effect or track along the course of the nerve roots. (C) Presence of fluid within the root sleeve does not necessarily reflect avulsion injury; however, pooling of fluid and abrupt interruption of the root sleeve are findings indicative of an avulsion injury. (D) A spinal cord hematoma may be seen in the setting of trauma but does not necessarily reflect avulsion injury. Focal edema may be seen in the spinal cord at the site of the avulsion.

3.
B Beta activity over temporal areas

The periodic discharges seen with herpes encephalitis typically occur over the temporal regions. Slow waves, rather than sharp waves, may be evident over the temporal lobes in many patients with severe disease. Seizures occur early in the course of herpes encephalitis, and electroencephalographic recordings can be very disrupted. (E) Periodic sharp wave complexes are seen in Creutzfeldt-Jakob disease.

4.
B Arachnoid cyst

Arachnoid cysts are lined by arachnoid cells, resulting in accumulation of cerebrospinal fluid. They are extra-axial and displace the brain parenchyma away from the calvaria. The displaced cortex in this case can be seen on both T2 and FLAIR sequence images. Arachnoid cysts follow cerebrospinal fluid signal on all sequences and, therefore, suppress on FLAIR, although they may show pulsation artifacts, as in this case, particularly when they are large. Arachnoid cysts do not show contrast enhancement, and most do not grow but sometimes can enlarge. They can result in mass effect and scalloping/thinning of the inner table of the calvaria (as seen on the T2 image accompanying the question). If symptomatic, arachnoid cysts can be shunted, fenestrated/marsupialized, or resected. (A) Porencephalic cysts are intra-axial (not extra-axial as in this case), and usually present as a cavity filled with cerebrospinal fluid; therefore, they also follow cerebrospinal fluid signal on all sequences and do not enhance. They typically are surrounded by dysplastic white matter (compared with the displaced cerebral cortex in this case). (C) Neurenteric cysts are lined by endodermal epithelium. The great majority of these cysts are extra-axial, but in rare cases can be intra-axial. They do not communicate freely with the subarachnoid space; therefore, they do not necessarily follow cerebrospinal fluid signal. They usually show variable signal intensities, depending on the degree of proteinaceous contents. (D) Schizencephaly is a neuronal migration disorder resulting in a cleft extending from the ventricular (ependymal) surface to the cortical (pial) surface. The cleft is lined with dysplastic gray matter and may be filled with cerebrospinal fluid.

5.
D Hyperphosphorylated tau protein

The image accompanying the question shows a neuron with a neurofibrillary tangle (NFT). NFTs are intracytoplasmic aggregates of hyperphosphorylated tau protein that can be found in various neurodegenerative processes, the most common being Alzheimer disease.

6.
E Striae medullaris thalami

The striae medullaris thalami connect the anterior thalamic and septal nuclei to the habenula. The inferior layer of the tela choroidea attaches to the striae medullaris thalami and forms the floor of the velum interpositum. (C) The internal medullary lamina runs longitudinally through the thalamus, separating the medial and lateral nuclear masses. (D) The thalamic fasciculus joins the ansa lenticularis and lenticular fasciculus with the basal ganglia and the ventral lateral nucleus of the thalamus.

7.
A Lack of weakness in the deltoid and latissimus dorsi

The radial and axillary nerves are terminal branches of the posterior cord. Lack of weakness in the deltoid (axillary nerve innervated) and latissimus dorsi (thoracodorsal nerve) indicates injury to the radial nerve and not the posterior cord in the presence of a wrist drop. (B) The long thoracic nerve innervates the serratus anterior and originates from the roots of C5 through C7. (C) The rhomboids are innervated by the dorsal scapular nerve, which originates from the C4 and C5 nerve roots before they form the superior trunk. (D) The medial antebrachial cutaneous nerve is derived from the C8 and T1 nerve roots and branches from medial cord. (E) Brachioradialis involvement would occur in a radial nerve injury, but this finding alone does not rule out a posterior cord injury.

8.

C Associated with atlantoaxial subluxation

Periodontoid panniculi can be seen in the setting of various etiologies, including rheumatoid arthritis, calcium pyrophosphate deposition disease, and psoriatic arthritis. They frequently are associated with atlantoaxial subluxation, and it is thought that chronic craniocervical instability may play a role in their development. (A) Various reports have shown periodontoid panniculi to resolve gradually after posterior stabilization without actual tissue resection. (B) Chordomas arise from notochordal elements. Although they can occur at the tip of the clivus, they usually are very bright on T2 sequences. (D) Meningiomas arise from arachnoid cap cells. The lesion in this case is periodontoid rather than dural based.

9.

A Amoebiasis

The organisms shown in the image accompanying the question morphologically are consistent with amoeba. *Naegleria* often is associated with primary amoebic encephalitis classically presenting in patients exposed to contaminated water. *Acanthamoeba* and *Balamuthia* can cause granulomatous amoebic encephalitis often in immunocompromised individuals.

10.

B *Herpes simplex*

Herpes simplex causes temporal encephalitis and temporal epileptiform discharge on electroencephalogram.

11.

C *Cryptococcus*

Central nervous system *Cryptococcus* infection can manifest with multiple focal mass lesions called cryptococcomas. The opening pressure during a lumbar puncture is high, cryptococcal antigen titer is positive, and cerebrospinal fluid India ink staining is also positive with this condition, which is common in patients with HIV. Treatment is with amphotericin B and flucytosine.

12.

A *Tenia solium*

Tenia solium is a tapeworm found in pigs that causes neurocysticercosis. Symptoms include seizures, decreased vision, papilledema, and parkinsonism. Although the pork supply in the United States is free of the organism, pork in Central and South America may be colonized. (D) Toxoplasmosis is one of the most common neurologic complications of AIDS. Patients present with fever, headaches, seizures, and possibly focal neurologic deficits. Multiple ring-enhancing lesions are seen in 70% of patients with toxoplasmosis. Distinguishing toxoplasmosis from lymphoma can be difficult, but a trial of antitoxoplasmosis medications for two weeks can confirm the diagnosis. (E) West Nile virus causes poliomyelitis and meningitis, with poliomyelitis being the more common manifestation. Patients typically have fever, myalgias, and encephalopathy, along with asymmetric weakness that quickly can progress to quadriplegia. Cerebrospinal fluid studies show pleocytosis and elevated protein. (F) JC virus leads to progressive multifocal leukoencephalopathy (PML). This fatal disease has no effective treatment. Symptoms develop over several weeks, and include clumsiness, progressive weakness, and visual, speech, and personality changes. Characteristic imaging findings include multifocal hypointense T1 and hyperintense T2 lesions.

13.

B Ependymoma

The tumor cells form perivascular pseudorosettes, a classic feature of ependymoma. Perivascular pseudorosettes are formed by the perivascular arrangement of tumor cells with an intervening fibrillary-rich, acellular area.

14.

D Sexual dysfunction

The incidence of sexual dysfunction is reported to occur in 0.4 to 20%, whereas retrograde ejaculation occurs in 5 to 22% of patients undergoing an anterior lumbar interbody fusion (ALIF) procedure. These injuries are assumed to be due to injury to the bilateral sympathetic chains contributing to the superior hypogastric plexus. Of note, ureteral injuries, deep venous thrombosis, hernias, and lumbar sympathetic dysfunction may be more common with ALIF procedures. Other complication rates are similar between ALIF and extreme lateral interbody fusion (XLIF) procedures. (A) Vascular injuries are seen in 0.5 to 15% (average 6.6%) of patients undergoing an ALIF procedure. (B) Neurologic injuries are seen in 5% of patients undergoing an ALIF procedure. In contrast, transient neurologic complaints can occur in up to 25% of patients undergoing an XLIF.

15.

C Surgical decompression

The CT scan shows tension pneumocephalus with a large amount of air underlying a left craniotomy.

There is resultant mass effect on the brain, shift of midline structures, and entrapment with early dilatation of the contralateral lateral ventricle. Tension pneumocephalus is a surgical emergency. Treatment includes surgical decompression and administration of 100% oxygen. (A) A lumbar puncture would be contraindicated in an acute herniation syndrome. (B) Hypertonic saline solutions are sometimes used in the treatment of cerebral edema and may lower increased intracranial pressures acutely. (D) Mannitol is a widely used osmotic diuretic that decreases cerebral edema and intracranial pressures by reducing water content in cerebral tissue.

16.

C After the peak of sodium conductance but before hyperpolarization

Potassium conductance peaks as some voltage-gated potassium channels begin to close at the peak of depolarization of the action potential (after sodium conductance peaks). (A) Before the peak of sodium conductance, the conductance of both sodium and potassium is increasing, with the former increasing at a greater rate. (B) During the peak of sodium conductance, the potassium conductance still is increasing. (D, E) Potassium conductance decreases throughout the remainder of the action potential through the hyperpolarization phase.

17.

C Miller Fisher syndrome

The patient has Miller Fisher syndrome, a variant of Guillain-Barré syndrome. It is characterized by the triad of areflexia, ataxia (usually without limb weakness), and ophthalmoplegia, and can occur with ascending facial diplegia. The condition is more common in middle-aged men and often follows a viral illness. (A) Although all of the symptoms fit with multiple sclerosis, the most likely diagnosis given the patient's symptoms and presentation is Miller Fisher syndrome. (B) A cerebellar stroke can result in an ataxic gait, but the other symptoms cited are not typical. (D) Diplopia and ataxia can be seen in ethanol intoxication, but it does not explain the facial diplegia. (E) Myasthenia gravis is characterized by muscle fatigue, which may manifest in ophthalmoplegia and facial weakness. In severe forms, there may be general muscle weakness (not found on the physical exam), resulting in an ataxic gait, but the mention of a recent viral illness makes Miller Fisher much more likely.

18.

C Somatosensory evoked potential

Somatosensory evoked potentials (SSEPs) in the upper extremities measure impulses in the posterior columns, whereas in the lower extremities, SSEPs are carried by the dorsolateral fasciculi, which receive their blood supply from the anterior spinal artery. (A) Motor evoked potentials are performed by stimulating the motor cortex and recording responses in the peripheral musculature. (E) Electromyography involves three phases of testing: insertional activity, spontaneous activity, and volitional activity as recorded by needle electrodes.

19.

D Shunt externalization

Shunt externalization at the chest or neck level should be the next step to allow resolution of the pseudocyst while monitoring cerebrospinal fluid content and cultures for a possible shunt infection and the need for complete shunt removal.

20.

D Neurohypophysis

The tissue shown in the image accompanying the question represents neurohypophyseal tissue. The occasional round eosinophilic bodies represent Herring bodies.

21.

B Type 2

Modic type 2 and 3 changes are chronic changes. A Modic type 2 change shows high signal on T1 and iso- to hyperintensity on T2, and is thought to be due to replacement of bone marrow by fat. (A) A Modic type 1 change is associated with hypointense T1 and hyperintense T2 signals, and is thought to represent bone marrow edema from acute/subacute inflammation. (C) A Modic type 3 change is hypointense on T1 and T2 sequences due to reactive osteosclerosis. (D) There are no Modic type 4 changes.

22.

A Provides special visceral efferent fibers to the stylopharyngeus and the laryngeal, pharyngeal, and palatine musculature

(B) Special visceral afferent fibers from the posterior one third of the tongue are derived from the solitary nucleus. (C) General visceral efferent fibers to the otic ganglion arise from the inferior salivatory nucleus. (D) General visceral efferent fibers going through the greater superficial petrosal nerve are derived from the superior salivatory nucleus. (E) Special visceral efferent fibers to the stylohyoid, stapedius, and posterior belly of the digastric originate in the facial motor nucleus.

23.

B The results are not clinically significant.

(A–E) All of the answer choices are potential issues with the study, but only one error is obvious from the information given. Researchers often confuse clinical and statistical significance. Although statistical significance means that there is an actual mathematical difference between two groups, clinical significance determines if this difference has meaningful clinical applications. In the example study, 2 weeks of extended life is clinically insignificant when electrodes last for decades. The authors' conclusion thus has little clinical applicability.

24.

D Shortens

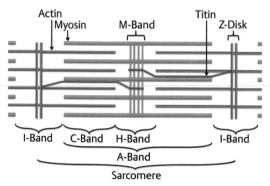

The H band is the region of the sarcomere composed of myosin thick filaments that do not overlap with actin thin filaments. The center of the H-band is the M-band. During sarcomere contraction, the myosin heads move along the actin thin filaments away from the M-band, thus shortening the H- and I-bands. (B) The A-band remains the same size during sarcomere contraction.

25.

D Foraminal/extraforaminal extrusion

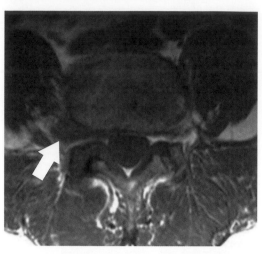

This image demonstrates a foraminal/extraforaminal disk extrusion, with dark disk material obliterating the foraminal and extraforaminal zones *(arrow)*. (A) A diffuse bulging disk is not considered a herniation and is defined as disk tissue circumferentially extending beyond the edges of the ring apophyses. (B) A protrusion is a herniation in which the base of the disk material extending beyond the margins of the disk space is greater than its height. It involves less than 25% of the circumference of the disk. There are no central or paracentral herniations in this case. (C) In an extrusion, the base of the herniated disk material is smaller than its height. (E) An asymmetrically bulging disk is not completely circumferential but involves greater than 25% of the circumference of the ring apophysis.

26.

E *Streptococcus pneumoniae*

In the elderly, the majority of community-acquired cases of meningitis are due to *Streptococcus pneumoniae*. This acute bacterial meningitis is characterized by acute inflammatory cells (neutrophils) in the leptomeninges.

27.

A Presence of β_2-transferrin

β_2-transferrin is not found in tears, saliva, nasal exudates, or serum. Besides the cerebrospinal fluid (CSF), the only other place it is found is in the vitreous fluid of the eye. (B) Testing fluid for glucose can be helpful, as normal CSF has a glucose content of about 67% (50 to 80 mg/100 mL) of the serum glucose content, whereas lacrimal secretions and mucus have glucose concentrations less than

5 mg/100 mL. Glucose testing, however, has a 45 to 75% false-positive result. (C) The ring sign test entails dripping CSF onto clean linen. A ring of blood with a larger concentric ring of clear fluid (double ring or halo sign) suggests CSF, but this finding is unreliable. (D) A reservoir sign occurs when a gush of fluid occurs with certain head positions and is thought to be due to pooled CSF in the sphenoid sinus. This also is an unreliable test. (E) Reliance on patients to report a salty taste has a high false-negative rate because taste is highly subjective.

28.
D Weakness of plantarflexion and ankle inversion

The tibial nerve is a branch of the sciatic nerve and gives motor branches to the gastrocnemius, popliteus, soleus, and plantaris muscles. It also innervates the tibialis posterior, flexor digitorum longus, and flexor halluces longus. Injury to the tibial nerve causes weakness of plantarflexion and ankle inversion.

29.
B Weakness of plantarflexion and ankle eversion

An S1 radiculopathy causes weakness of plantarflexion and ankle eversion. (A) An L5 radiculopathy is characterized by weakness in extension of the hallucis and potentially can result in a footdrop as well. Numbness and pain can be felt on the superior aspect of the foot. (C) The common peroneal nerve is derived from the L4 to S2 roots and innervates the short head of the biceps femoris by a motor branch that exits close to the gluteal cleft. The remainder of the common peroneal nerve innervates muscles through the deep and superficial peroneal nerves. The deep peroneal nerve innervates the tibialis anterior, extensor digitorum longus, peroneus tertius, and extensor hallucis longus. Damage to the deep peroneal nerve results in footdrop. The superficial peroneal nerve innervates the peroneus longus and brevis. Injury to this nerve results in an inability to evert the foot and loss of sensation over the dorsum of the foot, with the exception of the first web space. Injury to the common peroneal nerve results in footdrop and weakness of ankle eversion, with loss of sensation along the dorsal surface of the foot as described.

30.
D Associated with ankylosing spondylitis

Ossification of the posterior longitudinal ligament (OPLL) has been associated with diffuse idiopathic hyperostosis, ankylosing spondylitis, and other spondyloarthropathies. (A) OPLL is seen most frequently in the Asian population (particularly in Japan) with an incidence of 2.5%. (B) OPLL is more common in men and presents in patients between 50 and 70 years of age. (C) Meningiomas arise from arachnoid cap cells and are more common in women. Spinal meningiomas occur most frequently in the thoracic spine.

31.
C Demyelination

Optic neuritis causes unilateral decreased visual acuity over hours to days and is associated with globe tenderness and eye pain exacerbated by eye movement. The most common cause is multiple sclerosis. (A) Nonarteritic anterior ischemic optic neuropathy presents as a sudden, painless, monocular visual loss usually with an altitudinal deficit. It is associated with atherosclerosis and other general cardiovascular risk factors. (B) Temporal arteritis often is accompanied by systemic symptoms, temporal headaches, jaw claudication, and an elevated erythrocyte sedimentation rate. (D) Vision loss can be due to transient monocular blindness (amaurosis fugax), which usually is associated with embolism into the retinal arteries. The event occurs over seconds and resolves within minutes. (E) Increased intracranial pressure is associated with bilateral papilledema, which is painless.

32.
C Lumbar region

The cleft in diastematomyelia is located in the lumbar region in 47%, thoracolumbar region in 27%, thoracic region in 23%, and sacral or cervical region in 1.5% of cases.

33.
C Hawthorne effect

The Hawthorne effect is the tendency of a study population to affect outcomes due to its awareness of being studied. (A) Sample distortion bias occurs when the estimates of exposure and outcomes are biased because the sample is not representative of the target population. (B) Information bias occurs due to inadequate assessment of associations between the exposures and outcomes as a result of errors in measurement. (D) Observer bias (also known as the observer expectancy effect) is seen in nonblinded studies. This bias stems from researchers tending to influence consciously or unconsciously the participants in studies. (E) Lead time bias occurs when there is an incorrect assumption that a screening test improves disease prognosis. This happens when a screening test leads to the early detection of a disease, therefore possibly increasing survival from time of diagnosis.

34.

C Largest width of the frontal horns divided by the maximal biparietal diameter of the skull from the inner table to the inner table

The Evans ratio is the ratio of the frontal horn (FH) width to the maximal biparietal diameter (BPD) from the inner table to the inner table, with a value over 3 suggesting ventriculomegaly/hydrocephalus. If the temporal horns are more than 2 mm wide and the FH width to internal diameter of the skull at that level is more than 0.5, ventriculomegaly/hydrocephalus may be present. Other signs that suggest ventriculomegaly/hydrocephalus include ballooning of the FHs/third ventricle, transependymal absorption, and bowing of the corpus callosum on a sagittal MRI. Occipital-frontal circumference is followed for every growing child, and abnormal growth, such as rapid growth, measurements crossing growth curves, growth more than two standard deviations above normal, and a head circumference out of proportion to length/weigh, should prompt clinicians to look for underlying conditions (e.g., ventriculomegaly/hydrocephalus).

35.

C Anterior inferior cerebellar artery

36.

A EPSP decreases and IPSP increases

An increase in the sodium flux increases the membrane potential of a neuron, bringing it closer to the threshold membrane potential. With less of an electrochemical drive (the more positive membrane potential is less conducive to allowing positive ions to enter the cytoplasm), the magnitude of each excitatory postsynaptic potential (EPSP) decreases, whereas the reverse is true of each inhibitory postsynaptic potential (IPSP). The end result on membrane potential is due to the summation of all of the EPSPs and IPSPs within a certain temporal window.

37.

C Urgent craniotomy and resection of lesion

Clinical history, imaging, and lab work are consistent with a cerebral abscess. There are multiple reasons to consider surgical resection: young age, large size of the lesion, and lesion proximity to the ventricle. Needle aspiration is an option, although given the size of the lesion, resection may be beneficial. Systemic workup including blood cultures, antibiotics, and a search for an infectious source is indicated. (A) Lumbar punctures generally are con-traindicated in patients with large supratentorial lesions and a risk of downward herniation. (B) A ventriculostomy may be indicated in the event of hydrocephalus or intraventricular rupture. (E) Medical treatment without surgical management likely would not shrink the abscess and would put the patient at risk for the abscess rupturing into the ventricle, which is associated with a high rate of mortality.

38.

E Hypertonicity, no muscle fasciculations, hyperreflexia, and a positive Babinski response

In an upper motor neuron lesion, one can find depressed superficial reflexes and disuse atrophy over time. (A) Hypotonicity, muscle fasciculations, hyporeflexia, and a negative Babinski response are found in a lower motor neuron lesion, which may exhibit prominent muscle atrophy.

39.

A Succinylcholine

Succinylcholine is a depolarizing paralytic with a time to onset of less than 1 minute and a duration of action of 5 to 10 minutes. It is plasmacholinesterase dependent and has many side effects. (B) Among nondepolarizing paralytic agents, rocuronium is the shortest acting with the shortest time to onset. Rocuronium is the preferred agent in the setting of major burns and trauma.

40.

A Persistence of the accessory neurenteric canal

The axial T2 image shows a type 1 split spinal cord malformation (diastematomyelia) with two hemicords and a bony septum separating the spinal canal (thought to develop due to the persistence of the accessory neurenteric canal). In this type of malformation, each hemicord is surrounded by its own thecal sac, and features dorsal and ventral horns only on the lateral sides. This condition may be associated with other vertebral anomalies. A type 2 split spinal cord malformation is a milder form in which there is a single thecal sac and spinal canal. The accessory neurenteric canal is usually resorbed but may persist as a fibrous band. (B) Failure of closure of the rostral neuropore would result in anencephaly. (C) In utero infarction is not known to be associated with diastematomyelia. (D) Infection is not known to be associated with diastematomyelia. (E) The neurenteric canal is a transient structure connecting the amniotic cavity and yolk sac. Its persistence may result in anomalies in the development of the notochord.

22   Practice Exam Answers

41.

A Posterior vertebral body, pedicle, and superior articular facet

42.

C Secondary active transport

In secondary active transport (also known as ion-coupled transport), the movement of one molecule along its concentration or electrical gradients is coupled with the movement of another molecule against its concentration or electrical gradients. With the sodium-glucose cotransporter, one glucose molecule and two sodium ions are transported into the cell. The movement of the sodium ions along their electrical and concentration gradients is coupled with the movement of glucose against its concentration gradient. (A) Facilitated diffusion uses either electrical or concentration gradients to drive molecules and ions across a cellular membrane through a protein channel. (B) Simple diffusion is seen with lipophilic molecules that diffuse across cell membranes without the assistance from channel proteins. (D) Primary active transport involves the transport of molecules across a cellular membrane using direct metabolic energy (e.g., ATP). An example is the sodium-potassium pump seen in neuronal membranes, where the hydrolysis of one molecule of ATP enables three sodium ions to move extracellularly and two potassium ions to move intracellularly against their concentration gradients. (E) Gap junctions are protein pores connecting the cytoplasms of cells, which enable the free passage of ions and small molecules. They are abundant in cardiac tissue.

43.

A Lower apparent diffusion coefficient values

Although location and imaging features may overlap, recent studies suggest that chordomas, particularly when poorly differentiated, have significantly lower apparent diffusion coefficient values (greater restricted diffusion) compared with chondrosarcomas. (B) Well-circumscribed lesion margins can be seen on MRI in chordomas and chondrosarcomas. Ill-defined erosive changes are common on CT. (C) Marked T2 hyperintensity can be seen in chordomas and chondrosarcomas. (D) Enhancement pattern is not a reliable discriminator between chordomas and chondrosarcomas. (E) Location at the petroclival synchondrosis is typical of chondrosarcomas, although the chondroid subtype of chordomas has an increased tendency to arise laterally at this site. Most chordomas occur at the midline.

44.

B Complete resection

To obtain a cure for osteoblastoma/osteoid osteoma, the lesion needs to be excised completely. (A) Osteoid osteomas are less than 1 cm in size, whereas osteoblastomas typically are considered of the same pathology but are larger. Curettage is associated with pain relief but with a high percentage of recurrence. (C) Radiation likely is ineffective in the treatment of an osteoblastoma/osteoid osteoma.

45.

A) Ulnar nerve palsy

The exam findings are consistent with a positive Froment sign, indicating ulnar nerve palsy. This test evaluates the action of the adductor pollicis. With an ulnar nerve palsy, patients experience difficulty maintaining a hold on a piece of paper and will compensate by flexing the flexor pollicis longus to maintain grasp pressure, which causes the pinching effect as shown in the image accompanying the question. (B) A median nerve palsy leads to loss of the ability to abduct and oppose the thumb due to paralysis of the thenar muscles. (C) A radial nerve palsy typically manifests as wrist drop. (D) The anterior interosseous branch of the median nerve innervates the flexor pollicis longus responsible for the pinching seen in testing for a Froment sign. If this nerve is injured, the patient will be unable to pinch. (E) Injury of the C5 nerve root leads to difficulty flexing the elbow.

46.

A Breast carcinoma

The lesion displayed in the image accompanying the question represents a meningothelial or syncytial meningioma (WHO grade I). There is a well-known association of meningiomas with breast and endometrial carcinomas. Meningiomas also are associated with a history of radiation and neurofibromatosis type 2.

47.

C C4-C5

(A) The angle of the mandible is at the level of C1-C2. (B) The hyoid bone is at the level of C3-C4. (D) The cricothyroid membrane is at the level of C5-C6. (E) The cricoid cartilage is at the level of C6-C7. The carotid tubercle (Chassaignac tubercle) is at the level of C6.

48.

E Enhancement following contrast administration

Enhancement following contrast administration indicates disruption of the blood–brain barrier and is seen in the subacute stage of stroke. As a general rule, enhancement starts at around day 3, peaks at 3 weeks, and may last up to 3 months after the stroke. (A) A hyperdense middle cerebral artery is the earliest sign that may be seen on CT in a patient with an acute stroke (as early as 90 minutes from ictus) and is produced by a highly attenuating thrombus lodged within the vessel. It appears even before any parenchymal changes are evident. (B–D) Decreased attenuation of the lentiform nucleus, loss of the insular ribbon, subtle sulcal effacement, and effacement of the cerebral sulci all are potential early signs of stroke on CT; however, the sensitivity of these signs in the first 3 hours is particularly low, in that they are seen in about 40 to 50% of patients, increasing to about 60% after 6 hours. Parenchymal hypoattenuation in the first 6 hours portends a poor prognosis, particularly when extensive. Virtually all strokes are visible on CT after 25 hours.

49.

A Ventral to the thalamus, dorsal to the substantia nigra, and medial to the internal capsule

(B) The subthalamic nucleus is deeper rather than posterior to the third ventricle and medial to the globus pallidus. (C) The subthalamic nucleus is ventral to the thalamus and dorsal to the substantia nigra. (D) The subthalamic nucleus is ventral to the quadrigeminal plate and deep to the thalamus. (E) The subthalamic nucleus is located dorsal to the red nucleus.

50.

B Minimize carbohydrates

The respiratory quotient (RQ) is the ratio of CO_2 production to O_2 consumption, and is a direct manifestation of ingested food. The RQ is 1.0 for carbohydrates and 0.7 for fats; therefore, minimizing carbohydrates can help a patient with hypercapnia.

51.

D Cochlear and vestibular damage

Vancomycin can cause cochlear and vestibular dysfunction.

52.

E Unpleasant taste

Side effects of temozolomide include nausea, vomiting, constipation, diarrhea, blurred vision, sleep problems, unusual or unpleasant tastes, and headaches. Patients also may have temporary hair loss. (A) Amphotericin B can lead to benign intracranial hypertension. (B) Penicillins and cephalosporins have been linked to aseptic meningitis, with the exact pathophysiology being unknown. Other medications linked to aseptic meningitis are trimethoprim-sulfamethoxazole, ciprofloxacin, metronidazole, and isoniazid. (C) Ethambutol is known for causing optic neuritis; however, another side effect of this antituberculous drug is cerebellar ataxia. Patients need routine ophthalmologic exams while on the medication.

53.

A Cerebral venous thrombosis

The CT scan presented in the image accompanying the question demonstrates an "empty delta" sign, which is typical for sagittal sinus thrombosis. Risk factors for cerebral venous thrombosis include thrombophilias, chronic inflammatory disease, pregnancy, use of estrogen containing hormonal contraception, direct injury to the sinuses, and dehydration. (D) Dural arteriovenous fistulas usually are seen on contrast-enhanced CT scans as enlarged and tortuous vessels in the subarachnoid space. An enlarged external carotid artery or transdiploic vessels also may be a clue for dural arteriovenous fistulas. (E) Except for some subtle findings, acute ischemic stroke usually does not appear on CT scan.

54.

D Periventricular leukomalacia

Periventricular leukomalacia (PVL) is the most common abnormality seen in premature infants with cerebral palsy. PVL is a white matter injury due to either ischemia/hypoxia or inflammation in the periventricular white matter. Intraventricular hemorrhage is a risk factor for its development but is a separate pathological process and etiology for cerebral palsy.

55.

C It is associated with developmental venous anomalies.

This lesion demonstrates multiple small locules of different signal intensities with foci that are hyperintense on both noncontrast T1- and T2-weighted images that correspond to blood products of different stages. Note the dark hemosiderin rim, tiny fluid–fluid levels on the T2 image, and "popcorn" appearance that is best seen on the T1 image. Such a constellation of findings is compatible with a cavernous malformation. Approximately 50% of cavernous malformations calcify, and 25%

are associated with developmental venous anomalies. Cavernomas usually are asymptomatic initially, but 50% of patients eventually present with seizures and 25% with focal neurologic deficits. (A) Cavernous malformations typically are occult on conventional angiography. (B) Cavernous malformations usually do not show restricted diffusion, and therefore, diffusion-weighted imaging is not useful for their detection. They usually are seen best on gradient echo or T2* sequences, particularly susceptibility-weighted imaging. (D) Cavernous malformations do not have normal interspersed brain as opposed to other vascular lesions such as capillary telangiectasias. (E) There is no arteriovenous shunting in cavernous malformations, and therefore no early venous drainage is seen.

56.

A IIH is self-limiting and will resolve with age regardless of weight and lifestyle changes.

Idiopathic intracranial hypertension (IIH) always eventually resolves despite weight and lifestyle; however, resolution may require a couple of decades or more. In the meantime, patients typically report headaches and other subjective complaints along with the more worrisome decrease in vision. The latter may not reverse with treatment and may progress as long as papilledema is present, so it is important to prevent it with therapy as soon as IIH is diagnosed.

57.

B Tyramine

The "cheese reaction" occurs when tyramine-rich foods (such as wine) are ingested along with monoamine oxidase inhibitors (MAOIs). MAOIs block the breakdown of dietary amines including tyramine (a breakdown product of tyrosine) in the liver, primarily by blocking the action of monoamine oxidase A. Accumulation of tyramine causes it to compete with tyrosine for transportation across the blood–brain barrier and into the neuronal cytoplasm. Tyramine then displaces norepinephrine from synaptic vesicles, causing a surge of norepinephrine release. This leads to blood pressure augmentation.

58.

C Paresthesias

Placement of a deep brain stimulation lead posterior to the ventral intermediate nucleus of the thalamus (VIM) would stimulate the ventral caudal nucleus of the thalamus, potentially causing intolerable paresthesias. (A) Lateral stimulation

would cause muscle contractions from contact with the internal capsule. (D, E) Facial contractions and dysarthria can be seen with aggressive stimulation of the subthalamic nucleus due to corticobulbar stimulation.

59.

C It occurs as a result of mutations in tumor-suppressor genes.

The CT scan *(left)* accompanying the question shows densely calcified subependymal nodules, which also are seen but are less conspicuous on the FLAIR sequence image *(right)*. The latter also demonstrates hyperintense cortical tubers bilaterally. These findings and the patient's history are typical for tuberous sclerosis. This condition develops as a result of mutations in the *TSC1* (hamartin) and *TSC2* (tuberin) genes, which encode proteins that are widely available in normal tissues. Several lines of evidence indicate that these genes function primarily as tumor suppressors, and mutations that prevent the formation of a functional TSC1/TSC2 protein complex lead to variable manifestations of the disease. The hallmark of tuberous sclerosis is hamartomatous formations in various tissues (e.g., cardiac rhabdomyomas, subependymal nodules, cortical tubers, and angiomyolipomas) and an increased risk of neoplasms (e.g., subependymal giant cell astrocytomas and renal cell carcinomas). (A) Eighty percent of cases of tuberous sclerosis are sporadic and arise de novo, and 20% are familial. (B) Neuropathological and advanced neuroimaging studies have shown various white matter changes in multiple sclerosis, which are present even in normal-appearing white matter on conventional MRI. White matter lesions include radial migration lines, parenchymal cysts, areas of dys/demyelination, and disorganized neuronal and glial elements with astrocytosis. (D) Both subependymal nodules and subependymal giant cell astrocytomas may enhance, calcify, and hemorrhage, and there is no pathological distinction between the two. The most useful criterion to establish the development of a subependymal giant cell astrocytoma is growth of a nodule on serial imaging, and the other major factors determining management are the presence of new symptoms or manifestations of increased intracranial pressure such as papilledema. Unresectable or incompletely resectable subependymal giant cell astrocytomas (e.g., multiple or infiltrative) may qualify for medical therapy with mammalian target of rapamycin (mTOR) inhibitors. Malignant transformation of subependymal giant cell astrocytomas has been reported but is rare.

60.

B Anterior atlanto-occipital membrane

(A) The apical odontoid ligament connects the tip of the dens to the foramen magnum. (C) The posterior atlanto-occipital membrane connects the posterior arch of C1 to the posterior part of the foramen magnum. (D) The tectorial membrane is the cephalad extension of the posterior longitudinal ligament.

61.

A Anaplastic

The medulloblastoma displayed is marked by scattered, very atypical-appearing tumor cells characteristic of the anaplastic variant. (B) The classic subtype has a monotonous appearance of small, densely packed cells with hyperchromatic nuclei. (C) The desmoplastic subtype is similar to the classic subtype except that there are pale islands of collagen bundles and a tendency for neuronal differentiation. (D) The large cell subtype has cells with large, round, pleomorphic nuclei with high mitotic activity. (E) The excessive nodularity subtype has a grape-like appearance on neuroimaging and demonstrates extreme nodularity on pathological examination with a fine fibrillary background.

62.

A Carbon monoxide intoxication

Carbon monoxide (CO) has a predilection for causing lesions in the globi pallidi bilaterally, although other basal ganglia regions may be affected particularly in the setting of hypoxic-anoxic injury. Patients also can have confluent abnormalities in their subcortical white matter. On MRI, CO poisoning produces low or high signal intensity lesions on T1 and high intensity on T2 in the globi pallidi. Restricted diffusion may be seen in the acute phase. Mechanisms of the pathology include acute demyelination, hypoxia and oxidative injury, excitotoxicity, and apoptosis. Positive CT findings herald long-term neurologic complications, occasionally following a period of lucidity that may last from days to weeks. (B) Abnormal accumulation of copper in Wilson disease may manifest with lesions in the lentiform nuclei and thalami. Neurologic manifestations are variable, ranging from subtle to rapidly progressive symptoms; however, the presentation usually is not as acute as described in this scenario unless the patient is unconscious due to seizures. (C) Lead encephalopathy is rare and can lead to cerebral and cerebellar white matter edema and demyelination. (D) Methanol is a constituent of various commercially available solvents.

Lesions are characterized by hemorrhagic necrosis and preferentially involve the putamina, hemispheric white matter, and, less commonly, the caudate nuclei.

63.

C Type 1 error only

A type 1 error occurs when the null hypothesis (that there is no difference in the clinical outcomes between the two drugs) is incorrectly rejected. (D) A type 2 error occurs when the null hypothesis is incorrectly accepted (typically due to a small sample size). This means that treatments would be interpreted as equal when in fact they are not. (E) A type 3 error occurs when the null hypothesis is rejected but for fallacious reasons.

64.

B A false-negative result when assessing prolactin levels for a suspected prolactinoma

The Hook (prozone) effect is a falsely low prolactin level during the assessment of very high concentrations of prolactin, usually in the setting of a prolactinoma. The prolactin assay must be repeated at 1:10 and 1:100 dilutions to determine if the actual concentration is higher. (A) Elevated prolactin levels secondary to pituitary stalk compression describe the stalk effect where the dopamine pathways that normally inhibit prolactin production are compressed and inhibited. (C) Infertility, sexual dysfunction, and amenorrhea are symptoms of hyperprolactinemia. (D) Hyponatremia and decreased extracellular fluid volume from the renal loss of sodium describe salt wasting. (E) High output of hypotonic urine due to insufficient release of antidiuretic hormone describes diabetes insipidus.

65.

A Capillary wedge pressure less than 18 mm Hg, bilateral chest infiltrates, and PaO_2/FiO_2 ratio less than 200

A capillary wedge pressure less than 18 mm Hg indicates the absence of pulmonary edema, whereas bilateral chest infiltrates indicate the presence of diffuse alveolar pathology. A ratio of PaO_2/FiO_2 less than 200 indicates reduced arterial oxygen content relative to the inhaled oxygen.

66.

A Upper trunk of the brachial plexus

Injuries to the upper trunk of the brachial plexus result in an Erb palsy and often occur secondary to birth trauma, a fall on the shoulder, and improper operative positioning. The C5 and C6 nerve roots are involved, and paralyzed muscles are the biceps, deltoid, and brachioradialis with weakness of the supraspinatus, infraspinatus, and supinator. (B) An injury of the middle trunk of the brachial plexus (Klumpke palsy) involves the C8 and T1 nerve roots. Paralyzed muscles are the intrinsic muscles of the hand and ulnar flexors of the wrist and fingers. Patients have a claw hand.

67.

B Variant

The history and clinical exam as well as electro-encephalographic and MRI findings are compatible with Creutzfeldt-Jakob disease (CJD). Abnormal signal in the dorsomedial thalamic nuclei ("hockey stick" sign) and pulvinar nuclei ("pulvinar" sign) is typical and thought to be highly specific for the variant form (vCJD), although it also can be seen in the sporadic form (sCJD), particularly the MV2 molecular subtype. (A) Sporadic CJD accounts for 85% of cases of the disease. MRI usually shows bilateral and less commonly unilateral basal ganglia abnormalities with preferential involvement of the corpus striatum as well as increased diffusion-weighted imaging (DWI) and FLAIR signal intensity in the cerebral cortex that result in "cortical ribboning." DWI is the most sensitive sequence for early findings. (C) Familial CJD (fCJD) accounts for 10% of cases. The clinical presentation and MRI findings are similar to the sporadic form. (D) Iatrogenic CJD is rare and constitutes less than 5% of cases. The clinical presentation and MRI findings are similar to those of the sporadic form.

68.

E Smaller Z-band width

Type 2A fibers have the largest Z-band width and type 2B fibers having the smallest. Type 1 fibers have an intermediate Z-band width. In general, type 1 fibers are considered the fibers of endurance muscles requiring prolonged and frequent contraction. Type 2B fibers are designed to undergo quick, forceful, nonsustained contractions. Type 2A fibers can be thought of as a compromise between type 1 and type 2B. (A) Both type 1 and type 2A muscle fibers are relatively fatigue resistance due to their oxidative nature. Type 2B (fast glycolytic) fibers have a low resistance to fatigue but a fast twitch speed. (B) Type 1 fibers have more acidic

ATPase activity than type 2A fibers, which have more activity than type 2B fibers. (C) Type 2B fibers have a greater twitch force than type 2A fibers, which have a greater twitch force than type 1 fibers. (D) The myoglobin levels in type 1 and type 2A fibers are relatively similar. Type 2B fibers contain little myoglobin and large amounts of glycogen.

69.

D 70% and 30%

The incidence of radiographic or clinical vasospasm after aneurysmal subarachnoid hemorrhage is substantially greater than the risk after traumatic subarachnoid hemorrhage.

70.

B 30%

A Chiari 2 malformation occurs in almost all patients with a myelomeningocele. Although only 25 to 30% of cases of Chiari 2 malformation become clinically relevant, it remains a significant contributing factor for secondary disability and mortality.

71.

E Inferolateral

The porus trigeminus is the entrance to the Meckel cave and is contained within the inferolateral triangle. (A) The oculomotor triangle, also known as the medial or Hakuba triangle, contains the oculomotor nerve and horizontal segment of the internal carotid artery. It is the triangle by which access to most intracavernous aneurysms and tumors is gained. (B) Historically, the Parkinson triangle was accessed to treat carotid-cavernous fistulas. It also contains the abducens nerve. (C) The Glasscock triangle (posterolateral) contains the middle meningeal artery in the floor of the triangle as it exits the foramen spinosum, horizontal petrous internal carotid artery, and infratemporal fossa. The triangle is useful as it enables the surgeon to gain proximal control of the internal carotid artery for more distal vascular procedures. Approximately 10 mm of the carotid artery is accessible through this triangle. (D) The Kawase (posteromedial) triangle contains the petrous apex, internal carotid artery, cochlea, and vertebrobasilar junction. It can be used to perform an anterior petrosectomy so that the posterior fossa, anterior brainstem, and root of the trigeminal nerve can be visualized.

72.

B Neuronal ceroid lipofuscinosis

The neuronal ceroid lipofuscinoses are a group of autosomal recessive disorders characterized by neurologic deterioration and by the accumulation of lipofuscin-like products. Ultrastructurally, these accumulations may manifest as granular osmiophilic deposits, curvilinear bodies, or fingerprint bodies. (A) Fucosidosis is an autosomal recessive disease due to a deficiency of the enzyme α-L-fucosidase, which is involved in the metabolism of complex sugars and not lipofuscin. (C) Schindler disease is an autosomal recessive lysosomal storage disease caused by a deficiency of α-N-acetylgalactosaminidase causing a buildup of glycosphingolipids. (D) Sialidosis is a lysosomal storage disease caused by a deficiency of α-N-acetyl neuraminidase, which leads to the accumulation of mucopolysaccharides and mucolipids. (E) Wolman disease is due to a deficiency of lysosomal acid lipase, which leads to an accumulation of fats in various body tissues.

73.

A Thoracic outlet syndrome and Pancoast tumors

Horner syndrome arises from pathology of the sympathetic nervous system in the neck, upper thoracic spine, and skull base. It is characterized by miosis, ptosis, and anhidrosis with or without enophthalmos. Horner syndrome can be due to first-order neurons being disrupted by central nervous system lesions affecting the hypothalamospinal tract (e.g., spinal cord lesions). Preganglionic lesions are also known as second-order neuron disorders and can result from compression of the sympathetic chain by a lung tumor (Pancoast tumor). Third-order neuron pathology (postganglionic Horner syndrome) results from lesions at the level of the internal carotid such as cavernous sinus lesions. (B, C) Shoulder dislocations are associated with axillary nerve injuries. (D, E) Second-order preganglionic pupillomotor fibers exit the spinal cord around the T1 level to enter the cervical sympathetic chain. A lesion at the T5 level would not affect the sympathetic pathways involved in Horner syndrome.

74.

C Diskitis/osteomyelitis

Differentiation of infection from tumor can be difficult, but disk space involvement/destruction strongly favors infection. (B) A disk herniation does not enhance, but there may be peripheral enhancement if the herniation is surrounded by scar. (D) Tuberculosis often characteristically spares the disk space.

75.

D Elevated choline and myoinositol

The patient's history and imaging findings of increased FLAIR signal involving the corticospinal tracts bilaterally are consistent with amyotrophic lateral sclerosis (ALS). Of note, imaging studies are frequently normal. On MR spectroscopy, patients may have elevated choline and myoinositol in the precentral gyrus and increased glutamate/glutamine in the medulla. There also may be low signal intensity in the motor cortex on T2 or gradient echo based sequences (particularly on susceptibility-weighted imaging) due to iron accumulation. (A) There is no contrast enhancement in ALS. (B, C) Diffuse tensor imaging (DTI) studies have shown increased mean diffusivity (MD) and decreased fractional anisotropy (FA) in the white matter of patients with ALS due to degeneration.

Section 4

1.

C Cisternal

Because the visualization of a structure on MRI depends primarily on its intrinsic signal properties and those of the surrounding structures, non-contrast steady-state free precession (SSFP)-based sequences are most useful for the evaluation of the cisternal segments of the cranial nerves due to the bright signal of cerebrospinal fluid. (A, B) Overall, CISS or FIESTA-C imaging does not allow good parenchymal differentiation. In particular, visualization of the cranial nerve nuclei generally is not possible on conventional imaging, although it has been reported in the research setting using diffuse tensor imaging. (D, E) The interdural and foraminal segments of the cranial nerves are not visible on conventional CISS or FIESTA-C sequences, which do not routinely use contrast. The recently described use of contrast material with SSFP sequences enables delineation of the interdural and foraminal segments of the cranial nerves due to enhancement of the surrounding blood.

2.

A Sphingomyelinase; sphingomyelin

Sphingomyelinase is the enzyme deficiency in Niemann-Pick disease that causes a buildup of sphingomyelin. (B) Sphingomyelinase is the enzyme deficiency in Niemann-Pick disease, but glucocerebroside is the metabolite that accumulates in Gaucher disease. (C) Hexosaminidase A and GM2 ganglioside are the enzyme deficiency and accumulating metabolite, respectively, in Tay-Sachs disease. (D) Hexosaminidase A is the enzyme deficiency in Tay-Sachs disease, whereas glucocerebroside is the metabolite that builds up in Gaucher disease. (E) Glucocerebrosidase and glucocerebroside are the enzyme deficiency and accumulating metabolite, respectively, in Gaucher disease.

3.

C Spinal cord stimulation

Spinal cord stimulation is useful in treating neuropathic leg pain following failed back surgery mainly in cases where imaging does not show a compressive lesion impinging on any neural structures. The most appropriate level for implantation is at T10-T11.

4.

A Dorsal root entry zone lesioning

Dorsal root entry zone lesioning is most beneficial in nerve avulsion pain such as that of the brachial plexus or in transitional zone pain following spinal cord injury. The procedure should be reserved for cases where patients have shown no evidence of functional recovery of the affected nerve. (B) The spinothalamic tract is divided at the level of C1-C2. A cordotomy at this level is reserved for intractable severe upper extremity pain due to cancer. Side effects include dysesthesia, urinary retention, sleep apnea, and weakness. (D) A selective dorsal rhizotomy is performed on the lower spinal cord and is best for diplegic spasticity. It is used primarily in treating children with cerebral palsy with lower extremity spasticity who have borderline ambulation abilities. (E) Visceral cancer pain in the pelvic and rectal area is relayed through a midline pathway in the dorsal columns. Punctate midline myelotomies have been shown to alleviate visceral cancer pain.

5.

C Palmar sensation

The superficial sensory branch of the median nerve (providing sensation to the base of the palm) branches proximal to the carpal tunnel and travels more superficially; thus, palmar sensation is lost in more proximal median nerve injuries but preserved in carpal tunnel syndrome.

6.

C Pulmonary embolism

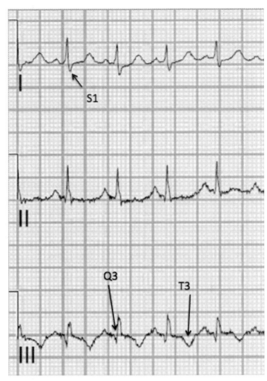

The most sensitive finding associated with a pulmonary embolism is sinus tachycardia, as shown in this image. In addition, the waves S1, Q3, and T3 are typical findings and are secondary to right ventricular stress.

7.

C Typical antipsychotic

The patient described likely has Lewy body dementia. Individuals with this condition are at an increased risk for neuroleptic malignant syndrome, and therefore antidopaminergic medications such as the typical antipsychotics should be avoided. (A) Anticholinergics may worsen dementia in patients with Lewy body dementia. (B) Dopamine agonists do not cause neuroleptic malignant syndrome but their abrupt cessation can. (D) Atypical antipsychotics can cause neuroleptic malignant syndrome, but the risk is much lower than the risk associated with typical antipsychotics. (E) Nonsteroidal anti-inflammatory agents are not associated with neuroleptic malignant syndrome.

8.

D Characterized by β-amyloid peptide deposits

The constellation of a lobar hemorrhage (as opposed to one centered in the deep gray nuclei, brainstem, or cerebellum), the distribution of the microhemorrhages (in a cortical/subcortical location as seen around the right sylvian fissure in this case), and evidence of superficial siderosis are most compatible with cerebral amyloid angiopathy. This entity is seen most commonly in elderly individuals (older than 70 years of age) and is related to the deposition of β-amyloid peptide in small to medium-sized cerebral vessels and leptomeninges. It may be accompanied by leptomeningeal enhancement due to inflammation. Hemorrhage may extend into the subarachnoid space (sometimes isolated to the central sulcus even in the absence of visible parenchymal hemorrhages) and is a common cause of superficial siderosis. (A) Although there may be some overlap, hypertensive hemorrhages typically show a central distribution and occur in the putamen, thalami, brainstem, and cerebellum. (B) Cerebral cavernous malformations can show foci of increased susceptibility and can be multiple when they occur as sequelae of radiation or when they are related to mutations in the *CCM* gene family. They usually have a more random distribution. (C) Microhemorrhages in sickle cell disease usually are smaller and often punctate and distributed at the gray matter–white matter junctions or diffusely throughout the brain and cerebellum.

9.

D Chi-square

The chi-square test is used to compare proportions of two categorized outcomes (observed frequencies to expected frequencies). In this case, back pain is compared to no back pain. (A) The z-test is used to compare the means of two samples and assumes a normal distribution of data. It typically is used for larger data samples. Of note, the z-test would not be useful in this data sample as there are two groups (weight lifting and no weight lifting) that are being compared based on two variables (no back pain and back pain). (B) The t-test is used to compare the means of two samples when the standard deviation is not known. The test compares the difference between two groups on some variable of interest. A normal distribution of data is not assumed but does provide for a more accurate test. The z-test typically is preferable to the t-test, but the latter is preferable with smaller data samples. Of note, the t-test would not be use-

ful in this data sample as there are two groups (weight lifting and no weight lifting) that are being compared based on two variables (no back pain and back pain). (C) The rank-sum test (also known as the Mann-Whitney U test) is the nonparametric equivalent of t-test. (E) The analysis of variance (ANOVA) test is used to compare the means of three or more variables. The test determines if there is a difference between groups but does not tell which group is different.

10.

D Geniculate

The geniculate ganglion receives the fibers from the chorda tympani subserving taste from the anterior two thirds of the tongue. (A) The pterygopalatine ganglion is a parasympathetic ganglion largely innervated by the greater petrosal nerve. (B) The gasserian (trigeminal) ganglion receives the three trigeminal nerve branches. (C) The otic ganglion is a parasympathetic ganglion that innervates the parotid gland. (E) The nodosal ganglion is the inferior ganglion of the vagus nerve and is concerned chiefly with visceral afferent information.

11.

A Mobius syndrome

Mobius syndrome is a rare, congenital disorder characterized by facial palsy and an inability to move the eyes laterally. Other findings seen in Mobius syndrome include the occasional palsies of cranial nerves V and VII, limb abnormalities, and corneal erosions. (B) Duane syndrome is characterized by congenital strabismus, most commonly with limitation of abduction of the affected eye. Other symptoms include retraction of the eyeball into the socket on adduction, narrowing of the palpebral fissure, poor convergence, and a head turn to the affected side to compensate for movement limitation and to maintain binocular vision. (C) Kallmann syndrome is characterized by delayed or absent puberty and an impaired sense of smell. (D) A Poland anomaly is characterized by underdevelopment or absence of the chest muscle on one side of the body. It can be associated with Mobius syndrome. (E) A Klippel-Feil anomaly is characterized by the congenital fusion of any two of the seven cervical vertebrae.

12.

E 3 pounds per cervical vertebral level, 5- to 10-pound incremental increases not to exceed 5 to 10 pounds per vertebral level

When attempting to reduce facet dislocations with cervical traction, the initial weight applied is 3 pounds multiplied by the cervical vertebral level. The weight is increased in 5- to 10-pound increments with plain radiographs and a neurologic exam performed after each addition of weight. The total weight applied should not exceed 10 pounds multiplied by the cervical vertebral level in order to avoid overdistraction. Weight additions should be stopped if any disk height exceeds 10 mm.

13.

E Wilson disease

The changes of Alzheimer type 2 astrocytes are associated with hepatic encephalopathy as first was described in Wilson disease.

14.

D Shunt placement

History of infection is considered a risk factor for endoscopic third ventriculostomy (ETV) failure. Recent studies suggest ETV along with choroid plexus coagulation (CPC) can have success rates up to 60% in the setting of postinfectious and posthemorrhagic hydrocephalus; however, shunt placement remains the gold standard for the management of this condition.

15.

A Free nerve endings

Free nerve endings transmit information about pain. (B) Merkel disks are nonencapsulated and are found in the center of papillary ridges. (C) Hair follicle receptors are nonencapsulated and are found around sebaceous glands and hair follicles. (D, E) Meissner and Pacinian corpuscles are encapsulated, with the former being found in the dermal papillae, especially the palms and soles of the feet. The latter is found widely distributed throughout the dermis, subcutaneous tissues, joint capsules, pleura, pericardium, and nipples.

16.

B Toxoplasmosis

The two major differential diagnoses in an immunocompromised patient with HIV who has a ring-enhancing lesion are toxoplasmosis and lymphoma. The eccentric "target" sign on contrast-enhanced T1 images is related to infolding of inflamed vessels into the lesion and is thought to be highly suggestive of toxoplasmosis (present in 30% of patients). The concentric "target" sign has been described on T2 FLAIR images and is present in 30% of patients with toxoplasmosis. Patients who have CD4 counts greater than 500 are only very mildly impaired and essentially have the same risk as the general population for the development of opportunistic infections. (A) *Cryptococcosis* results in a meningoencephalitis with lesions characteristically spreading along the perivascular spaces. Patients may have enhancing granulomas most commonly seen in the basal ganglia and medial cerebellum. Enlarged perivascular spaces and formation of gelatinous pseudocysts also can be seen. (C) A "target" sign has not been described for lymphoma, although the imaging features of lymphoma and toxoplasmosis may overlap. (D) Cytomegalovirus infection presents with nonspecific imaging findings, and the diagnosis mainly is clinical. Patients can have ventriculitis, encephalitis, myelitis, and/or peripheral neuropathies with the condition.

17.

B Decamethonium

Succinylcholine is an agonist of nicotinic acetylcholine receptors and provides neuromuscular blockade through persistent motor end-plate depolarization. By binding to receptors, succinylcholine prevents the binding of acetylcholine, and once calcium is depleted from the muscle cell cytoplasm, the muscle no longer can contract. As plasma concentrations of the agent accumulate, there also is a desensitization of the muscle cell, so that depolarization and contraction do not occur following repolarization. It is degraded by butyrylcholinesterase and not by acetylcholinesterase. (A) Tubocurarine is a nondepolarizing neuromuscular blocking agent that works by antagonizing nicotinic acetylcholine receptors. It has the side effect of causing histamine release. (C) Vecuronium acts in a similar manner to tubocurarine by antagonizing nicotinic acetylcholine receptors without muscle end-plate depolarization but has a much more rapid onset and shorter duration of action. (D) Although acetylcholinesterase will diminish the effects of acetylcholine at the motor end plate, it does not block or activate the postsynaptic nicotinic acetylcholine receptors. (E) Diazepam is not a neuromuscular blocking agent and acts by activating $GABA_A$ receptors.

18.

C 29%

The risk of recurrence after meningioma resection is based on the Simpson classification of the resection. A Simpson grade 1 resection entails a macroscopically complete tumor resection with removal of the affected dura and underlying bone and has a recurrence rate of 9%. A grade 2 resection is a gross total resection with coagulation of the affected dura, and it has a recurrence rate of 16%. A grade 3 resection is a gross total resection without removal of the dura or bone, and it has recurrence rate of 29%. A grade 4 resection equates to a subtotal resection, and it has recurrence rate of 39%. A grade 5 resection consists of only a decompression and biopsy.

19.

E Werdnig-Hoffmann disease

Infantile spinal muscular atrophy or Werdnig-Hoffmann disease is most likely to present as described in this patient. (A, C, D) These options usually do not present with fascicular atrophy on a muscle biopsy. (B) Kugelberg-Welander disease represents a later onset version of spinal muscular atrophy.

20.

A "Tigroid" pattern

Metachromatic leukodystrophy results in extensive bilateral white matter abnormalities that spare the U fibers. Sparing of the perivascular white matter sometimes results in a "tigroid" pattern. (B) A leading edge of enhancement in the periventricular parietooccipital white matter is characteristic of adrenoleukodystrophy. (C) Symmetric basal ganglia lesions have an extensive differential diagnosis but are not a characteristic feature of metachromatic leukodystrophy. (D) T2 hyperintensity in the dorsomedial and pulvinar thalamic nuclei may result in the "pulvinar" and "hockey stick" signs that are seen most commonly in the variant form of Creutzfeldt-Jakob disease. In metachromatic leukodystrophy, there may be decreased T2 signal in the thalami in severe cases.

21.

B Inferior oblique

The inferior oblique originates from the maxillary bone. All other muscles originate from the annulus of Zinn.

22.

B Breaths are patient- or time-triggered, flow limited, and volume cycled; breaths taken by patients are not assisted.

Synchronized intermittent mandatory ventilation is similar to assist control ventilation except that patient-initiated breaths are not supported. (A) Assist control ventilation is patient-triggered. If a patient fails to breathe, the ventilator machine will take over at a specified rate. Each breath taken has a preset tidal volume. (C) Pressure support ventilation can be a stand-alone ventilation mode or combined with synchronized intermittent mandatory ventilation. The concept is to deliver additional pressure for patient initiated breaths. (D) This represents continuous positive airway pressure (CPAP) ventilation, in which the patient must breathe independently of the ventilator.

23.

A 3 mm

The distance between the dorsal margin of the anterior arch of C1 and the dens (in the fully flexed position) should measure less than 3 mm in an adult and less than 5 mm in a child. The causes of atlantoaxial subluxation are varied, and include congenital conditions, trauma, and degenerative changes. In patients with Down syndrome, the cause of the instability is uncertain and may be related to ligamentous laxity or possibly congenital absence of the transverse ligament, although this is controversial.

24.

E Cranial nerve XI

The brain death exam involves assessing for pupil reaction (cranial nerves II and III), corneal reflex (cranial nerves V and VII), vestibulo-ocular reflex (cranial nerves III, VI, and VIII), cough and gag reflexes (cranial nerves IX and X), and doll's eyes (cranial nerves III, VI, and VIII). Cranial nerves I, IV, XI, and XII are not assessed directly during a brain death exam.

25.

B 20%

Children with neurofibromatosis type 1 (NF1) have an increased propensity to develop WHO grade I and grade II astrocytomas in the visual (optic) pathways. Approximately 20% of all patients with NF1 develop an optic pathway glioma.

26.

C Electromyography

The patient presents with upper and lower motor neuron signs and an MRI suspicious for cervical spondylotic myelopathy (CSM). Given the patient's upper and lower motor neurologic findings, his age, and the absence of sensory findings, amyotrophic lateral sclerosis (ALS) should be on the differential. ALS typically spares sensation, which also may be diminished only minimally in CSM. In addition, atrophy of the hands can be associated with both conditions as well. One tool to distinguish between the two diagnoses is electromyography, which demonstrates positive sharp waves in ALS.

27.

D Sturge-Weber

Unilateral congenital glaucoma occurs in 30 to 70% of patients with Sturge-Weber, and cavernomas of the choroid occur in half of affected individuals. The condition often occurs sporadically. (A) Neurofibromatosis type 1 has the ocular findings of Lisch nodules (iris hamartomas) and optic nerve gliomas. (B) Neurofibromatosis type 2 has the ocular finding of posterior subcapsular cataracts. (C) Tuberous sclerosis is associated with retinal astrocytic hamartomas that appear white/yellow and can calcify. (E) Von Hippel–Lindau can include findings of bilateral and multiple retinal angioblastomas.

28.

C Poor communication skills

Poor communication skills have been shown to be the leading cause of lawsuits and sentinel events in health care. A root cause analysis performed by the Joint Commission determined that a breakdown in communication is the most common cause of multiple sentinel events including wrong-site and wrong-level surgeries. (A) Poor medical knowledge has been linked to poor outcomes; however, it is not the most common cause of lawsuits. (B) Substandard patient care has also been linked to poor outcomes, but it is not the most common cause of lawsuits. (D) Unprofessional behavior also can lead to an increased rate of lawsuits. (E) Quality of hospital food has not been linked to an increased rate of lawsuits.

29.

A Recurrent artery of Heubner

The recurrent artery of Heubner arises from the proximal anterior cerebral artery, and it supplies the anteromedial head of the caudate nucleus, the anterior limb of the internal capsule, and the anterior portion of the lentiform nucleus. (B) The anterior choroidal arteries arise lateral and distal to the posterior communicating arteries. They supply the posterior limb of the internal capsule, lateral geniculate nucleus, optic tract and chiasm, hippocampus, amygdala, and choroid plexuses, among other structures. (C) The posterior choroidal arteries arise from the P2 segments of the posterior cerebral arteries. They most commonly are involved as part of larger posterior circulation strokes, but when posterior choroidal artery infarcts occur in isolation, infarcts may be seen in the pulvinar nuclei, geniculate body, hippocampus, and parahippocampal gyrus. (D) The lateral lenticulostriate arteries are branches of the middle cerebral artery and supply the external capsule, lateral aspect of the putamen, and upper half of the internal capsule.

30.

E Phenylephrine

Phenylephrine is an α-agonist, and it elevates blood pressure through peripheral vasoconstriction. It has an immediate onset and lasts for 20 to 40 minutes. It preferably is used in vasospasm patients because it has essentially no β-adrenergic activity at clinically used dosages. Although α-receptors exert a vasoconstrictor effect, β-receptors exert a vasodilatory effect.

31.

C Distance from source

The distance from a radiation source is extremely important, as exposure is proportional to the inverse square of the distance. Conventional wisdom is to try to keep at least 6 feet from sources like fluoroscopy. Lead aprons reduce radiation exposure equivalent to moving about 6 inches further from a radiation source. Remember that doubling the distance from a source reduces the exposure by 75%.

32.

A Arylsulfatase A; Sulfatide

Arylsulfatase A is the enzyme deficiency in metachromatic leukodystrophy that causes a buildup of sulfatide. (B) Sphingomyelinase is the enzyme deficiency in Niemann-Pick disease that causes a buildup of sphingomyelin. (C) Hexosaminidase A is the enzyme deficiency in Tay-Sachs disease that causes a buildup of GM2 ganglioside (not glucocerebroside [D]). (E) Glucocerebrosidase is the enzyme deficient in Gaucher disease that causes a buildup of glucocerebroside.

33.

D There is a high incidence of concurrent abdominal injuries.

The sagittal CT image accompanying the question demonstrates acute compression fracture of an anterior thoracic vertebra with a horizontal fracture component extending posteriorly through the pedicles (not shown) and spinous process, which is compatible with a Chance fracture. These fractures involve all three spinal columns and are secondary to a flexion-distraction injury. They are characterized by compression of the anterior column and distraction of the middle and posterior columns of the spine. Chance fractures occur as a result of injury from lap seat belts without a shoulder strap or from a fall from a height. They are associated with a high incidence of concurrent abdominal injuries (up to 80% in some series) and can lead to progressive kyphosis. (A) The underlying mechanism of injury in a Chance fracture is flexion-distraction. (B) Chance fractures occur most commonly from T11 to L3. (C) Chance fractures are secondary to flexion-distraction and not a shear injury. Shear injuries also can result in the disruption of all three columns and may present with variable degrees of lateral, anterior, or posterior listhesis. In contrast to Chance fractures, they are associated with disruption of the anterior longitudinal ligament (not compression of the anterior column) and vertebral translation/displacement. (E) Chance fractures less commonly are associated with neurologic deficits compared with other serious spine injuries.

34.

A $V_{eq} = (RT/zF)\ln([X]out/[X]in)$

This is the Nernst equation. Thinking of the sodium ion with a large extracellular compared with intracellular concentration, and knowing that it has a positive equilibrium potential, one can determine that the equation must incorporate the natural log of the extracellular divided by the intracellular concentration. The inverse would yield a negative equilibrium potential. In addition, increasing temperature increases diffusion rates and thus would enable increased passage of ions across a membrane through facilitated diffusion. This would create an equilibrium potential of a greater magnitude, meaning that the temperature component should go in the numerator of the equation.

35.

D Kawase

The Kawase (posteromedial) triangle contains the petrous apex, internal carotid artery, cochlea, and vertebrobasilar junction. It can be used to perform an anterior petrosectomy so that the posterior fossa, anterior brainstem, and root of the trigeminal nerve can be visualized. (A) The oculomotor triangle, known as the medial or Hakuba triangle, contains the oculomotor nerve and horizontal segment of the internal carotid artery. It is the triangle by which access to most intracavernous aneurysms and tumors is gained. (B) Historically, the Parkinson triangle was accessed to treat carotid-cavernous fistulas. It also contains the abducens nerve. (C) The Glasscock triangle (posterolateral) contains the middle meningeal artery in the floor of the triangle as it exits the foramen spinosum, the horizontal petrous internal carotid artery, and the infratemporal fossa. The triangle is useful as it enables the surgeon to gain proximal control of the internal carotid artery for more distal vascular procedures. Approximately 10 mm of the carotid artery is accessible through this triangle. (E) The porus trigeminus is the entrance to the Meckel cave and is contained within the inferolateral triangle.

36.

B *FGFR2*

FGFR2 is the most commonly involved gene in syndromic craniosynostosis. In Apert and Crouzon syndromes, the inheritance of the *FGFR2* mutations is autosomal dominant. The independent mutations found in different genes in syndromic craniosynostosis are most prevalent in *FGFR2*, followed, in decreasing order, by *FGFR3*, *TWIST1*, and *FGFR1*. The P250R mutation in *FGFR3* (Muenke syndrome) is the single most common craniosynostosis mutation observed.

37.

B Anterior communicating artery aneurysm

The coronal postcontrast T1-weighted image accompanying the question shows a large, suprasellar mass that demonstrates both areas of avid enhancement and prominent T2 hypointensity. This, together with the presence of pulsation artifact in the phase-encoding direction (evident in the image by "ghosting" propagated along a horizontal plane at the level of the lesion), cinches the diagnosis of a giant (larger than 2.5 cm) intracranial aneurysm. Depending on the amount of thrombosis and the stage of blood products, aneurysms can show varied signal intensities. Given the location in this case, there likely is compression of the optic nerves and chiasm along with compression of the hypothalamus, pituitary gland, and infundibulum, which can result in pituitary dysfunction. (A) Sheehan syndrome constitutes a rare cause of hypopituitarism secondary to infarct of the pituitary gland following postpartum hemorrhage. (C) Lactotroph adenomas (prolactinomas) arise within the pituitary gland and constitute the most common hormone-secreting pituitary tumors (about 30%). (D) Pituitary apoplexy refers to the clinical syndrome defined by the sudden onset of headache, visual symptoms, altered mental status, and endocrine dysfunction due to hemorrhage or infarction of the pituitary gland commonly in the setting of a preexisting adenoma. (E) A normal physiological decrease in lactation would not explain the presence of this suprasellar mass.

38.

B Nitrous oxide

Nitrous oxide is 34 times more soluble than nitrogen. As it emerges from a solution in a closed space (e.g., the cranial cavity), it can convert pneumocephalus to tension pneumocephalus. Nitrous oxide markedly increases cerebral blood volume and mildly increases the cerebral metabolic rate. (A, C, D) These halogenated inhalation agents suppress electroencephalographic activity.

39.

C Bradycardia and hypotension

The carotid sinus reflex is activated as the carotid sinus senses a pressure elevation and responds by ultimately inducing a lowering of the blood pressure and heart rate.

40.

C Intravenous nicardipine

Nicardipine improves angiographic vasospasm without resulting in a significant improvement in long-term clinical outcomes and does not seem to prevent the developmental of neurologic deficits and/or strokes. (A) Prior to large studies like the IMASH trial, intravenous magnesium was thought to improve long-term outcomes and reduce cerebral infarctions much more than offer any benefit regarding angiographic vasospasm. Following these large investigations, magnesium therapy plays no role in the management of aneurysmal subarachnoid hemorrhage except to normalize serum magnesium levels. (B) Some studies have shown long-term outcome improvements with erythropoietin administration but no effects on angiographic vasospasm. (D) There is no definitive benefit to using oral verapamil in aneurysmal subarachnoid hemorrhage patients. (E) Nimodipine has not been proven to reverse angiographic vasospasm but has been shown to reduced morbidity, poor outcomes, and progression of neurologic deficits over the long term in aneurysmal subarachnoid hemorrhage patients.

41.

D Hemangiopericytoma

The pathological description is most consistent with a hemangiopericytoma. These tumors are locally aggressive with a high incidence of recurrence, but they sometimes can be small and indistinguishable from meningiomas by imaging, as in this case. Hemangiopericytomas usually avidly enhance and sometimes can show a small dural tail. On MR spectroscopy, an alanine peak that may be seen in meningiomas is absent in hemangiopericytomas. (A) Neurosarcoid can present with lesions involving the leptomeninges, parenchyma, and infundibular/pituitary region. They are characterized by the presence of noncaseating granulomas. (B) Primary dural lymphomas are rare and more commonly are seen in middle-aged women. They can present as avidly enhancing dural masses and mimic other neoplasms. (C) The postcontrast MRI scans accompanying the question show an avidly enhancing dural-based mass along the right tentorium cerebelli. The imaging findings are indistinguishable from those of meningiomas, but the pathological description is consistent with a hemangiopericytoma.

42.

D Symptomatic carotid artery stenosis 70 to 99%

The NASCET found that for patients with symptomatic carotid artery stenosis less than 30%, the best medical management is indicated, with a stroke risk reduction of 0.8% at 5 years. NASCET recommended carotid endarterectomy (CEA) for symptomatic carotid artery stenosis of 70 to 99%, with a stroke risk reduction of 16.5% at 2 years. CEA also was thought to be moderately beneficial when carotid artery stenosis was 50 to 69%, with a stroke risk reduction of 10.1% at 5 years. Performing a CEA in this group of patients requires a low surgical complication rate to justify the procedure. (A) The Asymptomatic Carotid Atherosclerosis Trial (ACST) recommends CEA for patients younger than 75 years of age with an asymptomatic carotid artery stenosis greater than 60%, and this is associated with a stroke risk reduction of 5.4% at 5 years. (B) The surgical recommendations of the European Carotid Surgery Trial (ECST) are to perform a CEA for patients with symptomatic carotid artery stenosis greater than 60%. Operating on these patients is associated with a stroke risk reduction of 11.6% at 3 years. (C) The surgical recommendations of the Veterans Administration Cooperative Study (VACS) are to perform a CEA for patients with asymptomatic carotid artery stenosis greater than 50%; however, the results from this study are considered equivocal.

43.

D Carbamazepine

The gold standard of treatment for partial seizures is carbamazepine, although phenytoin also is a good medication. A study in 2007 found that lamotrigine has a lower incidence of treatment failure compared with carbamazepine for partial seizures. (A) Topiramate is a second-line drug for any seizure type and is associated with cognitive impairment and weight loss. (B) Phenobarbital is an effective medication for seizure control or abatement, but its adverse effects limit its attractiveness for long-term use. (C) Valproic acid is the drug of choice for absence seizures (ethosuximide also may be used) and myoclonic seizures, and often is the drug of choice for primary generalized seizures. Phenytoin also can be the drug of choice for partial or generalized seizures. (E) Levetiracetam is increasingly use as a substitute for phenytoin due to its lower rate of severe side effects, but it is not as well studied at this point.

44.

A Melanin-stimulating hormone (MSH) overproduction

The patient has Nelson syndrome, which, following bilateral adrenalectomy (a treatment for Cushing syndrome and not Cushing disease), is a rapid enlargement of a pituitary adenoma that secretes ACTH. Without the negative feedback from cortisol (adrenal gland produced), there is overproduction of proopiomelanocortin (POMC) from which MSH and ACTH are derived. It is the high levels of MSH that induce skin hyperpigmentation. Nelson syndrome is a complication of total bilateral adrenalectomies for Cushing disease that affects 10 to 30% of treated patients. It usually manifests between 1 and 4 years following surgery. These patients present with a triad of hyperpigmentation, increased serum ACTH, and progression of the pituitary tumor.

45.

B Aneurysmal bone cyst

Aneurysmal bone cysts are rare benign tumors that may be locally aggressive. They most commonly occur in the lumbar spine in children and adolescents, and characteristically involve the posterior elements. The appearance of an expansile mass with thin osseous rims and fluid–blood levels due to repeated hemorrhage is near pathognomonic. (A) Spinal metastases can have a variety of appearances, but this presentation would be unusual. (C) About 10% of osteoid osteomas are found in the spine, usually in young patients. They typically are small, lucent lesions with surrounding sclerosis and sometimes with central nidal calcifications. (D) Osteoblastomas histologically are similar to but larger (more than 1 cm) than osteoid osteomas and more commonly are located in the axial skeleton. About 20% may have an associated aneurysmal bone cyst. (E) Eosinophilic granuloma is often used to refer to the benign, localized form of Langerhans cell histiocytosis. It presents as a lytic lesion and most commonly occurs in the skull, ribs, long bones, and, rarely, spine, where it may result in a vertebra plana.

46.

B Retinal hemorrhages

The most common cause of retinal hemorrhages in an infant is head trauma, and a dilated ophthalmologic exam should be a part of any nonaccidental trauma workup. (A) Retinal detachment can occur with acute ocular trauma but is not used as a screening tool for nonaccidental trauma. (C) Cherry red spots typically are seen in lipid storage disorders or retinal artery occlusions rather than in nonaccidental trauma. (D, E) Ophthalmoplegia and ptosis are not sensitive enough to detect non-accidental trauma.

47.

B Chronic subdural hematomas

Extra-axial fluid collections commonly are associated with macrocrania. A clinical history, thorough examination, and MRI can distinguish between benign cerebrospinal fluid hygromas and subdural hematomas. Note that the extra-axial fluid collections shown in the image accompanying the question are hyperintense relative to the cerebrospinal fluid.

48.

B B

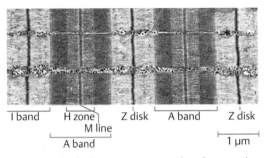

I band   H zone   Z disk   A band   Z disk
M line
A band   1 μm

Letter B in the image accompanying the question is the H zone, which is the region of the sarcomere where myosin thick filaments do not overlap actin thin filaments. The H zone shortens during sarcomere contraction. (A) Letter A is the I band, which contains only actin thin filaments. (C) Letter C is the M line, which is an anchoring point of the myosin thick filaments composed of cross-connecting cytoskeletal elements occurring in the middle of the H zone. (D) Letter D is the Z disk, which is in the middle of the I band and defines the border of each sarcomere. The protein titin anchors the Z disk to the M line. (E) Letter E is the A band, which is composed of the H zone plus the region of overlap of the myosin thick filaments and actin thin filaments.

49.

C V3

The vertebral artery is divided into four sections. The first section (V1) runs from the subclavian artery to the foramen transversarium (usually at the level of C6). V2 runs through the foramen transversarium to the transverse process of the axis (C2). V3 exits the axis and curves posteromedially around C1 and enters the foramen magnum. V4 pierces the dura and enters the subarachnoid space. The image accompanying the question shows the vertebral artery running along the groove of the posterior arch of C1 prior to entering the foramen magnum. Note the large posterior meningeal/muscular artery.

50.

E Sporadic mitochondrial

The disease described is Kearns-Sayre syndrome, characterized by chronic progressive external ophthalmoplegia (weakness of the levator palpebrae, orbicularis oculi, extraocular muscles, and some facial muscles), pigmentary retinopathy, cerebellar dysfunction, and heart block. Various endocrinopathies also can occur. The disease is thought to arise through sporadic mutations in the autosomal mitochondrial DNA.

51.

D May show a lactate peak on MR spectroscopy

The images accompanying the question show an avidly enhancing, extra-axial, dural-based mass in the right cerebellopontine angle, most consistent with a meningioma. The mass is only mildly hyperintense on T2 relative to gray matter (e.g., the dentate nuclei and cerebellar folia). Overall, meningiomas represent the most common intracranial, extra-axial tumors in adults. In the cerebellopontine angle, however, about 80% of tumors are schwannomas, 10% are meningiomas, and 5% are epidermoid tumors. Meningiomas may show heterogeneous signal and enhancement depending on their degree of calcification (relatively frequent) and rarely have cystic changes or hemorrhage. An elevated alanine peak is characteristic of meningiomas on MR spectroscopy, although it does not typically play a role in diagnosis. (A) Schwannomas demonstrate avid enhancement, which usually is heterogeneous in larger tumors where cystic degeneration is frequent. Most schwannomas originate within the internal auditory canal with variable extension into the cerebellopontine angle; however, note that 20% of meningiomas can show extension into the internal auditory canal. (B) Meningiomas derive from arachnoid cap cells, whereas epidermoid tumors arise from the inclusion of ectodermal rests during neural tube closure. Epidermoid tumors do not enhance and usually demonstrate very bright signal on diffusion-weighted images and a "dirty" appearance on FLAIR images. (C) Most meningiomas are sporadic and discovered in middle-aged women. They also are associated with neurofibromatosis type 2 (not type 1) and may be induced by radiation.

52.

A Carmustine

Carmustine is a nitrosourea that works by carbamylating amino groups and cross-linking DNA strands. This agent is seen incorporated into implantable wafers. (B) Tamoxifen inhibits protein kinase C. (C) Temozolomide is a DNA methylating agent that interferes with protein synthesis through alkylation. (D) Cyclophosphamide is a nitrogen mustard that works through DNA alkylation and carbonium ion formation. (E) Cisplatin forms DNA strand cross-links and subsequent chelation.

53.

B Branches of the internal carotid, anterior cerebral, and anterior communicating arteries

(D) The ophthalmic artery provides the blood supply to the orbit, with collaterals to the face and meninges.

54.

D Posterior to the trochlear nerve

55.

B 10 cc/kg; 2 to 3 g/dL

56.

B Disk extrusion

Herniation is defined as focal or localized displacement of disk material beyond the margins of the intervertebral disk space. In this case, the greatest craniocaudal dimension of the herniated disk is larger than that of its base, making this a disk extrusion. (A) In a disk protrusion, the height of the herniated disk material is smaller than its base. (C) A disk bulge occurs when disk tissue extends beyond the margins of the ring apophyses throughout the circumference of the disk. An asymmetric disk bulge is defined as tissue extending more than 25% beyond the circumference of the disk. These bulges are not considered forms of herniation. Although no axial images are presented in this case, the amount of disk material outside of the disk space (which is larger than at its base) makes this a disk herniation. (D) In a sequestered disk, a portion of the herniated disk loses is connection with the parent disk. (E) Migration sometimes is used to indicate displacement of disk material away from the site of extrusion.

57.

D There is reduced interictal metabolism in the epileptogenic region.

Positron emission tomography (PET) with 18-fluoro-2-deoxyglucose (FDG) shows reduced interictal metabolism in the epileptogenic region. (A) In most patients, the area of hypometabolism usually is larger than the epileptogenic zone, and therefore FDG-PET contributes to lateralization and general localization but cannot precisely delineate the seizure focus. (B) Studies are performed in the interictal phase in the great majority of patients. Ictal scanning with FDG-PET is challenging due to the short duration and unpredictability of seizures and the long period of cerebral uptake of FDG after injection. (C) Single photon emission computed tomography (SPECT) provides a measure of cerebral perfusion by injection of a lipophilic radiopharmaceutical that is taken up in proportion to cerebral blood flow. With this technique, there is increased blood flow in the epileptogenic focus if the radiopharmaceutical is injected shortly after seizure onset (ictal scan) and decreased blood flow in this region, and frequently in other areas of the affected lobe in interictal scans. FDG-PET, on the other hand, measures glucose metabolism, which is associated closely with neuronal activity.

58.

A Left posterior cerebral artery stroke

Pure alexia is secondary to an infarct in the left posterior cerebral artery territory, causing ischemia of the splenium of the corpus callosum and left visual cortex.

59.

A The 95% confidence interval range

The stacked horizontal lines in a forest plot represent individual studies included in a meta-analysis, as shown in the image accompanying the question. The horizontal line length refers to the 95% confidence interval of each study. An arrow at one end of the line indicates that the confidence interval extends beyond the scale of the plot.

60.

E Phosphorylase

The condition described is concerning for glycogen storage disease type V, also known as McArdle disease. In this condition, a defect in the skeletal muscle-specific phosphorylase enzyme causes insufficient glycogen phosphorylation in skeletal muscles. The liver and heart are unaffected. Patients typically present with early fatigue and cramping of skeletal muscles, which are relieved by rest. (A) Glucose-6-phosphatase is the enzyme deficiency responsible for glycogen storage disease type I, also known as Von Gierke disease. (B) Alpha-1,4 glucosidase is the enzyme deficiency responsible for glycogen storage disease type II, also known as Pompe disease. (C) Alpha-1,6 glucosidase is the enzyme deficiency responsible for glycogen storage disease type III, also known as Cori disease. (D) Branching enzyme is the enzyme deficiency responsible for glycogen storage disease type IV, also known as Andersen disease.

61.

C Left optic tract

A left optic tract disruption would produce a right homonymous hemianopsia as shown in the image accompanying the question. The incongruity of the deficits points to an optic tract lesion, as the fields become more congruous as lesions are closer to the occipital cortex. By convention, the visual fields are displayed from the patient's point of view, with the left eye represented on the left. The region with the hash marks on the left image represents the blind spot, which is not seen on the right image as it is in the region of visual loss. (A) A lesion causing complete disruption of the left optic nerve would result in a normal visual field in the right eye, with a complete loss of vision in the left eye. (B) A lesion affecting the optic chiasm classically would produce a bitemporal hemianopsia. (D) A lesion of the left Meyer loop (temporal optic radiation) would produce a right superior quadrantanopsia. (E) A left occipital lobe lesion would produce a congruous left homonymous hemianopsia with macular sparing. Only an occipital lobe lesion to the occipital pole would cause a deficit in the macula.

62.

A Autoclaving for 1 hour at 132°C

The most effective sterilization procedure involves autoclaving for 1 hour at 132°C and immersion in 1 N NaOH for 1 hour at room temperature. (B, C) Partially effective sterilization procedures involve autoclaving for 15 to 30 minutes at 121° to 132°C, immersion in 1 N NaOH for 15 minutes, and

immersion in sodium hypochlorite (undiluted) for 1 hour. (D) Standard operative room sterilization procedures (e.g., ultraviolet light, ethylene oxide, alcohol, formalin) are considered ineffective against Creutzfeldt-Jakob disease.

63.

B It can be associated with Klippel-Feil syndrome.

The images accompanying the question show inferior displacement of peg-like cerebellar tonsils below the foramen magnum and formation of a syrinx in a patient with a Chiari 1 malformation. Several osseous abnormalities may be seen with any of the Chiari malformations such as platybasia, atlas assimilation, Klippel-Feil syndrome, and atlantoaxial subluxation among others. (A) An open myelomeningocele is the sine qua non for development of a Chiari 2 malformation. This patient has a Chiari 1 malformation. (C) Failure of diverticulation of the brain can result in the holoprosencephaly spectrum. (D) A Blake pouch cyst can result from persistence of the embryonic Blake pouch.

64.

B Todd paralysis

Todd paralysis also is known as postictal paralysis and describes a persistent but self-limited weakness following a seizure. (A) Cerebral vasospasm usually occurs between 3 and 21 days following subarachnoid hemorrhage. (C, E) Extension of the edema or hemorrhage would have been detected on the CT scan.

65.

B Stria medullaris

The stria medullaris carries fibers from the septal nuclei of the hypothalamus to the habenula. (A) The stria terminalis connects fibers from the amygdala to the hypothalamus and separates the thalamus from the caudate nucleus. (C) The tract of Vicq d'Azyr arises from the mammillary nuclei and connects to the anterior thalamic nuclei. (D) The field of Forel H1 is the thalamic fasciculus, composed of the ansa lenticularis, lenticular fasciculus (field of Forel H2 from the pallidum through the internal capsule to the thalamus), and cerebellothalamic tracts. (E) The ansa lenticularis passes from the lentiform nucleus (globus pallidus and putamen) inferior to the internal capsule to terminate in the thalamus.

66.

E It may be associated with callosal abnormalities.

The axial T2 image accompanying the question demonstrates subependymal nodules that are iso-intense to gray matter and more numerous along the left lateral ventricle. This is compatible with subependymal nodular heterotopia, which represents neuronal rests along white matter migration pathways. Note decreased white matter volume, particularly in the right posterior hemisphere. Subependymal nodular heterotopia, particularly the posterior predominant type, may be associated with callosal abnormalities, decreased white matter volumes, and mid- or hindbrain malformations. (A) Glioneuronal hamartomas (also known as cortical tubers) are part of the tuberous sclerosis complex (TSC). Most patients with TSC have subependymal nodules. (B) Subependymal nodular heterotopia does not enhance and follows gray matter signal intensity on all sequences. Subependymal nodules in TSC may show enhancement. (C) Heterotopias do not calcify, but subependymal nodules in TSC do. (D) Subependymal nodular heterotopia does not cause ventricular obstruction. The subependymal nodules of tuberous sclerosis can grow and become subependymal giant cell tumors and eventually obstruct the foramina of Monro.

67.

D Adrenal glands

Primary hypercortisolism resulting from excessive release of cortisol from the adrenal glands (usually from tumors) suppresses the hypothalamic-pituitary-adrenal axis and results in suppression of the of adrenocorticotropic hormone (ACTH) released by the pituitary gland. (A) In Cushing disease of hypothalamic origin, corticotropin-releasing hormone is secreted in elevated amounts, resulting in elevated levels of ACTH in the presence of hypercortisolism. (B) In Cushing disease of pituitary origin, ACTH is released in elevated amounts. (C) In hypercortisolism of lung origin (usually small cell carcinoma), there is ectopic production of ACTH. (E) Renal disease may results in hypokalemic alkalosis, but ACTH levels should be unaffected.

68.

D Usually presents as a dilated median prosencephalic vein draining through a persistent falcine sinus

A vein of Galen malformation develops due to arteriovenous shunting from various possible feeders (commonly choroidal, thalamostriate, and pericallosal arteries) into the embryonic median prosencephalic vein (of Markowski). The term *vein of Galen malformation* actually is a misnomer, and the dilated vessel represents the median prosencephalic vein, which typically drains through a persistent dilated falcine sinus (as seen in this case) or through the straight sinus. (A) A proximal high-flow arteriovenous malformation draining into the true vein of Galen would result in secondary dilatation of this vessel; however, this is a separate phenomenon, in essence a "pseudomalformation," and not a "true" vein of Galen malformation, which is characterized by arteriovenous shunting into and dilation of the median prosencephalic vein. (B) The inferior sagittal sinus is not a usual drainage pathway for a vein of Galen malformation. (C) A vein of Galen malformation typically drains through a persistent falcine sinus in which the straight sinus does not form (as in this patient) or through the straight sinus. (E) The occipital sinus is not a usual drainage pathway for a vein of Galen malformation.

69.

B 3 months

(C, D) Radiation necrosis most often occurs 6 to 12 months following radiosurgery, but it even has been reported to emerge several years later.

70.

E Atlantoaxial instability

Atlantoaxial instability (AAI) affects 10 to 20% of individuals with Down syndrome (DS). The condition mostly is asymptomatic and diagnosed on radiography by an enlarged anterior atlanto-odontoid distance. Symptomatic AAI affects 1 to 2% of individuals with DS, manifests with spinal cord compression, and requires surgical decompression and fusion.

71.

C 20 mL per 100 g of tissue/min

A cerebral blood flow under 20 mL per 100 g of tissue/min is associated with ischemia and will lead to cell death if it is prolonged. (A) A cerebral blood flow under 10 mL per 100 g of tissue/min is associated with cell death/stroke and alterations in cell membrane transport. These effects are not reversible. (B) A cerebral blood flow under 15 mL per 100 g of tissue/min is associated with physiological paralysis and a "flat" electroencephalogram. (D) A cerebral blood flow of 20 to 30 mL per 100 g of tissue/min is the normal flow for white matter, whereas 45 to 60 mL per 100 g of tissue/min is the blood flow in a normal brain at rest. (E) A cerebral blood flow of 75 to 80 mL per 100 g of tissue/min is the rate in a normal brain.

72.

D Abducens nerve

The arrow in the image accompanying the question indicates the abducens nerve, which typically is small in caliber and can be seen exiting the brainstem at the level of the pontomedullary junction. It courses cranially and anteriorly and reaches the cavernous sinus through the Dorello canal. (A) The oculomotor nerves are relatively thick and can be identified exiting the brainstem at the level of the pontomesencephalic junction. They course between the posterior cerebral and superior cerebellar arteries on coronal images. (B) The trochlear nerve generally is not seen on CISS or FIESTA images due to its small caliber unless thinner slices (e.g., 0.4 mm) are acquired. (C) The trigeminal nerves exit the lateral aspects of the pons and have a characteristic shape with fibers that appear to spread out before piercing the dura and entering their corresponding Meckel caves. (E) The glossopharyngeal nerve is part of the cranial nerve IX, X, and XI complex. It exits the upper medulla and leaves the skull through the pars nervosa of the jugular foramen.

73.

B The retinal area for vision during good light

The retinal area for central fixation vision during good light is the macula. (A, D) The optic disk represents the optic nerve and corresponds to a small blind spot in each eye. (C) Within the macula, the fovea is a small, central pit with densely packed cones responsible for high-resolution color vision. (E) The hyaloid canal is a transparent canal running through the vitreous body extending from the optic disk to the lens.

74.

B Dystrophin

The gene for dystrophin is located on the X chromosome and is mutated in Duchenne muscular dystrophy. This disease usually affects young boys and is progressive over the course of years. Affected children usually do not survive past adolescence.

75.

A Ipsilateral, monocular, inferior nasal quadrantanopsia

Ophthalmic aneurysms classically produce a nasal quadrantanopsia due to the aneurysm pressing on the lateral inferior fibers. This initially causes a superior nasal field cut, and as the aneurysm increases in size it pushes against the falciform ligament, causing an inferior nasal field cut. The aneurysms typically do not cause temporal field cuts. (B) Bitemporal field cuts often are associated with sellar pathologies such as macroadenomas. (C) A cranial nerve III palsy is characteristic of posterior communicating artery aneurysms.

Section 5

1.

B Hemangioblastoma

Approximately two thirds of hemangioblastomas present as cystic masses with an avidly enhancing mural nodule (which usually abuts the pial surface), and one third is completely solid. Their walls should not enhance, and they typically do not incite significant adjacent edema. They are very vascular, and flow voids often are identified on MRI. Sporadic hemangioblastomas usually are solitary, but up to 20% may be multiple particularly when associated with von Hippel–Lindau syndrome. Hemangioblastomas histologically are benign, but recurrence rates range from 8 to 25% depending on the histological subtype (note that this patient has had surgery in the left cerebellum). (A) Ependymomas are heterogeneous tumors due to the presence of calcifications, cystic changes, and sometimes hemorrhages. They would not form a clean cyst with a discrete enhancing mural nodule. Ependymomas have a "plastic" configuration and typically extrude through the foramina of the posterior fossa. (C) Medulloblastomas are the most common malignant brain tumors of childhood. They can arise at the midline or in the cerebellar hemispheres and generally enhance heterogeneously. (D) Juvenile pilocytic astrocytomas occur more commonly in children and represent the most common cerebellar tumor. They also typically do not incite significant parenchymal edema, and their walls sometimes may enhance. (E) Metastases can be cystic, and a lesion of this size usually would result in a higher degree of edema.

2.

C High-grade glioma

A decrease in N-acetylaspartate (NAA) is a reflection of neuronal loss, and choline (Cho) is a marker of cellular membrane turnover. As the grade of a tumor increases, NAA decreases, and Cho, lipids, and lactate tend to increase (the last two are markers of severe tissue damage and necrosis). The MR spectroscopy profile shown in the image accompanying the question demonstrates elevation of Cho, which resonates at 3.2 ppm, and the near absence of NAA (2.0 ppm), a pattern that is consistent with a high-grade glioma. Note that there also is a tiny lactate peak at 1.3 ppm. Lactate usually is superimposed on lipids, but appears inverted when using an intermediate TE, which allows their distinction. (A) In radiation necrosis, Cho, creatine (Cr), and NAA are markedly decreased. Lactate and lipids may or may not be elevated. (B) In an abscess, as in any process that results in neuronal destruction, NAA is reduced. The central necrotic portion of the abscess may show elevated lactate, alanine, acetate, amino acids, and other metabolites. Cho would not be elevated. (D) Infarction usually produces a larger lactate peak (not the minimal elevation seen in this case) and would not be expected to increase Cho. NAA decreases in infarcted tissue.

3.

D LL = Pelvic incidence + 10

The sacral slope approximates the pelvic incidence (PI); thus, as the PI increases, so does the sacral slope. This means that patients with a small PI have a small sacral slope and typically flattened lordosis. Patients with this relationship presenting with kyphosis have an increased positive sagittal imbalance compared with patients with large PI.

4.

E Epithelial membrane antigen and vimentin

Transthyretin can be seen in choroid plexus papillomas, which tend to be negative for epithelial membrane antigen. CD45 reactivity can be found in central nervous system lymphomas. S-100 reactivity is observed in melanoma, schwannomas, neurofibromas, and malignant peripheral nerve sheath tumors. S-100 and epithelial membrane antigen reactivity can be seen in melanoma.

5.

A Choriocarcinoma

Choriocarcinomas are germ cell tumors that are associated with high levels of β-HCG. Following the cerebrospinal fluid β-HCG levels can yield information about treatment response and recurrence. (C, D) Pure germinomas and teratomas usually present with negative markers (no cerebrospinal fluid β-HCG or α-fetoprotein [AFP] detected), although low levels of β-HCG sometimes can be detected. (E) Yolk sac tumors are germ cell tumors that are associated with high levels AFP. Checking the cerebrospinal fluid AFP levels can yield information about treatment response and recurrence.

6.

A Chorioretinitis

Other neurologic problems seen in prenatal *Cytomegalovirus* infection include microcephaly, developmental delays, seizures, and hearing deficits. (B) Microaneurysms are seen in diabetic neuropathy. (C) Hemorrhages are more typical of hypertensive disorders. (D) Cotton wool spots develop in the retinae secondary to ischemic or infectious processes. (E) Macular cherry red spots are seen in lipid storage disorders and central retinal artery occlusion.

7.

C Respiratory alkalosis with metabolic compensation

The pH > 7.40 indicates an alkalosis. Compensation never completely normalizes the pH. The P_aCO_2 of 26 (< 40) indicates a respiratory alkalosis. It could not be respiratory compensation, as the pH would remain in the acidotic range. The fact that the HCO_3^- is reduced from its normal of 26 indicates some metabolic compensation. This also rules out metabolic alkalosis. Finally, an accompanying metabolic acidosis is not seen as a proper metabolic compensation for a respiratory alkalosis, and it results in approximately a 4 mEq/L reduction in HCO_3^- for every 10 mm Hg reduction in P_aCO_2. In this case, 40 − 26 = 14, 14/10 = 1.4, 1.4 × 4 = 5.6, 26 − 5.6 = 20.4. This indicates that the patient has an adequate and expected metabolic compensation and not an additional metabolic acidosis.

8.

B Lewy body

Intracytoplasmic, round, eosinophilic inclusions, which are classic Lewy bodies, are found typically in pigmented neurons of the substantia nigra of patients with Parkinson disease. (A) Cowdry bodies are eosinophilic nuclear inclusions composed of nucleic acid and protein found in *Herpesvirus* infections. (D) Negri bodies are eosinophilic intracytoplasmic bodies found in rabies. (E) Neurofibrillary tangles are found in neurodegenerative disorders such as Alzheimer disease and occur both within the cytoplasm and outside affected neurons.

9.

A Ventral posterior medial nucleus

The principal trigeminal nucleus receives information about light touch. Pain and temperature information is received by the spinal nucleus of cranial nerve V. Proprioception is received by the mesencephalic nucleus of cranial nerve V. All three nuclei synapse on the ventral posterior medial nucleus of the dorsal thalamus. (B) The ventral posterior lateral nucleus receives sensory fibers from the body. (C) The ventral anterior nucleus is involved in motor relay functions. (D) The dorsal medial nucleus is involved in memory and emotions. (E) The ventral medial nucleus is a nucleus of the hypothalamus and frequently is referred to as a "satiety" center. Damage to the nucleus results in hyperphagia and obesity.

10.

A NMO-IgG antibodies are found only in NMO, not in MS.

NMO-IgG antibodies are not found in patients with multiple sclerosis (MS) but are seen in 70% of patients with neuromyelitis optica (NMO). (B) MS typically progresses to a secondary progressive phase. NMO does not, and presents with disabilities from acute attacks. (C) Contiguous spinal cord lesions on MRI extending at least three vertebral levels are required for the diagnosis of NMO, but these also may be seen in MS. (D) MS is not considered an autoimmune disease, as no antibodies have been identified, whereas the NMO-IgG antibodies are present in most cases of NMO. (E) Brain lesions on MRI are not part of NMO, whereas they help to characterize MS.

11.

B The use of intermittent pneumatic compression with or without graduated compression stockings is recommended in all patients undergoing intracranial neurosurgery.

There is level 1A evidence to recommend thromboprophylaxis in patients undergoing major neurosurgery and the use of intermittent pneumatic compression with or without graduated compression stockings in patients undergoing intracranial neurosurgery. (C) There is level 2 evidence supporting the use of low-dose unfractionated heparin and postoperative low molecular weight heparin in patients undergoing intracranial neurosurgery. (D) There is level 2 evidence supporting the combi-

nation of mechanical prophylaxis (graduated compression stockings and/or intermittent pneumatic compression) in high-risk neurosurgery patients. Patients on low molecular weight heparin after surgery had bleeding rates that were twice as high as those who received mechanical prophylaxis alone. (E) Thromboprophylaxis should be used in patients undergoing major neurosurgery and not just those undergoing spine procedures.

12.

A X-linked recessive

In the images accompanying the question, the sagittal CISS image (*left*) shows stenosis of the cerebral aqueduct due to what appears to be a transverse web. Note a defect along the floor of the third ventricle from an endoscopic ventriculostomy. The second MR phase contrast image (*right*) shows a white jet through the location of the third ventriculostomy, indicating that it is patent. Aqueductal stenosis represents the most common cause of congenital hydrocephalus. Approximately 5 to 7% of patients have a congenital form (X-linked hydrocephalus) seen in males and determined by mutations in the *L1CAM* gene. (B, C, D) These modes of inheritance are not seen in congenital hydrocephalus.

13.

D Metencephalon

The pons and cerebellum arise from the metencephalon. It is a division of the rhombencephalon. (A) The medulla arises from the myelencephalon. It is a division of the rhombencephalon. (B) The epithalamus, thalamus, hypothalamus, subthalamus, pituitary gland, pineal gland, and third ventricle arise from the diencephalon. It is one of two divisions of the prosencephalon. (C) The telencephalon yields the cerebral cortex, amygdala, basal ganglia, hippocampus, and lateral ventricles. It is a division of the prosencephalon. (E) The mesencephalon yields the midbrain, cerebral peduncle, pretectum, tectum, and cerebral aqueduct.

14.

D Lacunar infarct; posteroventral nucleus of the thalamus

Pure sensory strokes usually are lacunar strokes affecting the posteroventral nucleus of the lateral thalamus. They present with contralateral numbness and tingling. Pure motor strokes also are mostly secondary to lacunar infarcts. They occur when the lacunar stroke affects the internal capsule, causing isolated hemiplegia.

15.

D Sinonasal carcinoma

The image accompanying the question is a fat-saturated, contrast-enhanced, T1-weighted MRI that shows a relatively ill-defined mass involving the ethmoid sinuses and nasal cavity (not shown). The lesion can be distinguished from the much more avidly enhancing mucosal thickening in the remaining ethmoid sinuses and right sphenoid sinus. Of the given options, the findings are most consistent with a sinonasal carcinoma, which accounts for 50 to 80% of all sinonasal malignancies, with squamous cell carcinoma being the most common subtype by far. Sinonasal carcinoma is more common in males who have chronic exposure to wood dust, which is a recognized risk factor. In contrast to other head and neck malignancies, smoking does not play a major role in the development of sinonasal carcinoma but does increase the risk of lesion development two- to threefold. (A) Mucoceles are expansile lesions that are well circumscribed. They originate most commonly in the frontal sinuses, followed by the ethmoid sinuses. (B) The patient does have background sinusitis as seen by extensive mucosal enhancement in the ethmoid and sphenoid sinuses, but this is not the most important diagnosis. (C) Juvenile nasopharyngeal angiofibroma occurs in children and young adults (almost exclusively in males) and is rare in patients older than 25 years of age. These lesions are highly vascular tumors that enhance markedly following contrast administration. Flow voids often are seen on MRI, particularly on T2 images. Juvenile nasopharyngeal angiofibromas originate in the sphenopalatine foramen. (E) Ninety percent of rhabdomyosarcomas occur in individuals younger than 25 years of age, with presentation in older adults being unusual. These tumors usually enhance avidly, and hemorrhage is a frequent finding in the alveolar and pleomorphic subtypes.

16.

E Type 2b

The cortical section shown in the image accompanying the question demonstrates atypical-appearing neurons (dysmorphic neurons) and occasional large balloon cells. These findings are characteristic of type 2b focal cortical dysplasia. (A–C) Cortical architectural abnormalities in a horizontal and/or vertical orientation in the absence of dysmorphic neurons and balloon cells define type I patterns. (D) The presence of dysmorphic neurons without balloon cells represents type 2a dysplasia.

17.

E Decrease in peak amplitude more than 50% and increase in latency more than 10%

During somatosensory evoked potential (SSEP) recordings, the criteria for monitoring personnel to notify the surgeon include a decrease in peak amplitude more than 50%, increase in latency more than 10%, and complete loss of the waveform. In the event of SSEP deterioration, multiple considerations need to be made: technical factors (e.g., operating room interference, electrode placement, anesthesia), hypotension/anemia, and spinal alignment (check radiographs). The surgeon must retrace his or her last steps following an SSEP change to see if it can be reversed. Readjusting hardware, repositioning retractors, administering steroids, performing a "wake up" test, and terminating the surgery are reasonable maneuvers.

18.

C Lundberg C waves

Lundberg C waves are characterized by variable intracranial pressure (ICP) elevations with a frequency of four to eight per minute. High-amplitude waves may represent a pre-terminal state and are suggestive but not pathognomonic of increased ICP. (A) Lundberg A waves are known as plateau waves, and are characterized by ICP elevations more than 50 mm Hg lasting 5 to 20 minutes. These waves often indicate uncontrollable ICP. (B) Lundberg B waves, also known as pressure pulses, are characterized by ICP elevations of 10 to 20 mm Hg lasting for 30 seconds to 2 minutes. Lundberg B waves also vary with periodic breathing and are seen with increased ICP, but this relationship is not entirely consistent. (D) Lundberg D waves do not exist.

19.

A Immune reconstitution inflammatory syndrome

The axial T2-weighted image accompanying the question shows confluent white matter abnormalities bilaterally that extend peripherally to involve the subcortical U fibers and also involve the corpus callosum. Many immunosuppressive drugs have been associated with progressive multifocal leukoencephalopathy (PML), including cyclophosphamide, corticosteroids, mycophenolate mofetil, and monoclonal antibodies such as natalizumab, rituximab, and brentuximab. PML should not show contrast enhancement or mass effect, which suggests the diagnosis of immune reconstitution inflammatory syndrome (IRIS). (B) Acute disseminated encephalomyelitis (ADEM) can show very similar imaging findings to PML-IRIS. Although the corpus callosum can be involved in ADEM, the abnormality almost always is asymmetric. The clinical history in this case favors PML-IRIS. (C) Tumefactive demyelination usually is more focal that the findings in this case and would be highly suggested by an incomplete rim of enhancement. (D) Secondary central nervous system lymphoma more commonly is leptomeningeal and usually shows avid enhancement and restricted diffusion.

20.

C 60%

The specificity is 60%. This value is obtained by dividing the number of true negatives (30) by the sum of the number of true negatives and false positives (30 + 20).

21.

D 80%

The sensitivity is 80%. This value is obtained by dividing the number of true positives (40) by the sum of the number of true positives and false negatives (40 + 10).

22.

B 67%

The positive predictive value is 67%. This value is obtained by dividing the number of true positives (40) by the sum of the number of true positives and false positives (40 + 20). (C) The negative predictive value is 75%. This value is obtained by dividing the number of true negatives (30) by the sum of the number of true negatives and false negatives (30 + 10).

	Positive Test	Negative Test
Have Disease	True positive	False negative
No Disease	False positive	True negative

23.

D Ethmoidal encephalocele

Recurrent bacterial meningitis in children necessitates a search for an underlying cause, which usually is either an altered immune status or a craniospinal defect. In the absence of an immunodeficiency, anatomic anomalies must be investigated thoroughly to rule out an intranasal encephalocele, as it is one of the most common causes of recurrent bacterial meningitis.

24.

C The adamantinomatous subtype more commonly calcifies.

Calcification is much more common in adamantinomatous craniopharyngiomas, in which it is present in 95% of cases. (A) Papillary craniopharyngiomas are more commonly solid and usually lack the characteristic cystic changes described in adamantinomatous ones. (B) Papillary craniopharyngiomas more commonly present in older individuals. (D) Both papillary and adamantinomatous craniopharyngiomas commonly arise at the infundibulum. Occasionally, they may be purely intrasellar or even infrasellar. (E) There is no evidence that either tumor subtype shows more avid enhancement, although the papillary subtype is more commonly solid and therefore may have more enhancing components.

25.

E Wilson disease

The changes of Alzheimer type 2 astrocytes are associated with hepatic encephalopathy, as first described in Wilson disease.

26.

A Tryptophan

Melatonin is produced through a two-step enzymatic process beginning with serotonin. Serotonin synthesis begins with tryptophan as a precursor. (E) Tyrosine is involved in the synthesis of dopamine, norepinephrine, and epinephrine.

27.

B Anterior spinothalamic tract

The anterior spinothalamic tract carries nociceptive sensory information to the thalamic reticular formation. This slowly conducting tract crosses in the anterior white commissure. It comprises the spinal lemniscus along with the lateral spinothalamic tract. (A) The lateral spinothalamic tract carries pain and temperature sensory information. The fibers of the tract cross a few levels above where the nerve roots synapse on them, thus ultimately ascending the spinal cord contralateral to their origin. The tract is composed of fast-conducting myelinated A-delta fibers and slow-conducting unmyelinated C fibers. (C) The dorsal spinocerebellar tract carries proprioceptive sensory information from ipsilateral muscle spindles and Golgi tendon organs and runs parallel to the anterior spinocerebellar tract. This two-neuron tract has its synapses in the Clarke nuclei. (D) The dorsal columns carry fine touch and proprioceptive sensory information in an ipsilateral manner until fiber decussation occurs in the inferior medulla.

28.

C Glomus jugulare tumor

The constellation of symptoms including motor paralysis of cranial nerves IX through XII is known as Collet-Sicard syndrome and is seen with lesions at the jugular foramen, such as a glomus jugulare tumor or schwannoma. A variant of Collet-Sicard syndrome is Vernet syndrome, which consists of motor paralysis of cranial nerves IX through XI. (A, B, D, E) These pathologies include sensory deficits as well.

29.

B Use a starting point 2 mm medial and 1 to 2 mm superior to the center of the lateral mass, and aim 20 to 25 degrees laterally and 30 degrees superiorly (parallel to facet joint)

(A) This is the An technique. (C) This is the Roy-Camille (transarticular screw) technique. (D) This is the technique for the placement of a translaminar screw. (E) This is the technique used for the placement of a thoracic spine pedicle screw.

30.

D A sentinel headache usually is absent.

The imaging findings, and in particular the negative conventional angiograms, are consistent with nonaneurysmal, perimesencephalic subarachnoid hemorrhage. Note that obtaining a second angiogram is controversial in the presence of a negative initial high-quality study, and a repeat exam is not performed in many places. Sentinel headaches usually are absent with perimesencephalic, non-aneurysmal hemorrhage, in contrast to aneurysmal hemorrhage, in which headaches may be seen in 40% of patients. (A, B) Perimesencephalic, non-aneurysmal subarachnoid hemorrhage has a low incidence of re-hemorrhage and hydrocephalus, and it is thought that the source of the hemorrhage may be venous. Sometimes an underlying lesion, such as a cavernous malformation, may be identified on MRI of the brain or cervical spine. (C) Aneurysms may be difficult to identify on angiography in the setting of vasospasm. In this case, vasospasm likely would have resolved by the time the second angiogram was performed.

31.

D Rasmussen encephalitis

The findings shown in the section accompanying the question, which is from the cortex, are foci of chronic inflammatory cells. This finding is most suggestive of Rasmussen encephalitis. Additionally, some cases are marked by nodules of microglial cells. This entity, albeit rare, is a well-known cause of medically intractable epilepsy and affects only a single cerebral hemisphere.

32.

E Potentiation of $GABA_A$ receptors, sodium channel blockade, and the endocannabinoid system

33.

E Both the receptors at rest and the tonically active receptors begin firing and increase the frequency of action potentials.

Baroreceptors in the carotid sinus, vena cava, and aortic arch all fire action potential at variable frequencies while at baseline/rest. The frequencies can be as low as zero. As pressure increases, the rate of action potentials of the entire system increases, whereas it decreases with decreasing pressure. Tonically firing baroreceptors even may stop firing action potentials as the pressure falls below baseline. (A) Increasing the amplitude of a signal through a neuron involves increasing the frequency and not the amplitude of action potentials. An action potential can be thought of as a digital signal with an "all-or-none/off-or-on" coding.

34.

C Improper neuronal migration

The cleft of schizencephaly can be unilateral or bilateral, but it usually involves the region near the central sulcus. Patients can present with seizures or focal deficits. Schizencephaly means "split brain," referring to abnormal clefts lined with heterotopic gray matter. This is in contrast to porencephaly, in which the clefts are lined with white matter.

35.

D T4

(A) There is often no C1 dorsal root and therefore often no C1 dermatome. (B) The middle finger is in the C7 dermatome. (C) The T2 dermatome is across the upper part of the chest. (E) The umbilicus is at T10.

36.

C Type C

Type C shunts are indirect dural shunts between the meningeal branches of the external carotid artery and the cavernous sinus. (A) Type A shunts are direct, high-flow shunts between the internal carotid artery and the cavernous sinus. (B) Type B shunts are indirect dural shunts between the meningeal branches of the internal carotid artery and the cavernous sinus. (D) Type D shunts are indirect dural shunts between the meningeal branches of both the internal and external carotid arteries and the cavernous sinus. Indirect fistulas require placement of coils on the venous side.

37.

E Engorged pituitary gland

The most common cause of intracranial hypotension is a persistent cerebrospinal fluid leak, commonly occurring after spinal procedures or craniotomy, and patients are at risk virtually any time the dura has been violated. The Monro-Kellie hypothesis states that the volume of intracranial blood, cerebrospinal fluid, and brain is constant. A decrease in one of these components must be accompanied by a compensatory increase in one or both of the other two, and vice versa. With intracranial hypotension, there is a decrease in cerebrospinal fluid that is accompanied by a compensatory increase in intracranial blood volume. This is reflected by engorgement (not collapse) of the venous sinuses, engorgement of the pituitary gland, and diffuse dural (not leptomeningeal) thickening and enhancement. Subdural effusions and even subdural hematomas may occur. (B, C) In intracranial hypotension, the brainstem sags, and the distance between the mammillary bodies and pons decreases. The pons also can become flattened against the clivus, and the angle between the upper surface of the pons and rostral mesencephalon decreases. Patients can develop tonsillar herniation.

38.

C SIADH has no effect on cerebral edema.

The syndrome of inappropriate antidiuretic hormone secretion (SIADH) has no effect on cerebral edema. The reasons for this are unknown, but it is hypothesized that cerebral edema should increase as serum sodium decreases due to free water reabsorption in the distal renal tubule.

39.

A –90 mV

This is near the equilibrium potential for potassium, as voltage-gated sodium channels are closed regardless of membrane potential, and the cell is most permeable to potassium ions. This membrane potential is slightly greater than the equilibrium potential for potassium because there is some flux and "leaking" of other ions.

40.

A *Candida*

(A–E) All these agents are well-recognized causes of maternally transmitted infections that can cause significant damage in the developing fetus (the "TORCH" infections: *t*oxoplasmosis, *r*ubella, *c*ytomegalovirus, *H*IV). Although rare, *Candida* can be transmitted to the fetus and results in a papulovesicular to pustular disseminated dermatitis. (B) Cytomegalovirus is the most frequent congenital central nervous system infectious agent. It is transmitted transplacentally, and results in periventricular calcifications and necrosis, and damages the brain, liver, and spleen. (C) HIV is transmitted perinatally and results in brain atrophy and basal ganglia calcifications. Most infected newborns dies within 1 year. (D) Rubella is transmitted transplacentally and can cause congenital rubella syndrome (chorioretinitis, cataracts, glaucoma, microphthalmia, microcephaly, mental retardation, and deafness). (E) Toxoplasmosis is the second most common congenital central nervous system infection. It is transmitted hematogenously through the placenta, and causes seizures, microcephaly, and spontaneous abortions, with the classic symptoms triad being hydrocephalus, chorioretinitis, and cranial calcifications.

41.

B Sacral insufficiency fracture

The CT image shown in the image accompanying the question demonstrates an irregular vertical lucency through the right sacral ala with surrounding sclerosis, with the typical appearance of an insufficiency fracture. These are more common in postmenopausal women with osteoporosis, and occur from normal physiological stress upon weakened bone. They may be unilateral or bilateral with or without a transverse component, and may produce the so-called Honda sign on a nuclear bone scan. They can be difficult to detect on plain films and are most conspicuous on fat-saturated T2-weighted or short tau inversion recovery (STIR) MRI sequences, depending on the degree of edema. They rarely occur in isolation, and patients commonly have associated fractures of the pubic rami or iliac crests. (A) The linear, vertical distribution of the lesion in the right sacrum is typical of a sacral insufficiency fracture. The surrounding sclerosis develops during the healing phase and is not related to blastic metastases, which would demonstrate a random distribution. The two focal radiodensities in the middle and left upper sacrum correspond to small bone islands. (C) The presence of sclerosis indicates some healing, ruling out an acute traumatic fracture (although acute stress/edema on chronic fractures can be present). Traumatic fractures also usually are associated with other fractures of the pelvis. (D) No discrete lesion, cortical destruction, or mass is appreciated to suggest a chordoma. (E) Sacroiliitis would be centered in the sacroiliac joint and not the sacral ala. Additionally, a fracture line would not be expected in sacroiliitis.

42.

B Cranial nerve VII

The superior salivatory nucleus gives rise to parasympathetic axons that project along cranial nerve VII to the submandibular and sublingual glands. Additional parasympathetics from cranial nerve VII course along the greater superficial petrosal nerve to the sphenopalatine ganglion. (A) Cranial nerve V projects sensory information to the chief sensory, spinal trigeminal, and mesencephalic nuclei, whereas motor information is relayed to the trigeminal motor nucleus. (C) The inferior salivatory nucleus projects to the parotid gland along cranial nerve IX. (D) The nucleus ambiguus gives rise to branchial efferents through cranial nerves IX, X, and XI. (E) The solitary nucleus has tracts involved with cranial nerves VII, IX, and X.

43.

D Hexosaminidase A

Tay-Sachs disease is secondary to the accumulation of gangliosides in neurons secondary to a deficiency of hexosaminidase A. Usually, the *HEXA* gene on chromosome 15 encoding the α-subunit of the enzyme is mutated. (A) Glucocerebrosidase is deficient in Gaucher disease. (B) Alpha-galactosidase is deficient in Fabry disease. (C) Sphingomyelinase is deficient in Niemann-Pick disease. (E) Phosphofructokinase is deficient in glycogen storage disease type 7 (Tarui disease).

44.

D Injury to the sphenopalatine artery

The sphenopalatine artery is found in the inferolateral corner of the sphenoid sinus. When enlarging the sinus and removing tissue inferolateral, it is important to strip the mucosa so that the artery is protected. Injury leads not only to devascularization of the nasal septal flap but also to the potential for delayed bleeding and epistaxis. For bleeding not controlled with packing, an external carotid injection should be performed to look for possible internal maxillary artery embolization options.

45.

C Vesicles at 400 mm per day in the orthograde direction

(A) Maximum retrograde transport speeds are around 250 mm per day for vesicles and are mediated by dynein. (B) Cytoskeletal proteins move in the orthograde direction much slower than vesicles and have a maximal speed of less than 8 mm per day. Orthograde transport is mediated by kinesin along microtubules. (D) Retrograde transport speeds vary but generally are fast (on the order of 50 to 250 mm per day).

46.

D Hypoplastic or absent infundibulum

Approximately 60% of patients with septo-optic dysplasia present with endocrine dysfunction due to hypoplasia of the pituitary gland or infundibulum. The posterior pituitary gland may be translocated. (A) A monoventricle characteristically is seen in alobar holoprosencephaly. (B) A high-riding third ventricle is seen in patients with dysgenesis of the corpus callosum. (C) "Viking helmet" or "moose head" appearance of the lateral ventricles is described in dysgenesis of the corpus callosum, in which there is eversion of the cingulate gyrus and Probst bundles.

47.

A Adenoma sebaceum

The pathology demonstrated in the image accompanying the question is marked by gliosis, large balloon cells, and a focal microcalcification (the purple lesion). These are features seen in a cortical tuber of tuberous sclerosis. The adenoma sebaceum skin lesion, often involving the nasolabial folds, commonly is encountered in this setting. (B) Nevoid basal cell carcinomas are associated with Gorlin syndrome as are medulloblastomas. (C) Café-au-lait spots are associated with neurofibromatosis type 1 and McCune-Albright syndrome. (D) Epidermal inclusion cysts are formed by the dermal entrapment of epidermal elements. (E) Tricholemmomas are benign, cutaneous neoplasms associated with Cowden syndrome.

48.

D Papilledema

Papilledema is seen in the image accompanying the question as indicated by the venous engorgement, blurring of the optic disk margins, and elevation of the optic disk (appearing as a white "donut" in the image). The image also shows Paton lines at the 7 and 11 o'clock positions, cascading in a radial pattern from the optic disk. (A) Drusen are accumulations of white extracellular material typically in the macula and occasionally in the optic disk. They are associated with advancing age, and individuals with pseudopapilledema (i.e., small cup-to-disk ratio) are prone to excess drusen. Drusen can be indicative of macular degeneration. (C) Pseudopapilledema is any scenario where the optic disk appears swollen but is not, and it is not associated with elevations in intracranial pressure. Causes can be a small cup-to-disk ratio (normal variant) and an optic nerve that enters the eye at such an angle as to elevate the edge of the optic disk. (E) Neuroretinitis is inflammation of the optic nerve and retina, and is classified as either infectious or idiopathic. It is characterized by disk edema and inflammation and erythema of the disk and retina. Radial exudates in the macula ("macular star") provide further support for the diagnosis.

49.

C Administer dantrolene.

The patient in this case has malignant hyperthermia, which is characterized by an acute onset of a high-grade fever, tachycardia, and rigidity. It has a very high mortality rate if left untreated. The condition may be caused by volatile anesthetics, especially halothane, and by depolarizing neuromuscular blockers, such as succinylcholine. Treatment consists of discontinuation of anesthesia, administration of dantrolene, and supportive measures. (A) Although cooling blankets may be helpful, attention should be turned to discontinuing the anesthesia and administering dantrolene. (B) Hydration is assumed to be adequate in this elective case. (D) Phenobarbital administration does not help with malignant hyperthermia. (E) Succinylcholine may precipitate malignant hyperthermia.

50.

D Posterior inferior cerebellar artery; vertebral artery

Wallenberg syndrome (also known as lateral medullary syndrome) is characterized by loss of pain and temperature sensation on the contralateral side of the body and ipsilateral side of the face. Dysphagia, slurred speech, ataxia, vertigo, nystagmus, and Horner syndrome can occur. Although occlusion of the posterior inferior cerebellar artery is sufficient to produce a Wallenberg syndrome, most cases are diagnosed following the occlusion of the more proximal vertebral artery.

51.

C A2

The recurrent artery of Heubner originates from A2 about 60% of the time, from the junction of the anterior communicating artery (ACOM) and anterior cerebral artery (ACA) about 32% of the time, and from A1 about 8% of the time. It overwhelmingly originates within 2 mm either proximal or distal of the ACOM and ACA junction.

52.

A High-grade, non-Hodgkin B-cell neoplasm

High-grade, non-Hodgkin B-cell neoplasms are primary central nervous system lymphomas. They are seen in increasing frequency in immunocompetent patients, in immunocompromised patients such as those with HIV/AIDS, and in posttransplant patients. (C) Burkitt lymphoma is a secondary B-cell central nervous system lymphoma that originates in germinal centers and spreads to the central nervous system. It is associated closely with the Epstein-Barr virus. (D) Leptomeningeal lymphoma usually is due to secondary central nervous system lymphoma spread from a disseminated lymphoma relapse. The prognosis is poor.

53.

C Cushing disease

In Cushing disease (excess ACTH production by the pituitary gland), the pituitary gland retains some feedback control and suppresses ACTH production with high but not low doses of dexamethasone. The interpretation of dexamethasone suppression test results is detailed in the table below. (A) Cushing syndrome is the overproduction of cortisol by the adrenal glands. The pituitary gland senses the high cortisol levels and suppresses ACTH production; therefore, dexamethasone cannot further suppress ACTH production or alter cortisol levels. (B) Ectopic ACTH production by an ACTH-producing tumor yields a clinical picture similar to that of Cushing syndrome. (D) Addison disease is adrenal insufficiency, and it results in low cortisol production by the adrenal glands regardless of ACTH level.

Pathology	ACTH	Cortisol (during dexamethasone suppression test)
Cushing syndrome	Undetectable or low	Not suppressed by high or low doses
Ectopic ACTH-secreting tumor	Elevated	Not suppressed by high or low doses
Cushing disease	Normal to elevated	Suppressed by high but not low doses
Addison disease	Elevated	Low

54.

A Inhibits apoptosis

Bcl-2 is an anti-apoptotic factor that is inhibited by p53 activation of the pro-apoptotic factor Bax. Bcl-2 inhibits Smac and cytochrome C activation by apoptotic stimuli. The *Bcl-2* gene is considered an oncogene, as its mutation causes excessive apoptosis.

55.

A Aberrant regeneration of the facial nerve

Following injury to the facial nerve, regenerating fibers may be misdirected. Fibers intended for the periorbital region may end up innervating the perioral muscles. This process most likely is responsible for this patient's symptoms. (B) A transient ischemic attack in unlikely in this patient in the absence of any acute neurologic deficits. (C) Steroid side effects include infections, poor wound healing, weight gain, mood changes, and weakening of connective tissues. (D) New injury

to the facial nerve would lead to facial weakness. (E) Trigeminal neuralgia is a sensory syndrome, with patients feeling pain in a trigeminal nerve territory.

56.

B Atlantoaxial instability

An increased atlantodental interval is indicative of atlantoaxial instability or dislocation due to disruption of the transverse ligament, which is the primary restraint against anteroposterior translation. The interval is measured by drawing a line from the most anterior aspect of the dens (at the midpoint of the thickness of the anterior C1 arch) to the posterior aspect of the anterior C1 arch. It is considered abnormal if the interval is greater than 3 mm in men, 2.5 mm in women, or 5 mm in children. When dislocation occurs, it almost always is due to anterior displacement of C1 over C2, with potential compression of the spinal cord between the dens and the posterior arch of C1. (A) The atlantodental interval evaluates the relationship of the atlas (C1) and dens (C2) and not the atlas and skull. Among other possible abnormalities, anterior atlanto-occipital dislocation would present with an increased basion-axial interval, but the atlantodental interval will be normal if the transverse ligament is intact. (C) The atlantodental interval is a measure of atlantoaxial instability or dislocation, not atlanto-occipital dislocation. (D) An atlantodental interval of 5 mm is an abnormal finding in an adult, but this is the upper limit of normal in a child. (E) An accompanying alar ligament injury may occur with an increased atlantodental interval, particularly when the interval is greater than 6 mm. Nevertheless, an increased atlantodental interval primarily is due to disruption of the transverse ligament.

57.

E External capsule and extreme capsule

(A–E) The order, from medial to lateral, of these structures is as follows: internal capsule, globus pallidus, putamen (the lentiform nucleus is the combination of the globus pallidus and putamen), external capsule, claustrum, extreme capsule, and insular cortex.

58.

A Posterior reversible encephalopathy

The mechanism of posterior reversible encephalopathy syndrome is not entirely certain but appears to be related to impaired cerebral regulation and endothelial dysfunction. The distribution of cortical and subcortical signal abnormalities is relatively characteristic and frequently involves the posterior circulation and the region around the superior frontal sulci. Approximately 90% of abnormalities are reversible, but some cases may be complicated by infarction or hemorrhage. (B) Superior sagittal sinus thrombosis may result in venous infarctions that often are bilateral and can mimic the posterior cerebral abnormalities seen in this case; however, it would be rare for a superior sagittal sinus thrombosis also to show the patchy abnormalities along the superior frontal sulci and the expected flow void of the superior sagittal sinus that is present on both FLAIR images accompanying the question. (C) Infarct of the posterior circulation would have a distinct arterial distribution. (D) Hypoxic ischemic encephalopathy may show signal abnormalities (particularly on diffusion-weighted imaging in the acute setting) in the cerebral cortex (particularly in the perirolandic and occipital cortices), basal ganglia, thalami, cerebellum, and sometimes the brainstem.

59.

B Retinitis pigmentosa

Nyctalopia is night blindness, which may be degenerative, congenital, traumatic (e.g., following the LASIK procedure), or due to vitamin A deficiency. Retinitis pigmentosa is a condition in which rod photoreceptors progressively degenerate and is the most common cause of nyctalopia. (A) Xeroderma pigmentosum is an autosomal recessive condition that results in the inability to repair DNA damage caused by ultraviolet light. (C) De Morsier syndrome (septo-optic dysplasia) is a congenital malformation resulting in the underdevelopment of the optic nerve, pituitary dysfunction, and absence of the septum pellucidum. (D) Wyburn-Mason syndrome is a phakomatosis characterized by arteriovenous malformations of the brain, retinae, visual pathways, and facial structures. (E) Balint syndrome is characterized by simultanagnosia, oculomotor apraxia, and optic apraxia resulting from bilateral watershed strokes in the parieto-occipital regions.

60.

E Diffuse axonal injury

Diffuse axonal injury is a result of traumatic shear forces related to acceleration/deceleration. Most cases occur after high-speed motor vehicle collisions or direct blows to the head but also can be seen in nonaccidental trauma. MRI can show small foci of susceptibility artifact reflecting microhemorrhages usually located at the gray matter–white matter junction and in the corpus callosum and brainstem in more severe cases. Hemorrhages commonly follow white matter tracts as seen in the frontal lobes in this case. (A) Chronic hypertensive encephalopathy may present with centrally located micro- or macrohemorrhages that tend to occur in the basal ganglia, brainstem, and cerebellar hemispheres. (B) Cortical contusions are more superficial and are commonly associated with extra-axial hemorrhage. (C) Fat embolism most commonly is a result of long bone fractures, but it also can be seen following orthopedic procedures. MRI gradient echo sequences, particularly susceptibility-weighted imaging, show fine petechial hemorrhages distributed randomly in the supratentorial brain and posterior fossa, sometimes with foci of restricted diffusion. Lesions would not follow white matter tracts as seen in the frontal lobes in this case. (D) Septic emboli can result in foci of microhemorrhage usually located in the gray matter–white matter junction or cerebellum.

61.

C Percutaneous aspiration of pneumocephalus

Symptomatic tension pneumocephalus always should be considered in patients with an abnormal mental status following posterior fossa surgery that was performed with the patient in the sitting or prone positions. During infancy, emergent aspiration of air can be performed through the anterior fontanelle.

62.

B Orbital wall fracture

Unique to the transseptal approach (as compared with an endoscopic endonasal approach), aggressive distraction of the Hardy speculum can cause fractures of the medial orbital wall or orbital floor that extend into the optic foramen and cause injury to the optic nerve.

63.

C Ipsilateral; contralateral; ipsilateral; ipsilateral

The affected structures in Wallenberg syndrome include the spinothalamic tract, causing contralateral loss of pain and temperature in the body; the trigeminothalamic tract, causing loss of pain and temperature sensation in the ipsilateral face; the nucleus ambiguus, causing hoarseness, dysphagia, and loss of the gag reflex; the descending sympathetic tract, causing an ipsilateral Horner syndrome; the vestibular nucleus, causing vertigo, nystagmus, and nausea/vomiting; and the inferior cerebellar peduncle, causing ipsilateral cerebellar defects.

64.

B 305.5

Serum osmolarity is estimated by the following equation:

$$\text{Serum osmolarity} = 2(\text{Na} + \text{K}) + \text{BUN}/28 + \text{Glucose}/18$$

65.

C Sigma receptor

Sigma receptors once were classified as an opioid receptor subtype but now are thought to be an independent type of receptor. Activation of sigma receptors is seen with phencyclidine and cocaine and causes hallucinations, increased muscle tone, tachycardia, tachypnea, and mydriasis. (A) Delta opioid receptors are responsible for analgesia (to a lesser extent than kappa opioid receptors) and use enkephalins as their endogenous ligands. (B) Mu opioid receptor activation produces analgesia, sedation, decreased blood pressure, euphoria, and respiratory depression. Mu opioid receptors have enkephalins and beta-endorphins as their endogenous ligands with a low affinity for dynorphins. (D) The nociceptin receptor (orphan opioid receptor) is a newly classified receptor thought to be involved in instinctive and emotional behavior modulation. The receptor has many endogenous ligands including nociceptin, and activation is thought to antagonize dopamine transport. (E) Kappa opioid receptors have dynorphin as their endogenous ligand and produce analgesia, dysphoria, and hallucinations with activation. Kappa receptors tend to antagonize the effects of mu opioid receptor activation.

66.

C Superior cerebellar artery

The superior cerebellar artery supplies blood to most of the cerebellar cortex, dentate and other cerebellar nuclei, and superior cerebellar peduncle. (B) The posterior inferior cerebellar artery supplies the medulla, lower cranial nerve nuclei, spinal trigeminal nuclei, and inferior cerebellar peduncle. (D) The anterior inferior cerebellar artery supplies the middle cerebellar peduncle and cranial nerves VII and VIII.

67.

B Oriented posteriorly and arising from the posterior wall

Posterior communicating artery aneurysms usually point posteriorly toward cranial nerve III.

68.

B Meperidine

Meperidine induces histamine release and can cause seizures through the neuroexcitatory effects of its metabolite. (A) Morphine induces histamine release and may raise intracranial pressure through cerebral vasodilation. It has difficulty crossing the blood–brain barrier. (C) Fentanyl reduces intracranial pressure through reduction in cerebral oxygen consumption and cerebral blood volume. It crosses the blood–brain barrier. It does not cause a histamine release. (D) Sufentanil can raise intracranial pressure. It does not cause a histamine release. (E) Alfentanil can raise intracranial pressure. It does not cause a histamine release.

69.

C *HLA-B27*

The CT images accompanying the question show fusion of the sacroiliac joints and formation of marginal syndesmophytes between adjoining vertebrae in a patient with ankylosing spondylitis. Additional findings that may be seen include the Romanus lesion (erosive, inflammatory changes involving the end-plate corners ("shiny corner" sign) and the Andersson lesion (diskitis). The presence of *HLA-B27*, a variation of the *HLA-B* gene, results in a markedly increased risk of developing the disease. Additional genes that may be involved include *ERAP1*, *IL1A*, and *IL23R*, although most have not been identified. (A) The *PTPN22* gene has been associated with an increased risk of developing rheumatoid arthritis. (B) The *HLA-DRB1* gene is the major genetic susceptibility locus in rheumatoid arthritis. (D) Mutations in the *PHEX* gene can lead to X-linked hypophosphatemic rickets.

70.

B Renal transplantation

Neuropathy in the setting of dialysis mostly is attributed to the presence of neurotoxins in the blood that are not eliminated by dialysis. Although vitamin replacement can help with symptoms, patients are much more likely to improve if they receive kidney transplants.

71.

D Tay-Sachs disease

The clinical presentation described and the identified enzyme deficiency represent Tay-Sachs disease. The neurons shown in the photomicrograph accompanying the question are distended with their cytoplasm stuffed with ganglioside material.

(A) Individuals with Fabry disease present with diffuse pain (especially gastrointestinal pain), renal failure, angiokeratomas, and neuropathy. (B) Neuronal ceroid lipofuscinosis results in a permanent loss of motor and psychological abilities as lipofuscin accumulates. (C) Niemann-Pick disease is characterized by a retinal cherry red spot, hepatosplenomegaly, and progressive motor decline. (E) Wolman disease is caused by lysosomal acid lipase deficiency and manifests with feeding difficulties, hepatosplenomegaly, and failure to thrive.

72.

D Origin at the glial–Schwann cell junction

The images accompanying the question show an avidly enhancing mass in the right cerebellopontine angle with both cisternal and canalicular components and small cystic changes compatible with a vestibular schwannoma. These lesions represent the most common posterior fossa tumor in adults, and they most commonly arise from the superior division of the vestibular nerve. Between 5 and 20% of vestibular schwannomas may present with cystic or necrotic changes and may be associated with peritumoral arachnoid cysts, particularly when large. Vestibular schwannomas arise from the glial–Schwann cell junction (Obersteiner-Redlich zone). (A) Vestibular schwannomas are diagnostic of neurofibromatosis type 2 if they occur bilaterally. (B) Tumors that have a propensity for perineural spread include adenoid cystic carcinoma, squamous cell carcinoma, mucoepidermoid carcinoma, melanoma, and lymphoma (usually advanced non-Hodgkin lymphoma). (C) Schwannomas commonly have cystic or necrotic changes. (E) Meningiomas originate from arachnoid cap cells.

73.

D Point of maximal stress

The point of maximal stress can vary depending on how the screws and other elements are combined in a construct. Maximal stress often occurs at the fulcrum of a lever arm.

74.

C Tuberous sclerosis

Subependymal giant cell astrocytomas (SEGAs) are found in 6 to 14% of patients with tuberous sclerosis. It is debatable if SEGAs occur in the absence of the tuberous sclerosis. SEGAs can present with worsening epilepsy or signs of hydrocephalus (obstructive in nature). SEGAs positively stain for glial acidic fibrillary protein. (B) Patients with neurofibromatosis type 2 are prone to developing bilateral vestibular schwannomas and meningiomas. (D) Patients with von Hippel–Lindau disease are prone to developing hemangioblastomas and endolymphatic sac tumors. (E) Patients with Osler-Weber-Rendu syndrome are prone to developing telangiectasias and arteriovenous malformations.

75.

D Mucopolysaccharidoses

Mucopolysaccharidoses such as Morquio and Hurler syndromes are associated with diffuse scalloping of the posterior vertebral bodies, although the mechanism is uncertain. Vertebral scalloping usually is secondary to a slow-growing process at a time of active osseous remodeling and can be produced by various masses. Scalloping can be secondary to dural ectasia, such as that seen in collagen vascular diseases (e.g., Marfan and Ehlers-Danlos syndromes). It also has been described in achondroplasia and acromegaly. (A) Multiple myeloma presents as lytic, destructive lesions and does not result in scalloping. (B) Neurofibromatosis type 1 is associated with vertebral body scalloping and other distinctive osseous abnormalities such as sphenoid wing dysplasia and deformities involving the long bones. (C) Diskitis is an inflammatory process that results in the destruction of the vertebral end plates.